ALLE ZEIT WACH 1842

F. Kubli D. von Fournier
H. Junkermann M. Bauer M. Kaufmann (Eds.)

Breast Diseases

Breast-Conserving Therapy, Non-Invasive Lesions, Mastopathy

With Contributions by
J.A. Andersen, H.W. Anton, H. Becker, J.D. Boice, J.A. van Dongen
K. Engel, G.E. Feichter, M. Friedrich, J.F.H. Gauwerky, F. Harder
J.R. Harris, J. Hayward, S. Hellmann, I.C. Henderson, R. Hünig
G. Kindermann, D.W. Kinne, W. Kübler, W. Leucht, H. Maass
R.E. Mansel, R.G. Margolese, A. Müller, K. Prechtel, P.E. Preece
M. Reitzenstein, K. Rotte, M. Säbel, R. Sauer, A. Schauer
V. Schirrmacher, J.M. Spitalier, J.S. Spratt, A. Staffen, H.E. Stegner
A.H. Tulusan, U. Veronesi

With 247 Figures

Springer-Verlag Berlin Heidelberg New York
London Paris Tokyo Hong Kong

F. KUBLI †
University of Heidelberg
Women's Hospital
Voßstr. 9
D-6900 Heidelberg, FRG

M. BAUER
University Women's Hospital
Department of Gynecological
Radiology
Hugstetterstr. 5
D-7800 Freiburg/Brsg., FRG

M. KAUFMANN
University of Heidelberg
Women's Hospital
Voßstr. 9
D-6900 Heidelberg, FRG

D. VON FOURNIER
University of Heidelberg
Women's Hospital and
Clinic of Radiology
Voßstr. 9
D-6900 Heidelberg, FRG

H. JUNKERMANN
University of Heidelberg
Women's Hospital and
Clinic of Radiology
Voßstr. 9
D-6900 Heidelberg, FRG

ISBN-13:978-3-642-73525-7 e-ISBN-13:978-3-642-73523-3
DOI: 10.1007/978-3-642-73523-3

Library of Congress Cataloging-in-Publication Data
Breast diseases. Includes bibliographies and index. 1. Breast–Cancer–Treatment. I. Kubli, F. II. Fournier, D. von III. Andersen, J. A. [DNLM: 1. Breast Neoplasms–radio-therapy. 2. Breast Neoplasms–surgery. 3. Mammography. WP 870 B82795] RC280.B8B718 1989 616.99'44906 89-6073
ISBN-13:978-3-642-73525-7 (U.S.: alk. paper)

Softcover reprint of the hardcover 1st edition 1989

Typesetting: International Typesetters, Inc., Manila, Philippines

2121/3145-543210 – Printed on acid-free paper

Preface

Breast cancer is the commonest cause of cancer death (18%) in women in Germany, and is still on the increase. The incidence rate in the USA is comparably high, although recently the incidence rate of colorectal and bronchial carcinomas has caught up with that of breast cancer. There is every indication that the life-style in the industrial countries is to some extent responsible for the increase in these cancers.

In this book we present contributions on the current understanding of the treatment of malignant breast diseases and precancerous lesions by prominent experts from various European countries and North America. The difficulties involved in early detection and the increasing fear women have, not only of breast cancer but also of benign breast diseases, have prompted us to include the problem of fibrocystic diseases (mastopathy) as a whole. However, in so doing we have confined ourselves to dealing with methods of clinical relevance, at the same time aiming for an adequate degree of scientific reliability. We have tried to avoid premature conclusions, as there are still many areas of uncertainty in the field of breast cancer. Accordingly, we have sought to display alternative opinions without comment: the reader is to judge for himself where the better arguments lie.

Undoubtedly, more research has been carried out and more has been written on breast cancer than on any other malignant disease. Research into breast diseases has become a pacemaker for modern oncology and has led to valuable developments: hormone receptors, epithelial growth factors, oncogenes, etc. Although the cure rate for breast cancer has only improved in small steps, despite the enormous research efforts, great strides have been made as regards disease-free survival, quality of life, and the psychological well-being of the patient. Also, the design of randomized trials, modeled on those used in studying detection and treatment of breast cancer, has shown a decisive improvement.

Sadly, the untimely death of F. KUBLI prevented him from completing his contributions personally. He was a motivating force and played a key role in winning many contributions for this book. We have done our utmost to prepare the topics as F. KUBLI would have wished, based on our 18 years' work together and a joint book on breast diseases[a].

We would like to extend our thanks, in particular, to the many distinguished authors whose contributions have been invaluable in providing a balanced picture of the state of the art in the field of breast cancer.

DIETRICH VON FOURNIER

---

[a] F. Kubli, D. von Fournier (1984) Neue Konzepte de Diagnostik und Therapie des Mammakarzinoms. Springer, Berlin, Heidelberg, New York, Tokyo

Acknowledgements

The editors are greatly indebted to the following companies and private donors without whose generous contributions this book could not have been published:

Nourypharma, ICI-Pharma, Winthrop, Cyanamid/Lederle, Asta-Werke, Kali-Chemie, Upjohn, Hormonchemie, Boehringer, Sandoz, Frau M. Pericone/Italia

We also have pleasure in thanking the staff of Springer Verlag for the infinite patience they showed in helping the editors compile this book. We wish to thank them for their invaluable technical guidance and excellent publishing know-how. We are also extremely grateful to colleagues from the University of Heidelberg, Women's Hospital and Clinic of Radiology, especially Mrs. C. H. Bittner, for taking care of the many painstaking tasks entailed in the preparation of the book.

DIETRICH VON FOURNIER

Table of Contents

I. Biology, Morphology, Growth Behavior

Epidemiology of Breast Cancer 8
J.F.H. GAUWERKY, R. FRENTZEL-BEYME, D. VON FOURNIER

Breast-Cancer Biology and Breast-Preserving Surgery 24
A. SCHAUER, H. ROTHE, J. BALZER, R. BREHLER, M. BERGHOLZ

S Phase Fractions and DNA Ploidy as Prognostic Factors in Breast Cancer 43
G.E. FEICHTER, D. VON FOURNIER, M. KAUFMANN

Multicentricity in Breast Carcinoma 48
H.W. ANTON, A. GUHR, A. MÜLLER, U. ABEL

The Contralateral Breast: Bilateral Primary Breast Cancer 56
A.H. TULUSAN, G. RONAY, R. ADAM, M. REITZENSTEIN

Cell Biology of Tumor Metastasis Formation 62
V. SCHIRRMACHER

Prognostic Factors in Primary Breast Cancer 67
M. KAUFMANN, K. ENGEL, D. VON FOURNIER, F. KUBLI

Natural Growth Rate of Primary Breast Cancer and its Metastases 78
D. VON FOURNIER, W. HOEFFKEN, M. FRIEDRICH

Growth Rates and Cytokinetic Behavior of Breast Cancer 97
J.S. SPRATT, J.A. SPRATT

II. Diagnosis

The Value of Diagnostic Methods: Mammography, Screening and Other Imaging Techniques 112
M. FRIEDRICH, D. VON FOURNIER, W. HOEFFKEN

Standards in the Technique of Mammography 129
M. SÄBEL, H. AICHINGER

Current Status of Ultrasound Mammography 137
W. LEUCHT, DAGMAR RABE

Cytologic Diagnosis of Breast Cancer 143
W. KÜBLER, W. KÜHN, H.H. RUMMEL

III. Primary Treatment

Growth Behavior and Implications for Staging and Therapy 156
D. VON FOURNIER

Rationale for the Choice of Treatment 174
D. VON FOURNIER, F. KUBLI

Perioperative Clarification of Diagnosis 189
D. VON FOURNIER, F. KUBLI, E. KRAPFL

Surgical Treatment 201
D. VON FOURNIER, F. KUBLI

Breast-Conserving Therapy or Amputation with Reconstruction:
The Patient's View 209
K. ENGEL, D. VON FOURNIER, F. KUBLI, M. KAUFMANN

Surgical Techniques of Breast Preservation for Early Breast Cancer 218
D.W. KINNE

Conservation Trials in Early Breast Cancer 222
J. HAYWARD

Surgical Complications After Conservative Treatment of Breast
Cancer 227
F. HARDER, N. LÜSCHER, U. LAFFER, R. HÜNIG, E. WALTHER,
A. ALMENDRAL, J. TORHORST

IV. Radiology

Status of Radiotherapy after Ablative and Breast-Preserving
Treatment of Breast Cancer 240
D. VON FOURNIER, A. MÜLLER, H. JUNKERMANN,
W. SCHLEGEL

Treatment of Breast Cancer with Breast Preservation ... 262
S. HELLMAN

First Experiences in Würzburg of Interstitial Low-Dose Afterloading for Breast-Conserving Therapy with the Microselectron ... 267
K. ROTTE, E. LÖFFLER

V. Results

Long-Term Survival Following Breast-Conserving Therapy in Comparison to Radical Surgical Treatment: An Overview ... 276
J.M. SPITALIER, J.M. KURTZ, R. AMALRIC, H. BRANDONE, Y. AYME, C. BRESSAC, D. HANS

Breast-Conserving Treatment: Experience Derived from the National Surgical Adjuvant Breast Project ... 285
R.G. MARGOLESE

Local Recurrence After Breast-Conserving Treatment: Results from the Harvard Joint Center for Radiation Therapy ... 292
J.R. HARRIS, A. RECHT, S.J. SCHNITT, B. SILVER, J.L. CONNOLLY

Local Recurrence and New Primary Ipsilateral Carcinomas After Conservative Treatment of Breast Carcinoma ... 301
U. VERONESI, A. LUINI, M. DEL VECCHIO

Pathoanatomical Characteristics of Local Treatment Failure Following Breast-Conserving Therapy ... 308
A. MÜLLER, D. VON FOURNIER

Selective Issues in the Evaluation of the Efficacy of Breast-Conserving Therapy ... 313
J.A. VAN DONGEN, N.K. AARONSON, H. BARTELINK

VI. Complications

Long-Term Complications of Surgery and Associated Irradiation as Breast-Conserving Therapy ... 324
G. KINDERMANN, T. GENZ

Long-Term Complications of Breast-Conserving Treatment: Experience with the Basel Lumpectomy Protocol ... 329
R. HÜNIG, E. WALTHER, F. HARDER, A.C. ALMENDRAL, J. TORHORST, J. ROTH

The German Breast Cancer Study I: Preliminary Results of Breast-Conserving Treatment Dependent on Radiation Technique 343
R. SAUER, J. DUNST, H. RAUSCHECKER, A. SCHAUER, M. SCHUMACHER

Long-Term Results and Late Complications After Breast-Preserving Therapy of Breast Cancer in Vienna 358
A. STAFFEN

Possible Risk of Second Primary Cancers Associated with Irradiation in Breast-Conserving Therapy 363
J.D. BOICE

Psychological Problems of Women with Carcinoma of the Breast and Possible Means of Treatment 376
H. BECKER

Side Effects and Major Complications of Breast-Conserving Therapy 389
K. ENGEL, D. VON FOURNIER, M. KAUFMANN, F. KUBLI

Cosmetic Aspects of Breast-Conserving Therapy for Carcinoma of the Breast 402
K. ENGEL, A. MÜLLER, D. VON FOURNIER, F. KUBLI

VII. Adjuvant Chemotherapy and Hormonal Therapy – Results and Complications

The Integration of Radiotherapy and Chemotherapy in the Treatment of Early Breast Cancer 416
I.C. HENDERSON, D. HAYES, M.A. ROSE, S. COME, J. HARRIS

Adjuvant Endocrine Treatment With and Without Simultaneous Adjuvant Chemotherapy 436
H. MAASS

Complication Rates of Radiotherapy with Adjuvant Chemotherapy for Conservative Treatment 445
M. BAUER, D. VON FOURNIER, F. KUBLI, H. SCHMID, R. SCHULZ-WENDTLAND

VIII. Strategies for the Prevention of Invasive Breast Cancer: Treatment of Mastopathic, Precancerous and Non-Invasive Lesions

Diagnosis and Classification of Benign Breast Diseases 464
H. JUNKERMANN, D. VON FOURNIER, E. WEBER, B. ARABIN

Fibrocystic Disease, Precancerous Lesions, and Carcinoma In Situ: Characteristic Morphology and Risk of Malignant Degeneration 474
K. PRECHTEL

Multicentricity of Ductal Carcinoma In Situ 479
M. REITZENSTEIN, A.H. TULUSAN, N. BAUER, G. RONAY

Precancerous Lesions and Carcinoma In Situ: Problems of Treatment from the Morphological Viewpoint 481
H.-E. STEGNER

Endocrinological Profiles in Benign Breast Disease 488
R.E. MANSEL

Endocrinology of Benign Breast Disease in Relation to the Severity of Radiological Dysplasia 494
H. JUNKERMANN, K. KLINGA, E. WEBER, D. VON FOURNIER

Hormonal and Non-Hormonal Medical Therapy of Benign Breast Disease 499
D. VON FOURNIER, H. JUNKERMANN, U. WARENDORF, E. WEBER, E. KRAPFL, U. ABEL

Medical Treatment of Benign Breast Disease 507
P.E. PREECE

In Situ Carcinoma of the Female Breast: Frequency, Growth Pattern and Biologic Significance 513
J.A. ANDERSEN, J.M. NIELSEN, G.L. OTTESEN, J.L. THOMSEN

DNA Synthesis Rate and Ploidy in Precancerous and Non-Invasive Lesions of the Breast 523
G.E. FEICHTER, I.A. BORN

Pathoanatomical Findings in Subcutaneous Mastectomy Specimens Referred to the Indications for Surgery 527
A. MÜLLER

Subject Index 537

List of Contributors

AARONSON, N.K.
Department of Psychosocial Research
Cancer Institute
Amsterdam, The Netherlands

ABEL, U.
German Cancer Research Center
D-6900 Heidelberg, FRG

ADAM, R.
Universitätsfrauenklinik Erlangen
Universitätsstraße 21–23
D-8520 Erlangen, FRG

AICHINGER, H.
Medical Engineering Group
Siemens AG
D-8520 Erlangen, FRG

ALMENDRAL, A.
Department of Gynecology
Spitalstraße 21
University of Basel
CH-Basel, Switzerland

AMALRIC, R.
Department of Radiotherapy
Cancer Institute
Marseille, France

ANDERSEN, J.A.
Institute of Pathology
University of Odense
Odense, Denmark

ANTON, H.W.
University Hospital for Women
D-6900 Heidelberg, FRG

ARABIN, B.
Universitätsfrauenklinik u.
Deutsches Krebsforschungszentrum
D-6900 Heidelberg, FRG

AYME, Y.
Department of Surgery
Cancer Institute
Marseille, France

BALZER, J.
Pathologisches Institut
der Universität Göttingen
Robert-Koch-Str. 40
D-3400 Göttingen, FRG

BARTELINK, H.
Department of Radiotherapy
Cancer Institute
Amsterdam, The Netherlands

BAUER, M.
Universitätsfrauenklinik
Abt. Gynäkologisch-Geburtshilfliche Radiologie
Hugstetterstraße 5
D-7800 Freiburg/Brsg., FRG

BAUER, N.
Universitätsfrauenklinik Erlangen
Universitätsstraße 21–23
D-8520 Erlangen, FRG

BECKER, H.
Department of Psychosomatic Medicine
Heidelberg University Hospital
Thibautstr. 2
D-6900 Heidelberg, FRG

BERGHOLZ, M.
Pathologisches Institut

der Universität Göttingen
Robert-Koch-Str. 40
D-3400 Göttingen, FRG

BOICE, J.D.
National Cancer Institute
Landow Building, Room 3A22
Bethesda, MD 20892, USA

BORN, I.A.
Institute of Comparative
and Experimental Gynecology
University of Heidelberg
D-6900 Heidelberg, FRG

BRANDONE, H.
Department of Surgery
Cancer Institute
Marseille, France

BREHLER, R.
Pathologisches Institut
der Universität Göttingen
Robert-Koch-Str. 40
D-3400 Göttingen, FRG

BRESSAC, C.
Department of Surgery
Cancer Institute
Marseille, France

COME, S.
Beth Israel, Hospital Boston
Boston MA 02115, USA

CONNOLLY, J.L.
Department of Pathology
Beth Israel Hospital and
Harvard Medical School
Boston MA 02115, USA

DEL VECCHIO, M.
Instituto Nazionale per lo Studio
e la Cura dei Tumori
Via Venezian, 1
I-20133 Milano, Italy

DONGEN, J.A. VAN
Department of Surgery
Cancer Institute
Amsterdam, The Netherlands

DUNST, J.
Strahlentherapeutische
Universitätsklinik
Universitätsstr. 27
D-8520 Erlangen, FRG

ENGEL, K.
Universitäts-Frauenklinik
Voßstraße 9
D-6900 Heidelberg, FRG

FEICHTER, G.E.
Institute of Comparative and
Experimental Pathology
Institute of Pathology
University of Heidelberg
D-6900 Heidelberg, FRG

FOURNIER, D. von
University of Heidelberg Women's
Hospital and
Clinic of Radiology
Voßstr. 9
D-6900 Heidelberg, FRG

FRENTZEL-BEYME, R.
German Cancer Research Center
D-6900 Heidelberg, FRG

FRIEDRICH, M.
Krankenhaus am Urban
Röntgenabteilung
Dieffenbachstraße 1
D-1000 Berlin 61, FRG

GAUWERKY, J.F.H.
Department of Obstetrics and
Gynecology
University of Heidelberg
D-6900 Heidelberg, FRG

GENZ, T.
Universitätsfrauenklinik
Charlottenburg
der FU Berlin
Pulsstr. 4–14
D-1000 Berlin 19, FRG

GUHR, A.
University Hospital for Women

Voßstr. 9
D-6900 Heidelberg, FRG

HANS, D.
Department of Surgery
Cancer Institute
Marseille, France

HARDER, F.
General Surgical Clinic
Department of Surgery
University of Basel
CH-Basel, Switzerland

HARRIS, J.R.
Joint Center of Radiation Therapy
Department of Radiation Therapy
Harvard Medical School
50 Binney Street
Boston, MA 02115, USA

HAYES, D.
Dana-Farber Cancer Institute
Boston, MA 02115, USA

HAYWARD, J.
Breast Unit, Guy's Hospital and
London Bridge Hospital
27 Tooley Street
London, S.E., 1, England

HELLMAN, S.
Memorial Sloan-Kettering Cancer
Center
1275 York Avenue
New York, NY 10021, USA

HENDERSON, I.C.
Dana-Farber Cancer Institute
Boston, MA 02115, USA

HOEFFKEN, W.
Strahleninstitut
Machabäerstr. 19–27
D-5000 Köln 1, FRG

HÜNIG, R.
Department of Radiooncology
University of Basel
Spitalstr. 21
CH-Basel, Switzerland

JUNKERMANN, H.
University of Heidelberg Women's
Hospital and
Clinic of Radiology
Voßstr. 9
D-6900 Heidelberg, FRG

KAUFMANN, M.
Universitäts-Frauenklinik
Voßstraße 9
D-6900 Heidelberg, FRG

KINDERMANN, G.
1. Universitätsfrauenklinik
Maistraße 11
D-8000 München 2

KINNE, D.W.
Breast Service
Memorial Sloan-Kettering Cancer
Center
New York 10021, USA

KLINGA, K.
Universitätsfrauenklinik
u. Deutsches
Krebsforschungszentrum
D-6900 Heidelberg, FRG

KRAPFL, E.
University of Heidelberg Women's
Hospital and
Clinic of Radiology
Voßstr. 9
D-6900 Heidelberg, FRG

KUBLI, F.
Universitäts-Frauenklinik
Voßstraße 9
D-6900 Heidelberg, FRG

KÜBLER, W.
Department of Gynecological
Morphology
University Women's Hospital
Voßstraße 9
D-6900 Heidelberg, FRG

KÜHN, W.
Department of Gynecological
Morphology

University Women's Hospital
Voßstraße 9
D-6900 Heidelberg, FRG

KURTZ, J.M.
Division of Radiation Oncology
University Hospital, Basel
Switzerland

LAFFER, U.
General Surgical Clinic
Department of Surgery
University of Basel
Basel, Switzerland

LEUCHT, W.
Universitätsfrauenklinik
Voßstraße 9
D-6900 Heidelberg, FRG

LÖFFLER, E.
Department of Radiotherapy
University Women's Hospital
Josef-Schneider-Str. 4
D-8700 Würzburg, FRG

LÜSCHER, N.
General Surgical Clinic
Department of Surgery
University of Basel
CH-Basel, Switzerland

LUINI, A.
Instituto Nazionale per lo Studio
e la Cura dei Tumori
Via Venezian, 1
I-20133 Milano, Italy

MAASS, H.
Universitätsfrauenklinik
u. Poliklinik
Martinistraße 52
D-2000 Hamburg 20; FRG

MANSEL, R.E.
University Department of Surgery
University of Wales, College of
Medicine
Heath Park
Cardiff CF4 4XN, U.K.

MARGOLESE, R.G.
McGill University
Jewish General Hospital
3755 Chemin de la Côte, St. Catherine
Montreal, Quebec H3T1E2, Canada

MÜLLER, A.
University Hospital for Women
D-6900 Heidelberg, FRG

NIELSEN, J.M.
Institute of Pathology
Frederiksberg Hospital
Copenhagen, Denmark

OTTESEN, G.L.
Institute of Forensic Medicine
University of Odense
Odense, Denmark

PRECHTEL, K.
Am Fuchsengraben 3
D-8190 Starnberg, FRG

PREECE, P.E.
Ninewells Hospital
and Medical School
Dundee, Scotland DD19SY, U.K.

RABE, DAGMAR
Universitätsfrauenklinik
Voßstraße 9
D-6900 Heidelberg, FRG

RAUSCHECKER, H.
Chirurgische Universitätsklinik
Robert-Koch-Str. 40
D-3400 Göttingen, FRG

RECHT, A.
Joint Center for Radiation Therapy
Department of Radiation Therapy
Harvard Medical School
50 Binney Street
Boston MA 02115, USA

REITZENSTEIN, M.
Universitätsfrauenklinik Erlangen
Universitätsstraße 21–23
D-8520 Erlangen, FRG

RONAY, G.
Universitätsfrauenklinik Erlangen
Universitätsstraße 21–23
D-8520 Erlangen, FRG

ROSE, M.A.
Joint-Center for Radiation Therapy
Boston, MA 02115, USA

ROTH, J.
Department of Radiation Physics
University Hospital Basel
CH-Basel, Switzerland

ROTHE, H.
Pathologisches Institut
der Universität Göttingen
Robert-Koch-Str. 40
D-3400 Göttingen, FRG

ROTTE, K.
Department of Radiotherapy
University Women's Hospital
Josef-Schneider-Str. 4
D-8700 Würzburg, FRG

RUMMEL, H.H.
Department of Gynecological
Morphology
University Women's Hospital
Voßstraße 9
D-6900 Heidelberg, FRG

SÄBEL, M.
University Women's Clinic
D-8520 Erlangen, FRG

SAUER, R.
Strahlentherapeutische
Universitätsklinik
Universitätsstraße 27
D-8520 Erlangen, FRG

SCHAUER, A.
Pathologisches Institut
der Universität Göttingen
Robert-Koch-Str. 40
D-3400 Göttingen, FRG

SCHIRRMACHER, V.
Institute of Immunology
and Genetics
German Cancer Research Center
D-6900 Heidelberg, FRG

SCHLEGEL, W.
Deutsches Krebsforschungszentrum
D-6900 Heidelberg, FRG

SCHMID, H.
Department of Obstetrics
and Gynecology
University of Heidelberg
D-6900 Heidelberg, FRG

SCHNITT, S.J.
Department of Pathology
Beth Israel Hospital
and Harvard Medical School
Boston MA 02115, USA

SCHUHMACHER, M.
Institut für Medizinische Biometrie
und Informatik
Stefan-Meier-Straße 19
D-7800 Freiburg

SILVER, B.
Joint Center for Radiation Therapy
Department of Radiation Therapy
Harvard Medical School
50 Binney Street
Boston MA 02115, USA

SPITALIER, J.M.
Department of Surgery
Cancer Institute
Marseille, France

SPRATT, J.A.
Department of General and Thoracic
Surgery
Duke University Hospital
Durham, NC 17712, USA

SPRATT, J.S.
Division of Health Systems
James Graham Brown Cancer Center
University of Louisville
529 S. Jackson
St. Louisville, KY 40202, USA

STAFFEN, A.
Second Department of Surgery
University of Vienna
Spitalgasse 23
A-1090 Wien, Austria

STEGNER, H.E.
Abt. für gynäkologische
Histopathologie
und Elektronenmikroskopie
Universitätsfrauenklinik
Martinistr. 52
D-2000 Hamburg, FRG

THOMSEN, J.L.
Institute of Forensic Medicine
University of Copenhagen
Copenhagen, Denmark

TORHORST, J.
Spitalstraße 21
University of Basel
Ch-Basel, Switzerland

TULUSAN, A.H.
Universitätsfrauenklinik Erlangen
Universitätsstraße 21–23
D-8520 Erlangen, FRG

VERONESI, U.
Instituto Nazionale per lo Studio
e la Cura dei Tumori
Via Venezian, 1
I-20133 Milano, Italy

WARENDORF, U.
Deutsches Krebsforschungszentrum
D-6900 Heidelberg, FRG

WALTHER, E.
Department of Radiooncology
Spitalstraße 21
University of Basel
CH-Basel, Switzerland

WEBER, E.
Deutsches Krebsforschungszentrum
D-6900 Heidelberg, FRG

Introduction: In Memory of Joseph Hirsch (1876–1947)

D. VON FOURNIER

From 1914 onward, JOSEPH HIRSCH, working in the "*Israelitisches Krankenheim*" in Berlin, performed breast-conserving therapy in those of his breast cancer patients whose disease was not too advanced. In 1927, he published his results [10] with a 13-year period of meticulous follow-up. HIRSCH appears to be one of the first surgeons – if not the very first – to publish a controlled study or breast-conserving therapy in combination with radiotherapy for carcinoma of the breast.

Breast-Conserving Therapy – A New Strategy in Oncology

The greater possible degree of radicality, with removal of the breast cancer accompanied by the surrounding tissue (breast, pectoral muscle, axillary lymph nodes) was accepted as standard until about 1970 in the Western industrialized countries. Very recently, eminent surgeons [16] were still issuing warnings to the effect that the long-term survival following breast-conserving therapy could not be anything but poorer than that obtained with the modified radical operation, and this opinion is still voiced today. In Germany, modified radical mastectomy is the standard method of treatment for breast carcinoma even when the tumor is small, breast-conserving therapy being recommended only within the confines of controlled studies. Nonetheless, the proportion of cases of small cancerous tumors (clinical size up to 3 cm) treated by breast-conserving therapy seems to be increasing slowly but steadily in Germany and in other Western countries.

One must question why, especially in Germany, most surgeons continue with the conservative option of modified radical mastectomy especially since the pioneering studies of HIRSCH have been reinforced by numerous studies around the world [BLUMING 1986]. MARGULESE [14] has offered the following answer to this question: "Careful doctors just are conservative: they naturally keep on with well-tried techniques, because experience has proved their work and they obviously want their patients to have the benefit of the method that is safest in the long term." ENGEL et al. (this volume), however, report that 98% of women questioned some years after breast-conserving therapy say they would still select this form of treatment in preference to mastectomy. Breast-conserving therapy with partial resection of the breast and radium implantation was described in England as long ago as 1908 by FINZI [5] (results reported October 1927). KEYNES [12] has hitherto been accepted in literature [9] as the initiator of conservative surgery with irradiation, starting in London in 1924.

It is mainly BLUMING [2] of Los Angeles that we have to thank for reminding us of JOSEPH HIRSCH, who had been completely forgotten, at least in the German literature. The new emphasis on HIRSCH'S role is not in any way a matter of nationalistic pride; before World War I new ideas in medicine were passed around within Europe very quickly, so that a great many new developments can be considered the fruits of joint efforts. It is strange, however, that the medical community in each large country has to gather its own experience, even at the cost of duplicating studies, before a new treatment is accepted as standard.

Breast-conserving therapy is thus still a controversial rather than a well-established method of treatment because it reflects a new way of thinking in medicine and oncology. After 1900 the tendency toward maximum local radicality became established in the form of the standard Halsted mastectomy. However, the "new" tenet of organ conservation is increasingly gaining ground, with retention of the organ and of its function combined with high-dose local radiotherapy, e.g., in brain tumors or in tumors of the face and neck. HIRSCH was one of the first in oncology to adopt this concept, which is now considered modern.

Biographical Data Relating to J. Hirsch

JOSEPH HIRSCH was born in Halberstadt (south of Berlin) in 1876. He took his medical degree in Munich, attaining his doctorate in 1901 with the research topic: syphilis of the lung. He then took specialist training in obstetrics and gynecology in Landau (1902–1907) and in Vienna with SCHAUTA (1906–1907). From 1908 to 1933 he was head of the Department of Gynecology and Obstetrics at the *Israelitisches Krankenheim* (Fig. 1) under the auspices of the Adass Isroel Synagogue in Berlin [18]. In 1933, as the period of terror under HITLER gathered force, he emigrated to Jerusalem, where he worked until his death in 1947 as Medical Director and Head of Gynecology and Obstetrics at Bikur Scholim General Hospital [13,4].

In Germany HIRSCH had published scientific papers on the following topics: physiological weight loss in neonates, treatment of puerperal fever, pregnancy after artificial insemination, treatment with hormone extracts from the hypophysis and ovaries, and radium surgery of breast cancer [18]. The latest of these papers was published in 1927, after which HIRSCH'S name did not appear in the German literature again until his work was cited in 1983 [by VON FOURNIER] and 1985 [by BELLER].

Hirsch's Experience with Breast-Conserving Therapy

Between 1914 and 1924, HIRSCH had performed breast-conserving therapy in 22 patients (Steintal grading: 16 grade I, five grade II, one grade III). He published his results in 1927, when the follow-up period in the 19 patients still alive amounted to 3–13 years. Recurrence-free survival (RFS) for 5–13 years was recorded in 18 of these 19 cases. The patient with Steintal stage III disease died in the first year with generalized cancer. A further patient died of a stroke while locally disease-free.

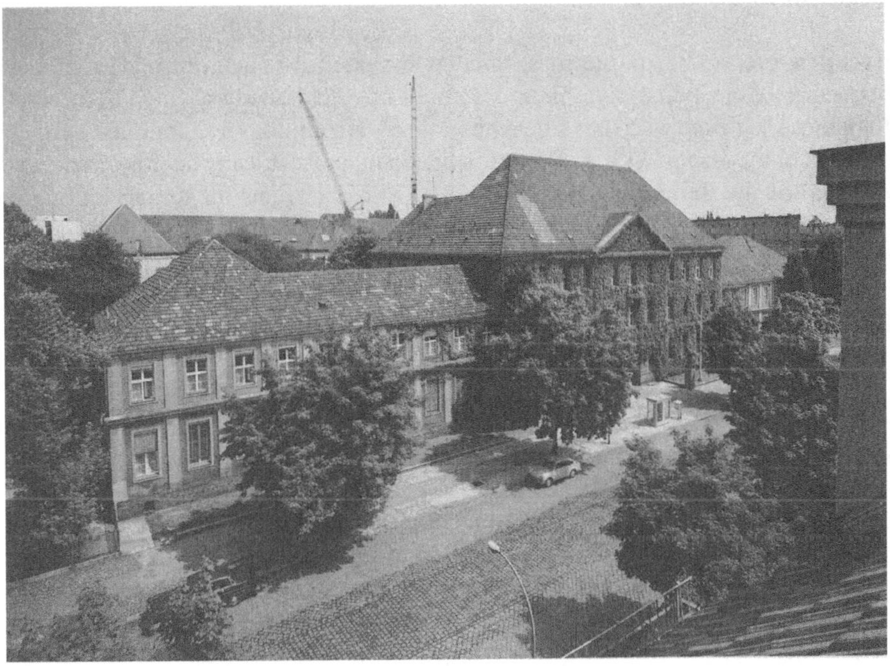

Fig. 1. The *Israelitisches Krankenheim* in Berlin (photograph taken in 1977 and supplied by the *Landesbildstelle Berlin*

Three early scar recurrences were treated by second excision and radiotherapy. All three of these patients were subsequently free of local and distant recurrence at 5 years or longer of follow-up.

J. Hirsch's Method

Operation. The operation technique used by HIRSCH consisted of wide excision of the tumor leaving grossly free margins, removal of the underlying pectoral fascia and, if necessary, of the underlying part of the pectoral muscle. The incision was extended toward the axilla to allow inspection of the lymph nodes and irradiation of the axillary area, and removal of any large axillary nodes found to be involved, but without axillary clearance.

Irradiation. Two rubber drains were positioned, one in the axillary region and one in the tumor bed. Each was filled with 30 mg radium (total of 60 mg). The duration of radiation was 12 h per session, and five sessions were given at intervals of 3–4 days. Thus, the total radium dose per patient was 2600–3600 milligram radium-element hours (mg Elh).

Treatment Strategy

HIRSCH wrote: "(The) question (is) whether less extensive operation and less radical dissection of the axillary lymph nodes might not yield results as good as or better than those achieved with the radical operation." His strategy was complete surgical excision of the tumor, with the resection line in macroscopically healthy tissue, and removal of the underlying pectoral fascia. Thus, it seems his understanding of radicality was closer to quadrantectomy reported by VERONESI [17] than to wide excision or lumpectomy. The subsequent irradiation was delivered to the remaining breast tissue and the uncleared axilla, in the form of brachytherapy with a fractionated low dose rate technique. The radiation dose at a tissue depth of 1 cm was at least 50 Gy according to present-day methods of dose calculation.

Recognition of J. Hirsch's Scientific Achievement

It is not possible to assess with certainty what effect the techniques pioneered by JOSEPH HIRSCH have had on the development of breast-conserving therapy. It is probable, however, that his ideas were widely discussed and incorporated in attempts at breast-conserving therapy, which were then continued in England. These ideas were never completely forgotten in Berlin. A. LAX was the first to reintroduce breast-conserving therapy in Germany, employing it in Berlin from 1963 onward [7].

As long ago as 1927, HIRSCH provided Germany with the opportunity to explore a treatment concept that is considered modern today, by building on his 13 years of clinical experience. This chance was wasted as a result of the discrimination that led to isolation and ultimately exile. Even today, HIRSCH'S work remains the only German contribution of international importance to the topic of breast-conserving therapy.

It is painfully obvious that JOSEPH HIRSCH'S story (Fig. 2) reflects the destruction of the basis of a person's life and, with this, of an important scientific idea. HIRSCH stands for many Jews and others who were persecuted in Germany's dark days and whose scientific or medical achievements have been forgotten. During his lifetime he did not receive due recognition for his contributions to medicine. He had improvement of the patient's quality of life in mind when he wrote: "I should like to recommend this method especially to those of my colleagues who have a larger number of cases of breast cancer available for treatment." The style of his publications betrays the modesty that current philosophical thinking suggests is essential if scientific research is to be pursued at all [6].

It should be borne in mind that HIRSCH was able to devise an astonishingly innovative scientific approach that remained current for a very long period with very simple scientific equipment and a small patient population. As an assimilated Jew he found the German liberalism prevailing before World War I a fertile ground for scientific ideas. At that time it was possible for Jewish people to achieve a "felicitous assimilation" [LEO BECK 1959, cited by KELLER 1973] in German-speaking areas, and this led to the high scientific standard exemplified by HIRSCH'S achievements.

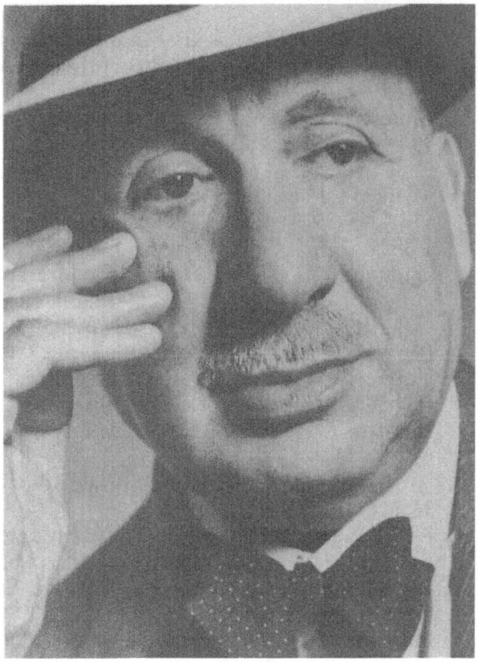

Fig. 2. Doctor Joseph Hirsch (born 1876 in Halberstadt, died 1947 in Jerusalem)

The agony following World War I in Germany led to the loss of liberal principles and thus to a discontinuation of the constructive dialogue with the Jewish culture. This was disastrous for all concerned: it meant not only an end to the assimilation of Jewish people in Germany but also the definitive self-destruction of the state that had made this acceptance possible. It is said that inside the arch of Titus (Forum Romanum) the following words are scrawled: "Evil Titus is dead, the nation of Israel lives." In the history books covering more than 1000 years of German culture there are many memorable examples of inextinguishable German-Jewish assimilation: Isaak of Aachen, the ambassador (797) of Charlemagne, Spinoza (Baruch, who did not accept a professorship in Heidelberg in 1673–6), Theodor Herzl, Albert Einstein, etc. In the natural way of things, only succeeding generations can fully appreciate all this. Consequently, scope must once again be given to those in the German community who wish the continuation of a "felicitous assimilation." This book is dedicated, in belated recognition, to JOSEPH HIRSCH, whose photograph was kindly supplied by Benjamin Feuchtwanger, his grandson in Jerusalem.

References

1. Beller FK (1985) Atlas der Mammachirurgie. Schattauer, Stuttgart
2. Bluming AZ (1982) Treatment of primary breast cancer without mastectomy. Am J Med 72:820–828
3. Bluming AZ (1986) Treatment of primary breast cancer without mastectomy. Ann Surg 204:136–147
4. Feuchtwanger M (1987) Personal report, Ben Gurion University of the Negev, Soroka Medical Center, Beer-Sheva, Israel
5. Finzi NS (1927) X-rays and radium in the treatment of carcinoma of the breast. Br Med J 2:728–733
6. Gadamer HG (1986) Ceremonial address at commemoration of 600th anniversary of University of Heidelberg (in German). Rektorat, Universität Heidelberg
7. Genz T, Schmidt-Gollwitzer M, Pachaly J, Meyer KD, Lax H, Kindermann G (1986) Die brusterhaltende Carcinomtherapie. Geburtshilfe Frauenheilkd 46:567–572
8. Haffner S (1987) Von Bismarck zu Hitler. Kindler, München
9. Harris JR, Hellman S (1987) Conservative surgery and radiotherapy. In: Harris JR, Helmann S, Henderson IC, Kinne DW (eds) Breast diseases. Lippincott, Philadelphia, pp 299–324
10. Hirsch J (1927) Radiumchirurgie des Brustkrebses. Dtsch Med Wochenschr 34:1419–1421
11. Keller W (1973) Und wurden zerstreut unter alle Völker. Droemer-Knaur, Munich
12. Keynes G (1937) Conservative treatment of cancer of the breast. Br Med J 2:643–647
13. Landesverwaltungsamt Berlin, Abt. III, Entschädigungsbehörde, Potsdamer Straße (1986) Gesch Z: III 7 31–161967
14. Margulese RG (1986) Personal report. Mc Gill University, Jewish General Hospital, Montreal, Canada
15. Speer A (1984) Der Sklavenstaat. Ullstein, Frankfurt, pp 354–355
16. Urban JA (1985) Conservative treatment of potentially curable minimal, occult and early breast cancer. In: Zander J, Baltzer J (eds) Early breast cancer. Springer, Berlin Heidelberg New York, pp 231–241
17. Veronesi U (1981) Comparing radical mastectomy with quadrantectomy, axillary dissection and radiotherapy in patients with small cancer of the breast. N Engl J Med 305:6–11
18. Winau R (1987) Letter, October. Institut für Geschichte der Medizin, Freie Universität Berlin

I. Biology, Morphology, Growth Behavior

Epidemiology of Breast Cancer

J.F.H. GAUWERKY, R. FRENTZEL-BEYME and D. VON FOURNIER

Frequency of Breast Cancer

Incidence and Mortality

In 1976, 88 000 patients with a breast carcinoma were registered in the USA and 33 000 died of breast cancer [81]. In 1982, 112 000 new cases and 37 000 deaths were estimated [55]. In the Federal Republic of Germany (FRG) in 1978, 11 790 women

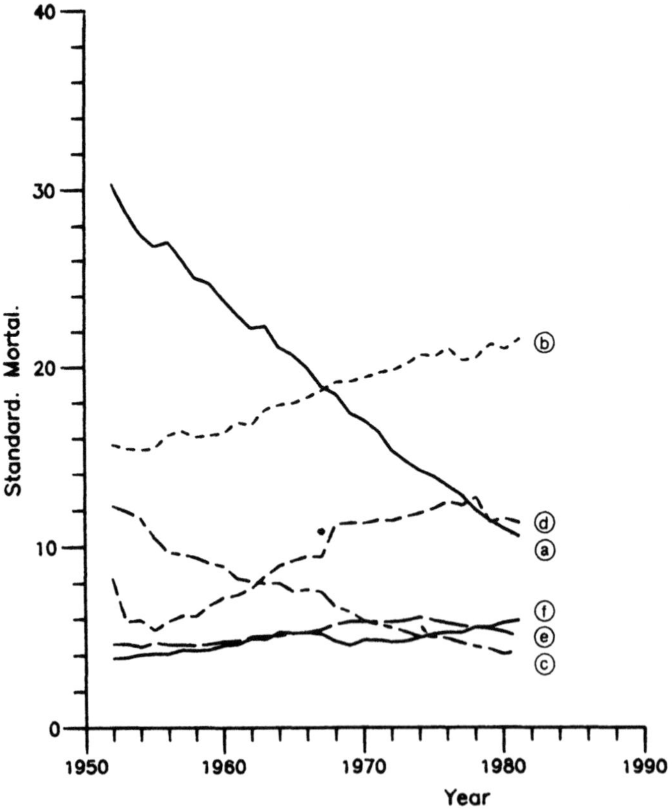

Fig. 1. Temporal trend of age-adjusted mortality for different cancers (women) in the Federal Republic of Germany. *a*, stomach; *b*, breast; *c*, corpus uteri; *d*, colon; *e*, rectum; *f*, lung. (Data from: BECKER et al. [4])

died of breast cancer, corresponding to 36/100 000 or 15.1% of all female cancer deaths [4]. By 1985, the number of breast cancer deaths had increased to over 15 000, representing 18% of all cancer deaths in women [75] (Fig. 1). In Central and Western Europe, from 1956 until 1975, the frequency of breast cancer has increased by 20%, i.e., by 1% per year. A decrease in mortality has only been observed in some Far Eastern countries and in Norway [4]. In the FRG, mortality is increasing continuously in almost all age groups. Between 1952 and 1982, there was a marked increase in mortality among those over 50 and especially over 70 (Fig. 2).

The frequency of breast carcinoma shows considerable regional and national differences (Fig. 3). Israel and Japan have the lowest incidence, Switzerland and certain regions of the USA and Canada the highest.

Age and Frequency

Below 30 years of age, and particularly below 20, breast cancer is very rare. PIRQUET [60] found 7/70 247 patients to be younger than 20 in a literature survey. As to age-related incidence, national differences can be observed. While there is a

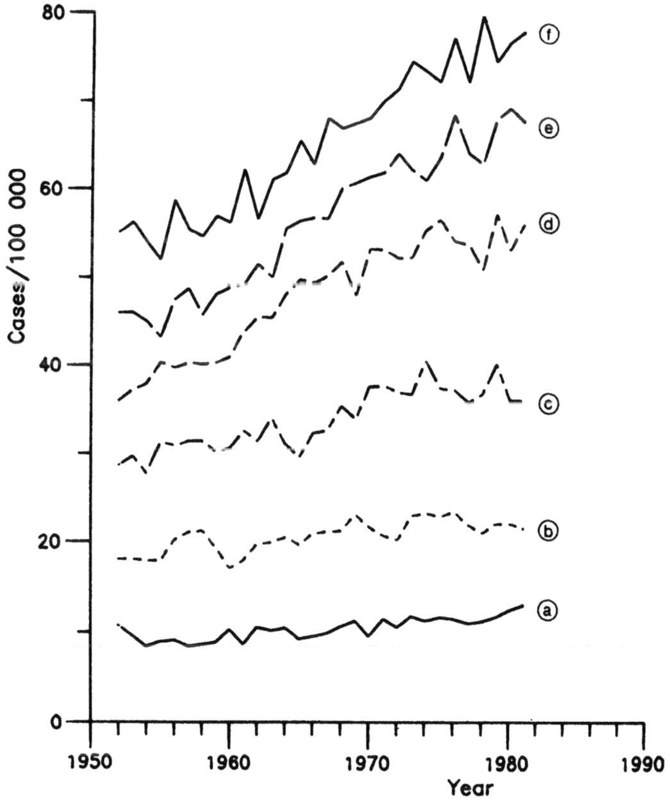

Fig. 2. Time trend of mortality in individual age groups, Federal Republic of Germany. Age groups: *a*, 35–39; *b*, 40–44; *c*, 45–49; *d*, 50–54; *e*, 55–59; *f*, 60–64. (Data from BECKER et al. [4])

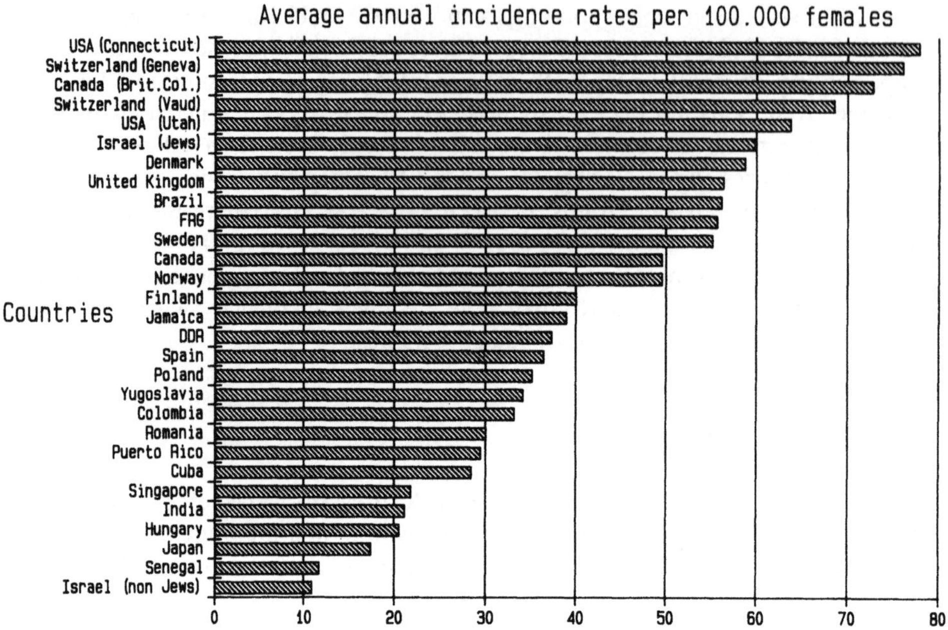

Fig. 3. Average annual incidences of carcinoma of the breast per 100 000 females in different countries. (From: WATERHOUSE et al., [81])

continuous increase of frequency with advancing age in Canada and Switzerland, in some other countries there is flattening with plateau formation, and in yet others, e.g., Japan, a decrease is observed (Fig. 4).

Plateau formation around 50 years of age is shown extremely clearly in the Scandinavian cancer registers ("Clemmesen's hook," Fig. 5). Premenopausal and postmenopausal risk groups, risk factors and constellations can be differentiated. Thus, for instance, the premenopausal cancer risk is higher for slim women, while there is an increased postmenopausal risk for obese women [32]. MYERS et al. [54] indicated a lowering of the breast cancer risk by breast-feeding for premenopausal cancers, but not after the menopause.

Regional Aspects

Taking the FRG as an example, one can show especially high cancer death rates in industrialized regions (Fig. 6), and cancer incidence and death rates are also higher in urban regions. This is also true for many other West European countries [79]. In the FRG there is an additional north-south difference, and on the European level higher standardized rates are observed in Western Europe and England than in Southern Europe, especially Italy (Fig. 7).

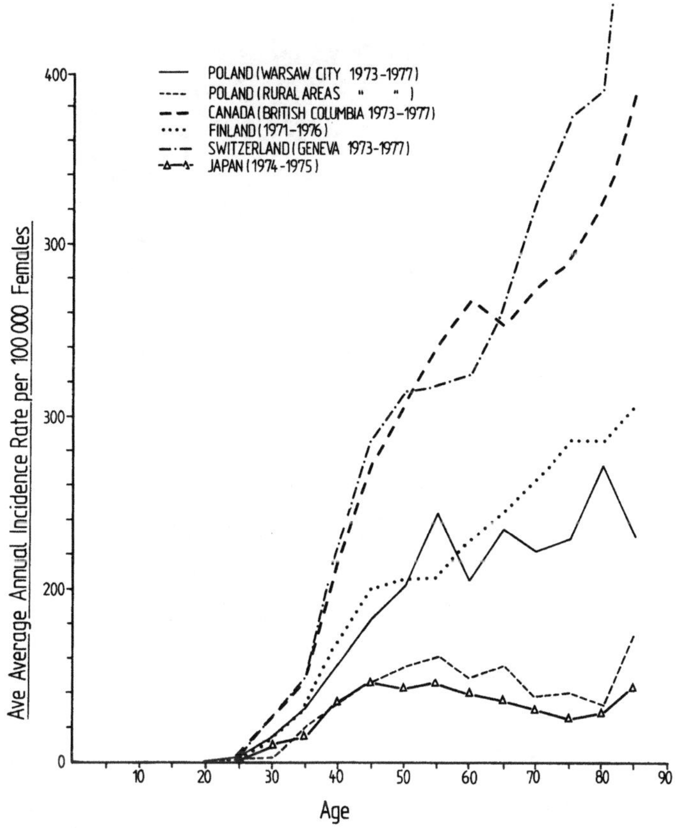

Fig. 4. Average annual incidence rates of breast carcinoma. (From WATERHOUSE et al. [81])

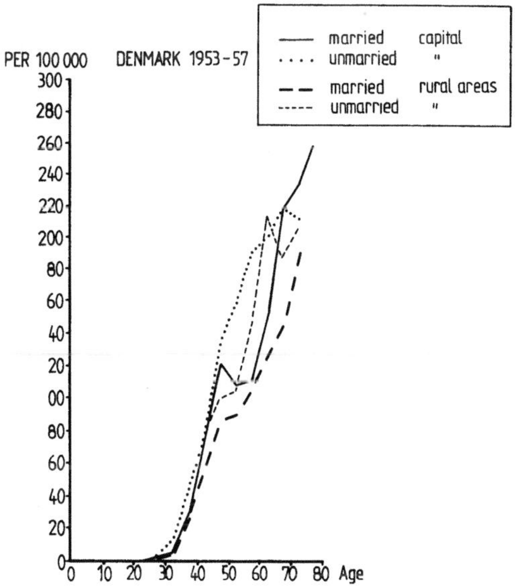

Fig. 5. Age specific incidences of breast carcinoma in Danish women. (From CLEMMESEN [12])

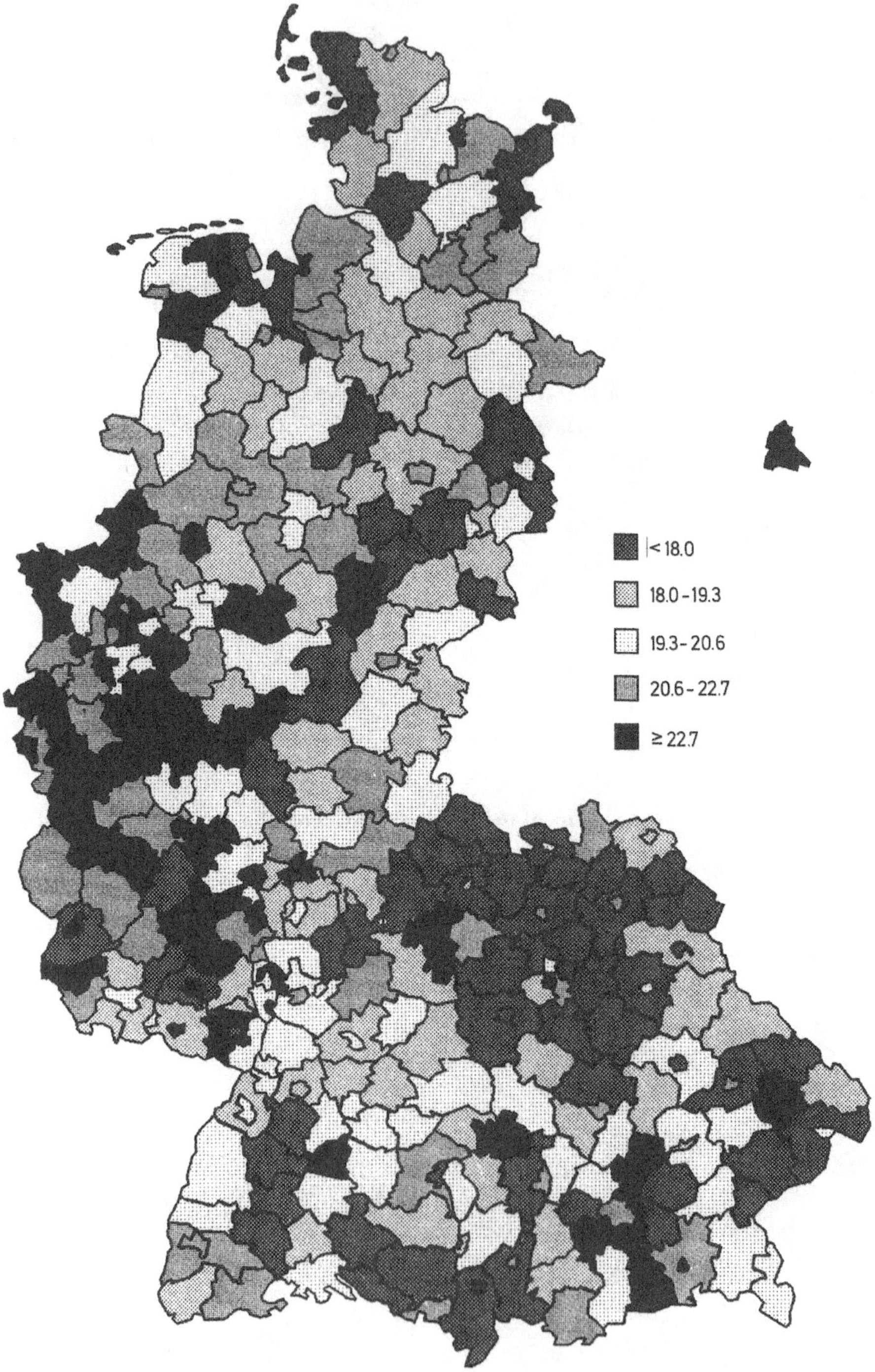

Fig. 6. Average annual mortality from 1976 to 1982 in the Federal Republic of Germany: cartographic presentation. Figures indicate age-standardized rates per 100 000 (From BECKER et al. [4])

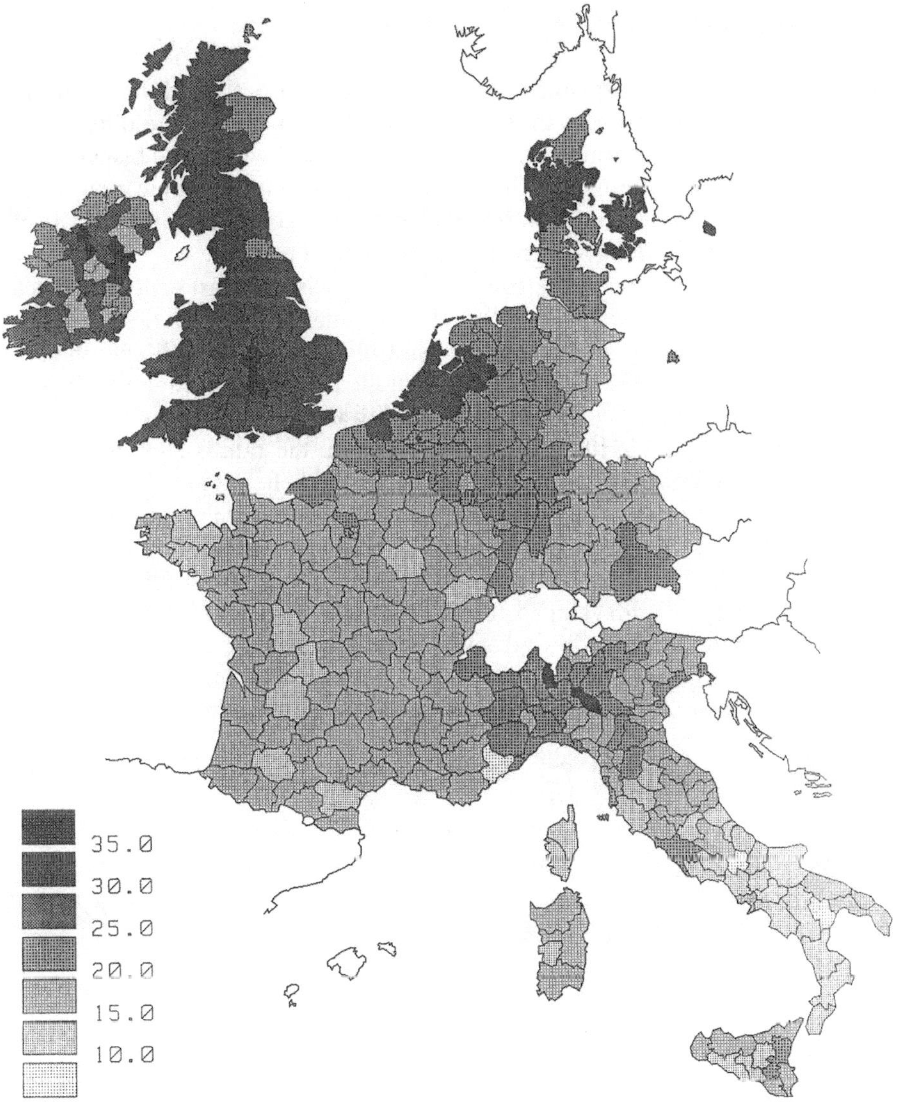

Fig. 7. Mortality from breast cancer in the European Community, 1970–1980, age-standardized, per 100 000 female population. (To appear in: SMANS et al. European Atlas of Cancer Mortality. IARC, Lyon, [74])

Risk Factors

Genetic Factors

Racial differences of breast cancer incidence have been described, but environmental factors and differences in way of life could also explain the differences. SEIDMANN et al. [68] found only small differences between whites and blacks in the USA (Fig. 8). Table 1 summarizes the incidence rates of various ethnic groups and geographic areas. These data show that socioeconomic conditions and the way of life connected with them have a greater influence than race.

In the black population of Detroit and San Francisco, breast cancer occurs 5 times more frequently than in that of Nigeria or Rhodesia. Similarly, the frequency of breast cancer in San Francisco and British Columbia is 2 times higher than in Poland [81]. The same tendency can be seen in the breast cancer rates of first and second generation Japanese women living in Hawaii (Table 2). In contrast to the annual incidence of 13.0/100 000 women in Japan, the rate is 35.9 in the first generation of Japanese in Hawaii, 57.2 in the second generation and 66.2 in the remaining population. According to KATZ et al. [29], the frequency of breast cancer among Israeli Jews is highest among those who have immigrated to Israel from highly industrialized regions of Europe and America and lowest for those from socioeconomically underdeveloped countries in Asia or Africa (Table 3).

However, there is a certain agreement regarding genetic predisposition for breast cancer. The higher breast cancer rate associated with Klinefelter's syndrome and a hereditary predisposition for breast cancer in certain families support this notion.

Breast cancer in men with Klinefelter's syndrome occurs 66 times more often than in healthy men, thus reaching the same frequency as in women. Approximately 3.3% of all men with Klinefelter's syndrome (XXY) will develop breast cancer [52]. The disease is thus possibly connected to the additional X chromosome.

According to JACOBSEN [26] and WYNDER et al. [82] the risk of developing breast cancer is 2–3 times higher for mothers and sisters of breast cancer cases. However,

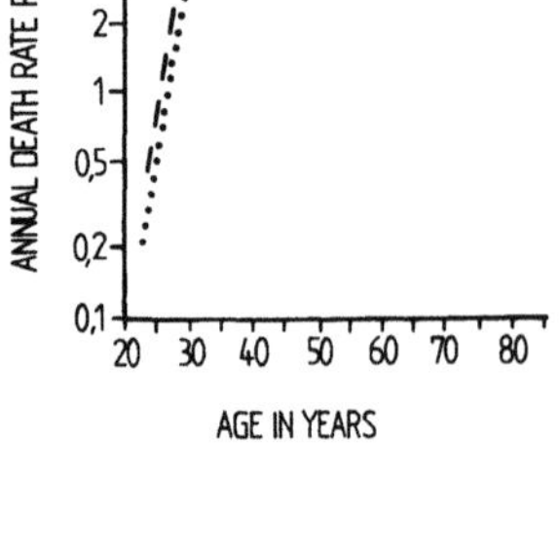

Fig. 8. Breast cancer death rates, United States 1966–1968. (From SEIDMANN [67])

Table 1. Age-standardized incidences of carcinoma of the breast by ethnic group and geographic area. Data adjusted to world population of Segi

Racial/ ethnic group	Geographic area	Incidence (per 100 000 females)
Caucasian (white)	Norway	49.6
	Denmark	58.8
	UK (Birmingham)	56.4
	Federal Republic of Germany (Hamburg)	55.7
	Poland (Cracow)	35.2
	Spain (Saragossa)	36.5
	USA	
	Alameda County	78.2
	San Francisco Bay Area	83.7
	Los Angeles	85.3
	New Mexico	78.7
	Hawaii	85.6
Latin American	Colombia (Cali)	33.2
	Cuba	28.5
	United States (New Mexico)	19.3
Negro (black)	Senegal (Dakar)	11.8
	USA	
	Alameda County	67.2
	San Francisco Bay Area	64.1
	Los Angeles	65.4
Indian	Singapore	28.2
	India (Bombay)	21.2
Israeli Jews	From European and American countries	61.7
	From Africa or Asia	34.3
East Asian	Japan	
	Miyaga Prefecture	17.5
	Osaka	12.7
	Singapore	21.9
	USA	
	San Francisco Bay Area	56.8/55.1[a]
	Los Angeles	42.7/57.3[a]
	Hawaii	53.3/47.1[a]

From WATERHOUSE et al. [81]
[a]Chinese/Japanese

no definite statement can be made as to the occurrence of breast cancer in distant relatives. ANDERSON [1,2] saw an especially high risk for first-degree relatives of premenopausal patients with a bilateral breast carcinoma (nine-fold risk, Table 4). BODIAN and HAAGENSEN [6] have found that daughters are on average 11 years younger at the time of diagnosis than their mothers had been; however, it must be said that there are major problems in the interpretation of data.

Table 2. Average annual incidence (world population as standard) of breast cancer: first and second generations of Japanese in Hawaii, compared with Japanese in Japan and Caucasians in Hawaii

	Number of cases	Annual incidence (per 100 000 females)
Japanese in Japan (1968–1971)	511	13.0
First generation Japanese in Hawaii (1973–1977)	41	35.9
Second generation Japanese in Hawaii (1973–1977)	407	57.2
Caucasians in Hawaii (1968–1972)	378	66.2

From KOLONEL et al. [35] and WATERHOUSE et al. [80]

Table 3. Incidence of breast carcinoma in Israel according to ethnic group and country of origin

	Number of cases and average annual incidence (per 100 000 females)			
	1969–1976		1972–1976	
Origin	Number	Rate	Number	Rate
Jews born in Israel	169	35.9	362	52.6
Jews born in Asia or Africa	485	22.2	825	34.2
Jews born in Europe or America	2596	55.5	280	61.9
All Jews in Israel	3250	44.9	4538	59.3
All non-Jews in Israel	44	8.1	76	10.9

Data from KATZ et al. [29]

Table 4. Familial breast cancer related to age at diagnosis and bilaterality in first-degree relatives. Relative risk as compared with controls (relative to the percent frequency of breast carcinoma among 699 first-degree relatives of patients with other types of carcinoma)

Characteristics	Number of relatives	Age-adjusted percent with breast carcinoma	Relative risk
Total	567	4.9	1.8
Age 20–49 at diagnosis	188	6.7	3.1
Age 50 and older at diagnosis	379	4.2	1.5
Unilateral	486	3.4	1.3
Bilateral	81	13.1	5.4
Age 20–49, unilateral	155	3.4	1.8
Age 50 and older, unilateral	331	3.5	1.2
Age 20–49, bilateral	33	17.1	8.8
Age 50 and older, bilateral	48	10.6	4.0

From ANDERSON [1,2]

Socioeconomic Factors, Way of Life

Studies on rats and mice have shown that the rate of spontaneous as well as chemically induced breast cancers is related to the fat content of their food.

In humans, CAROLL [10] showed a direct connection between fat consumption and breast cancer mortality in 39 countries (Fig. 9). WYNDER et al. [84] found high cholesterol and fat consumption in Western countries to be an additional cause for the high breast cancer rate. In Japan, fat consumption and breast cancer frequency are slowly increasing [83], as they are in Iceland [49]. Among Seventh Day Adventists (50% vegetarians), the rate of breast cancer is lower [18]. In a German Cancer Research Center study on 1046 female vegetarians [22], no deaths from breast cancer were noted in a 5-year follow-up period, though two deaths would have been expected on the basis of average mortality.

Table 5 shows that increased consumption of animal fats and lipids is accompanied by higher breast cancer mortality, while the consumption of vegetable fats seems to lower the death rate. One explanation for this might be a possible mechanism in obese women of better conversion of androstenedione into Estrane 1 and a lower tissue level of sex hormone-binding globulins [23,73].

Recently published evidence from USA and from Japan have challenged the contention that breast cancer could be importantly related with fat intake [27,71].

Various publications present data documenting a connection between higher education and breast cancer [24,40,57,17]. Especially the lower intensity of emotional reactions in these women is regarded as a psychosocial risk factor [3].

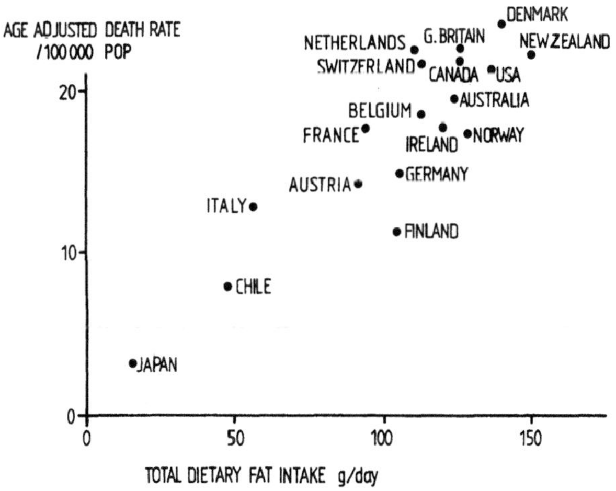

Fig. 9. Age-adjusted mortality and per capita consumption of dietary fat in different countries. (Data from CAROLL [10])

Table 5. Correlation coefficients for regional consumption of selected nutrients in 1973 and breast cancer mortality in Bavaria (1975) and the Federal Republic of Germany (1976–1980)

Nutrient	Bavaria	Federal Republic of Germany
Protein	0.74**	0.42
Lipids	0.57*	0.69**
Animal fat	0.76**	0.58*
Vegetable fat	-0.16	0.25
Carbohydrates	-0.01	-0.49
Polysaccharides	-0.29	-0.27
Disaccharides	0.38	-0.57*
Alcohol	0.35	0.14
Retinol equivalent	0.62*	0.58*
Vitamin B1	0.25	0.25
Vitamin C	0.49	0.81**
Crude fiber	0.12	0.64*
Iron	0.05	0.27
Calcium	0.85*	0.42
Cholesterol	0.84*	0.61*

From FRENTZEL-BEYME [21] and BÖING et al. [7]
*$0.01 < p < 0.05$; **$p < 0.01$

Reproduction

SHAPIRO et al. [69] conducted a 1.5-year follow-up study on a group of 20 211 women, among whom he diagnosed 111 new cases of breast cancer (Table 6). According to this study, the risk of developing breast cancer is extremely high for women who have never married (2.3-fold), for women with less than three pregnancies (2-fold) and for women with early menarche (1.7-fold). The risk is also increased for women with previous benign breast lesions or a history of breast cancer in their families. In contrast to the conclusions of certain retrospective studies, SHAPIRO could not prove any protective effect of breast-feeding or of an extended lactation period.

The earlier in life a pregnancy occurs, the lower the potential risk for breast cancer [46] (Fig. 10). An early marriage associated with multiparity thus results in a reduced risk for breast cancer. Therefore, early endocrine changes influence the risk of developing breast cancer later. It is postulated that carcinogenic effects take place early in life, so that protective mechanisms also have to be set into motion early. These observations are valid only for women whose pregnancies last for more than 5 months. For women with early and late abortions (less than 4–5 months) the cancer risk seems to be higher [11,32,41,85].

Prolonged cyclic ovarian function (early menarche or late menopause) increases the risk of breast cancer [30]. A break in this cyclic ovarian activity can distinctly lower the breast cancer risk. Early artificial menopause, for instance, lowers the risk [19]. This protection is lifelong, the effect seeming the clearer the earlier the time of castration [19,76]. Castration before 35 years of age lowers the cancer risk to one-third, but there is no protective effect of castration after 40 years of age [76].

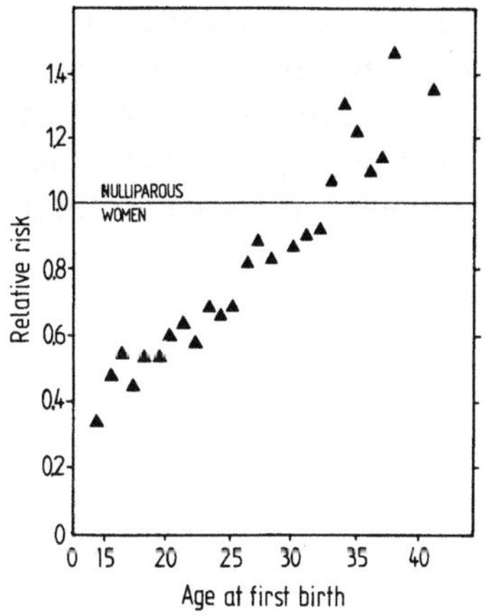

Fig. 10. Relative risk of breast cancer related to age at first birth. (Data from MACMAHON et al. [46])

Table 6. Reproductive variables: comparison of relative risks for breast cancer

Characteristics	Ratio of relative risk
Never married vs married	2.3*
One or two pregnancies vs three or more pregnancies	2.0*
Age at menarche: under 12 vs 15 or older	1.7
Aggregate years menstrual activity: 30 years or more vs less than 30 years	1.4
Breast conditions: one or more vs none	3.1*
Sisters, with breast cancer: one or more vs none	1.9

From SHAPIRO et al. [69]
*statistically significant increase

Hormones

Animal experiments have shown a carcinogenic effect of estrogens. The development of breast cancer can be influenced by estrogens and antiestrogens [30]. However, the importance of endogenous and exogenous estrogen substitution for the development of breast cancer has not yet been clarified. COLE and MACMAHON [14] postulated that the higher the relation of estriol E3 to estrone E1 and estradiol E3, the lower the cancer risk. Some clinical studies corroborate this hypothesis [47] but others do not [20,59].

The hypothesis that estrogens develop their carcinogenic effect only when there is no corresponding opposing progesterone influence (estrogen window) is still controversial [36]. The carcinogenic effect of progesterone shown in some animal experiments is also still unclear [51,61]. For women, progesterone seems to have a protective effect. A case study on patients with luteal insufficiency showed an increased cancer risk [16]. The importance of prolactin is not clear, the results of clinical studies being controversial. There is no evidence for the influence of prolactin on breast cancer occurrence [33,53]. No influence of ovulation inhibitors on breast cancer rates could be proven [77,78]. In contrast, benign breast lesions occur less frequently after a period of ovulation inhibition [8,9,31,38,56]. This protective effect seems to correlate with their progesterone content [9,63]. However, the protection may be exerted only in a subgroup with minimal epithelial atypia. In cases of major epithelial changes (which must be clarified by biopsy), ovulation inhibitors increase the cancer risk [13,34,42,58]. Further studies on this subject are necessary.

Ionizing Radiation

Exposure to ionizing radiation increases the risk of breast cancer in women. MCGREGOR et al. [48] observed in 63 275 female atomic bomb survivors of Nagasaki and Hiroshima a dose-response relationship to neutron and gamma radiation that yielded an overall absolute risk per rad of 1.9 excess cases per 1 million woman years. Women 10–19 years old at the time of exposure experienced much greater excess risk of breast cancer than did women older than 35 at the time of exposure.

In 1965, MACKENZIE found higher rates of breast cancer after multiple irradiation of pulmonary tuberculosis. SHORE et al. [72] found a higher occurrence of breast cancer after radiologically treated puerperal mastitis. Most studies on cancer risk after low exposure to radiation presume a linear relation between cancer risk and radiation dose, The cancer risk for low radiation exposure is calculated by linear extrapolation of the data obtained for higher exposures (e.g., A bombs, radiation therapy, radiation accidents). From a radiobiological point of view, it is improbable that this linear relation is valid for women over 30 years of age. The benefit of regular mammographies in a screening program has been demonstrated in various studies [15,25,50].

Predisposition Due to Previous Diseases

SCHOTTENFELD [64] reported a frequent association of diseases of the thyroid with breast cancer. The risk of a secondary carcinoma in the contralateral breast has been stated to be increased twofold [39], threefold [62] or even sevenfold [5] A contralateral secondary tumor is more likely the earlier the primary tumor has occurred. Other cancer forms, such as ovarian cancer [43], cancer of the corpus uteri [65] and cancer of the colon and rectum [44,66] are said to be associated with increased breast cancer risk. The influence of benign breast diseases on breast cancer is dealt with elsewhere in this volume [28].

References

1. Anderson DE (1972) A genetic study of human breast cancer. JNC'I 48:1029
2. Anderson DE (1975) Familial and genetic predisposition to breast cancer. In: Stoll B (ed) Risk factors in breast cancer, vol 2. Heinemann, London
3. Bahnson CB (1981) Stress and cancer: the state of the art. Part 2. Psychosomatics 22:207
4. Becker N, Frentzel-Beyme R, Wagner G (1984) Atlas of cancer mortality in the Federal Republic of Germany. Springer, Berlin Heidelberg New York

5. Berendt H, Borrmann C, Klein K (1976) Zweitkarzinom der Brustdrüse. Arch Geschwulstforsch 36:55
6. Bodian C, Haagensen CD (1986) Family history of breast carcinoma predisposing to the disease. In: Haagensen CD (ed) Diseases of the breast, 3rd edn. Saunders, Philadelphia, pp 409–423
7. Böing H, Martinez L, Frentzel-Beyme R, Oltersdorf U (1985) Regional nutritional pattern and cancer mortality in the Federal Republic of Germany. Nutr Cancer 7:121
8. Boston Collaborative Drug Surveillance Program (1973) Oral contraceptives and venous thromboembolic disease, surgically confirmed gallbladder disease, and breast tumours. Lancet 1:1399
9. Brinton LA, Vessey MP, Flavel R (1981) Risk factors for benign breast disease. Am J Epidemiol 113:203
10. Caroll KK (1975) Experimental evidence of dietary factors and hormone dependent cancers. Cancer Res 35:3374
11. Choi NW, Howe GR, Miller AB (1978) An epidemiologic study of breast cancer. Am J Epidemiol 107:510
12. Clemmesen J (1965) Statistical studies in malignant neoplasms, vol 1. Munksgard, Copenhagen
13. Cole P, Elwood JM, Kaplan SD (1978) Incidence rates and risk factors of benign breast neoplasms. Am J Epidemiol 108:112
14. Cole P, MacMahon B (1969) Oestrogen fractions during early reproductive life in the etiology of breast cancer. Lancet 1:604
15. Colette HJA, Day NE, Rombach JJ, de Waard F (1984) Evaluation of screening for breast cancer in a non-randomized study by means of a case-control study. Lancet 2:1224
16. Cowan LD, Gordis L, Tonascia JA et al. (1981) Breast cancer incidence in women with a history of progesterone deficiency. Am J Epidemiol 114:209
17. Devesa SS, Diamond EL (1980) Association of breast cancer and cervical cancer incidence with income and education among white and blacks. JNCI 65:515
18. Enstrom JE (1979) Cancer mortality among low risk population. CA 29(6):352
19. Feinleib M (1968) Breast cancer and artificial menopause: a cohort study. JNCI 41:315
20. Fishman J, Fukushima D, O'Connor J et al. (1978) Plasma hormone profiles of young women at risk for familial breast cancer. Cancer Res 38:4006
21. Frentzel-Beyme R (1986) The Federal Republic of Germany. In: Howe GM (ed) Global geocancerology. A world geography of human cancers. Livingstone, Edinburgh
22. Frentzel-Beyme R, Claude J, Eilbar U (1988) Mortality among German Vegetarians: First results after five years of follow-up. Nutr Cancer 11:117–126.
23. Grodin JM, Siiteri PK, MacDonald PC (1973) Source of estrogen production in postmenopausal women. J Clin Endocrinol Metab 36:207
24. Hliang T, Myint TM (1978) Risk factors of breast cancer in Burma. Int J Cancer 21:432
25. Holmberg LH, Adami HO, Tabar L, Bergström R (1986) Survival in breast cancer diagnosed between mammographic screening examinations. Lancet 2 p 27
26. Jacobsen CO (1946) Heredity in breast cancer: a genetic and clinical study of 200 probands. Nyt-Nordisk, Copenhagen
27. Jomes Y, Schatzhin A, Green S, Block G, Bruitzi L, Ziegler R, Hoover R, Taylor PR (1987) Dietary fat and breast cancer in the NHANESI epidemiologic follow-up study. J Natl Cancer Inst 79:465–471
28. Junkermann H, von Fournier D, Weber E, Arabin B, Diagnosis and classification of benign breast disorders (mastopathy). This volume, Chap VIII, pp 464–472
29. Katz C, Steinitz R, Sela T (1981) Epidemiological review of breast cancer in Israel. Isr J Med Sci 17:810
30. Kelsey JL, Hildreth NG (1983) Causative factors in breast cancer. In: Margolese R (ed) Breast cancer. Livingstone, Edinburgh
31. Kelsey JL, Lindfors KK, White C (1974) A case-control study of the epidemiology of benign breast diseases with reference to oral contraceptive use. Int J Epidemiol 3:333

32. Kelsey JL, Fischer DB, Holford TR (1981) Exogenous estrogens and other factors in the epidemiology of breast cancer. JNCI 67:327
33. Kleinberg DL (1987) Prolactin and breast cancer. N Engl J Med 316:269
34. Kodlin D, Winger EE, Morgenstern NL (1977) Chronic mastopathy and breast cancer. A follow-up study. Cancer 39:2603
35. Kolonel CN, Hinds MW, Hankin JH (1980) Cancer patterns among migrant and native-born Japanese in Hawaii in relation to smoking, drinking and dietary habits. In: Gelboin F et al. (eds) Genetic and environmental factors in experimental and human cancer. Japan Scientific Societies Press, Tokyo, p 327
36. Korenman SG (1980a) Oestrogen window hypothesis of the etiology of breast cancer. Lancet 1:700
37. Korenman SG (1980b) The endocrinology of breast cancer. Cancer 46:874
38. Lees AW, Burns PE, Grace M (1978) Oral contraceptives and breast disease in premenopausal Northern Alberta women. Int J Cancer 22:700
39. Lewison EF, Neho AS (1971) Bilateral breast cancer at the Johns Hopkins Hospital. Cancer 28:1297
40. Lin RS, Kessler II (1980) Epidemiologic findings in female breast cancer. Proc Am Assoc Cancer Res 21:72
41. Lin TM, Chen KP, MacMahon B (1971) Epidemiologic characteristics of cancer of the breast in Taiwan. Cancer 27:1497
42. LiVolsi VA, Stadel BV, Kelsey JL (1978) Fibrocystic breast disease in oral contraceptive users: a histopathologic evaluation of epithelial atypia. N Engl J Med 299:381
43. Lynch HT, Krush AJ (1971) Carcinoma of the breast and ovary in three families. Surg Gynecol Obstet 133:644
44. Lynch HT, Krush AJ, Guirgis H (1973) Genetic factors in families with combined gastrointestinal and breast cancer. Am J Gastroenterol 1:131
45. MacKenzie I (1965) Breast cancer following multiple fluoroscopies. Br J Cancer 19:1
46. MacMahon B, Cole P, Brown J (1973) Etiology of human breast cancer: a review. JNCI 50:21
47. MacMahon B, Andersen AP, Brown J et al. (1980) Urine estrogen profiles in European countries with high or low breast cancer rates. Eur J Cancer 16:1627
48. McGregor DH, Land CE, Choi K (1977) Breast cancer incidence among atomic bomb survivors, Hiroshima and Nagasaki, 1950–1969. JNCI 59:799
49. Miller AB (1977) Role of nutrition in the etiology of breast cancer. Cancer 39:2704
50. Moskowitz M, Gartside PS (1982) Evidence of breast cancer mortality reduction: aggressive screening in women under age 50. AJR 138:911
51. Mühlbock O, Boot LM (1967) The mode of action of ovarian hormones in the induction of mammary cancer in mice. Biochem Pharmacol 16:627
52. Mulvihill JJ (1975) Congenital and genetic diseases. In: Fraumeni JF (ed) Persons at high risk of cancer. Academic, New York
53. Musey VC, Collins DC, Musey PI, Martion-Saltzman D, Preedy JRK (1987) Long-term effect of a first pregnancy on the secretion of prolactin. N Engl J Med 316:229
54. Myers MH, Hankey BF, Steinhorn SC, Flannery JT (1982) Interrelationships of incidence and mortality and their effects on time trends. In: Magnus K (ed) Trends in cancer incidence. Causes and practical implications. Hemisphere, Washington, pp 79–87
55. National Center for Health Statistics (1984) Vital statistics in the United States, vol 2. Mortality, part B:1982 National Center for Health Statistics, Rockville
56. Ory H, Cole P, MacMahon B (1976) Oral contraceptives and reduced risk of benign breast diseases. N Engl J Med 294:419
57. Paffenbarger RS, Kampert JB, Chang HG (1980) Characteristics that predict risk of breast cancer before and after the menopause. Am J Epidemiol 112:258
58. Pastides H (1980) The epidemiology of fibrocystic breast disease with special reference to its histopathology. PhD dissertation, Yale University, New Haven
59. Pike MC, Gerkins VR, Casagrande JT et al. (1979) The hormonal basis of breast cancer. Natl Cancer Inst Monogr 53:187
60. Pirquet C (1930) Allergie des Lebensalters. Thieme, Leipzig
61. Poel WE (1968) Progesterone enhancement of mammary development as a causal

model of carcinogenesis. Br J Cancer 22:867

62. Prior P, Waterhouse JAH (1978) Incidence of bilateral tumors in a population-based series of breast cancer patients. I. Two approaches to an epidemiological analysis. Br J Cancer 37:620
63. Royal College of Practitioners (1977) Oral contraceptive study: effect on hypertension and benign breast disease of progestagen component in combined oral contraceptives. Lancet 1:624
64. Schottenfeld D (1968) The relationship of breast cancer to thyroid disease. J Chronic Dis 21:303
65. Schottenfeld D, Berg JW (1971) Incidence of multiple primary cancers. IV. Cancers of the female breast and genital organs. JNCI 46:161
66. Schottenfeld D, Berg JW, Vitsky B (1969) Incidence of multiple primary cancers. II. Index cancer arising in the stomach and lower digestive system. JNCI 43:77
67. Seidmann H (1972) Cancer of the breast, statistical and epidemiological data. American Cancer Society, New York
68. Seidmann H, Siverberg E, Holleb A (1976) Cancer statistics 1976. A comparison of white and black populations. American Cancer Society, New York
69. Shapiro S, Strax P, Venet L, Fink R (1968) The search for risk factors in breast cancer. Am J Public Health 58:820
70. Shapiro S, Venet W, Strax P, Venet L, Roeser R (1982) Ten-to-fourteen-year effect of screening on breast cancer mortality. JNCI 69:349
71. Shumizu H, Mack TH, Ross RK, Henderson BE (1987) Cancer of the gastrointestinal tract among Japanese and white emigrants to Los Angeles Country. J Natl Cancer Inst 78:223–228
72. Shore RE, Hempelmann LH, Kowaluk E (1977) Breast neoplasms in women treated with X-rays for acute postpartum mastitis. JNCI 59:813
73. Siiteri PK, Hammond GL, Nisker JA (1981) Increased availability of serum estrogens in breast cancer: a new hypothesis. In: Pike MC, Siiteri PK, Welsch CW (eds) Hormones and breast cancer. Cold Spring Harbor, Cold Spring Laboratory. Cold Spring Harbor (Banbury report 8)
74. Smans M, Boyle P, Muis CS (1989) Cancer Mortality in Nine European Countries. IARL Scientific Publications, Lyon, in preparation
75. Statistisches Bundesamt Wiesbaden (1986) Gesundheitswesen. Reihe 4: Todesursachen, 1985. Kohlhammer, Stuttgart
76. Trichopoulos D, MacMahon B, Cole P (1972) Menopause and breast cancer risk. JNCI 48:605
77. Vessey MP, Doll R, Jones K, McPherson K, Yeates D (1979) An epidemiological study of oral contraceptives and breast cancer. Br Med J 1:1755
78. Vessey MP, McPherson K, Doll R (1981) Breast cancer and oral contraceptives findings in Oxford – Family Planning Association contraceptives study. Br Med J 282:2093
79. Wagner G (1985) Epidemiologie und Ätiologie des Mammacarcinoms. Mitteilungsdienst der Gesellschaft zur Bekämpfung der Krebskrankheiten Nordthein-Westfalen e.v. 45:3
80. Waterhouse J et al. (eds) (1976) Cancer incidence in five continents, vol 3. IARC, Lyon (IARC scientific publication no 15)
81. Waterhouse J, Muir CS, Shanmugaratnom K, Powell JG (eds) (1982) Cancer incidence in five continents, vol 4. IARC, Lyon
82. Wynder EL, Bross IJ, Hirayama T (1960) The study of the epidemiology of cancer of the breast. Cancer 13:559
83. Wynder EL, MacCornack F, Hill P (1976) Nutrition and the etiology and prevention of breast cancer. Cancer Detect Prevent 1:293
84. Wynder EL, Chan P, Cohen C (1978) Die Ätiologie des Brustkrebses und ihre Bedeutung für Präventionsmaßnahmen. In: Grundmann E, Beck C (eds) Brustkrebs-Früherkennung. Methoden und Ergebnisse. Fischer, Stuttgart
85. Yuasa S, MacMahon B (1970) Lactation and reproductive histories of breast cancer patients in Tokyo, Japan. Bull WHO 42:195

Breast-Cancer Biology and Breast-Preserving Surgery*

A. Schauer, H. Rothe, J. Balzer, R. Brehler and M. Bergholz

Introduction

Interdisciplinary planning of therapy for patients with breast cancer increasingly requires evaluation of the biologic behavior of the individual tumor, using special histochemical and photometric methods. Our group is especially concerned with immunohistochemical investigations directed towards improved evaluation of essential prognostic factors. The quality of these rapidly developing methods could be increased very intensively in the last years, so that most of the morphologically based diagnostic techniques are applicable to typing, grading, evaluation of histiogenesis and growth activity, analysis of receptor status and staging of tumors.

Diagnostic Confirmation

The first and most important consideration in therapy is unequivocal diagnosis. It is sometimes practically difficult to distinguish between neoplastic and reactive processes of the female breast and between ductal and lobular cancer. In some certain cases it is not easy to delineate soft-tissue tumors and primary malignant lymphomas of the breast by histopathology. To resolve such difficulties, the malignant nature of a suspicious lesion can in most cases be confirmed by evaluation of normal hematoxylin- and eosin-stained sections. Cytophotometric evaluation as performed by some investigative groups is more useful in the evaluation of degree of malignancy or growth activity than in primary assessment of malignancy. This opinion is supported by most laboratories concerned with this problem [1,42]. Furthermore in difficult cases it is possible to definitely determine whether an anaplastic tumor is of epithelial or mesenchymal origin or to distinguish epithelial histiocytoid tumor cells from reactive histiocytes in the stroma. German, Swiss and American groups [2,26,34] have demonstrated that ductal and lobular breast cancers invariably contain cytokeratins (Fig. 1). In diagnosis of metastatic tumor tissue it is partly possible to distinguish breast cancer from other cancers by characteristic keratin patterns [24,25]. But it is impossible to distinguish between ductal and lobular types on the basis of cytokeratin patterns (Table 1). Generally all mesenchymal tumors can be identified using antibodies directed against vimentin.

*Supported by the Ministry for Research and Technology, Federal Republic of Germany

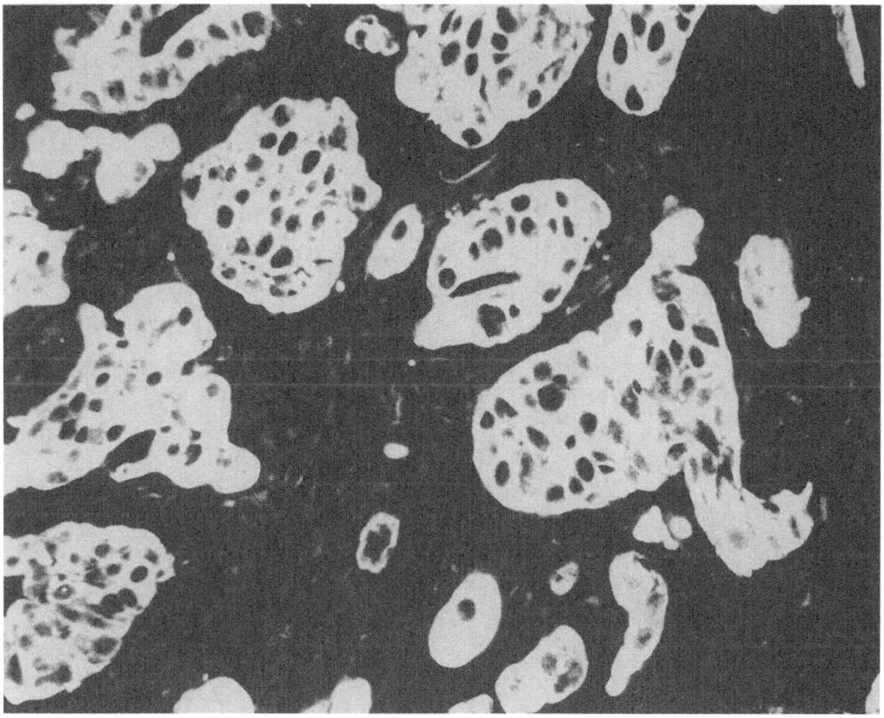

Fig. 1. Invasive ductal carcinoma of the breast. Tumor cells detected by antibodies against cytokeratins (indirect immunofluorescence)

Table 1. Cytokeratin patterns of epithelia and carcinomas of the female breast (MOLL and FRANKE 1985)

Cytokeratin No.	1	4	5	6	7	8	10 11	13	14	15	16	17	18	19
Mammary gland ducts			+		+	+				+	+	+	+	+
Invasive ductal carcinoma														
no. 1 primary tumor					+	+							+	+
lymph node metast.					+	+							+	+
no. 2					+	+							+	+
no. 3					+	+						+	+	+
no. 4					+	+							+	+
no. 5					(+)	+							+	+
no. 6						+							+	+
Invasive lobular carc.														
no. 1					+	+							+	+
no. 2					+	+							+	+
Medullar carcinoma						+							+	+

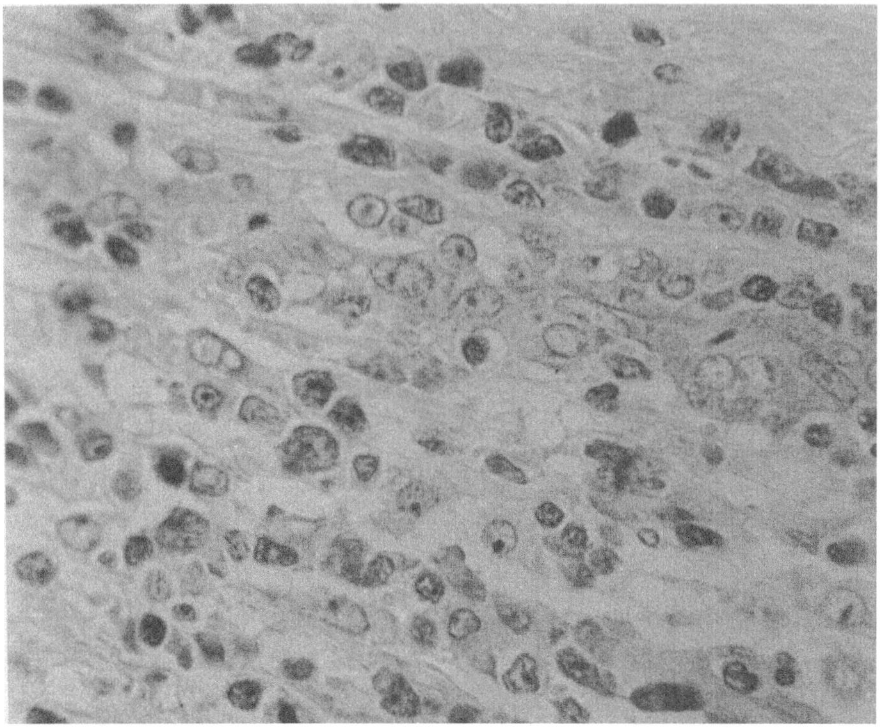

a

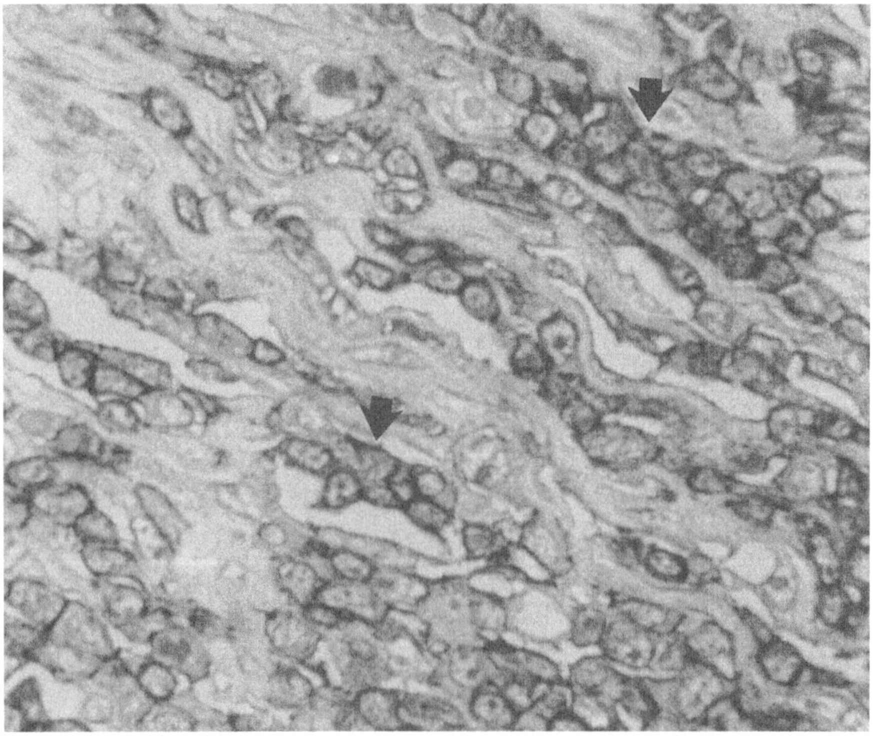

b

Furthermore lymphomas of the breast showing a pseudoepithelial cord-like growth pattern along collagen fibres can be diagnosed using antibodies directed to common leucocyte antigens and by the demonstration of characteristic lymphoma markers (Fig. 2a, b). On the other hand histiocytoid lobular carcinomas, histiocytomas and histiocytic reactions can be distinguished using immunohistochemical reactions directed against cytokeratin, on the one hand respectively α-antichymotrypsin, and lysozym on the other hand.

Early Stromal Invasion

Besides histogenetic studies and typing it is sometimes important to detect early stromal invasion from ductal carcinoma in situ (DCIS) and lobular carcinoma in situ (LCIS). In this context it must be pointed out that PAS-reactions and silver stains sometimes provide no truly satisfactory solution to this problem. However, according to the immunohistochemical investigations of EKBLOM et al. [9] and our own investigations using antibodies directed against laminin, structures such as the basement membrane are usually intact in sclerosing adenosis, whereas in tubular cancer ductal carcinoma and stromal invasion by lobular carcinoma show discontinuities or total loss of laminin (Fig. 3, 4). It seems to be important that although cancer cells destroy the matrix and basement membrane by enzymatic lysis, the laminin receptors of tumor cells are obviously at least partly preserved [18]. After preincubation of paraffin sections in acetic acid solution using 1 mg pepsin in 0.5 ml acetic acid, the continuity of the basement membrane can be evaluated very well, according to EKBLOM et al. [9] and our own experience. The loss of fibronectin parallels that of laminin when invasive carcinoma develops. Discussing the problem of myoepithelial proliferation in cancer development, one must ask whether proliferative processes of these cells are combined with the development of LCIS. Using actin as a marker, myoepithelial proliferation was not observed in LCIS foci, although in particular cases reactive proliferation or proliferation enhanced by special stimuli could not be completely ruled out.

Tumor Grading

After confirmed diagnosis of invasive breast cancer (IC), a further important point in cancer characterization is tumor grading, which is usually performed according to the basic scheme described by BLOOM and RICHARDSON in 1957 [5]. In this scheme, the extent to which glandular tissue is formed and the degree of polymorphism are both easy to evaluate, but the degree of hyperchromatism and also the exact evaluation of mitotic activity are very much dependent on the quality

◄

Fig. 2a. Malignant lymphoma of the breast with pseudoepithelial cord-like arrangement of tumor cells (lymphoblastic type) (GIEMSA) **b.** Lymphoblastic extranodal Non-Hodgkin-Lymphoma, antibodies against common leucocyte antigen (APAAP)

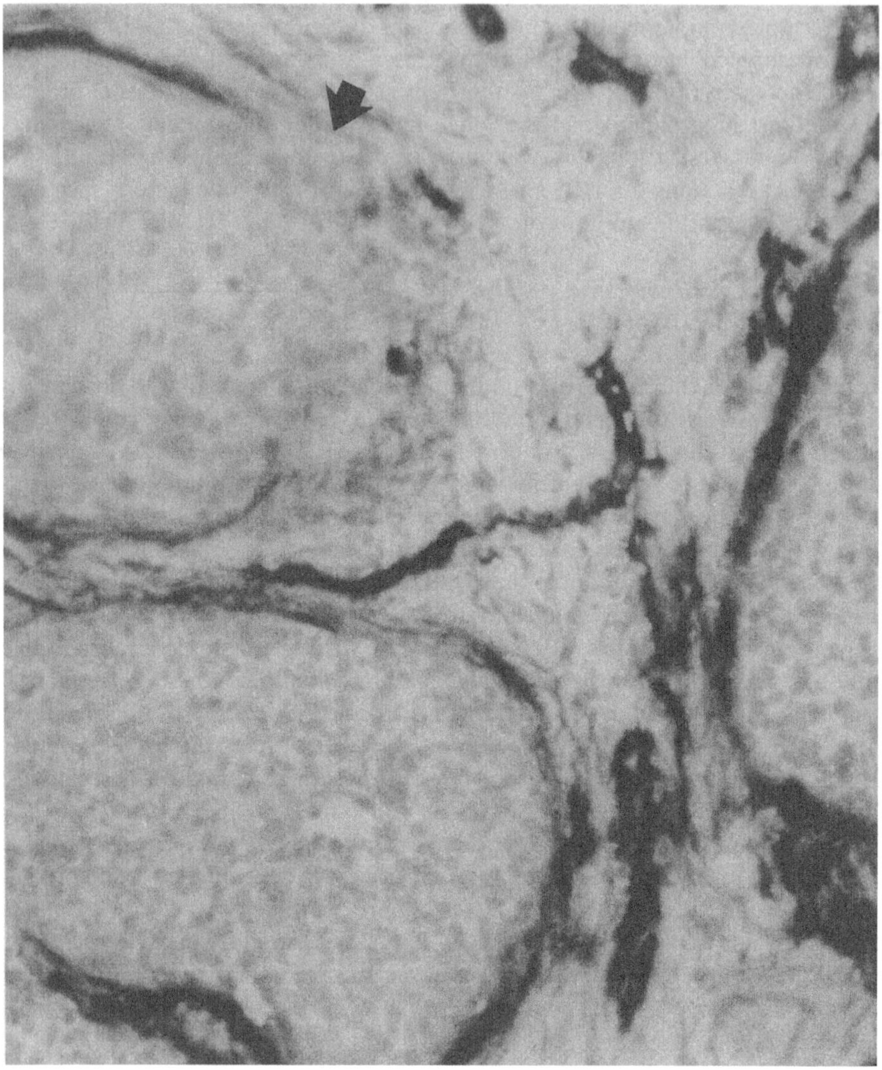

Fig. 3. Lobular carcinoma in situ (LCIS). Immunohistochemical reaction with antibodies against laminin, incomplete destruction of basal lamina (APAAP)

of histologic sections. Accordingly ongoing grading within a study can only be carried out when the sectioning and staining techniques are in the hands of a single highly qualified technician. In our National Breast Cancer study we evaluated the tumors using significant paraffin-blocks from every case in the study group. In most of the approximately 1050 cases, grading was performed using sections produced and stained by one and the same technician.

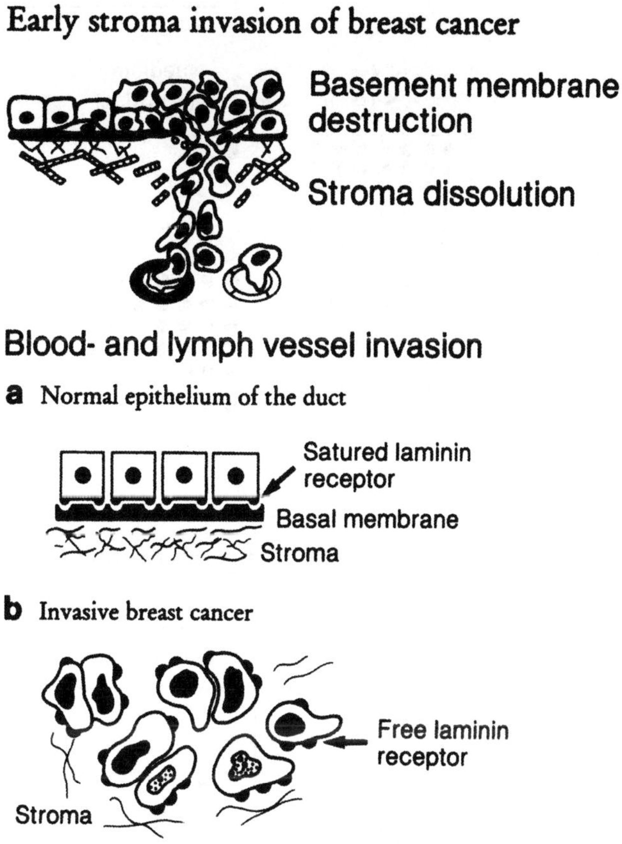

Fig. 4a,b. Basal membrane and adherent receptors for laminin **a.** Normal epithelium of the duct, **b.** Invasive cancer with free laminin receptors

Proliferative Activity

As mitotic cells are very sensitive, additional parameters to support the evaluation of proliferative activity are highly valuable. Recently available new techniques, introduced by GERDES et al. [11,12], allow immunohistochemical demonstration of a nuclear nonhistone protein associated with tumor-cell proliferation. This protein is expressed in the S-, G2-, and M-phases and also partly in G1. Nonproliferating cells do not express this antigenic nuclear protein. The significance of this protein has mainly been evaluated in normal and neoplastic lymphatic tissue. We have used this antibody – called Ki-67 – to evaluate the proliferation of breast-cancer cells. Our major interest concerning tumor grading has been whether there is a correlation between degree of malignancy and proliferative activity. Our results from 105 cases under investigation showed a good correlation of mitotic activity to Ki-67-measured proliferation (Fig. 5a). The proliferative activity was low in 55 cases, medium in 34 cases and high in 16 cases. The mean values were: for a low grade of proliferation 0.8 mitoses/high-power

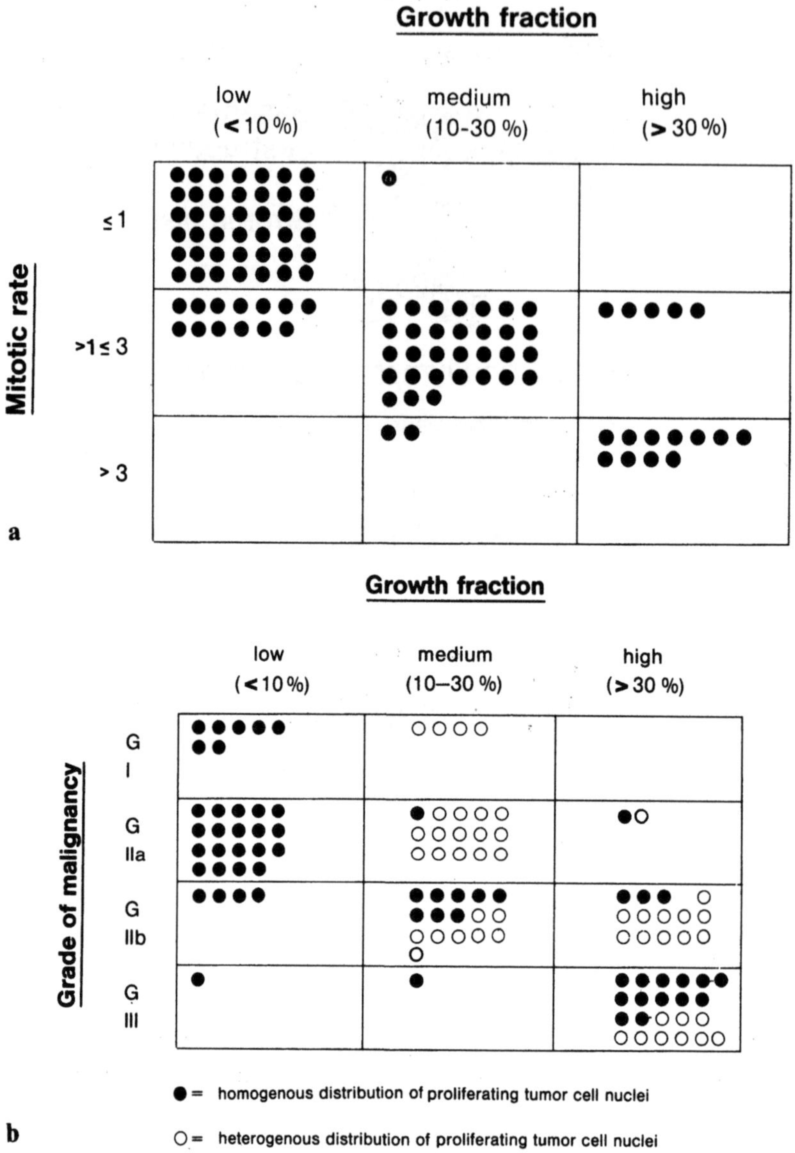

Fig. 5a. Correlation of growth fraction to mitotic rate measured by Ki-67-antibody (APAAP). **b.** Correlation of proliferative activity (growth fraction) and degree of malignancy (Grading) (Ki-67-antibody)

field, for medium grade proliferation 1.8 mitoses/high-power field and for tumors with high proliferation rates 3.2 mitoses/high-power field. Furthermore, there was a good correlation with the degree of malignancy according to the scheme of BLOOM and RICHARDSON [5] (Fig. 5b). When incorporating measures of proliferative activity into our scheme, which was worked out with WEISS [33], the proliferative activity was, with a few exceptions, low in nearly all grade-I and -IIa cases, whereas it was high in grade-IIb and -III cases. In summary, it seems at least possible to obtain additional information concerning the proliferative activity of breast cancers, although the question as to how these values can be incorporated in improved grading systems is unresolved. Data presented by our group at the Conference of the International Association of Breast Cancer Research, Miami, [38] agree with data given by GERDES et al. [13] (Fig. 6a,b).

In further agreement with GERDES et al. we found no clearcut correlation to the estrogen-receptor status as evaluated using the Abbott monoclonal antibody. There are cases with very high proliferative activity which have a strong and homogeneous response to tests for estrogen-receptor equipment. These findings somewhat elucidate why the growth of receptor-positive cases sometimes cannot be influenced by tamoxifen. From these results it must be realized that under special conditions such cases can be treated with cytostatics much more effectively than with hormone therapy. Protocols based on these considerations should be established as soon as possible.

Further investigations concerning the significance of the receptor for epidermal growth factor (EGFR) have demonstrated that this antigen is mainly localized on the tumor-cell membrane (Fig. 7a,b). Recently published data by NEAL et al. [27] for urinary bladder cancer, SAINSBURY et al. [31] for breast cancer and GULLICK et al. [15] for ovarian cancer demonstrate that tumors of these different origins with high levels of EGF-receptor are highly invasive and associated with a poor prognosis. In our preliminary evaluation of one hundred cases we found a close correlation between proliferative activity and levels of EGF-receptor, implying that tumors which are highly proliferative have abundant EGF-receptors (Table 2).

Table 2. Comparison of Epidermal Growth Factor Receptor – Estrogen Receptor- and Proliferation Activity in Breast Cancer (n 118)

EGFR		Estrogenreceptor positive		Estrogenreceptor negative		Tumors with high proliferation, measured with the antibody Ki-67	
n	%	n	%	n	%	n	%
positive							
67	56.8	45	67.2	22	37.8	46	68.7
negative							
51	43.2	45	88.2	6	11.8	14	27.5

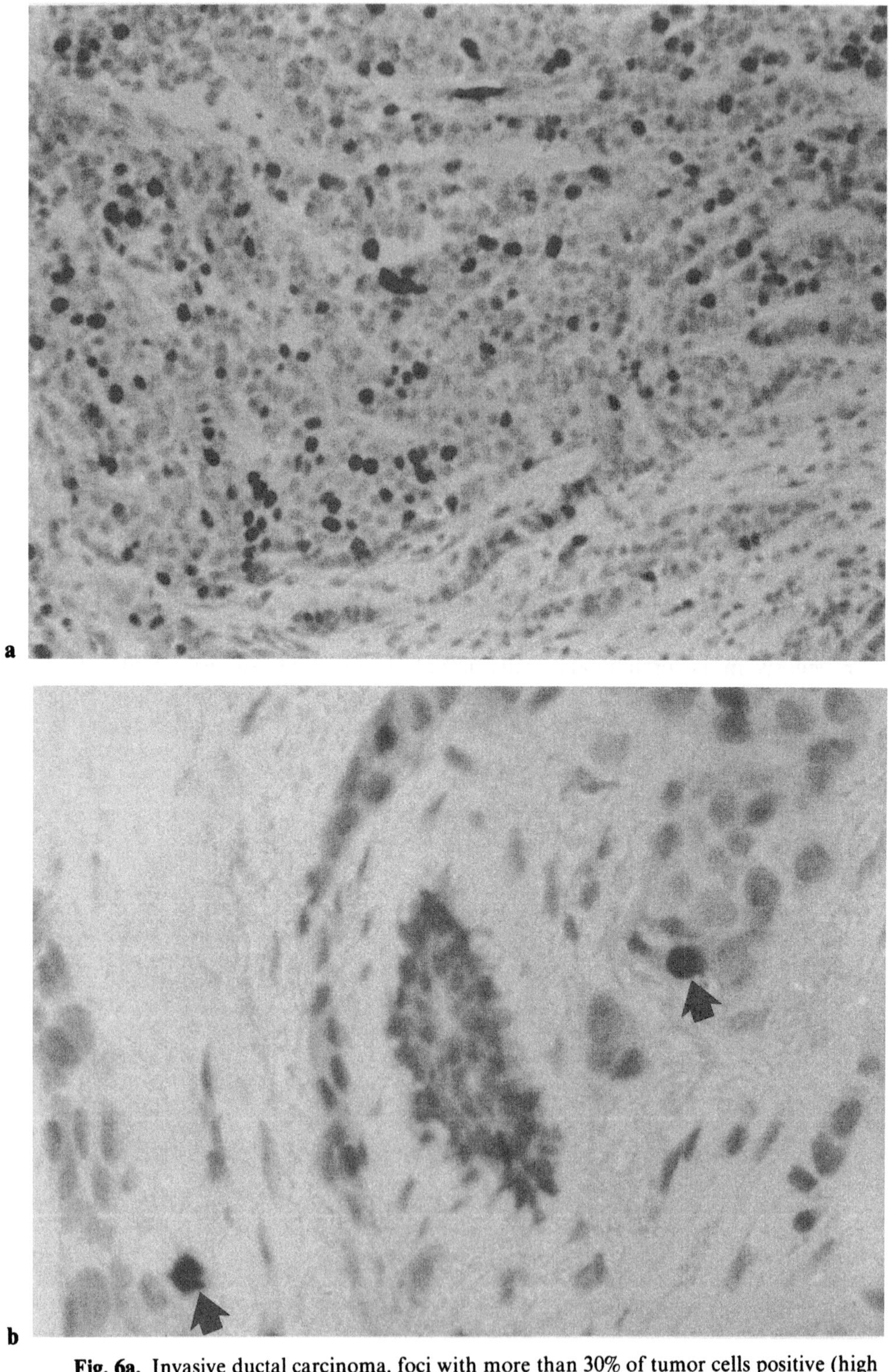

Fig. 6a. Invasive ductal carcinoma, foci with more than 30% of tumor cells positive (high proliferative activity) (APAAP). b Tumor cells surrounding a small duct, small cell lobular cancer. Only few tumor cells detected by monoclonal antibody Ki-67 (low proliferative activity) (APAAP)

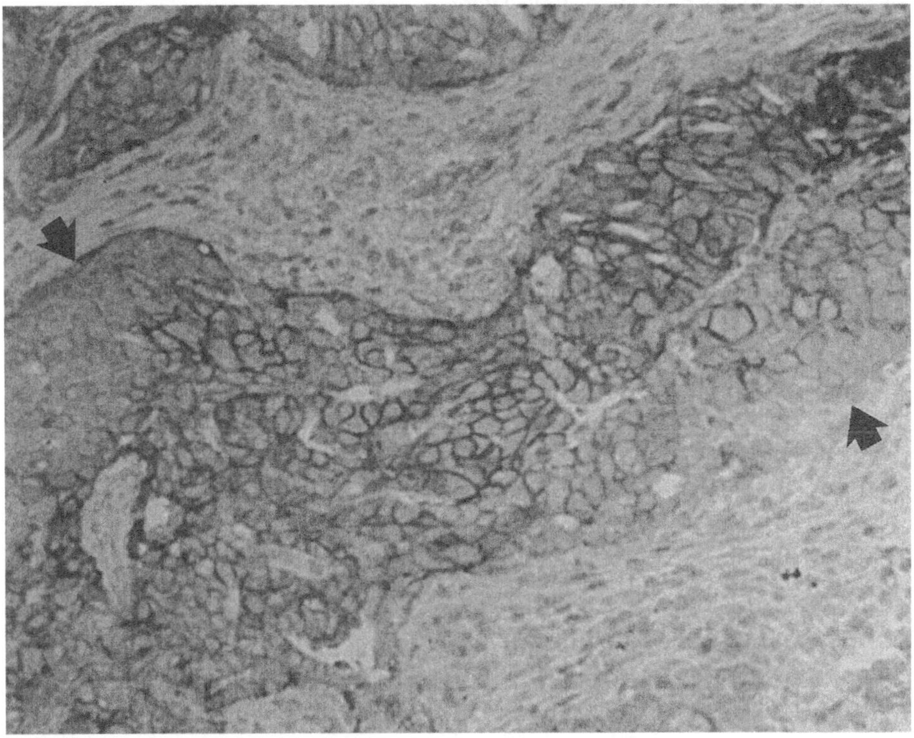

a

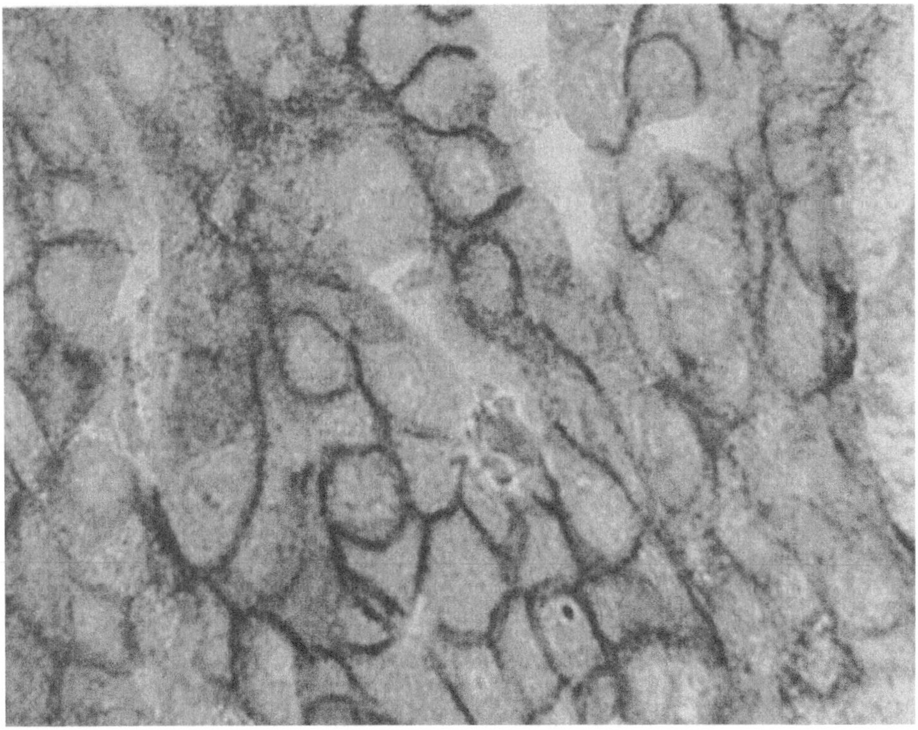

b

Fig. 7a. Invasive ductal carcinoma of the breast. Immunohistochemical detection of the Epidermal-Growth-Factor-Receptor (EGF-R), localized on cell-membranes; note distinction of receptor-negative and receptor-positive tumor cell areas. (APAAP) **b.** Invasive ductal carcinoma. Cell membranes positive for EGF-receptors

Immunohistochemical Steroid Receptor Analysis

Further improvement in the assessment of breast cancer biology has followed the development of monoclonal antibodies directed against nuclear estrogen receptor protein by GREENE et al. (1980). In our investigations using cryostat sections of 138 breast cancers, the probes were fixed for 10–15 min using 10% buffered formalin solution, followed by additional treatment with cold methanol at between 10° and 25°C and acetone fixation at the same temperature for 1–3 min. The immunohistochemical reaction was then performed, using the peroxidase anti-peroxidase technique with 3,3-Diaminobenzidine as substrate and 0,5% osmium acid solution for contrast staining. The antibody used was not helpful in the judgement of carcinogenesis respectively the start of malignant proliferation. The results for normal breast tissue and fibrocystic disease were very variable and showed no obvious pattern nor did they elucidate epithelial proliferation. In normal breast tissue sometimes only some focal ductal and acinar areas were positive. Similar results were demonstrated for fibrocystic disease (Fig. 8a,b). Fibroadenomas sometimes showed totally negative nuclei, but in some nearly all nuclei were strongly positive. In 138 breast cancers investigated so far, the results were quite different. There were cases that were fully receptor-negative and others with exclusively positive nuclei. Between the extremes, many different states could be found (Fig. 9a,b). From this it follows that there are cases with homogeneous, fully receptor-positive status and cases with heterogeneous positive status. It can also be deduced that in the latter cases the response to hormone therapy must be more or less incomplete. However, we do not know whether negative cells are negative all the time or only during certain phases of the cell cycle. The demonstration of highly proliferative tumors with the antibody Ki-67 with a simultaneous strongly homogeneous estrogen receptor status is in contrast to this opinion, sometimes expressed.

Compared with the charcoal method, the accordance was 78.3%. The biochemically positive cases showed positive reactions in 85.2%. In 58.3% of the estrogen-receptor-negative cases, the immunohistochemical reaction was also negative (Table 3). In case with a discrepant status, the immunohistochemical findings were mostly in accordance with the progesterone receptor status.

Parallel to these investigations, we also used the ER-D5 antibody supplied by Amersham, U.K.. This antibody does not directly stain the estrogen receptor protein. According to the results of KING's group in England, the antibody is directed against a cytoplasmic protein associated with the estrogen receptor [16]. This antibody has been tested in nearly one hundred cases of breast cancer. In comparison to the charcoal method results were concordant in 74.5%. More than 90% of biochemically positive results agreed with the immunohistochemical results,

Fig. 8a. Terminal ducts of cystic disease. ER-ICA: inhomogeneous positive reaction of different nuclei; immunohistochemical reaction with monoclonal antibody against estrogen-receptor-protein (Abbott, Chicago). **b.** Only single tumor cell clusters positive (ER-ICA)

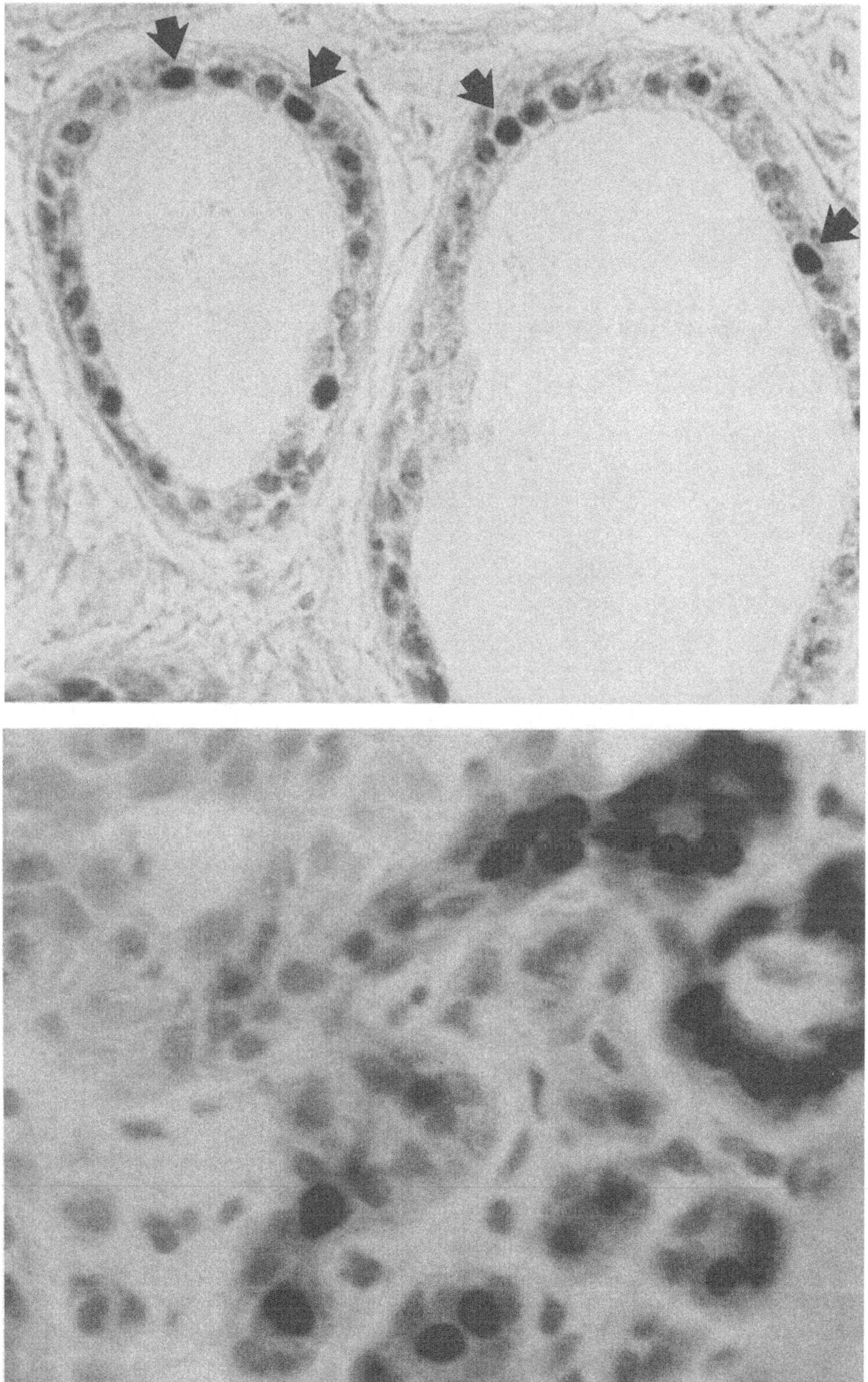

a

b

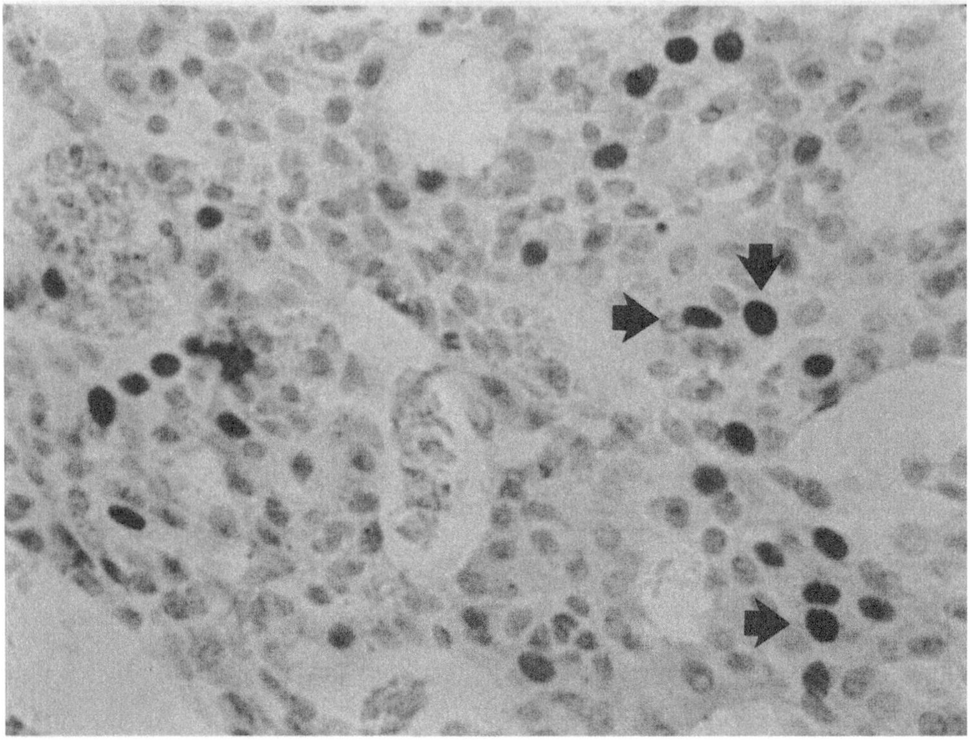
a

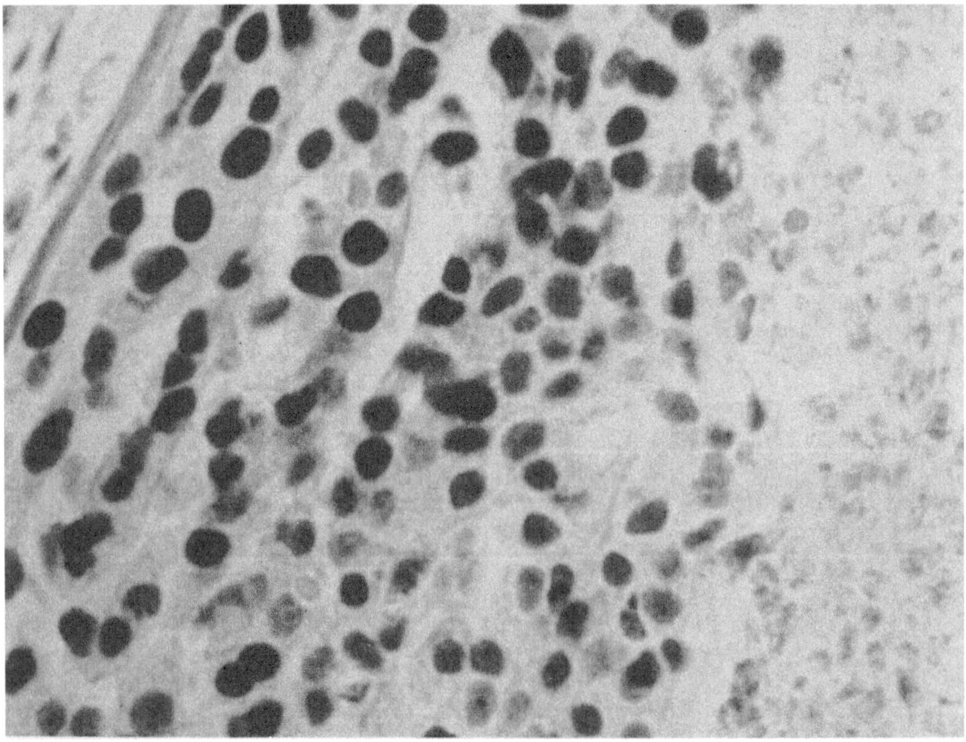
b

Table 3.

Comparison of Immunohistochemical ER-Status with Biochemical Results (138 Cases):

	immunohistochemical	
ER–5f mol/mg	receptor evaluation	
ER + 5f mol/mg	A = 78.3%	A = Accordance
	S = 85.2%	S = Sensivity
	Z = 58.3%	Z = Specifity

Comparison of Immunohistochemically ER-D5 – positive Cases with the Biochemical Receptor Status (98 Cases):

	immunohistochemical	
ER–5f mol/mg	ER - D5 evaluation	
ER + 5f mol/mg		
	A = 74.5%	A = Accordance
	S = 90%	S = Sensitivity
	Z = 28%	Z = Specifity

but estrogen-receptor-negative cancers were immuno-histochemically positive in 72% (Table 3, Fig. 10). At the present time many questions arise in connection with immunohistochemical receptor analysis as compared with cytoplasmic biochemical evaluation.

The advantages of immunohistochemical investigations are:

1. Receptor analysis is still possible for very small cancers and aspiration biopsies of metastases.
2. The receptor status of individual tumor cells can be explored, which is relevant to the question of homogeneity and heterogeneity of receptor status.
3. Receptor analysis is not interfered with by endogeneous estrogen binding.

At present, immunohistochemical receptor analysis is in progress; antibodies directed against progesterone receptor protein have not yet been extensively used in comparative immunohistochemical investigations. However, antibodies of this type have already been prepared by MILGROM et al. [22] and the Abbott Company. Some results were already demonstrated by FIEBIG and SCHAUER [10].

The final question is whether immunohistochemical reactions can help to detect early metastases for instance in lymph nodes. The answer is clearly positive. With antibodies directed against cytokeratins, which can also be used for paraffin sections, single epithelial tumor cells or small clusters of them in lymph-node tissue can be detected (Fig. 11a,b). This method seems useful for exact studies based on the TNM system. In summary, all the groups of antibodies used are helpful in exact studies of breast cancer and also in diagnosis and therapy of single cases.

◄

Fig. 9a. Cribriform intraductal carcinoma. Only few tumor cells are positive for nuclear estrogen (ER-ICA). **b.** Comedo intraductal carcinoma of the breast with homogeneous estrogen receptor equipment near to central detritus

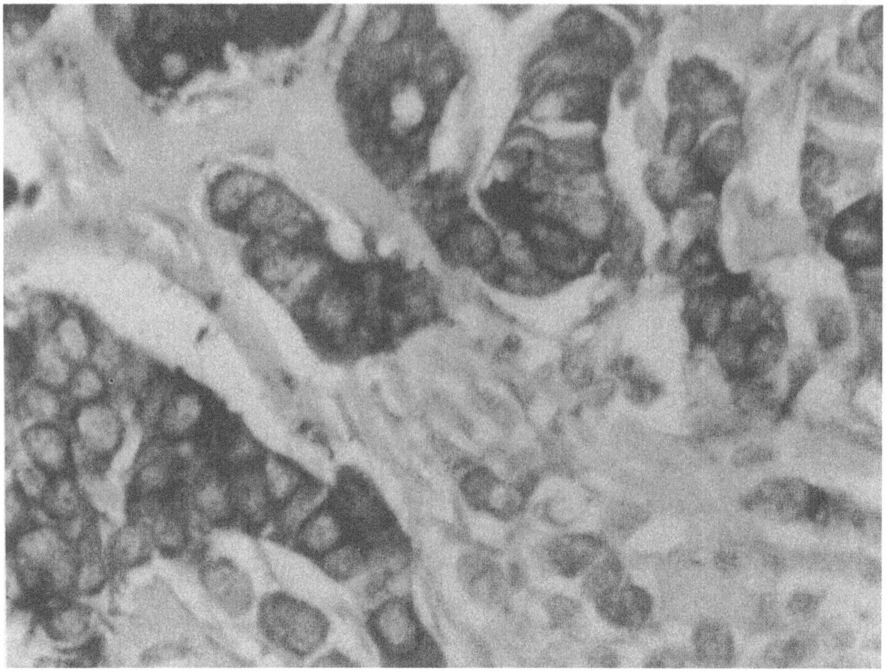

Fig. 10. Invasive ductal carcinoma. Immunohistochemical reaction of tumor cells with antibodies against cytoplasmic estrogen-receptor-associated protein (ER-D5)

Addendum

In the German Breast Cancer Study in about 70% of 1050 pTl NO MO Cases breast conserving surgery has been performed.

In all cases tumor grading according to Bloom and Richardson, modified by Schauer and Weiss (1981) has been carried out.

When deep frozen tumor tissue was available from our clinic or by special delivery from outside the Ki-67-proliferative compartment, the Epidermal Growth Factor Receptor (EGFR), the C-erb-B2-oncogene and the Er- and Pr-receptor status have been evaluated by immunohistochemical methods. In the period between Oct. 1983 to December 1988 952 cases have been observed. Up to the end of 1988 52 locoregional and distant recurrences (5,25% in the cases with breast conserving surgery and 5,94% in cases with mastectomy) were reported.

The preliminary results demonstrate that one of the most reliable prognostic factors is tumor-grading.

It shows a strong correlation to age, tumor size and the receptor status, but furthermore it is an indicator for the risk of tumor recurrence. Whereas in the whole group about 37% were grade I tumors, the recurrence rate was only 23%.

Fig. 11a. Easy detection of single tumor cells in a lymph node with cytokeratin antibodies. **b.** Axillary lymph node, metastases in random sinus, detection with antibodies against cytokeratin

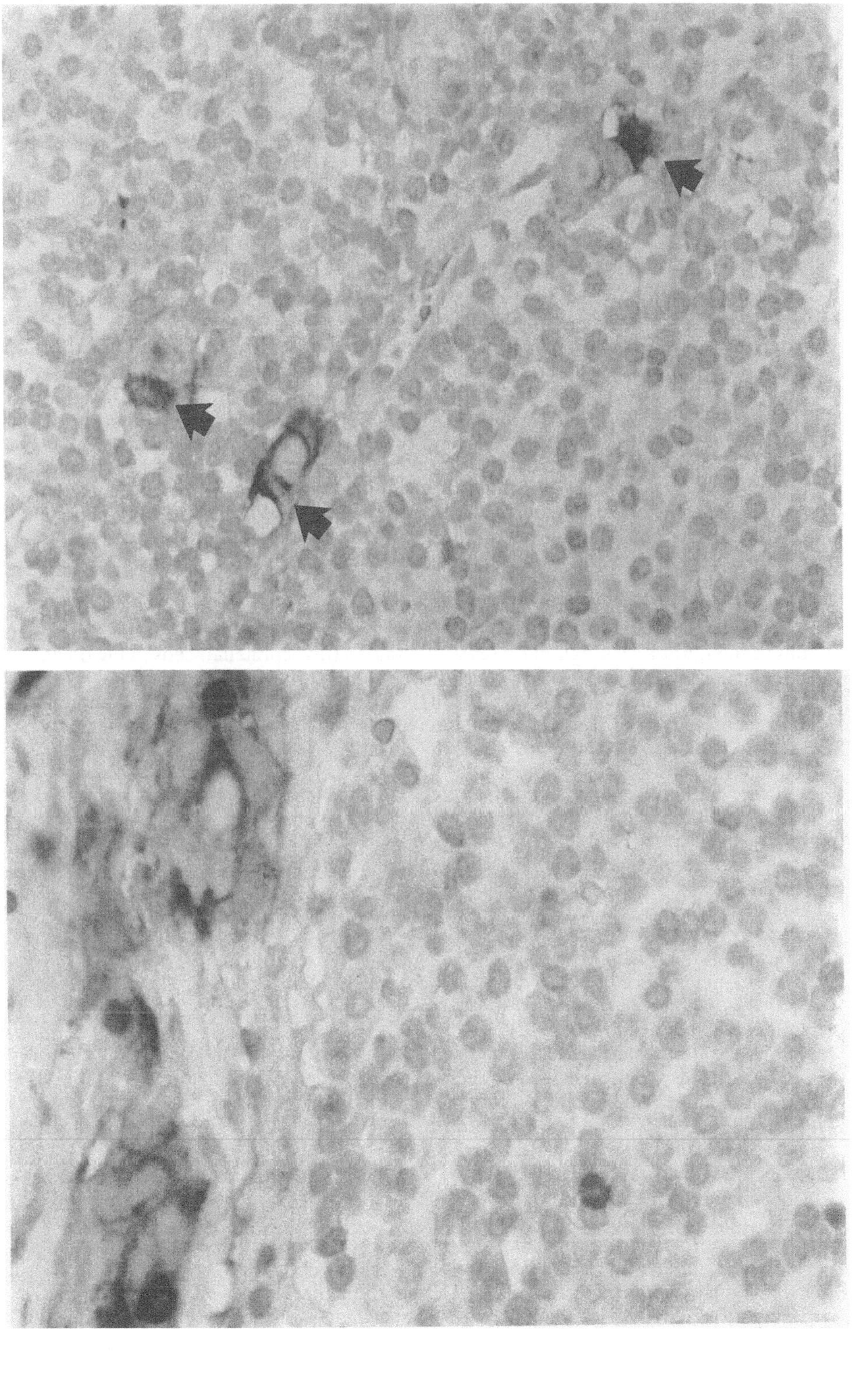

a

b

On the other hand grade III tumors amounted only to 12% but nearly 20% of the recurrences. These preliminary results were elaborated by the German Breast Cancer Study Group (GBSG).

Ref. Center Pathology: Prof. Dr. A Schauer and L. Ummenhofer, Univ. Göttingen
Ref. Center Surgery: Dr. H. Rauschecker, Dr. W. Gatzemeier, Univ. Göttingen
Ref. Center Radiology: Prof. Dr. R. Sauer, Dr. M.H. Seegenschmiedt, Univ. Erlangen
Ref. Center Doc. and Statistics: Prof. Dr. M. Schumacher, W. Sauerbrei, Univ. Freiburg

References

1. Auer GU, Arrhenius E (1980) Comparison of DNA distribution in primary human breast cancers and their metastases. Eur J Cancer 16 (2):273-278
2. Altmannsberger M, Osborn M, Hölscher A, Schauer A, Weber K (1981) The distribution of keratin type intermediate filaments in human breast cancer. An immunhistological study. Virchows Arch (B) 37:277-284
3. Azzopardi JG (1979) Problems in breast pathology. Saunders, Philadelphia (Major problems in pathology, Vol 11)
4. Balzer I, Rothe H, Brehler R, Schauer A (in press) Epidermal growth factor-receptor. Immunhistochemische Untersuchungen an Mammakarzinomen. In: W Jonat (ed) Aktuelle Aspekte in der Diagnostik des Mammakarzinoms. Stuttgart (Enke) (in press)
5. Bloom HJG, Richardson WW (1957) Histologic grading and prognosis in breast cancer. A study of 1409 cases of which 359 have been followed for 15 years. Br J Cancer 11:359-377
6. Bussolati G (1985) Markers of mammary cell types and their use in tumor diagnosis. Verh Dtsch Ges Pathol 69:187-193
7. Bussolati G, Botta G, Gugliotta P (1980) Actin rich (myoepithelial) cells in the ductal carcinoma in situ of the breast. Virchows Arch (B) 34:251-259
8. Bussolati G, Gugliotta P, Fulcheri E (1984) Immunhistochemistry of actin in normal and neoplastic tissue. In: de Lellis RA (ed) Advances in immunohistochemistry. Masson, Paris pp 325-341
9. Ekblom P, Miettinen M, Forsman L, Andersson LC (1984) Basement membrane and apocrine epithelial antigens in differential diagnosis between tubular carcinoma and sclerosing adenosis of the breast. J Clin Pathol 37:357-363
10. Fiebig I, Schauer A (1988) Immunhistochemische nucleare Progesteronrezeptor-analyse mit dem Antikörper Transbio 1 bei Mammakarzinomen. Verh Dtsch Ges Path 72:388-389
11. Gerdes J, Schwab U, Lemke H, Stein H (1983) Production of a mouse monoclonal antibody reactive with a human nuclear antigen associated with cell proliferation. Int J Cancer 31:13-20
12. Gerdes J, Lemke H, Baisch H, Wacker HH, Schwab U, Stein H (1984) Cell cycle analysis of a cell proliferation associated human nuclear antigen defined by the monoclonal antibody Ki-67. J Immunol 133:1710-1715
13. Gerdes J, Pileri S, Bartels H, Stein H (1986) Der Proliferationsmarker Ki-67: Korrelation zur histologischen Diagnose, zur histologischen Einschätzung des Malignitätsgrades und zum klinischen Verlauf. Verh Dtsch Ges Path 70:152-158
14. Greene GL, Nolan C, Engler JP, Jensen EV (1980) Monoclonal antibodies to human estrogen receptor. Proc Natl Acad Sci USA 77:515-519
15. Gullick W; Downward DJH, Marsden JJ, Waterfield MD (1984) Radioimmunassay for human epidermal growth factor receptor. Anal Biochem 141:253-261
16. King WJ, Jensen EV, Miller L, Greene GL (1982) Immunocytochemical detection of estrogen receptor in frozen sections of human breast tumors with monoclonal anti-receptor antibodies (abstract). Endocrinology (Suppl) 110:258
17. Lellé RJ, Heidenreich W, Stauch G, Gerdes J, Peter HH (1985) Determination of proliferative activity in carcinoma and benign changes of the breast by a monoclonal

antibody. 11th World Congress of Gynecology and Obstetrics, Berlin. Arch Gynaecol (Suppl) 237
18. Liotta LA, Rao CN, Barsky SH (1983) Tumor invasion and the extracellular matrix. Lab Invest 49:636
19. Liotta LA, Hand PH, Rao CN, Bryant G, Barsky SH, Schlom J (1985) Monoclonal antibodies to the human laminin receptor recognize structurally destruct sites. Exp Cell Res 156:117-126
20. McGurrin J, Doria MJ, Runyon-Hass A, Stein H, Franklin WA (1985) Demonstration of a proliferating cell antigen in breast carcinoma by immunhistochemistry using the monoclonal antibody Ki-67. 74th Annual Meeting of the International Academy of Pathology (United States-Canadian Division) Toronto. Lab Invest 52:1
21. Milgrom E (1985) Immunocytochemical study of mammalian progesterone receptor using monoclonal antibodies. Endocrinology 116:1473-1484
22. Milgrom E, Logeat F, Vu Hai MT, Fournier A, Legrain P, Buttin G (1983) Monoclonal antibodies to rabbit progesterone receptor: cross-reaction with other mammalian progesterone receptors. Proc Natl Acad Sci USA 80:6456-6459
23. Millis R (1984) Atlas of breast pathology. MTP Press, Lancaster
24. Moll R, Franke WW, Schiller D, Geiger B, Krepler R (1982) The catalogue of human cytokeratins: patterns of expression in normal epithelia, tumors and cultured cells. Cell 31:11-24
25. Moll R, Franke W (1985) Cytochemical cell typing of metastatic tumors according to their cytoskeletal proteins. Metastases Conference NIH 1985
26. Nagle RB, Mac Danie M, Clark VA, Payne CM (1983) The use of antikeratin antibodies in the diagnosis of human neo-plasma. Am J Clin Pathol 79:458-466
27. Neal DE, Marsh C, Bennett MK, Abel PD, Hall RR, Sainsbury JRC, Harris AL (1985) Epidermal growth factor receptors in human bladder cancer comparison of invasive and superficial tumors. Lancet 1:366-388
28. Papotti M, Gugliotta P, Ghiringhello B, Bussolati G (1984) Association of breast carcinoma and multiple intraductal papillomas: an histological and immunohistochemical investigation. Histopathology 8:963
29. Remberger K, Nerlich A (1985) Diagnostischer Wert der Darstellung von Basalmembranproteinen in benignen und malignen Mammaveränderungen. Verh Dtsch Ges Pathol 69:123-130
30. Rothe H, Brehler R, Balzer I, Schauer A (in press) Proliferationsaktivitäten in Mammakarzinomen – Immunhistochemische Untersuchungen mit dem monoclonalen Antikörper Ki-67. In Jonat W (ed) Aktuelle Aspekte in der Diagnostik des Mammakarzinoms. Stuttgart (Enke) (in press)
31. Sainsbury IRC, Malcolm AJ, Appleton DR, Farndon IR, Harris AL (1985) Presence of epidermal growth factor receptor as an indicator of poor prognosis in patients with breast cancer. J Clin Pathol 38:1225-1228
32. Schauer A (1989) Die Pathologie des invasiven Mammakarzinoms. In: Bohmert H (ed) Brustkrebs. Stuttgart (Thieme): 10-18
33. Schauer A, Weiss A (1981) Bedeutung des Tumorgrading und der Blutgefäßeinbrüche für die Verlaufsbeurteilung des Mammakarzinoms bei Stadium I-Patientinnen. Verh Dtsch Ges Pathol 65:382
34. Schauer A, Osborn M, Weber K, Altmannsberger M (1984) Antibodies to different intermediate filaments as histiogenetic tumor markers. Acta Histochem (Suppl) (Jena) 24:129-136
35. Schauer A, Bergholz M, Brehler R (1985a) Welchen Beitrag kann der Pathologe zur Verbesserung von Diagnostik und Therapie des Mammakarzinoms leisten? Verh Dtsch Ges Inn Med 91:235-247
36. Schauer A, Brehler R, Bergholz M (1985b) Immunhistochemische Brustkrebsdiagnostik. Verh Dtsch Ges Pathol 69:171-186
37. Schauer A, Brehler R, Bergholz M (1986) Morphologische Kriterien für die brusterhaltende Chirurgie. Langenbecks Arch Chir 369:427-436
38. Schauer A, Rothe H, Balzer I, Bergholz M, Brehler R, Fiebig I, Rauschecker H, Nagel G, Blossey HC, Weber K, Osborn M, Aus HM, Harms H, Sauer R, Scheurlen H,

Schumacher M (1988) Monoclonal antibodies for improved evaluation of breast cancer prognosis. In: Rich M, Hager J, Lopez D (eds) Breast Cancer: Scientific and Clinical Progress. Boston: 299–320

39. Schauer A, Rothe H, Balzer I, Fiebig I (1988) Immunhistochemische Tumordiagnostik beim Mammakarzinom – Einsatz zur Evaluiering von Stadium und Biologie des sogenannten "Kleinen Mammakarzinoms". Röntgenblätter 41:340–344
40. Schürch WT, Seemayer TA, Lagace R, Gabbiani G (1984) The intermediate filament cytoskeleton of myofibroblasts: an immun-fluorescence and ultrastructural study. Virchows Arch (A) 403:32–336
41. Stegner HE (1986) Histopathologie der Mammatumoren. Enke, Stuttgart
42. Tschahargane C (1988) DNS-Impulscytophotometrie zur Bestimmung der Proliferationsparameter beim Mammacarcinom In: Jonat W (ed) Aktuelle Aspekte in dev Diagnostik des Mammakarzinoms. Enke (in press)

S Phase Fractions and DNA Ploidy as Prognostic Factors in Breast Cancer

G.E. Feichter, D. von Fournier, and M. Kaufmann

Clinical experience has shown that mammary carcinomas can be classified according to their type of progression into slow-growing and fast-growing ones, where the terms "slow" and "fast" tend to reflect the subjective impression of the observing clinician. The biological explanation of the differences in tumor growth patterns, among other aspects of tumor aggression, is given by tumor cell cycle kinetic studies.

Human malignant tumors consist of non-synchronized cell populations. At any given time, different percentages of cells belong to the various cell cycle phases – G0, G1, S, G2, M. The fraction of cells in the S phase (S phase fraction, SPF) has been shown to be closely related to tumor growth and clinical course, and is therefore of major clinical interest [5,10,12,14].

The number of DNA-synthesizing cells can be assessed by different methods, but mainly by autoradiography and flow cytometry (FCM). The calculation of SPF by autoradiography is based on incorporation of radioactive-labeled ^{3}H-thymidine into the nuclear DNA of proliferating cells. In spite of its proven value, calculation of the thymidine labeling index (TLI) cannot be carried out during in vivo studies for ethical reasons. In vitro incubation of tumor samples with radioactive ^{3}H-thymidine as a routine clinical measure is limited by the long duration of the examinations. In in vitro incubation studies, ^{3}H-thymidine labeling has given evidence of the major importance of SPF as a prognostic factor in breast cancer [5,10,12,14].

The results of these examinations and of others have considerably stimulated the planning and execution of DNA FCM studies in breast cancer. DNA FCM measures the intensity of DNA proportional fluorescence of cellular nuclei in suspensions. The main advantages are the measurement of the DNA content of a high number of cells (up to 100 000) within a few minutes, the automated registration of the DNA histogram and, if required, automated evaluation of the histogram.

The evaluation of the histogram gives two basic types of informaion: (1) cell cycle analysis, from which the calculation of cells in the S phase has proved to be of importance, and (2) DNA ploidy, which is calculated from the position of the peak of tumor cells in G0/G1 phase in comparison to the peak produced by normal diploid cells such as test lymphocytes.

Since the term "ploidy" is reserved for results obtained by chromosome counting, flow cytometrists use either "DNA ploidy" or "DNA index." A normal diploid cell population has a DNA index of 1.00 (Fig. 1), whereas aneuploid cells in the G0/G1 phase have a DNA index other than 1.00 (Fig. 2).

DNA FCM examinations can be carried out on fresh tumor samples, on material after alcohol fixation and even on formalin-fixed and paraffin-embedded tumor material. The last-named method is known worldwide as the Hedley technique [9].

The percentage of DNA-diploid mammary carcinomas varies in the different studies, mainly depending on the quality of resolution and on the use of an internal standard, which is added to the sample for determination of the diploid peak. Studies in which an internal standard is used usually have higher DNA aneuploid distributions. Since nearly every mammary carcinoma contains a certain number of lymphocytes, which gives rise to a diploid peak, some authors do not use an additional internal standard for determination of DNA ploidy. In our material, currently including 300 evaluated mammary carcinomas, the rates of DNA diploid and aneuploid tumors are 37% and 63% respectively. These figures correspond to most data published on this subject in recent years [3,7]. Examples are given in Fig. 1–3.

Data from the literature, especially the publications by AUER et al. [1], TUBIANA et al. [14], SILVESTRINI et al. [13], and MCDIVITT et al. [10], supply strong evidence that aneuploidy and high numbers of SPF are both indicators of a poor prognosis in breast cancer. Similar data were obtained in our prospective study. Furthermore,

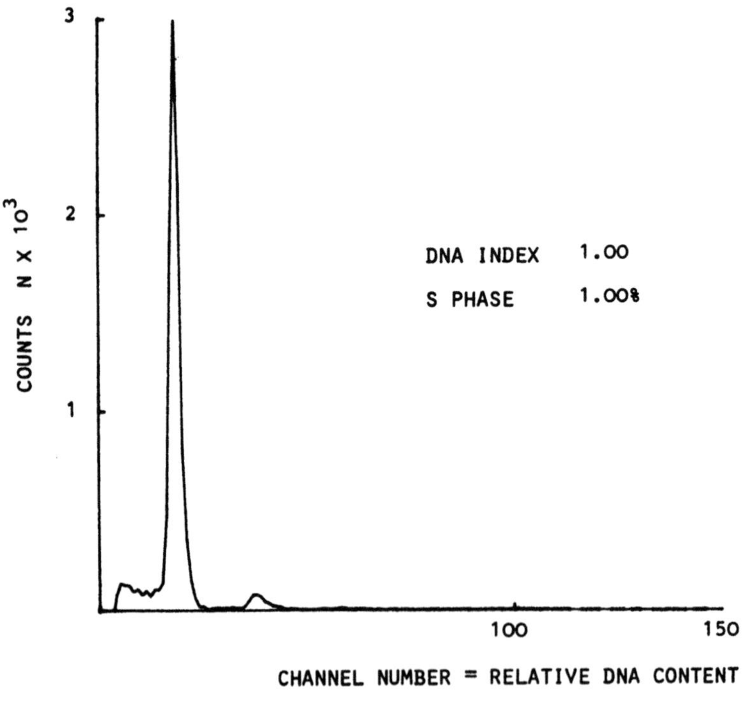

Fig. 1. DNA histogram with a DNA index of 1.00 (DNA diploid), and with a low percentage of cells in the S phase as an example of a DNA distribution of mammary carcinoma with a relatively favorable prognosis

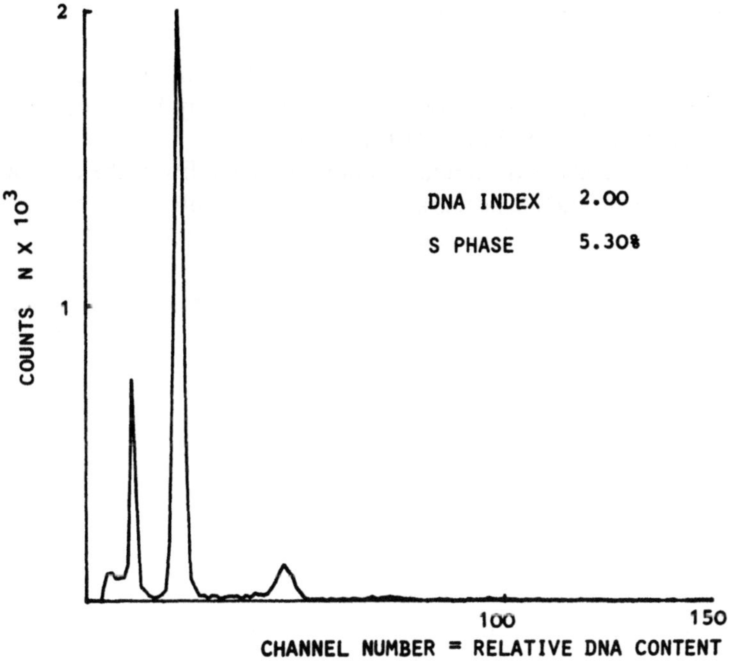

Fig. 2. DNA histogram with a DNA index of 2.00 (DNA tetraploid), and with a medium percentage of cells in the S phase from a mammary carcinoma with intermediate prognosis

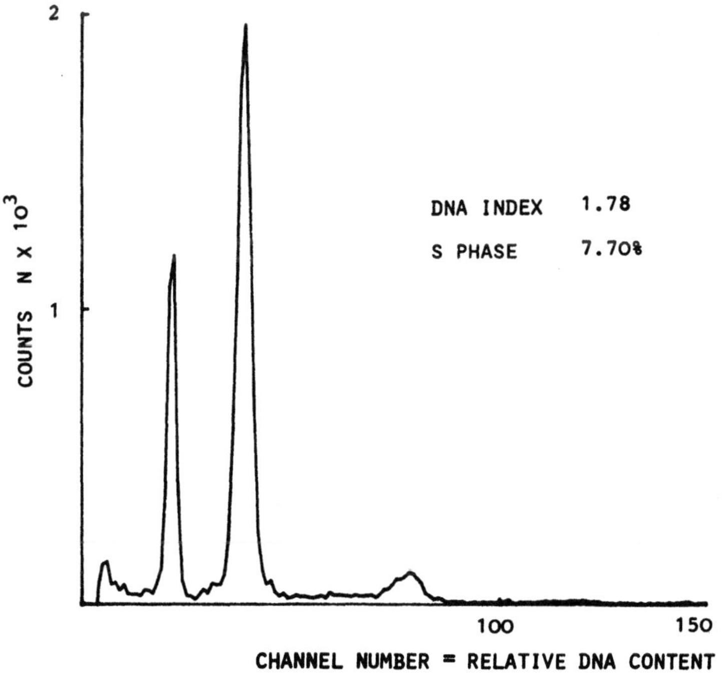

Fig.3. DNA histogram with a DNA index of 1.78 (DNA aneuploid), and with a high percentage of S phase fractions, corresponding to a mammary carcinoma with an unfavorable prognosis

in retrospective FCM examination of paraffin-embedded material from 68 mammary carcinomas, we found a significantly better course in patients with tumors with low SPF ($p < 0.01$) (Fig. 4).

Whereas there is agreement upon the reliability of the determination of DNA ploidy from DNA histograms, occasionally differences emerge concerning the calculation of SPF. The admixture of non-tumor cells such as lymphocytes and of varying amounts of cellular debris, caused by tumor necrosis and by preparation, certainly may negatively influence the preciseness of the SPF calculated from the DNA histogram. These sources of errors can be avoided by the application of special FCM techniques. Lymphocytes can be separated from the tumor cells by centrifugation with Lymphoprep. The false-positive pulses produced by the background debris can be eliminated using one of the known methods of background correction [2,6]. Background pulses do superpose on the DNA histogram and may cause a considerable "false-positive" elevation of the S-phase portion. This is probably the main reason for the differences which have been found between the SPF as measured by thymidine labeling and by FCM without background correction [11]. If background correction is performed, the SPF results as obtained by FCM are nearly identical with those of the TLI [8]. There is increasing evidence that only SPF which have been obtained after background correction should be used for studies of every kind and especially for clinical applications.

DNA FCM is actually the method of choice for the determination of both SPF and DNA ploidy from the same tumor sample. There is no doubt among researchers working in the field of DNA FCM that SPF and DNA ploidy give valuable information for the assessment of the individual prognosis in breast cancer. DNA FCM should be used as an additive examination, supplementing other methods such as histopathology and steroid receptor (estrogen receptor,

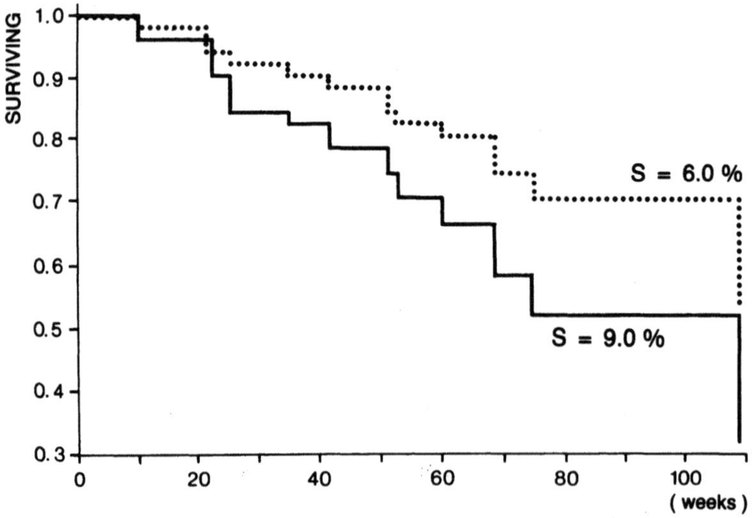

Fig. 4. Calculated survival times for patients with different types of mammary carcinomas containing 6% vs 9% S phase fractions. The better course in carcinomas with smaller S phase fractions is evident

progesterone receptor) determinations. However, it is not yet clear how the DNA data should be related in practice to other prognostic factors in breast cancer. One possibility, demonstrated recently, is compilation of the factors with prognostic importance into a prognostic score [4].

There has also not yet been sufficient examination of whether SPF can be used to predict tumor response to chemotherapy. Assessment of the implication of DNA parameters, especially SPF, on the efficacy of chemotherapy is probably the next main task for DNA FCM in breast cancer.

References

1. Auer G, Caspersson TO, Wallgren AS (1980) DNA content and survival in breast cancer. Anal Quant Cytol 2:161–165
2. Beck HP (1980) Evaluation of flow cytometric data of human tumours. Correction procedures for background and cell aggregations. Cell Tissue Kinet 13:173–181
3. Feichter GE, Mueller A, Kaufmann M, Haag D, Born I, Kubli F, Goerttler K (1985) DNA-ploidy, DNA synthesis, histological grading, stage and steroid receptor content of breast cancer. Verh Dtsch Ges Pathol 69:143–144
4. Feichter GE, Maier H, Adler D, Born IA, Abel U, Haag D, Goerttler K (1987) S-phase fractions and DNA-ploidy of oropharyngeal squamous epithelium carcinomas compared with histologic grade, stage, response to chemotherapy and survival. Acta Otolaryngol (Stockh), 104:377–384
5. Gentili S, Sanfillipo O, Silvestrini R (1981) Cell proliferation and its relationship to clinical features and relapse in breast cancer. Cancer 48:974–979
6. Haag D (1980) Flow microfluorometric deoxyribonucleic acid (DNA) analysis supplementing routine histopathologic diagnosis of biopsy specimens. Lab Invest 42:85–90
7. Haag D, Goerttler K, Tschahargane C (1984) The proliferative index (PI) of human breast cancer as obtained by flow cytometry. Pathol Res Pract 178:315–322
8. Haag D, Feichter GE, Goerttler K (1986) Systematical errors in evaluation of S-phase fractions from DNA-distributions of solid tumors. International Symposium on Clinical Cytometry and Histometry, Apr 20–26. Schloß Elmau
9. Hedley DW, Friedlander ML, Taylor IW, Rugg CA, Musgrove EA (1983) Method for analysis of cellular DNA content of paraffin-embedded pathological material using flow cytometry. J Histochem Cytochem 31:1333–1335
10. McDivitt RW, Stone KR, Craig RB, Palmer JO, Meyer JS, Bauer WC (1986) A proposed classification of breast cancer based on kinetic information. Cancer 57:269–276
11. McGuire WL, Meyer JS, Barlogie B, Kute TE (1985) Impact of flow cytometry on predicting recurrence and survival in breast cancer patients. Breast Cancer Res Treat 5:117–128
12. Meyer JS, Friedman E, McCrate MM, Bauer WC (1983) Prediction of early course of breast carcinoma by thymidine labeling. Cancer 51:1879–1886
13. Silvestrini R, Daidone MG, di Fronzo G (1979) Relationship between proliferative activity and estrogen receptors in breast cancer. Cancer 44:665–667
14. Tubiana M, Pejcevic J, Renaud A, Contesso G, Chavaudra N, Gioanni J, Malaise EP (1981) Kinetic parameters and the course of the disease in breast cancer. Cancer 47:937–947
15. von Fournier D, Weber E, Hoeffken W, Bauer M, Kubli F, Barth V (1980) Growth rate of 147 mammary carcinomas. Cancer 45:2198–2207

Multicentricity in Breast Carcinoma

H.-W. ANTON, A. GUHR, A. MÜLLER and U. ABEL

The concept of multicentricity of breast carcinoma in a single breast is generally recognized. Nonetheless, the strategy of breast-conserving therapy with the various techniques available (quadrantectomy, wide excision, lumpectomy, and subsequent radiotherapy) has found acceptance and is being applied in an increasing number of cases [2,3,5,16,17,20,36].

A major theoretical argument that has been and still is advanced against breast-conserving therapy is the possibility of multicentric disease [13]. It is not yet possible to make a prospective assessment of the biological significance of multicentric carcinomatous foci persisting in the breast remnant following treatment.

One autopsy study of all women to die in 1 year in one administrative district of Denmark [1] found that 25.4% had had invasive or non-invasive carcinoma of the breast. The lifelong cumulated incidence of invasive breast carcinoma recorded, however, was only 9.4%, suggesting that only about one-third of all cases of carcinoma or carcinoma in situ actually develop into clinically recognized carcinoma during the host's lifetime.

It has also been found that the same overall survival rates are achieved after breast-conserving therapy without radiotherapy as when a conventional mastectomy is performed [9].

Considering how topical the question of multicentricity is, it is amazing that the frequency rates given in the literature should vary so widely: between 13% [7] and 74% [10,11,12] (Table 1). Given the magnitude of the health problem posed by breast cancer and the possible therapeutic implications of multicentricity, it is important to resolve such discrepancies.

The differences are due partly to a lack of uniformity in the way the term "multicentric disease" is interpreted. GALLAGER and MARTIN, for example, extend the definition to include non-invasive carcinomas of the margin of the primary tumor and atypical ductal epithelial proliferation, ROSEN (1975) also lists residual tumors and axilliary lymph node metastases following quadrantectomy.

Most studies have not included any note of the sizes of primary tumors or the distances separating the tumor foci in multicentric disease.

Another important reason for the different frequency rates lies in the wide variation in preparation techniques used for the whole mammary gland. Some investigators concentrated mainly on central regions of the gland [GALLAGER and MARTIN 1969] while others made only two or three sections from each quadrant [29]. Still others selected tissue regions for histological preparation based on macroscopic examination or performed only a limited number of sections [9,23]. Since it

Table 1. Review of relevant publications on mammary carcinoma (as of 1987)

Author(s)	Year	Patients (*n*)	Sections/method	Multi-centric disease %
Qualheim et al.	1957	157	1-2 Large-area sections	54
Tellem et al.	1962	64	2-5 Sections per quadrant	26.5
Gallager/Martin	1970	70	Several sections, medial third, proliferative ductal epithelium, and tumor cavity included	74
Morgenstern et al.	1975	500	2 Sections per quadrant + any suggestive regions (11% in same quadrant)	42
Shah et al.	1973	508	Routine preparation	59
Fisher et al.	1975	904	1 Section from each quadrant	13
Rosen et al.	1975	203	2-3 Sections from each quadrant (tumor residue + axilla included)	65
Patchefsky et al.	1977	51	Lobular carcinoma in situ/ 2 sections per quadrant	47
Schwarz et al.	1980	52	1 Section per quadrant + suggestive regions	40
Westmann-Naeser et al.	1981	173	Approx. 12 sections per breast	30
Lagios et al.	1981	286	Several sections per quadrant/ radiography	28
Kalbfleisch	1982	432	2-3 Large-area sections	34
Egan et al.	1982	118	Multiple sections, radiography (tumor residue in biopsy cavity included)	60
Lesser et al.	1982	880	2 Sections per quadrant	30
Holland et al.	1985	282	Approx. 20 sections per breast radiographic	43
Fisher et al.	1986	426	12 Sections per breast	10
Sarnelli et al.	1986	100	5 Sections per breast	36
Tulusan et al.	1986	104	Large-area sections	33
Müller et al.	1987	131	Preparation of total mastectomy material as plastinated large-area sections	24

is not always possible to identify non-invasive carcinoma (in situ) or even small invasive carcinomata when the sections are selected by macroscopic examination, the results are neither complete nor easily comparable to other studies. In addition, even when malignant alterations are revealed by the detailed tissue examination with a relatively dense sequence of sections, accurate retrospective spatial reconstruction of the alterations is no longer possible in many cases. Thus, it is often difficult to ascertain whether the carcinomata detected are genuinely a manifestation of multicentric disease or whether one tumor has spread continuously by way of intraductal growth. Differentiating between these two possibilities will require the development of preparative techniques allowing greater architectural preservation than has previously been possible.

Recurrences, following breast-conserving therapy, have been consistently observed to arise either in the same quadrant or immediately adjacent to the primary tumor.

The following types of local recurrences have been observed:

1. Local recurrence in the same quadrant as the primary tumor (most common type)
2. Diffuse (usually inflammatory) recurrence throughout the mammary remnant (second most common type)
3. Locally circumscribed and spatially limited recurrence in one of the quadrants not affected by the primary tumor (rare)

One hypothesis is that multicentric tumorgrowth is not responsible for the recurrences, but that clinically and radiologically occult parts of the primary tumor extending beyond the surgical margins have persisted in the breast [MÜLLER, in this volume]. We now suggest that in inflammatory diffuse recurrences, which sometimes involve the entire breast, multicentric tumor development is already present throughout the mammary gland at the time of the primary diagnosis, which was not demonstrable with the diagnostic techniques available, and that because of the tumor's high level of aggressivity, it would have been incurable even had an ablation been performed. Local recurrences arising in other quadrants are relatively rare [36], and may actually represent a second carcinomata with multicentric development of disease.

Thus, in selecting patients for breast-conserving therapy, it is important to differentiate between the actual histological spread of invasive or non-invasive tumor structures beyond the region in which detection is possible by macroscopic and radiologic examination, and the genuine frequency of invasive and pre-invasive multicentric tumor development.

The true frequency of multicentric carcinomata cannot be ascertained without a complete histological examination of the entire body of mammary gland, which is extremely time-consuming. Two procedures which allow relatively rapid assessment of the entire gland while preserving three-dimensional architecture have been described in the literature: LAGIOS [22] and EGAN [4] cut the body of the gland into 2.5 mm and 5 mm sections respectively. The slices were then x-rayed in the form of section radiographs and after examination under magnification, any regions suspected of harboring malignancy on radiologic examination were prepared for thorough histologic examination. WELLINGS et al. [37] stained 2mm-thick tissue slices with hematoxylin and eosin (H&E) and then impregnated them with methylene salicylate, making the slices transparent. They were then sealed in plastic envelopes containing a fluid medium and examined at two- to four-fold magnification. Suggestive regions were excised, embedded in paraffin and further prepared for histologic examination. This sophisticated and demanding procedure allows the recognition and quantification of pathoanatomical changes in three-dimensional space.

Our Investigations

Working with colleagues at the Institute of Pathology in Heidelberg, we examined 131 mastectomy preparations from the period 1978–1981 by means of plastination techniques following simulated quadrantectomy [25]. Patient selection was based on the following criteria, which are also used in our own clinic in the selection of patients for breast-conserving therapy:

- The tumor must not exceed 3 cm in size on clinical or radiologic examination.
- The tumor must be at least 2 cm from the nipple.
- Neither clinical nor radiologic examination of the tumor must suggest the presence of multicentric disease.
- Carcinoma must be present as the primary tumor in one breast only.

For examination by the method used in this study, the glands are fixed, cut into 2.5-mm-thick slices and radiography performed on each slice (Fig. 1). The slices are then stained with Hämallaun, followed by plastination with epoxy resins. This makes the sections transparent and gives them a firm consistency [14] (Fig. 2). The stacks of sections cut in the same direction can be assessed in three dimensions on microscopic examination at 1:40 to 1:100 magnification. Tissue at any level can be brought into sharp focus. In addition, 5 μm-thick plastic sections of any regions that are particularly difficult to evaluate, can be prepared for microscopy. The firm tissue slices are numbered, allowing clear retrospective spatial reconstruction of the original shape of the breast.

This plastination technique has several advantages over conventional methods of histological preparation:

1. With plastination the *whole* female breast can be screened macroscopically and microscopically.
2. Plastination yields a three dimensional representation of the mammary gland.

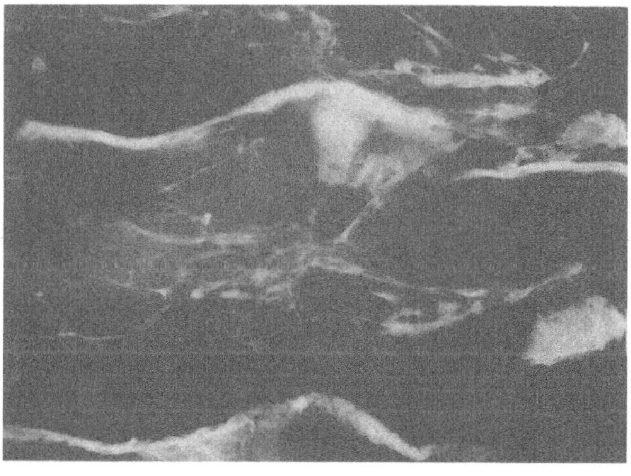

Fig. 1. Radiography of a 2.5 mm-thick slices after fixation

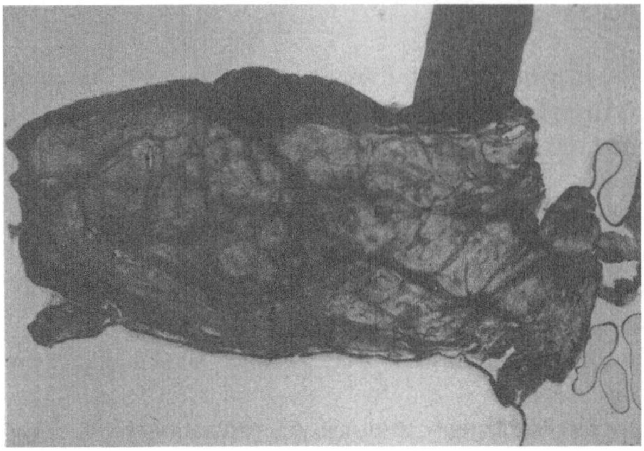

Fig. 2. Transparent slices with a firm consistence after plastination

3. Only 40–60 plastic slices are needed for a whole breast, instead of thousands of large paraffin sections.
4. Questionable regions can be cut into 5 μm-thick sections.
5. Magnification up to 100 times is possible with tissue slices 2.5 mm thick.

Figure 3 is a three-dimensional representation of a mammary gland with 2.5 mm thick plastinated slices with two tumors. Both are connected histologically by an intraductal tissue bridge, but this bridge does not appear in the normal large-area sections (5 μm). It is not possible to demonstrate its existence until after plastination and focusing of the entire thickness of the 2.5 mm-thick tissue stack.

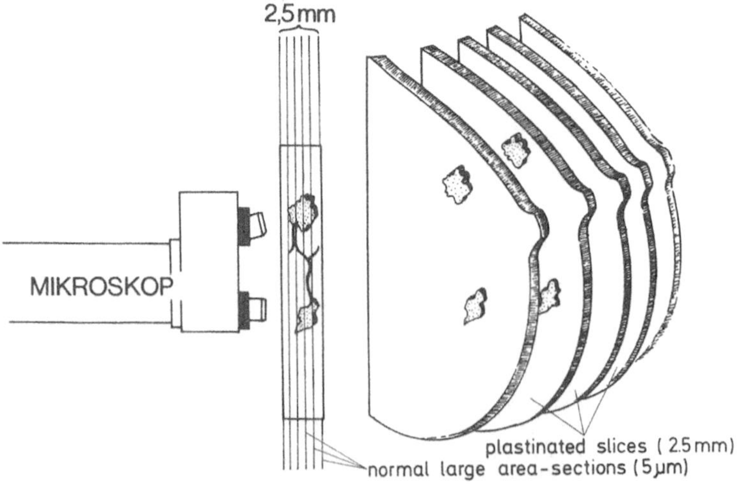

Fig. 3. Three-dimensional representation of a mammary gland with 2.5 mm thick plastinated slices with two tumors

Our own examination of preparation radiographs suggested a frequency of 40% for multicentric foci, approximately the mean of the frequencies reported in the literature. Further preparation of the same material by plastination allowed more precise examination of the spaces between the disease foci. We found that carcinomatous tissue infiltration was present in a considerable number of cases, suggesting that true multicentric disease was present in only *24%* of these cases.

Table 2 shows invasive carcinoma present in 15 cases (47%), ductal and/or lobular carcinoma in situ in 17 cases (53%).

Earlier studies on multicentric mammary carcinoma gave a mean frequency of 40%. This risk is countered by the observation that breast conserving therapy is followed by the absence of local recurrences in an acceptable proportion of cases and, in addition, by virtually the same overall survival rate as ablative therapy for carcinoma. The frequency of 24% which we found for multicentric disease with the plastination technique, seems to be closer to the true incidence. Even with a 24% frequency of true multicentricity, it must be assumed that a large proportion of these carcinomata can be sterilized by means of radiotherapy [MÜLLER, this volume]. The recurrences seen in the quadrants not affected by the primary tumor [36], probably arise from the few multicentric carcinomata that were already invasive at the time of the operation, leading to recurrence even after radiotherapy because of the tumor mass.

Table 2. Multicentricity

131 cases in total; of these:	
32 cases (24.4%) of multicentric disease (100%)	
16	cases of ductal carcinoma in situ (50%) (4 with concurrent lobular carcinoma in situ)
15	cases of invasive carcinoma (47%) (4 with concurrent lobular carcinoma in situ; 3 with concurrent ductal carcinoma in situ; 2 with concurrent lobular and ductal carcinoma in situ)
1	case of lobular carcinoma in situ

References

1. Andersen J, Nielsen M, Jensen J (1985) Essential Histological Findings in the Female Breast at Autopsy. Early Breast Cancer, Springer-Verlag 52–64
2. Atkins H, Hayward JL, Klingman HJ, Wayte AB (1972) Treatment of early breast cancer: a report after ten years of a clinical trial. Br Med J 2, 423
3. Crile G Jr (1975) Multicentric breast cancer: the incidence of new carcinomas in the homolateral breast after partial mastectomy. Cancer 35, 475
4. Egan RL (1982) Multicentric breast carcinoma. Clinical-radiographic-pathologic whole organ studies and 10-years-survival. Cancer 49:1123–1130
5. Fisher B, Montague E, Redmond C, Barton B, Borland D, Fisher ER, Deutsch M, Schwarz G, Margolese R, Donegan W, Volk H, Konvolinka C, Gardner B, Cohn I, Lesnick G, Cruz A, Lawrence W, Nealon T, Butcher H, Lawton R (1977) Comparison of radical mastectomy with alternative treatments of primary breast cancer: a first report of results from a prospective randomized clinical trial. Cancer 39:2827–2839

6. Fisher B (1981) A commentary on the role of the surgeon in primary breast cancer. Breast Cancer Res Treatm. 1, 17
7. Fisher ER, Gregorio R, Redmond C et al. (1975) Pathologic findings from the national surgical adjuvant breast project (Protocol no. 4). I. Observations concerning the multicentricity of mammary cancer. Cancer 35:247–254
8. Fisher ER, Palekar AS, Sass R, Fisher B (1983) Scar cancers: Pathologic findings from the National Surgical Adjuvant Breast Project (protocol 4). IX. Breast Cancer Res Treat 3:39–59
9. Fisher ER et al. (1986) Pathologic Findings from the national surgical adjuvant breast project (Protocol 6). II. Relation of Local Breast Recurrence to Multicentricity. Cancer 57:1717–1724
10. Gallager HS, Martin JE (1969) The study of mammary carcinoma by mammography and whole organ sectioning. Early observations. Cancer 4:855–873
11. Gallager HS, Martin JE (1969) Early phases in the development of breast cancer. Cancer 24:1170–1178
12. Gallager HS, Martin JE (1969) The study of mammary carcinoma by mammography and whole organ sections. Early observations. Cancer 23:855–873
13. Haagensen CD, MB (1986) Diseases of the Breast. WB Saunders Company Philadelphia, London, Toronto, Mexico City
14. von Hagens G (1979) Impregnation of soft biological specimens with thermosetting resins and elastomers. Anat Rec 194:247–256
15. von Hagens G (1985) Heidelberger Plastinationshefter. Sammlung aller Merkblätter zur Plastination (lokale Veröffentlichung). 1/1–9 bis 16/1–2. Anatomisches Institut I Universität Heidelberg, Im Neuenheimer Feld 307, 69 Heidelberg
16. Hayward JL (1985) Trials of Wide Excision and Radiation Therapy at the Breast Unit, Guy's Hospital, London. Early Breast Cancer Springer-Verlag Berlin Heidelberg New York Tokyo S. 253–264
17. Hirsch J (1927) Radiumchirurgie des Brustkrebses. DMW 53
18. Holland R et al. (1985) Histologic Multifocality of CIS, T 1–2 Breast Carcinomas. Cancer 56:979–990
19. Kalbfleisch H and Thomas C Histological Study on Multicentricity of Breast Carcinoma by Means of Whole-Organ Sections
20. Kubli F, v Fournier D (1984) Neue Konzepte der Diagnostik und Therapie des Mamma-Karzinomes. Springer-Verlag
21. Lagios MD (1977) Multicentricity of breast carcinoma demonstrated by routine correlated serial subcross and radiographic examination. Cancer 40, 1726
22. Lagios MD, Westdahl PR, Rose MR (1981) The concept and implications of multicentricity in breast carcinoma. Pathol Annu 16 (II), 83
23. Lesser ML, Rosen PP, Kinne DW (1982) Multicentricity and bilaterality in invasive breast carcinoma. Surgery 91:234–240
24. Morgenstern L, Kaufman PA, Friedman NB (1975) The case against tylectomy for carcinoma of the breast. The factor of multicentricity. Am J Surg 130:251–258
25. Müller A (1987) personal communication Univers. Frauenklinik Heidelberg, BRD
26. Patchefsky AS, Shaber GS, Schwarty GF et al. (1977) The pathology of breast cancer detected by mass population screening. Cancer 40:1659–1670
27. Pierquin B (1985) Conservative Treatment of Breast Cancer: Experience at the Mondor Hospital, Créteil. Early Breast Cancer Springer-Verlag Berlin Heidelberg New York Tokyo S. 276–285
28. Qualheim RE, Gall EA (1957) Breast carcinoma with multiple sites of origin. Cancer 10:460–468
29. Rojen PP, Fracchia AA, Urban JA, Schottenfield D, Robbins GF (1975) "Residual" mammary carcinoma following simulated partial mastectomy. Cancer 35:739–747
30. Sarnelli R, Squortini F (1986) Multicentricity in Breast Cancer: A submicroscopic Study Pathol. Annū 21:143–158
31. Spitalier JM, Amalric R, Brandone H, Ayme Y, Kurty JM (1985) Conservation Therapy of Potentially Curable Breast Cancer: Experience at the Marseille Cancer Institute. Early Breast Cancer. Springer Verlag Berlin Heidelberg New York Tokyo p 271–276

32. Schwartz GF, Patchefsky AS (1980) Clinically occult breast cancer. Multicentricity and implications for treatment. Ann Surg 191, 8
33. Tellein M, Prive L, Meranze DR (1962) Four quadrant study of breast removed for carcinoma cancer 15:10–17
34. Tulusan AH (1986) Multicentricity and Bilaterality of Ductal Carcinoma in situ and Microinvasive Cancer of the Breast: Pathology of Neoplastice and Endocrime Induced Diseases of the Breast: R Bössler, K Stübner, Gustav F Verlag p 297–302
35. Veronesi U, Saccozzi R, Del Vecchio M, Banfi A, Clemente C, De Lena M, Gallus G, Greco M, Luini A, Marubini E, Muscolino G, Rilke F, Salvadori B, Zecchini A, Zucali R (1981) Comparing radical mastectomy with quadrant ectomy, axillary dissection, and radiotherapy in patients with small cancers of the breast. N Engl J Med 305:6–11
36. Veronesi U, Zucali R, Luini A, Belli F, Crispino S, Merson M (1985) Conservative Treatment of Breast Cancer with the "QU.A.RT" Technique. Early Breast Cancer, Springer-Verlag Berlin Heidelberg New York Tokyo p 264–271
37. Wellings SR, Jensen HM, Marcum RG (1975) An atlas of subcross pathology of the human breast with special reference to possible precancerous lesions. J Natl Cancer Inst 55, 231
38. Westman-Naeser S, Bengtsson E, Eriksson O, Jarkrans T, Nordin B, Stenkvist B (1981) Multifocal breast carcinoma. J Natl Cancer Inst 67255

The Contralateral Breast: Bilateral Primary Breast Cancer

A.H. Tulusan, G. Ronay, R. Adam, and M. Reitzenstein

One of the most interesting phenomena in breast cancer is its bilaterality, which not only reveals the biologic nature and natural history of the disease, but is especially important because it allows the possibility of early detection of breast cancer in a high-risk population to be assessed. Although Foote and Stewart [2] had already defined patients with the greatest risk of breast cancer as those with a past history of the disease, interest in bilateral breast cancer was mainly stimulated by the investigative results of Urban. Recently Veronesi et al. [7] observed, in his study of conservative treatment for breast cancer, that 15 contralateral – and only 7 new ipsilateral – primary cancers arose. It is very interesting to consider the role of adjuvant prophylactic radiotherapy in preventing new primary contralateral tumors. Should the contralateral breast also be treated with radiotherapy? In fact, the difficulty of selecting patients at risk has led some authors to conclude that prophylactic mastectomy of the contralateral breast is sometimes justifiable [3]. It is, however, not certain that every breast cancer patient has, or will develop, a second primary in the contralateral breast.

The following report discusses the incidence of, and risk factors associated with, simultaneous bilateral breast cancer. Between 1969 and 1985, we operated upon 2400 patients with breast cancer. In 1048 patients, tissue from both breasts was examined. Figure 1 shows the various types of operation in the contralateral breast. During the past 5 years this procedure was carried out in about 85% of patients treated for breast cancer in our hospital.

When breast cancer was first diagnosed, 16.7% of the patients had a concomitant invasive cancer (6.1%) or carcinoma in situ (10.6%) in the contralateral breast (Table 1). In a further approximately 10% of patients, contralateral atypical proliferative mastopathy was detected. During the past 5 years the rate of benign findings in the biopsy of the contralateral breast has remained almost the same, about 75%. In search for predictive factors for the development of contralateral breast cancer, we compared the following 12 pathologic and clinical characteristics:

1. Patient age
2. Mammographic and clinical abnormalities
3. Mammographic pattern of the contralateral breast (Wolfe's type)
4. Family history
5. Weight of the tissue removed from the contralateral breast
6. Quadrant of ipsilateral and contalateral biopsies

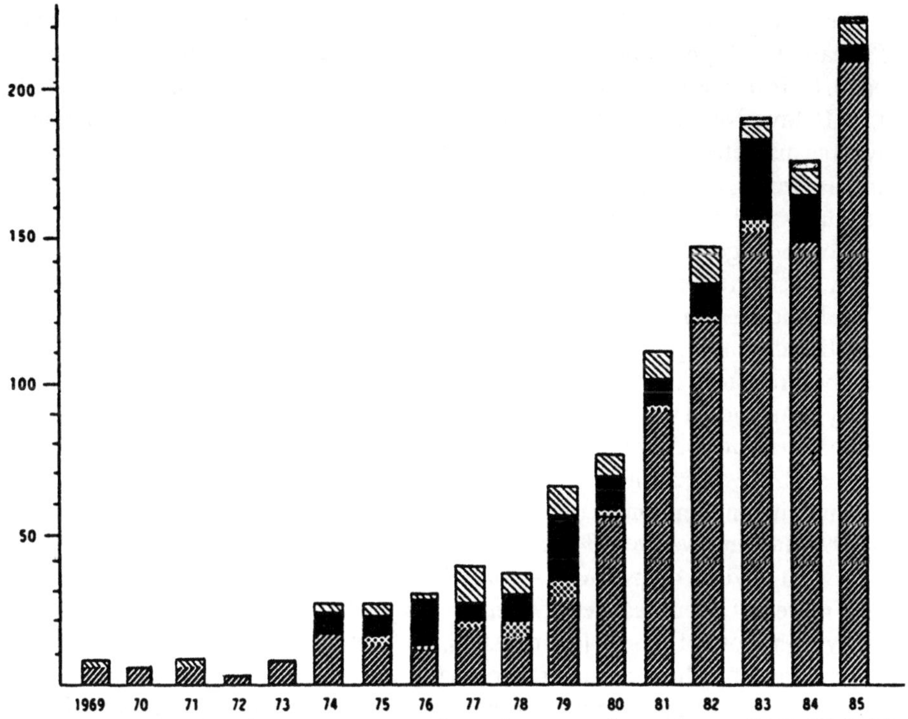

Fig. 1. Frequency of various operations performed on contralateral breast (1969–1985); ▩, quadrantectomy ($n=7$); ▧, mastectomy ($n=83$); ■, reduction mammaplasty ($n=116$); ▦, subcutaneous mastectomy ($n=19$); ▨, biopsy ($n=823$)

Table 1. Incidence of bilaterality among 1048 patients with invasive breast cancer treated at the Women's Hospital, Erlangen University 1969–1985

Ipsilateral breast	Opposite breast			
	Invasive cancer	Carcinoma in situ	Atypical proliferative mastopathy	Benign
Invasive cancer 1048 (100%)	64 (6.1%)	111[a] (10.6%)	101 (9.6%)	772 (73.7%)

[a]Ductal carcinoma in situ (DCIS), 38 patients; lobular carcinoma in situ (LCIS), 47 patients; DCIS with LCIS, 27 patients

7. Tumor size
8. Histologic type
9. Grade of malignancy
10. Axillary lymph-node status
11. Multicentricity of cancer in the ipsilateral breast
12. Receptors for estrogen and progesterone

The average age of patients with concomitant cancer in the contralateral breast (58 years) was higher than that of patients with a benign contralateral lesion (52 years). Of invasive cancers in the contralateral breast, 83% had a malignancy grade of I or II. Invasive cancer in the contralateral breast was diagnosed at an earlier stage (average diameter, 12.0 mm) than the ipsilateral neoplasm (average diameter, 25.3 mm). However, 26% of patients with concomitant contralateral tumors already had metastases in the axillary nodes.

Prior to surgery, all patients were subjected to bilateral mammography. The biopsy site in the contralateral breast was selected according to mammographic or clinical findings (microcalcification, asymmetric thickening of the breast tissue, etc.). If such findings – which can be very discrete were absent, the biopsy was usually taken from the upper-outer quadrant of the contralateral breast (random biopsy). As shown in Table 2, there was a high incidence of cancer in the contralateral breast among patients with clinical and mammographic abnormalities (22 invasive cancers, 9 carcinomas in situ, i.e., 31/64 or 48%). Of the 165 patients with only minimal contralateral mammographic abnormalities (M+C–), 48 (29%) had an invasive (8%) or noninvasive (21%) cancer. In those patients who underwent random biopsy (M–C–), only 9% had cancer, mostly noninvasive. These cases represent occult cancer. When we compared our observations of random biopsy with those of URBAN [6] or LEIS [3], we found *no difference* in the frequency of occult cancer in the contralateral breast (around 8%). This result was unexpected, as we *did not* perform such an extensive biopsy – removing 20%–25% of the breast parenchyma – as proposed by URBAN, but only a biopsy of about 10–50 g (average, 30–40 g) in order to obtain a better cosmetic result. However, this was combined with a very meticulous histologic examination of the whole biopsy specimen, not mere sampling or doing a biopsy from a biopsy.

We also investigated the radiologic appearance of the breast parenchyma [8] to assess its suitability as a method for determining the risk that contralateral cancer

Table 2. Detection of cancer in the contralateral breast in relation to presence or absence of mammographic and clinical signs; $n = 480$

Ipsilateral breast	Opposite breast			
	Invasive cancer	Carcinoma in situ	Atypical proliferative mastopathy	Benign
M+ C+ (64)	22	9	6	27
M+ C– (165)	14[a]	34	21	96
M– C+ (17)	–	1	1	15
M– C– (234)	1	19	20	194

n, no. of patients; M, mammographic signs; C, clinical signs; +, present; –, not present; figures in parentheses represent *n*

[a] Average diameter, 9 mm

will develop. Most contralateral breast cancers occur in WOLFE's type P2 breasts (46/193; 24%) and a smaller number in WOLFE's type DY (9/43; 21%). Another factor important in predicting bilaterality is the family history (Table 3). Among 72 patients with a strong family history of breast cancer, the incidence of cancer in the contralateral breast was 32% (23/72), nearly twice that of the group with no family history (17%; 66/378).

To determine the influence of histologic type, we distinguished three groups: ductal cancer, ductal cancer with lobular carcinoma in situ (LCIS) and invasive lobular cancer. As shown in Table 4, cancers with an LCIS component had a significantly higher frequency of bilaterality (33%–36%) than those without LCIS. In ductal cancer, the frequency was 18%.

One of the most important findings concerning bilaterality in breast cancer is the strong correlation between bilaterality and *multicentricity*. We defined multicentricity as the existence of at least two invasive or noninvasive cancers in different quadrants of the breast. To compile precise data on multicentricity, mastectomy specimens from patients with breast cancer were completely worked up according

Table 3. Correlation between family history and bilaterality; $n = 450$

Ipsilateral breast	Opposite breast			
	Invasive cancer	Carcinoma in situ	Atypical proliferative mastopathy	Benign
FH + (*n*, 72)	4	19	10	39
	23 (32%)			
FH – (*n*, 378)	24	42	37	275
	66 (17%)			

FH, family history

Table 4. Influence of histologic type on bilaterality of invasive breast cancer; $n = 475$ (Women's Hospital, Erlangen)

Ipsilateral breast	Opposite breast			
	Invasive cancer	Carcinoma in situ	Atypical proliferative mastopathy	Benign
Ductal cancer (418)	30 (7%)	47[a] (11%)	41 (10%)	300 (72%)
Lobular cancer + LCIS (24)	2 (8%)	6[b] (25%)	6 (25%)	10 (42%)
Ductal cancer + LCIS (33)	3 (9%)	9[c] (27%)	2 (6%)	19 (58%)

[a]LCIS, 17 patients; LCIS with DCIS, 11 patients; DCIS, 19 patients
[b]LCIS, 5 patients; LCIS with DCIS, 1 patient
[c]LCIS, 5 patients; LCIS with DCIS, 3 patients; DCIS, 1 patient

to a radial scheme. We divided the breast into four quadrants and a retromammillary area, and subjected the resected breast to total radial processing involving radiologic examination of each slice prior to embedding. We made only large-block sections so that we were able to determine the topographic location of each alteration found during the histologic examination (of 56 slides!). One hundred whole-breast specimens were analyzed for this purpose. In 33% of cases we found evidence of multicentric breast cancer in the ipsilateral breast. These cases had the highest incidence of bilaterality (Table 5). Of these patients, 45% had cancer in the contralateral breast (12% invasive, 33% in situ). In comparison, only 15% of the patients with unicentric cancer had bilateral disease. In other words, *positive biopsy results from the contralateral breast also indicate a strong possibility that the ipsilateral cancer is multicentric*. The same significant relationship was reported by LESSER et al. [4], analyzing 880 cases of breast cancer. This fact is important at a time when segmental resection is more frequently used for the treatment of breast cancer. Other factors such as tumor size, quadrant of location, grade of malignancy, hormone-receptor content, and presence of metastases in lymph nodes were not significantly correlated to the bilaterality of breast cancer.

During follow-up of 348 patients with negative findings on biopsy, 10 patients (2.8%) developed breast cancer in the contralateral breast within 3 years; 4 of these patients had metastases in lymph nodes. This fact emphasized the difficulty in detecting early breast cancer. Another example is that patients with asynchronous breast cancer in the contralateral breast have a high rate of lymph-node metastases even when monitored very closely: URBAN [6] reported 50%; FISHER et al. [1], 40%; our material yielded 35%. In contrast, simultaneously diagnosed, clinically occult breast cancer in the contralateral breast have a significantly lower rate of metastasis (URBAN 1985, 8%; our material, 10%). LEIS (1980) pointed out that, when a second primary breast cancer is detected some time after the first operation, the second lesion is often at *no* earlier stage than the first lesion. Some patients previously "cured" of breast cancer by their initial surgery may be lost through failure to recognize and treat a new primary lesion in the contralateral breast. We therefore agree with URBAN that biopsy of the contralateral breast at the time of mastectomy or quadrantectomy is *another method for early detection* of breast cancer.

Table 5. Relationship between multicentricity and bilaterality; $n = 100$

Ipsilateral breast	Opposite breast		
	Invasive cancer	Carcinoma in situ	Benign
Multicentric cancer ($n = 33$)	4 12(%)	11 (33%)	18 (55%)
Unicentric cancer ($n = 67$)	4 (6%)	6 (9%)	57 (85%)

In summary, the following *risk factors* are significantly predictive of bilaterality ($P < 0.025$):

1. Patient's age at diagnosis
2. Predominantly LCIS histology of primary tumor
3. Family history of breast cancer
4. Mammographic and clinical abnormalities of the contralateral breast
5. Wolfe's type P2 or DY parenchymal pattern
6. Multicentricity of ipsilateral cancer

References

1. Fisher ER, Fisher B, Sass R, Wickerham L (1984) Pathologic findings from the National Surgical Adjuvant Breast Project (protocol no 4). XI. Bilateral breast cancer. Cancer 54:3002–3011
2. Foote FW, Stewart FW (1945) Comparative studies of cancerous versus non cancerous breast I and II. Ann Surg 121:6, 197
3. Leis HP (1980) Managing the remaining breast. Cancer 46:1026–1030
4. Lesser ML, Rosen PP, Kinne DW (1982) Multicentricity and bilaterality in invasive breast carcinoma. Surgery 91:234–240
5. Tulusan AH, Egger H, Schneider M-L, Willgeroth F (1982) A contribution to the natural history of breast cancer. IV. Lobular carcinoma in situ and its relation to breast cancer. Arch Gynecol 231:219
6. Urban JA, (1985) Bilateral breast cancer revealed by biopsy of the opposite breast. In: Zander J, Baltzer J (eds) Early breast cancer, Springer, Berlin Heidelberg New York
7. Veronesi U, Zucali R, Luini A, Belli F, Crispino S, Merson M (1985) Conservative treatment of breast cancer with the "QU.A.R.T." technique. In: Zander J, Baltzer J (eds) Early breast cancer. Springer, Berlin Heidelberg New York
8. Wolfe JN, Albert S, Belle S, Salane M (1982) Breast parenchymal patterns: Analysis of 332 incident breast carcinomas. AJR 138:113–118

Cell Biology of Tumor Metastasis Formation

V. SCHIRRMACHER

It cannot be denied that progress has been made in the surgical techniques applied in the removal of local tumors or solitary metastases. The subject of this meeting, however, reflects the feelings that surgery is not always useful and that the surgeon's arch-enemies are micrometastases, which frequently prevent an operation from being successful and which determine the fate of the majority of patients. As little is known for sure about the basic processes involved in the formation of tumor metastases, and because surgical intervention can both inhibit and promote the process, it is of course important to familiarize ourselves with the main basic aspects of the cell biology in metastasis; most of our information is derived from experimental studies.

I should like to start by comparing two concepts used to explain and illustrate the formation of metastatic tumors in an experimental animal such as the mouse. The upper part of Fig. 1 shows a tumor-bearing mouse, with the same color used for both the primary tumor and the internal metastases. The purpose of this is to illustrate that the metastases derive from the primary tumor and that the individual cells of the metastases and those of the primary tumor are identical. According to this model, the whole process of metastasis formation is a random event, or in other words a process determined solely by the laws of probability. There is a certain probability that tumor cells that become detached from the localized tumor will either die or survive and grow into new tumors in internal organs.

The lower part of Fig. 1 illustrates an alternative interpretation. The make-up of the primary tumor is not uniform throughout; rather, it is heterogeneous, made up of various subpopulations of cells. The metastases deriving from this tumor and growing in the internal organs represent only specific individual subpopulations, and thus none of the metastases has a cell population identical with the total cell population of the initial tumor. This alternative concept has arisen mainly as a result of basic studies performed by FIDLER [1]. In these studies he isolated the individual cells of a primary tumor, which were then cloned; each individual clone was then tested in syngeneic animals for its capacity for metastasis formation after transplantation. This model suggests that the process of metastasis formation is a highly selective one, in which only subpopulations of the primary tumor cells with specific properties are capable of metastasis. The model illustrated in the lower part of Fig. 1 shows that the process of metastasis formation is a process of selection of subpopulations from the tumor. This model can now be regarded as largely accepted. The significance of this model for clinical practice lies in the fact that the cells of tumor metastases are different from those of the corresponding primary

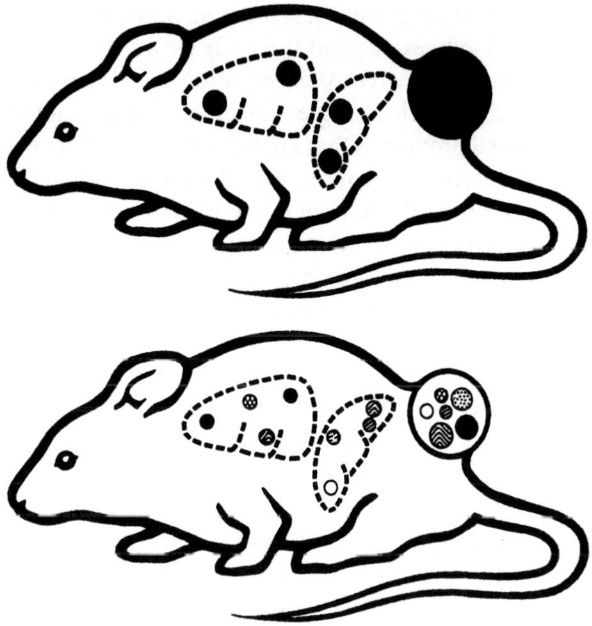

Fig. 1. Schematic illustration of two different ideas of how metastases are formed. *Above*, metastasis formation as a chance process; *below*, metastasis formation as a process of selection of metastatic subpopulations

tumor and that therefore the treatment of metastasis should differ from that of the primary tumor. Strategies for the therapy of metastases should thus recognize (a) the difference in disease localization (systemic versus localized) and (b) the difference in cellularity between a primary tumor and its metastases.

It can furthermore be stated that the process of metastasis formation is now seen as an extremely complex one, [2,3] though it can be dissected into steps with a cascade-type course in both the temporal and the spatial sense. Important steps in the metastatic process are:

1. Local invasive growth
2. Detachment of single cells or of cell clumps from the primary tumor
3. Infiltration into blood vessels or the lymphatic system
4. Survival in the circulation and adhesion in capillary vessels of internal organs
5. Extravasation, with cells leaving the vessels again
6. Resistance to the body's own defense mechanisms
7. Growth at a secondary site depending on the microenvironment of the internal organs
8. In the case of therapeutic intervention, development of tumor variants resistant to chemotherapeutic agents or radiotherapy

Thus, the formation of metastases proceeds in a sequence of steps. This is explained in part by the fact that the metastatic cells have to cross a series of barriers. Examples of such barriers are the basement membranes of the different tissues, in particular of the blood vessels, and the body's own defense system, which actually has the potential to prevent further extension everywhere and at any time. A further reason for the step-by-step progression of the disease might be seen in the absence of some tumor cell properties that are essential for further extension. The process of tumor progression cannot continue until suitable tumor cell variants have arisen. It is now thought probable that not every single tumor cell is capable of going through the whole process of metastasis formation from start to finish; rather, during the process, subpopulations can develop new capabilities for going through different steps in the metastatic cascade. Intensive research effort is currently devoted to studies in different models designed to reveal what cellular characteristics are important for metastasis formation and thus distinguish benign tumors from malignant ones: many factors with some importance for the overall process have been recognized. So far, however, no single factor has been found that could be the key determining factor for the overall process.

A few of these factors of importance are displayed in Table 1. They differentiate between properties of the tumor cells and properties influenced by the host organism. The following should be regarded as tumor cell factors with potential significance for metastatic capability: growth rate, tumor cell surface properties (which are connected with cell-cell interactions and cell-substrate interactions and also with signal reception, transmission and response), and then detachment and adhesion properties, migration properties, and deformability. In addition, the tumor cells' ability to prepare the surrounding tissue in such a way, with the aid of degradation enzymes, as to make it accessible to invasion also belongs in this group. Then come the more complex phenomena that are dependent on both the tumor and the host organism, e.g., angiogenesis, formation of a fibrous barrier, immune defense mechanisms, and tumor escape mechanisms.

Unfortunately it is impossible to discuss these cellular properties in more detail. I turn instead to the very important question of tumor diversification. How does tumor heterogeneity arise and how does progression to a higher level of malignancy come about? What are the driving forces behind this event? As far as the tumor cell is concerned, it was initially postulated that a certain genetic instability was the reason why further variants arose. A genetic instability of this kind was thought to

Table 1. Factors of potential importance for formation of metastases

	Properties of	
	Tumor	Host
Growth rate and mechanical pressure	+	–
Tumor cell surface properties	+	–
Adhesion properties	+	–
Migration capacity and deformability	+	–
Lytic enzymes	+	+
Angiogenesis	+	+
Antitumor immune reactions	–	+
Tumor-immune escape and resistance	+	–

be the explanation for a sudden change in the symptomatology in the course of a tumor's growth and extension. New tumor cell variants were first interpreted as mutants, i.e., cells in which certain genes have undergone structural changes. We are now also familiar with other genetic alterations that lead to the formation of variants, e.g., chromosomal alterations such as translocation, deletions, duplications and processes culminating in polyploidy of single chromosomes or entire chromosome sets. Finally, epigenetic mechanisms in tumor progression have lately also been the subject of lively discussions. If these were found to be implicated this would mean that tumor variants could be caused by all external influences that cause an alteration in the expression of genes. This is illustrated by experiments with 5-azacytidine, a drug that changes the degree of methylation of DNA (without itself directly causing mutations in the DNA) and in this way leads to a change in the expressions of genes in the cell. Gene regulation variants of this kind can be of high or low malignancy. Whether a particular tumor variant has a certain selective advantage allowing it to compete with the other cells and grow into a full-scale tumor will depend on the microenvironment in which it arises.

A further, completely new mechanism that could also be important in tumor diversification and formation of variants has been added recently: the process of somatic cell hybridization, the fusion of a tumor cell and a host cell. Hybridizations of this kind have been known from the literature for over 10 years, but they have not previously been considered in connection with the problems of metastasis formation. Experimental observations pointing to a potential importance of cell fusion for the development of metastatic variants have been published over the last 5 years from various tumor model systems, including the Eb/ESb animal tumor model, which we have been investigating in Heidelberg for some time. A schematic illustration of this process is shown in Fig. 2. First, it shows a tumor cell that is interacting with a cell that is part of the body's own defense mechanism, e.g., a macrophage or a lymphocyte. An activated macrophage or lymphocyte should normally be able to attack and destroy a tumor cell, i.e., lead to cell death of that tumor cell, as indicated by the arrow pointing upward. The scheme also shows that occasionally a fusion of a tumor cell and a host cell could take place at this time of this type of interaction, causing a tetraploid hybrid. Such cells are normally unstable, and the growth capacity of a hybridoma of this kind seems to be suppressed by the influence of the normal cell. It must be assumed that the instability of such hybrids may lead to the loss of individual chromosomes. This segregation process then leads to the development of variants with different chromosomal constitutions. If such variants lose for example chromosomes that have had a suppressive effect on growth, they can grow into new clones. It is conceivable that many hybrid cell segregation variants result from a single fusion, so that selective pressures from the microenvironment can filter out such cells which possess the appropriate properties enabling them to complete the next step in tumor growth and metastasis formation.

For some years we have been working intensively with a murine tumor model consisting of an original non-metastatic tumor cell line (T cell lymphoma, Eb) and a highly metastatic variant (ESb) that arose spontaneously in vivo. We have recently found that this variant expresses cell surface markers of both T cells and

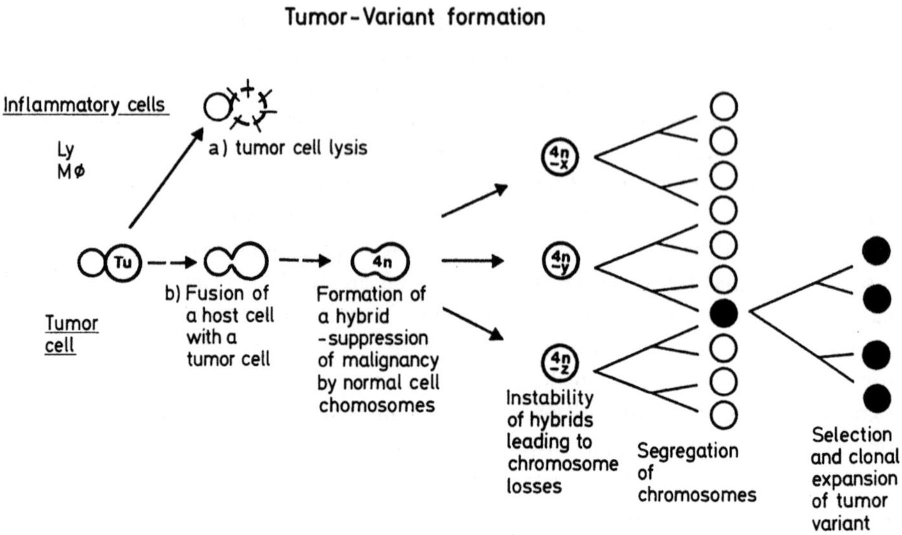

Fig. 2. Schematic illustration of tumor variant formation by way of somatic cell hybridization. *Ly*, lymphocytes; *Mφ*, macrophages; *Tu*, tumor cell; *4n*, tetraploid chromosome set

macrophages, leading us to suspect that it might be the result of a fusion between the original T lymphoma and a host macrophage. It was then possible to confirm this suspicion by in vitro fusion experiments [5]. We actually did obtained hybrid lines with highly metastatic properties, which we were able to characterize in some detail. We have discussed the potential significance of somatic cell fusion for the develcpment of metastatic variants in detail in a review [5].

A precise understanding of the cell-biological basis of tumor metastasis formation requires knowledge of causes of tumor cell variant formation, of the cell-biological properties of malignant cells, and of the routes of extension of the metastases. We cannot hope for a rational basis for a therapy of metastases without knowing the rules of this life-threatening process.

References

1. Fidler IJ, Gersten DM, Hart IR (1978) Adv Cancer Res *28*, 149–250
2. Nicolson GL (1982) Biochim Biophys Acta *695*, 113–176
3. Schirrmacher V (1985) Adv Cancer Res *43*, 1–73
4. Poste G (1982) Cancer Met Rev *1*, 141–199
5. Larizza L and Schrirrmacher V (1984) Cancer Met Rev *3*, 193–222

Prognostic Factors in Primary Breast Cancer

M. Kaufmann, K. Engel, D. von Fournier, and F. Kubli

The natural history of breast cancer is determined by patient and tumor characteristics and may be influenced by adjuvant and palliative treatment.

Numerous prognostic factors have been evaluated by a number of investigators [13]. However, to date only few prognosticators available for clinical routine work identify subsets of patients with biologically different aggressive breast carcinomas. Besides well-known and clinically established prognostic variables, common risk factors for breast cancer also play an important role for prognosis. A new generation of proposed prognostic markers may provide clinicians with new information. In principle, prognostic factors predict the natural course of the disease and/or the treatment outcome.

Risk Factors

There are reports about risk factors relevant for prognosis in breast cancer patients, but no general consensus exists. In general, the course of the disease may be influenced by patient factors, e.g., race, age, menopausal status, clinical history of the tumor, obstetric history, family breast cancer history and immunologic status.

Classic Prognosticators

At the time of diagnosis of breast cancer, clinical examination and TNM classification [11] provides useful information about prognosis. Poor prognosis is associated with increasing T, N and M stages.

The confirmed pathological axillary lymph node status is currently regarded as the most reliable prognostic factor, followed by tumor size, which is related to lymph node and distant metastasis. Other established prognostic factors are the morphologic type, nuclear and histologic grade of differentiation and steroid hormone receptor content.

Pathology

Tumor Size, Type and Histological grade

The clinical size of the primary tumor correlates well with the prognosis [8,19]. Axillary nodal involvement and the incidence of distant metastasis during the course of the disease are strongly related [16, 23].

Infiltrating duct carcinoma is the most common (≈ 70%) histologic type of breast cancer. Medullary carcinoma, a relatively uncommon tumor (≈ 6%) has been reported to have a better prognosis (Fig. 1) than other invasive carcinomas [17].

Histologic grade is an excellent prognosticator [3]. However, quantitation depends on the pathologist's subjective evaluation, which cannot be objective and reproducible. The feasibility of objective morphometry with prognostic value have been reported [1]. Other correlations between prognosis and microscopic information on blood vessel and lymphatic invasion or the presence of necrosis in the tumor and of elastosis in the stroma have been found.

Axillary Node Status

There is no question that to date the pathologic status of the axillary lymph nodes (Fig. 2) is the most important prognostic variable [27]. Four lymph node categories recently have been defined: negative, 1-3, 4-9 and 10 or more positive nodes [5].

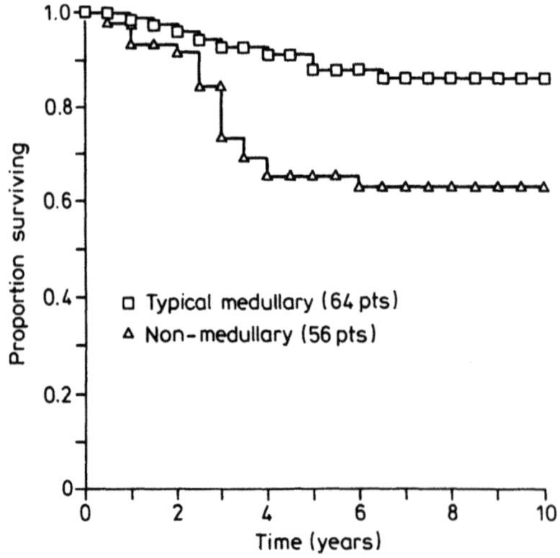

Fig. 1. Survival of 120 patients with typical medullary or non-medullary primary breast cancer [17]

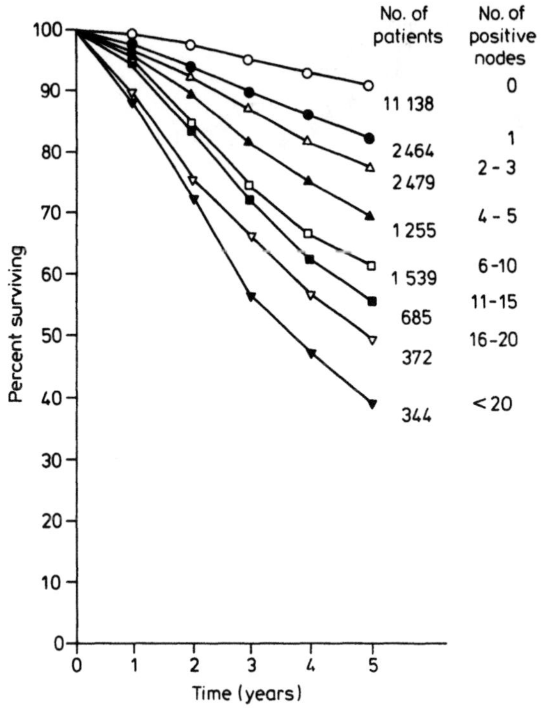

Fig. 2. Survival of 20 276 primary breast cancer patients according to the number of positive axillary lymph nodes [27]

Micrometastasis (lesion 2 mm or less in diameter) and macrometastasis (found as one lymph node metastasis in T1, N1, MO patients) yielded equal disease-free intervals (Fig. 3) after 2 years observation [20].

Steroid Hormone Receptors

Steroid hormone receptor determination has become a standard procedure in clinical routine work with prognostic and therapeutic relevance [15]. Biochemical assays [6] cannot yet be replaced by histochemical or immunohistologic methods [10], but the latter are already available and are using monoclonal antibodies against estrogen and progesterone receptor proteins for quantitation and localization of receptors.

Sensitivity to endocrine treatment is related to the presence and amount of both estrogen receptor (ER) and progesterone receptor (PR) proteins. In primary breast tumors with high levels of ER and/or PR, disease-free survival (DFS) and overall survival (OS) are better than in patients with receptor-negative tumors [13]. However, there are conflicting reports, especially on the prognostic value for survival and the importance of PR. Response and prognosis are directly correlated

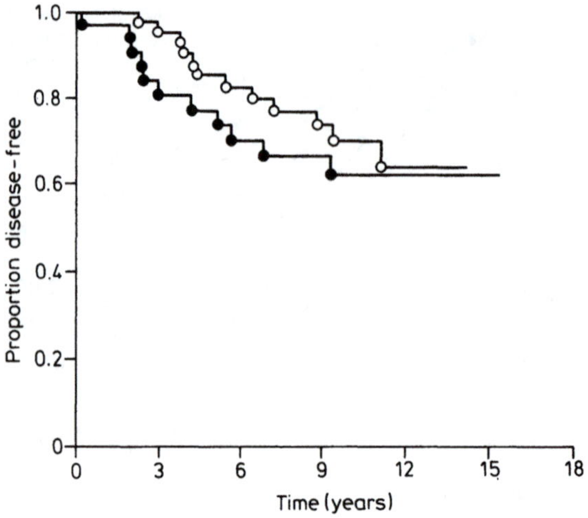

Fig. 3. Disease-free survival of 73 patients with primary T1 breast cancer and a single axillary lymph node metastasis. ○ micrometastases ($n = 41$) ● macrometastases ($n = 32$) [20]

to receptor density. In metastatic breast cancer, percent response decreases in the following order: ER+, PR+ (response ≈ 70%) >ER−, PR+ (≈ 40%) >ER+, PR− (≈ 30%) >ER− PR− (≈ 10%).

Although there is no general consensus, many data in the literature demonstrate correlation of prognosis with histopathology (well-differentiated tumors and elastosis-positive lesions show hormone receptor positivity) and also with proliferative activity (low proliferation shows hormone receptor positivity).

New Prognosticators: Tumor Proliferation and Growth

In recent years attempts have been made to examine and characterize proliferative activity and aggressiveness of breast tumors [12, 18, 24, 26].

The kinetic status of tumors can be calculated by measuring the fraction of cells actively synthesizing DNA, which is determined in vitro by tritiated thymidine labeling index (TLI) of native tumor samples. Proliferative activity is correlated with poor prognosis (Figs. 4, 5). There is also some evidence that highly proliferative tumors respond better to chemotherapy.

Discrimination between slowly and rapidly proliferating tumors has also been demonstrated using a chemoresistance short-term assay [12, 14]. DFS and OS (Fig. 6) were predicted to a significant degree of accuracy with this test system, which is thus suitable for routine clinical work. Analysis of two prognostic variables (hormone receptors and proliferative activity) together increased the prognostic significance.

Other new prognosticators can be obtained by the application of DNA flow cytometry [2]. This most promising technique can provide clinicians within 1 day

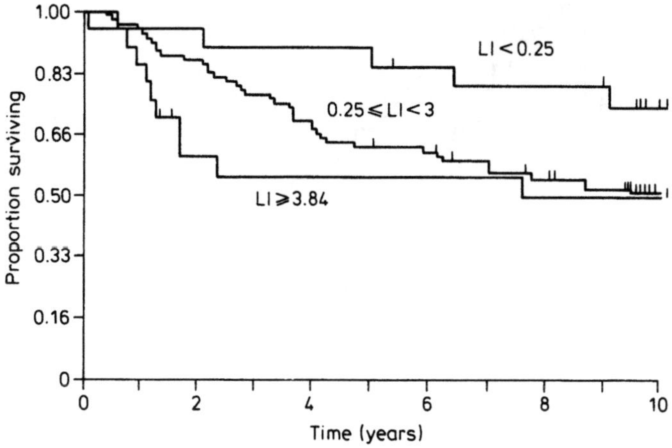

Fig. 4. Survival of 125 node-negative and -positive primary breast cancer patients according to different labeling indices (*LI*). No patient received adjuvant chemotherapy [26]

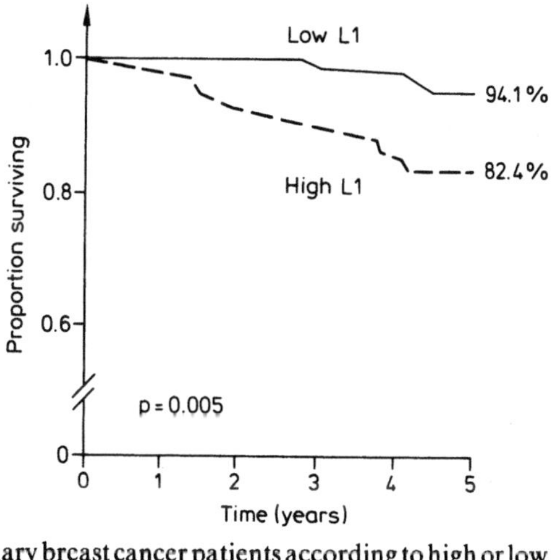

Fig. 5. Survival of 215 node-negative primary breast cancer patients according to high or low labeling index (*LI*). No patient received adjuvant chemotherapy [24]

with information on ploidy and S- phase fraction as prognostic factors of human tumors (Figs. 7,8). Aneuploidies show the amount of extra DNA in the tumor cell, whereas the percentage of cells in S- phase gives information on proliferation. There are data which show correlation between ploidy and S- phase fraction [7]. These two prognosticators seem to be independent factors and are considered to have better discriminative power than receptor studies, especially for node negative tumors.

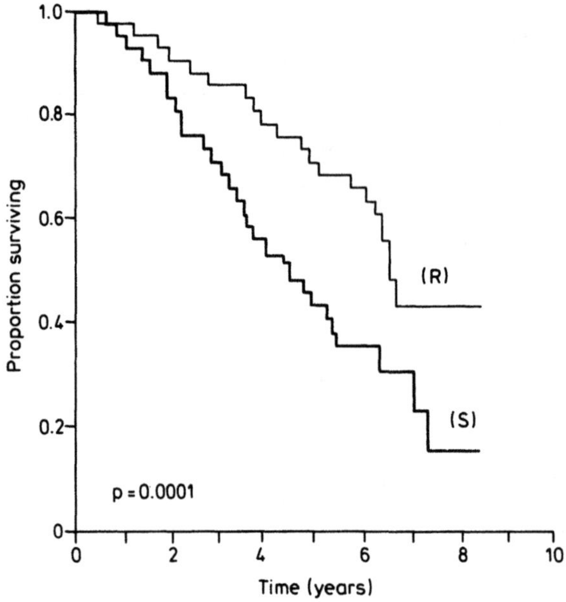

Fig. 6. Survival of 233 node-negative and -positive primary breast cancer patients according to proliferative activity (nucleic acid metabolic short-term assay). *R:* low proliferation; *S:* high proliferation (Kaufmann 1987, unpublished)

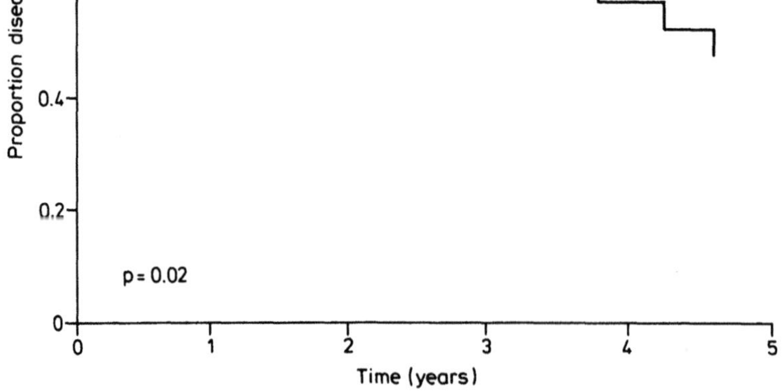

Fig. 7. Disease-free survival of 247 node-negative and -positive primary breast cancer patients according to ploidy status (Kaufmann and Feichter 1986 personal communication)

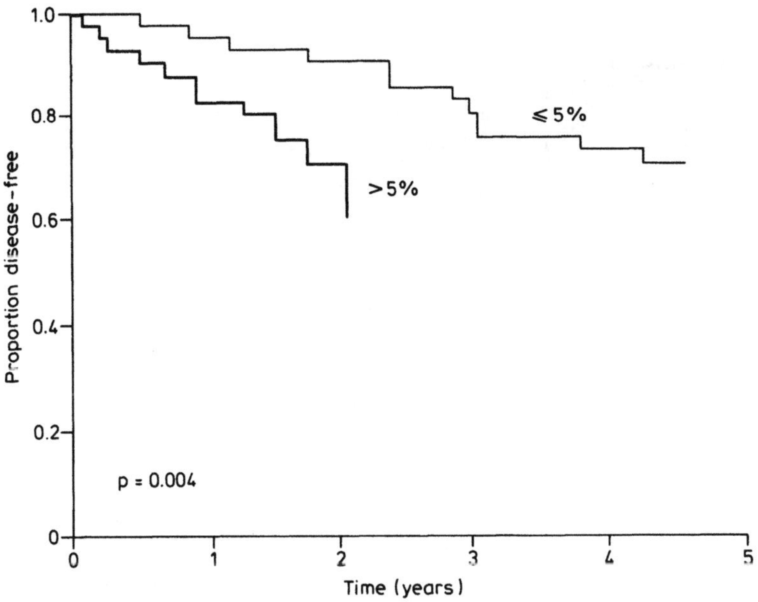

Fig. 8. Disease-free survival of 247 node-negative and -positive primary breast cancer patients according to the S-phase fraction (Kaufmann and Feichter 1986, personal communication)

Adjuvant Chemotherapy and Prognostic Factors

In 1985 a Consensus Conference was held in Washington, USA, to clarify the benefit of adjuvant chemotherapy in relation to DFS and OS [5]. The following statements concerning prognostic variables can be made for clinical routine practice:

1. Node-positive premenopausal women benefit from combination chemotherapy.
2. Node positive and hormone receptor-positive postmenopausal women benefit from tamoxifen treatment.

For certain pre- or postmenopausal women with node-negative tumors adjuvant chemotherapy should be considered.

The prognostic significance of hormone receptors or nuclear grade (Fig. 9) is demonstrated by the NSABP B-09 trial [9]. Positive effects of adjuvant chemotherapy in high-risk node-negative patients (Fig. 10) are shown by a recent Milan trial [4]. At our institution S- phase fraction is used to discriminate between high- and low-risk situations in node-negative women regardless of hormone receptor or menopausal status (Fig. 11).

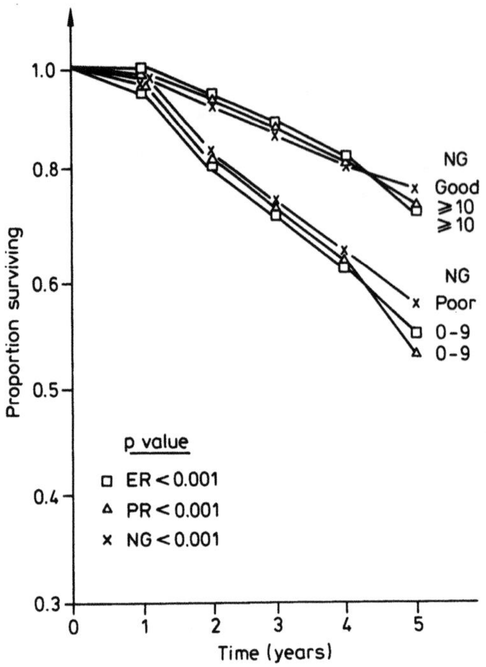

Fig. 9. Survival of 589 node-positive primary breast cancer patients treated with adjuvant chemotherapy (*L*-PAM, 5-FU, tamoxifen) according to estrogen receptor content (*ER*), progesterone receptor content (*PR*) and nuclear grade (*NG*). ER or PR 0–9 vs ≧ 10 fmol cytosol protein; NG poor vs good. (NSABP B09 Trial [9])

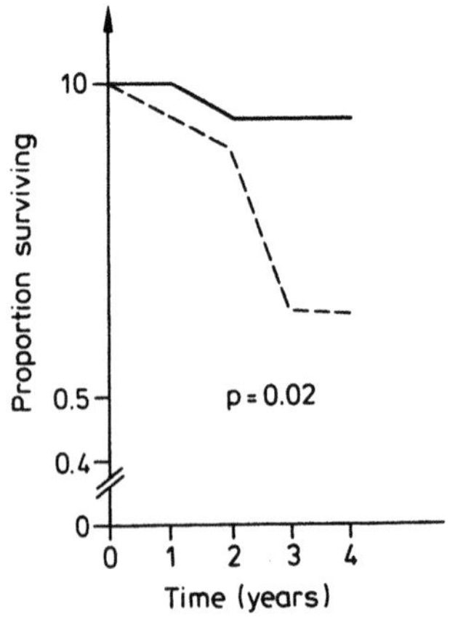

	Total	Death
CMF	45	2
Pre	27	2
Post	18	0
Control	45	10
Pre	27	6
Post	18	4

Fig. 10. Survival of 90 node-negative and ER-negative primary breast cancer patients with no adjuvant treatment or adjuvant CMF chemotherapy (12 cycles) [4] (pre- and postmenopausal)

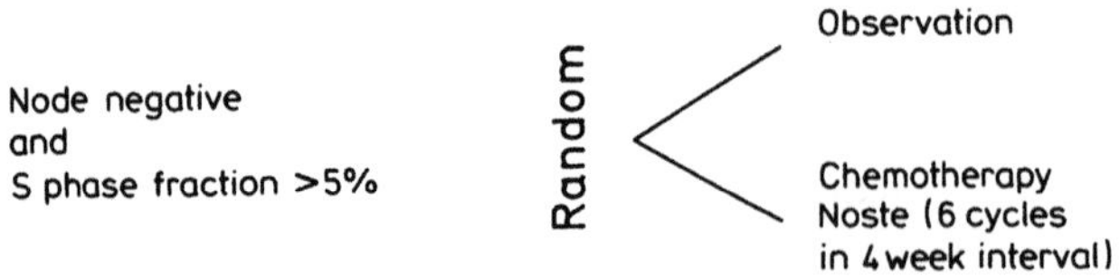

Fig. 11. Study design of the Heidelberg III randomized adjuvant chemotherapy trial in node-negative high-risk patients. *NOSTE*: mitoxantrone (Novantron) 12 mg/m² i.v. day 1 + prednimustine (Sterecyt) 100 mg/m² p.o. days 3–7, of four weeks for six cycles

Prognostic Factors for Local Recurrence in Patients with Breast Conservation Therapy

Since conservative surgery and irradiation became attractive and have been frequently employed in primary breast cancer management, many data have been reported which show risk factors for local recurrence [22]. Most workers seem to be of the opinion that recurrence will be induced by persistent disease rather than by new tumor cells. The following are relevant for local relapse:

1. Inadequate surgical excision of the primary tumor
2. Degree of intraductal components within the primary tumor
3. Non-invasive (in situ) carcinoma present adjacent to the primary tumor

No consensus exists about the relevance of high nuclear grade and/or high mitotic index, low age (less than 35 years) and family breast cancer history.

New Proposed Prognostic Factors

Recently published interesting data indicate that new factors may play an important role in the biologic behavior and pathogenesis of breast cancer. The presence of oncogene amplification (HER-2/neu oncogen) [25] and of epidermal growth factor receptors [21] have been directly correlated with DFS and OS (Figs. 12, 13), and these are thought by many to be the most important new prognostic variables.

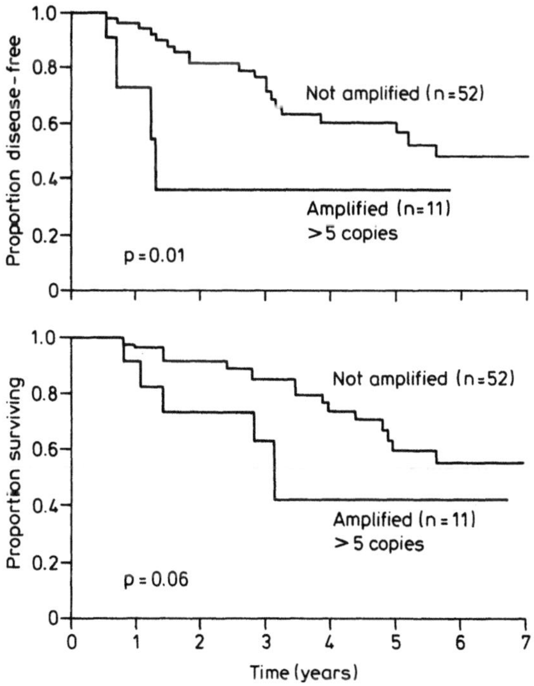

Fig. 12. Disease-free survival and total survival in 63 node-positive primary breast cancer patients. No amplification vs more than five copies of HER-2/neu oncogene [25]

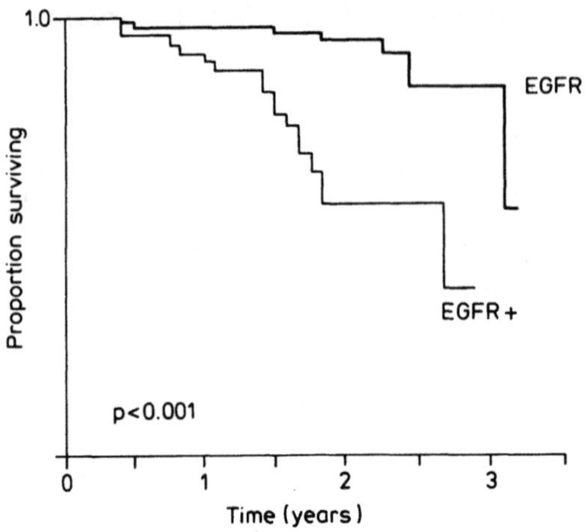

Fig. 13. Survival of 135 node-positive and -negative primary breast cancer patients. *EGRF*, epidermal growth factor receptor [21]

Besides lymph node status, hormone receptor determinations and the menopausal status of women with primary breast cancer, biochemical assays on proliferation and growth will become the most promising routine clinical measures to get further information with prognostic relevance for our treatment strategies.

References

1. Baak JPA, van Dop H, Kurver PH, Hermans J (1985) The value of morphometry to classic prognosticators in breast cancer. Cancer 56:374–382
2. Barlogie B, Raber MN, Schumann J, Johnson TS, Drewinko B, Swartzendruber DE, Göhde W, Andreeff M, Freireich EJ (1983) Flow cytometry in clinical cancer research. Cancer Res 43:3982–3997
3. Bloom HJG, Richardson WW (1957) Histological grading and prognosis in breast cancer: a study of 1409 cases of which 359 have been followed for 15 years. Br J Cancer 11:359–377
4. Bonadonna G, Zambetti M, Valagussa P, Bignami P, DiFronzo G, Silvestrini R (1986) Adjuvant CMF in node negative breast cancer. 22nd Annual Meeting of ASCO, Los Angeles
5. Consensus Conference (1985) Adjuvant chemotherapy for breast cancer. JAMA 254:3461–3463
6. EORTC Breast Cancer Cooperative Group (1973) Standards for the assessment of estrogen receptors in human breast cancer. Eur J Cancer 9:379–381
7. Feichter GE, Müller A, Kaufmann M, Haag D, Born J, Kubli F, Goerttler K (1985) DNA-ploidy, DNA synthesis, histological grading, stage and steroid receptor content of breast cancer. Verh Dtsch Ges Pathol 69:143–144
8. Fisher B, Slack MH, Bross DJ (1969) Cancer of the breast: size of neoplasm and prognosis. Cancer 24:1071–1080
9. Fisher B, Fisher E, Redmond C, Brown A, et al. (1986) Tumor nuclear grade, estrogen receptor, and progesterone receptor: their value alone or in combination as indicators of outcome following adjuvant therapy for breast cancer. Breast Cancer Res Treat 7:147–160
10. Greene GL, Nolan C, Engler JP, Jensen EV (1980) Monoclonal antibodies to human estrogen receptor. Proc Natl Acad Sci USA 77:5115–5119
11. Hermanek P, Sobin LH (eds) (1987) TNM classification of malignant tumors (UICC), 4th edn. Springer, Berlin Heidelberg New York

12. Kaufmann M, Klinga K, Runnebaum B, Kubli F (1980) In vitro adriamycin sensitivity test and hormonal receptors in primary breast cancer. Eur J Cancer 16:1609–1613
13. Kaufmann M (1983) Biochemische prognostische Faktoren beim Mammakarzinom. In: Kubli F, Nagel GA, Kadach U, Kaufmann M (eds) Neue Wege in der Brustkrebsbehandlung. Zuckschwerdt, München, pp 46–61 (Aktuelle Onkologie 8)
14. Kaufmann M (1984) Biochemical short-term predictive assay: results of correlative trials in comparison to other assays. Recent Results Cancer Res 94:151–160
15. Klinga K, Kaufmann M, Runnebaum B, Kubli F (1982) Steroidhormonrezeptoren beim Mammakarzinom. Dtsch Med Wochenschr 107:313–315
16. Koscielny S, Tubiana M, Lê MG, Valleron AJ, Mouriesse H, Contesso G, Sarrazin D (1984) Breast cancer: relationship between the size of the primary tumour and the probability of metastatic dissemination. Br J Cancer 49:709–715
17. Maier WP, Rosemond GP, Goldman LJ, et al. (1977) A ten year study of medullary carcinoma of the breast. Surg Gynecol Obstet 144:695
18. Meyer JS, Friedman E, McCrate MM, Bauer WC (1983) Prediction of early course of breast carcinoma by thymidine labeling. Cancer 51:1879–1886
19. Nemoto T, Vana J, Bedwani RN, Baker HW, McGregor FH, Murphy GP (1980) Management and survival of female breast cancer. Cancer 45:2917–2924
20. Rosen PP, Saigo PE, Braun WD Jr, Weathers E, Fracchia AA, Kinne DW (1981) Prognosis in stage II (T1, N1, M0) breast cancer. Ann Surg 194:585–591
21. Sainsbury JRC, Farndon JR, Needham GK, Malcolm AJ, Harris AL (1987) Epidermal-growth-factor receptor status as predictor of early recurrence and death from breast cancer. Lancet 1:1398–1402
22. Schnitt SJ, Connolly JL, Harris JR, Hellman S, Cohen RB (1984) Pathologic predictors of early local recurrence in stage I and II breast cancer treated by primary radiation therapy. Cancer 53:1049–1057
23. Schottenfeld D, Nash AG, Robbins GF, Beattie EJ (1976) Ten-year results of the treatment of primary operable breast carcinoma. Cancer 38:1001–1007
24. Silvestrini R, Daidone MG, DiFronzo G, Morabito A, Valagussa P, Bonadonna G (1986) Prognostic implication of labeling index versus estrogen receptors and tumor size in node-negative breast cancer. Breast Cancer Res Treat 7:161–169
25. Slamon DJ, Clark GM, Wong SG, Levin WJ, Ullrich A, McGuire WL (1987) Human breast cancer: correlation of relapse and survival with amplification of the HER-2/neu oncogene. Science 235:177–182
26. Tubiana M, Pejovic MH, Chavaudra N, Contesso G, Malaise EP (1984) The long-term prognostic significance of the thymidine labeling index in breast cancer. Int J Cancer 33:414–445
27. Wilson RE, Donegan WL, Mettlin C, Smart CR, Murphy GP (1984) The 1982 National Survey of Carcinoma of the Breast in the United States by the American College of Surgeons. Surg Gynecol Obstet 159:309–318

Natural Growth Rate of Primary Breast Cancer and its Metastases

D. VON FOURNIER, W. HOEFFKEN, and M. FRIEDRICH

Patients suffering from breast diseases generally die when metastatic spread into the bloodstream occurs. When distant metastases become clinically manifest the survival rates are about the same with various types of palliative therapy. Wide individual differences can be observed, however, in the interval between diagnosis of the primary tumor and development of local recurrences and detection of distant metastases. This interval varies from zero (distant metastases present at time of primary diagnosis) to more than 30 years. BRINKLEY and HAYBITTLE [6,7] showed that after a follow-up of 25 years, 81.5% of women had died after breast cancer, leaving only 18.5% still alive. As metastatic spread does not necessarily begin preoperatively, wide differences can be observed in the time the metastases take to reach a clinically detectable size. This is primarily due to the two following growth behaviors of the metastases:

1. The net metastatic growth varies; it may be extremely slow because of cell loss. As far as the speed of growth of the whole tumor is concerned, no significant changes can be observed; this behavior can be represented by a relatively uniform exponential function.
2. The growth behavior of metastatic cells is very heterogeneous. After a period of dormancy the cells may suddenly grow very rapidly because of a change in the host-tumor relation. This heterogeneity seems to be most important in the early stage of metastatic spread (100–1000 cells). At the time of detection (several hundred thousand cells), the differing growth behavior of individual cells is thought to play only a minor role.

The exact time before operation of the formation of the first metastasis is of decisive importance, as it largely determines the duration of the recurrence-free interval.

The clinical growth behavior of metastases is determined by the cell characteristics of the primary tumor in relation to the host, although propagation of the primary tumor is generally not fatal. The cell characteristics of the primary tumor are thus ultimately the key to overall survival.

Clinical and roentgenological measurements carried out in untreated tumors to determine the growth rate of the primary tumor and its metastases allow us to draw mathematical conclusions about the time of metastatic origin. Since it has already been demonstrated that the growth of metastases correlates with the growth of the primary tumor, though it is, clinically and radiologically, on average faster, we would first like to analyze the natural growth rate of the primary tumor.

The growth rate of the primary tumor allows us to assess the time of breast cancer formation, which in turn allows us to calculate both the period between tumor formation and tumor death and the influence of any therapy on the overall survival rate. The following can be stated about the growth behavior of the primary tumor:

1. The tumor growth rate can vary during the clinical history of an individual tumor. Whether this is important for the occurrence of "minimal cancer" or "carcinoma in situ" has yet to be examined. The change is of secondary importance for tumors of roentgenologically measurable size.
2. The metastatic potential of the cancer is largely determined by the tumor growth rate; nevertheless, in an individual tumor the correlation may be very weak.
3. The implantation of metastases disseminated by the primary tumor probably occurs at either a very early or a very late stage. Daily dissemination of tumor cells must always be expected in microscopically small tumors, but both implantation and growth of metastases can still vary widely. The implantation rate of metastases is presumably directly related to the growth behavior of the primary tumor.
4. An individual primary tumor consists of different cell compartments which induce the formation of different types of metastases that have different growth behaviors. The overall growth rate of the primary tumor as a net result of tumor growth and cell loss may be relatively low, while metastases of an aggressive cell line may grow very rapidly. In addition, disseminated cells may steadily develop characteristics different from those of the primary tumor, which is why the overall metastatic growth is determined by the cell compartment in which the growth is most rapid. Because this tumor growth behavior also characterizes the primary tumor, the growth behaviors of primary tumor and metastases seem to be largely related (see above). This seems to be the case for larger tumors at the time of primary therapy: HENDERSON and CANELLOS [16] demonstrated that in historic patient samples the survival rates of untreated patients after a follow-up period of 20 years were not significantly lower from 1805 to 1933 at the Middlesex Hospital than those after radical mastectomy carried out at Johns Hopkins Hospital between 1889 to 1931.
5. Very little is yet known about the exact growth behavior of very small tumors detected early (e.g., during screening programs or incidentally) and diagnosed as minimal cancer or intraductal carcinoma in situ. Because even tumors of 1 cm in diameter seem to consist of millions of cells, these tumors can obviously disseminate cells daily via the bloodstream. We assume that the probability of the implantation of metastases decreases if only a relatively small number of cells have been disseminated. DUNCAN and KERR [9] have reported that after a follow-up of 20 years the survival rate of patients with tumors 1 cm in diameter is significantly better than that of patients with tumors 2 cm in diameter, whereas among patients with large tumors (3–10 cm in diameter) there are no differences in survival rate (see Fig. 12).

Correspondingly, after studies carried out between 1954 and 1972 embracing 2648 patients with breast cancer, KOSCIELNY et al. [17] reported a direct relation between clinical tumor size and the probability of the occurrence of metastases during a follow-up period of 10–25 years. These findings confirm that not only the individual tumor growth but also the size of the tumor at the time of diagnosis determines the prognosis. These observations lead us to the assumption that small tumor volumes are commonly related to smaller metastatic volumes and therefore to longer survival.

Before they became clinically manifest the metastases had undergone a growth period in which their growth rate correlated with the growth rate of the primary tumor. Ultimately these metastases were the cause of death. Studies carried out with animals have revealed that even a few disseminated tumor cells can give rise to metastases.

The following questions are still unanswered:

- Is there a minimum tumor size below which disseminated tumor cells usually do not form metastases and are therefore not fatal?
- Do even these minute tumors constantly metastasize, or do they remain dormant for a long time before metastasizing, thus leading to the long survival times?

Natural Growth Rate of Mammary Carcinoma

BLOOM et al. [4] examined the survival rate in 250 untreated patients (1805–1933), all of whom had advanced tumors (stage IV 74%; stage III 23%; stage II 2%). Using a semilogarithmic mode of presentation, they revealed a constant death rate in these patients: 25% of all patients die every year. FOX [12] reported on two subgroups of treated patients suffering from breast cancer, with reference to the "force of mortality": in one subgroup (about 40% of all patients) the force of mortality was 25% per year. After a follow-up period of 10 years the patients with poor prognostic factors had already died. In the other, bigger subgroup (about 60%), the force of mortality was relatively constant at 2.5% per year. This leads to the assumption that in the subgroup of aggressive tumor types surgery had no influence on survival.

Over a follow-up period of 31 years, BRINKLEY and HAYBITTLE [7] examined 704 patients suffering from breast cancer who had been treated between 1947 and 1950. The survival rates were calculated according to life-table analysis and compared with the expected survival in the normal population. Even 25 years later the two curves were not parallel; that is to say, even after 25 years patients still die of breast cancer metastases. Among those who died, 26% (176/683) had had a "personal cure": they died of other illnesses with no symptoms of breast cancer.

BLOOM [3] estimated the growth rate of breast cancer on the basis of natural life expectancy in untreated patients. In untreated patients the mean duration of life was found to be 38.7 months (range 3 months to over 30 years). COLLINS et al. [8] suggested that the rate of doubling of a tumor mass reflects the rate of cell division and that volume-doubling time (T_V) is constant, resulting in exponential growth. All these authors supported their hypotheses with measurements of pulmonary metastases of various tumors.

GERSHON-COHEN et al. [13] determined T_V of human breast cancer from the increase in the tumor shadow in serial mammograms. SPRATT et al. [23], using the same method, observed a mean T_V of 325 days in 26 cases. FOURNIER et al. [10,11] observed a mean T_V of 202 days in 100 cases of breast cancer, also based on measurements from serial mammograms.

The gross T_V depends on (1) the duration of the mitotic cycle, (2) the fraction of proliferating cells compared to dormant cells, and (3) the rate of cell loss (hypoxia, necrosis, immunological defense). TUBIANA [25] and TUBIANA and KOSCIELNY [26] found that up to 50% of the cells in the tumor may die every day. Tumor growth is the net result of cell proliferation and cell loss in a given tumor.

In very advanced experimental tumors the growth rate slows as the tumors reach a certain size. In these cases tumor growth is best described by the Gompertz function:

$$V = k_0 \cdot \exp\,(k_1/k_2 \cdot (1 - \exp\,(-k_2 t)))$$

where k_0 = initial value, k_1 = acceleration factor and k_2 = deceleration factor (Fig. 1). In the early phase the Gompertz function is similar with an exponential function. There are indications that metastases of breast cancer correspond to the primary tumor in their speed of growth, but have a faster average growth rate [19,23].

There is very little in the literature about the relation between the growth rate of the primary tumor and histological parameters [24], but several reports suggest that histological findings correlate with survival rates [2].

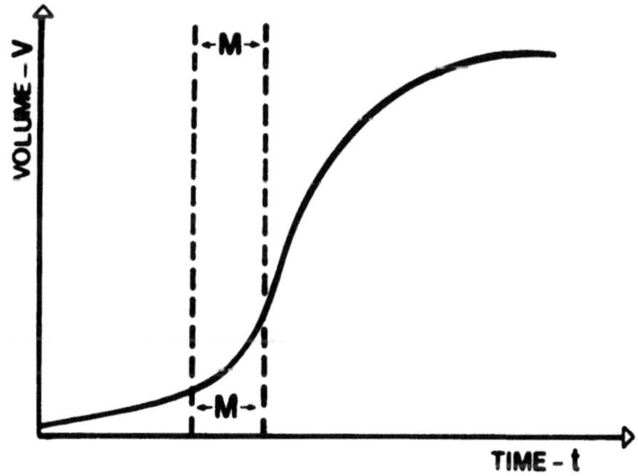

Fig. 1. The Gompertz function, a model describing tumor growth: $V = k_0 \times \exp\left|\frac{k_1}{k_2} \times (1 - \exp(-k_2 t))\right|$. k_0, Initial size; k_1, accelerating factor; k_2, inhibiting factor; M, interval between mammographies

Estimation of Growth Rate from Tumor Volume-Doubling Time

The T_V of 400 primary breast cancers were assessed by our team from mammograms. Serial mammograms were taken in this population before definite treatment of the cancer because of delay in the final diagnosis (neoplasm could be identified only retrospectively) and patients' refusal to undergo treatment, among other reasons. Between 2 and 11 mammograms were taken, the time between first and last examinations ranging between 0.2 and 16 years. Altogether, 528 patients with previous mammographies were collected from 28 clinics in Germany, but in 128 of them the tumor shadow was not measurable in previous screenings, so these cases could not be included.

SPRATT et al. [23] and FOURNIER et al. [11] discussed measurement of tumor diameter and its limitations. The method is as follows: First, the tumor diameter is normalized by measuring the tumor nucleus shadow in three places. The T_V is then calculated as follows:

$$T_V = \frac{t}{9.97 \times I_g \frac{d_2}{d_1}}$$

where t = time in days between two observations, d_1 = normalized diameter of tumor at the beginning of observation and d_2 = normalized diameter of tumor at the end of observation. An example of the scope for error: with a tumor size of 20–30 mm, inaccuracy of ± 0.75 mm in measurement yields an error of 11.3% in the doubling time.

Assuming that malignant growth begins with a single cell or a small cell cluster, and on the premise of a constant T_V, the number of volume doublings necessary to reach a given tumor size can be calculated. Using this method, growth rates and life spans of tumors can be projected. Based on an exponential growth model beginning with a primary tumor cell 10 μm in diameter, 21 doublings are needed to achieve a size of 0.5 cm (Fig. 2). At this point the tumor already has the potential ability to disseminate metastatic cells [1]. It takes the tumor more than half of its whole life to reach a size of 0.5 cm. To reach the clinically detectable size of 1 cm the tumor needs over 25 doublings. By the time the primary tumor achieves this size, detectable metastases have already been formed in 28% of patients with mammary carcinoma [15].

Figures 3 and 4 show two examples of tumor growth as seen on mammograms. Figure 5 shows the very slowly growing tumor of a patient who refused therapy from 1963 to 1974. As the tumor grew larger, T_V lengthened in accordance with the Gompertz function (see Fig. 1). Of all T_V observed, 95% were between 65 and 657 days. The shortest was 26 days, the longest 2400 days.

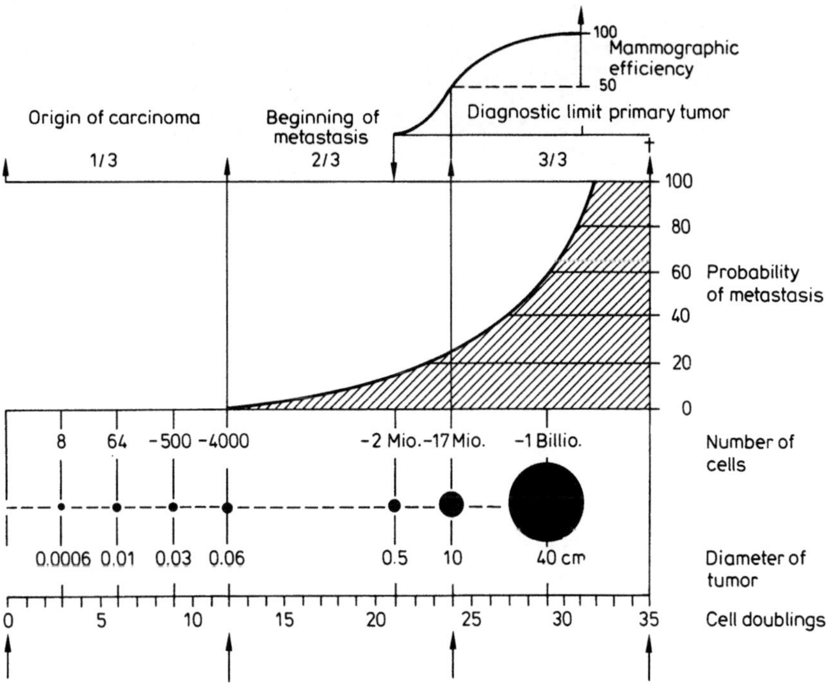

Fig. 2. Model of tumor growth behavior based on constant volume-doubling times [11]

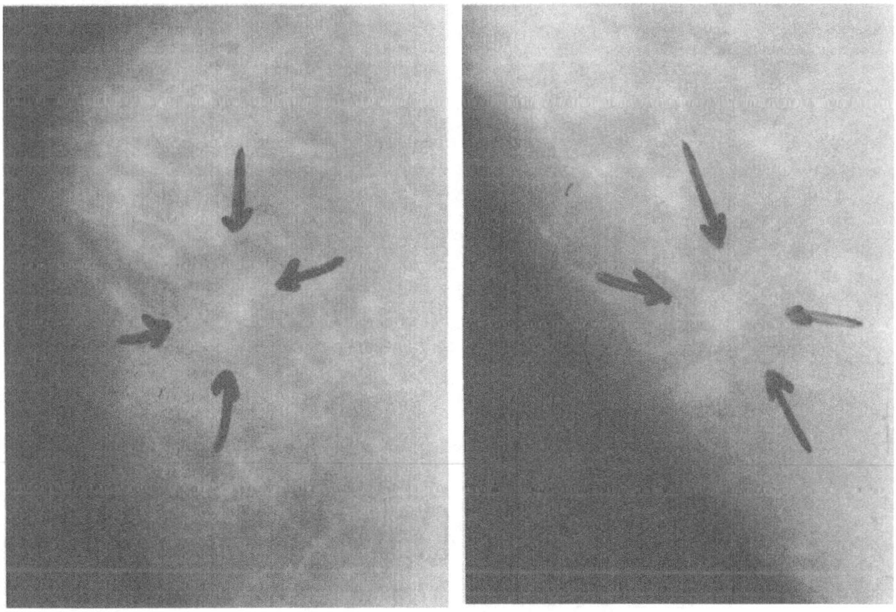

Fig. 3a,b. Growth of a solid tumor with a volume-doubling time of 300 days. **a** May 1981; **b** July 1983

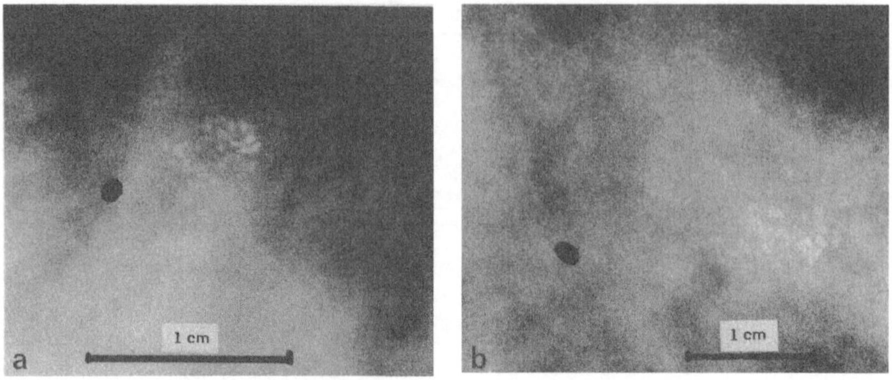

Fig. 4a,b. Growth of a carcinoma in situ. **a** Suspicion of carcinoma in situ. **b** Six years later: confirmed carcinoma in situ, incipient invasion (2 mm). Note different magnification

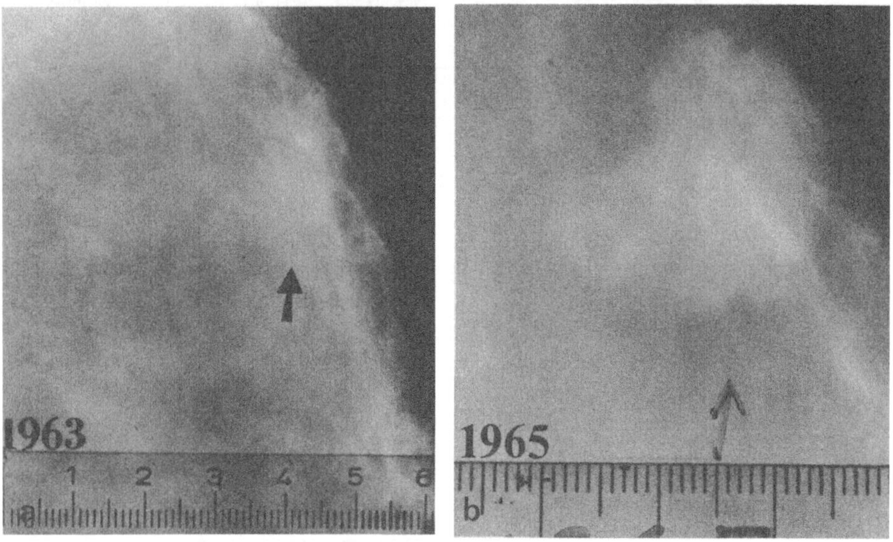

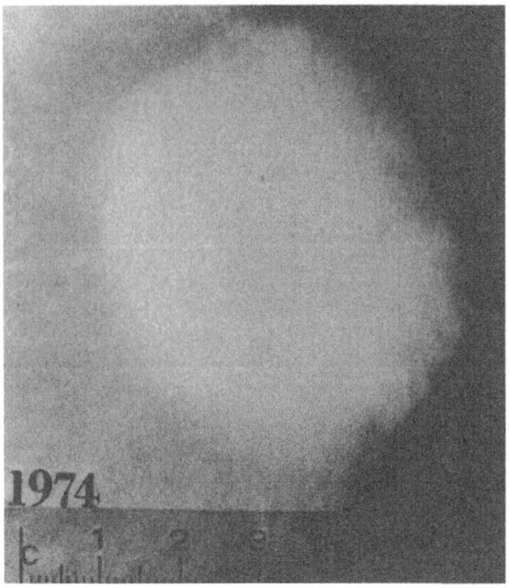

Fig. 5a-c. Growth of a tumor with a volume-doubling time increasing from 243 days between 1963 **(a)** and 1965 **(b)** to 922 days between 1965 and 1974 **(c)** Mammographic diameter of tumor increased from 13 mm in 1963 to 51 mm in 1974. Histology in 1974: solid duct carcinoma

Evaluation of 12 Cases with Five or More Mammographies per Case

Figure 6 shows the results in 12 patients with five or more single measurements from serial mammograms. The good fit of the observed growth to the estimated exponential growth curves indicates the applicability of the exponential growth model for the observation periods in most cases. Figure 7 shows the data from these 12 cases after logarithmic transformation so that the exponential growth curves are straight lines. Assuming constant doubling times from the beginning of neoplastic growth it is possible to extrapolate the time of the development of the first tumor cell. We estimated that on average it took more than 20 years for the tumor to reach a size of 20 mm (average $T_V = 308$ days in these 12 cases).

Different Tumor Diameters and Age of Patients

The T_V values were used to estimate at what age women would have a tumor of 0.01 mm (representing the first tumor cell), 0.1 mm, and so on up to 20 mm in diameter. It must be borne in mind that our hypothesis may not reflect the true situation in early cancer growth. Figure 8 shows the frequency distribution of estimated age at a tumor diameter of 20 mm (average 58 years). The mean estimated age of women with a 0.1-mm tumor was 44 years. The mean age for occurrence of the first cancer cell (tumor 0.01 mm across) was 35 years. This indicates that the average growth time for a palpable 20-mm tumor is close to 20 years and that in most of our cases the breast cancer will have originated at the age of 30–40 years. This may have important implications for the interval between screening mammographies, the age at which screening should be started and also the evaluation of therapeutic results.

Different Growth Rates

Table 1 shows different speeds of growth in the 400 cases of primary breast cancer. Figure 9 shows the different groups of breast cancers according to their growth behavior. Year by year we observe a 3% rate of extremely fast-growing tumors, those of the inflammatory type for instance. In these cases there is no measurable tumor shadow, and growth rates can be estimated only on the basis of personal reports from the patients. From the visible tumor enlargement as reported by the patient we estimated that it needed less than 3 years from the first cancer cell to the

Table 1. Different growth rates in 400 cases of mammary carcinoma

Speed of growth	T_V (days)	n	%
Very fast	< 100	45	12
Fast	101–150	36	9
Moderate	151–300	161	40
Slow	> 300	158	39

Growth Rate of Primary Mammary Carcinoma

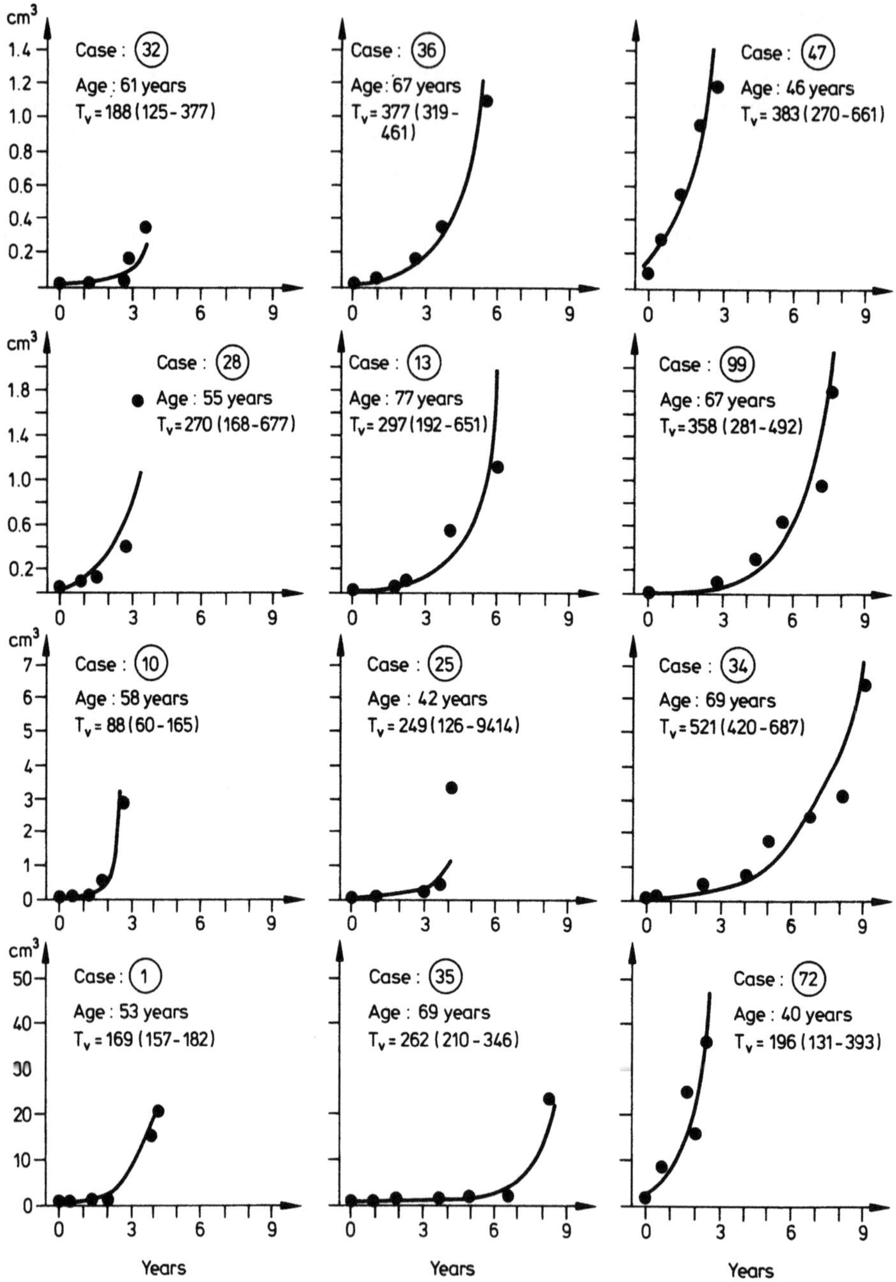

Fig. 6. Tumor growth as a function of time in 12 cases monitored by mammography. *Dots*, observed growth; *solid lines*, estimated exponential growth curves. T_v, tumor volume-doubling time (days)

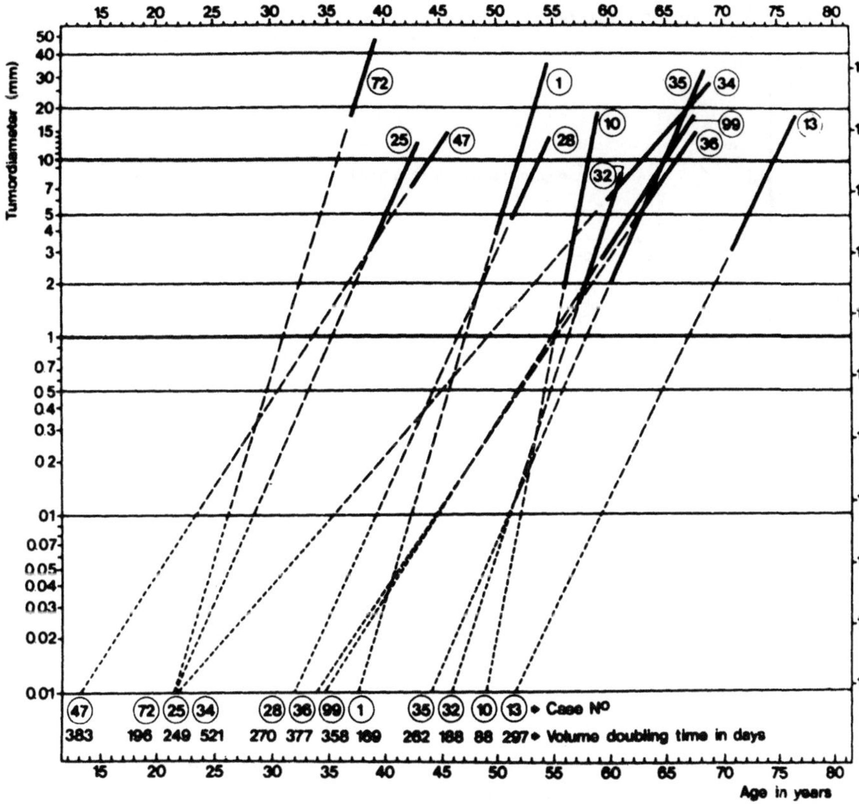

Fig. 7. Tumor function of same 12 cases as in Fig. 6 (five or more measurements with note of age at times of measurement). *Ordinates,* log tumor diameter/volume; *abscissa,* time in years; *solid lines,* exponential growth curves; *broken lines,* calculated development of first tumor cell

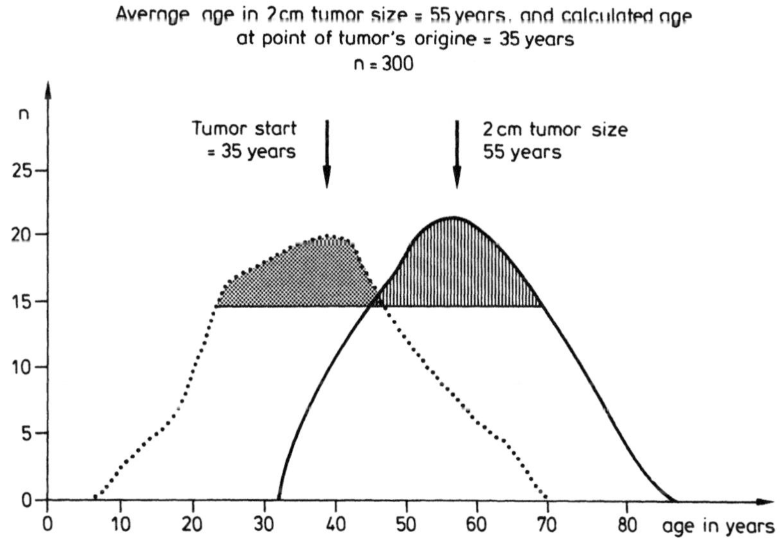

Fig. 8. Frequency distribution of estimated ages at tumor diameters of 0.01 cm (*dotted lines;* 35 years) and 2 cm (*solid line;* 55 years). $n = 300$

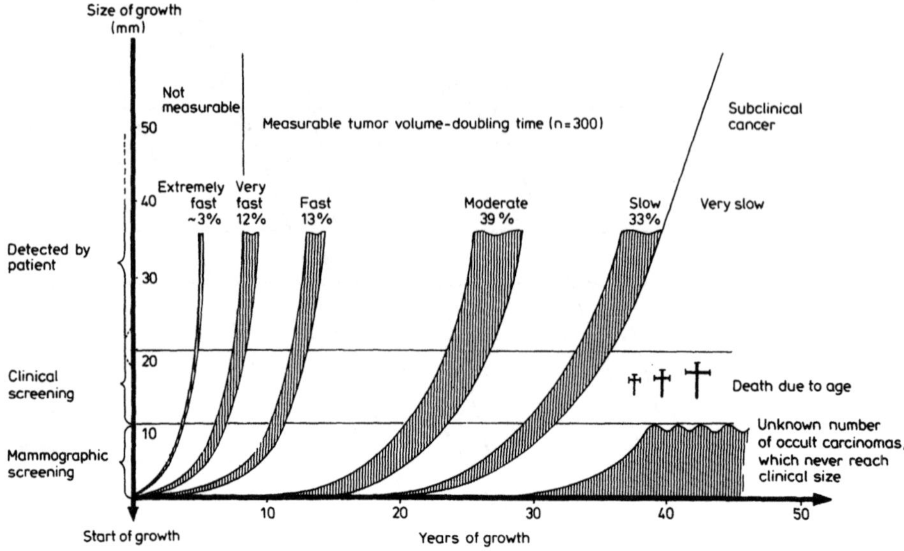

Fig. 9. Proportions of tumors with different growth rates [11]

clinical size in these inflammatory cases (left curve in Fig. 9). Very fast growth ($T_V \leqslant$ 100 days) was observed in 12% of the measurable cases, fast growth (T_V = 101–149 days) in 13%, moderately fast-growing tumors (T_V = 150–299 days) in 39%, and slow growth ($T_V \geqslant$ 300 days) in 33% of the 300 cases (Fig. 9).

An unknown number of breast cancers grow so slowly that they fail to reach a clinically detectable size during the patient's natural life span. These tumors can be found only by means of meticulous serial section methods, as described by ANDERSEN et al. (this volume), who report an incidence of about 25% for invasive and noninvasive carcinomas of the breast in all women who died within 1 year in a certain county of Denmark. According to ANDERSEN et al. most breast cancers never attain clinical relevance. In accordance with this, MÜLLER et al. [21], studying two comparable collectives of specimens from subcutaneous mastectomies, showed that carcinoma (in situ or invasive) was detected in 13.1% of cases using a conventional method and in 27.1% using a serial section method (Table 2). Many (probably around two-thirds) of these carcinomas will never reach a clinically relevant size ("academic cancers").

Table 2. Diagnosis of premalignant and malignant lesions in subcutaneous mastectomy. [21]

	Conventional workup (%) $n = 130$	Workup in serial 2.5-mm-thick sections (%) $n = 70$
Mastopathy with atypias	7.7%	24.3%
Lobular or ductal carcinoma in situ	10.8%	17.1%
Invasive carcinoma	2.3%	10.0%

Growth Rate of Primary Tumors and Histomorphological Characteristics of the Tumor

We found a correlation between the calculated tumor growth rate and the histological tumor grading [5] (Table 3).

Table 3. Histological grading and growth rates of 61 breast cancers

Type of tumor	*n*	Very fast	Fast	Moderate	Slow	Mean T_V (days)
Grade 1 Carcinoma	8	0	2	4	2	470
Grade 2 Carcinoma	32	3	2	19	8	270
Grade 3 Carcinoma	13	2	5	5	1	193
Lobular Carcinoma	3	0	0	3	0	200
Mucinous Carcinoma	1	1	0	0	0	90
Papillary Carcinoma	3	0	0	2	1	372
Ductal Carcinoma in situ	1	0	0	1	0	261

Grading according to BLOOM and RICHARDSON (1957)

Growth Rate of Primary Tumors and Hormone Receptor Status

In a group of our cases with slow average growth, we found that tumors positive for estrogen and progesterone receptors showed significantly slower growth rates than those that were receptor negative (Table 4).

Table 4. Growth rates and hormone (estrogen and progesterone) receptor status in 59 cases with slow average growth rates

Estrogen receptor and progesterone receptor	*n*	Average T_V (days)
Positive	39	580
Negative	20	203

Growth Rate and DNA Synthesis

Table 5 shows the correlation between primary tumor growth rate and fraction of cells in S-phase. Very fast-growing tumors (doubling time less than 100 days) had an S-phase fraction of 8%–16%, slowly growing tumors ($T_V \geq$ 300 days) only 2%. The differences were significant. There was also a significant correlation between fast growth and polyploidy.

Table 5. Speed of tumor growth according to DNA synthesis (preliminary results of a prospective study on unfixed tumor samples)

Tumor growth	T_V (days)	S-phase fraction (%)	*n*
Very fast	⩽ 100	8–16	8
Fast	101–149	6–10	6
Moderate	150–299	2–4	6
Slow	⩾ 300	2	9

Growth Rate of Primary Tumors and Growth Rate of Metastases

Table 6 shows the ages of 12 patients at operation, their calculated ages at the time of the origin of metastases and the T_V of the primary tumors and the metastases. All the metastases were measured from X-rays of the bones and the lung. The T_V of the metastases are related to that of the primary, but on average shorter.

Figure 10 and Fig. 11 show the T_V of the primary tumor and of one to three lung metastases in seven cases. The results indicate that most lung metastases originate many years before diagnosis of the primary tumor. In a survey of 70 cases, the findings were as follows:

Average age at origin of tumor: 35 years

Average age at operation: 58 years

Table 6. Doubling times of metastases in mammary carcinoma

Pt. no.	A	MA.	T_V (primary)	T_V (metastases)
1	59	56	237	68
		57		56
		51		173
		55		78
2	53	31	499	315
		22		508
3	71	64	102	99
		65		90
		67		59
4	74	71	114	63
5	63	33	97	459
6	65	52	896	166
7	52	42	66	140
		37		208
8	66	52	164	211
9	47	43	129	93
10	68	62	272	73
11	65	64	82	20
		65		8
12	66	64	83	48

A, Age at operation for primary tumor; MA.01, calculated age of patient at time of origin of metastases.

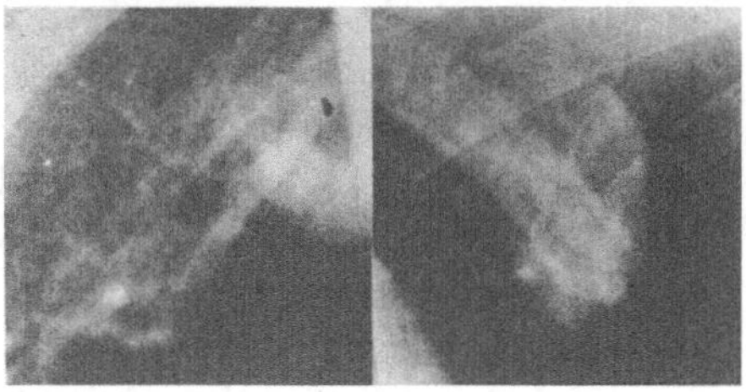

Fig. 10. Example of growth of lung metastases (untreated). *Left*, January 1983; *right*, December 1983

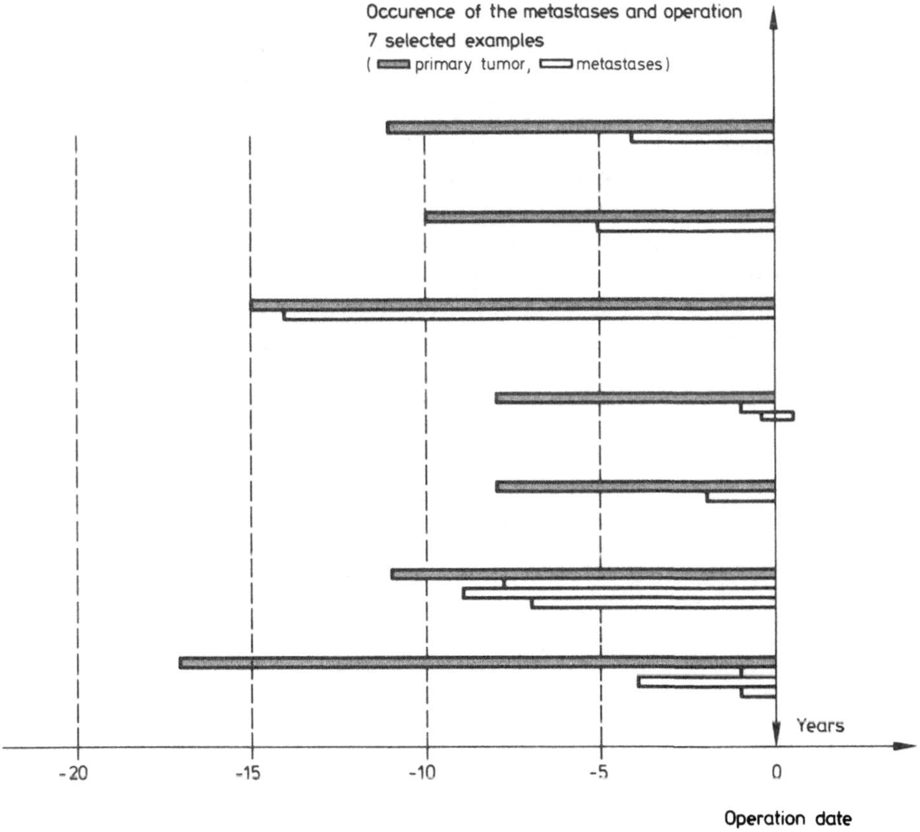

Fig. 11. Time span of growth of primary tumors before operation and of lung metastases ($n = 77$)

Average tumor diameter at operation: 2.8 cm

Average time between origin of metastases and operation: 12 years

In a group of 7 cases we found a correlation between the growth rate of the metastases and that of the primary tumor (Fig. 11). Fast-growing tumors seem to produce fast-growing metastases, and slowly growing tumors, slowly growing metastases.

After mean observation times of 2.5 years following operation we found that fast-growing tumors had a higher rate of distant metastases (22%) than moderately fast-growing (14%) or slow-growing tumors (6%). (Fig. 12). These data cannot necessarily be interpreted as indicating a higher metastatic potential of fast-growing tumors, because the already established metastases of slowly growing tumors need a longer time to reach a clinically detectable size. To determine conclusively whether there is a correlation between growth rate and metastatic potential a much longer observation time will be needed. Assuming that the tumor is able to disseminate metastatic cells before as few as 21 doublings (Fig. 2), the so-called early detection of breast cancer with the help of sophisticated methods (mammography) may actually be biologically late [20].

This is exemplified in the studies of [9], who showed that women with small tumors, up to 1 cm in diameter, die of metastatic disease even after 20 years (Fig. 13). In contrast to women with tumors 3 cm or more in size, then, women with small tumors cannot be called "cured" even if they have survived for 20 years. It is obvious that in the majority of cases, metastases start to spread by the time the tumor reaches 0.5 mm (see Fig. 2). In individual cases we are merely able to reveal the diagnosis to our patients a few years earlier; the remaining life span may already have been predetermined by the progressing occult metastases. For instance, diagnosis of a tumor 5 years earlier by mammography would be of no benefit if metastasis had already occurred. Though survival time from detection would be 5 years longer (Fig. 13), the actual life span would not be extended.

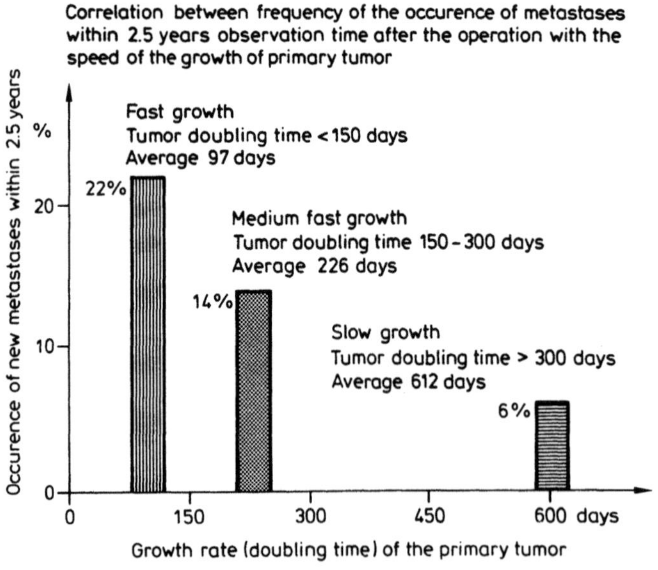

Fig. 12. Growth rates of primary tumors and probability of distant metastases. Observation period 2.5 years after operation ($n = 294$)

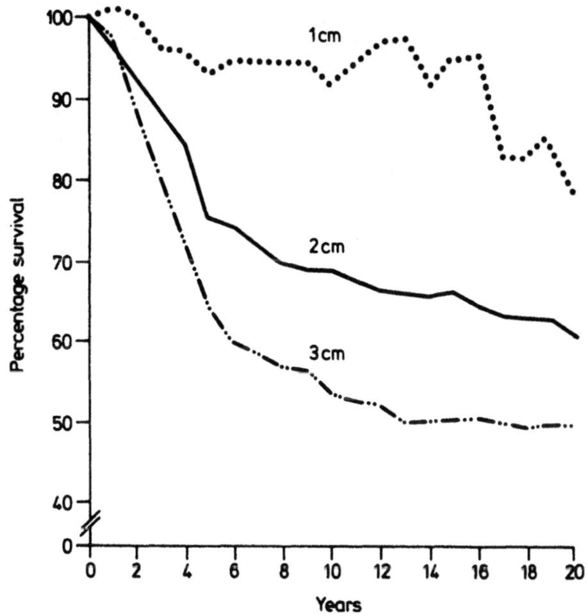

Fig. 13. Age-corrected survival rates for women treated for breast cancer 1–3 cm in diameter [9]

Discussion

The concept of constant tumor volume-doubling times, i.e., exponential growth up to the clinical phase of the tumor, yields a plausible explanation for some strange phenomena in the behavior of breast carcinoma (Fig. 14).

It can be demonstrated theoretically that the tumor takes about three-quarters of its life-span to achieve a size at which it can be detected clinically; this means that what we call "early diagnosis" actually takes place in a late phase of tumor growth. Metastases may have spread at a much earlier preclinical stage. The establishment of metastases before the diagnosis of the primary tumor predetermines the life span of the host. Local therapy does not cure the patient in this case.

The appearance of metastases many years after diagnosis of the primary breast cancer has been attributed to the possible existence of dormant cells. However, the existence of rather long doubling times explains the sometimes long latency period between primary tumor and detection of metastases, so that the hypothesis of dormant cells can be dismissed in the majority of cases (see Fig. 15).

Our knowledge of tumor growth behavior has implications for the clinical management of patients: The majority of mammary carcinomas grow at a moderate or a slow rate, needing, theoretically an average of 15–20 years to grow from the first malignant cell to a clinically detectable tumor 2 cm in diameter. As women are on average 35 years old when the growth of their breast carcinoma begins, methods for early detection of breast carcinoma should be first applied at

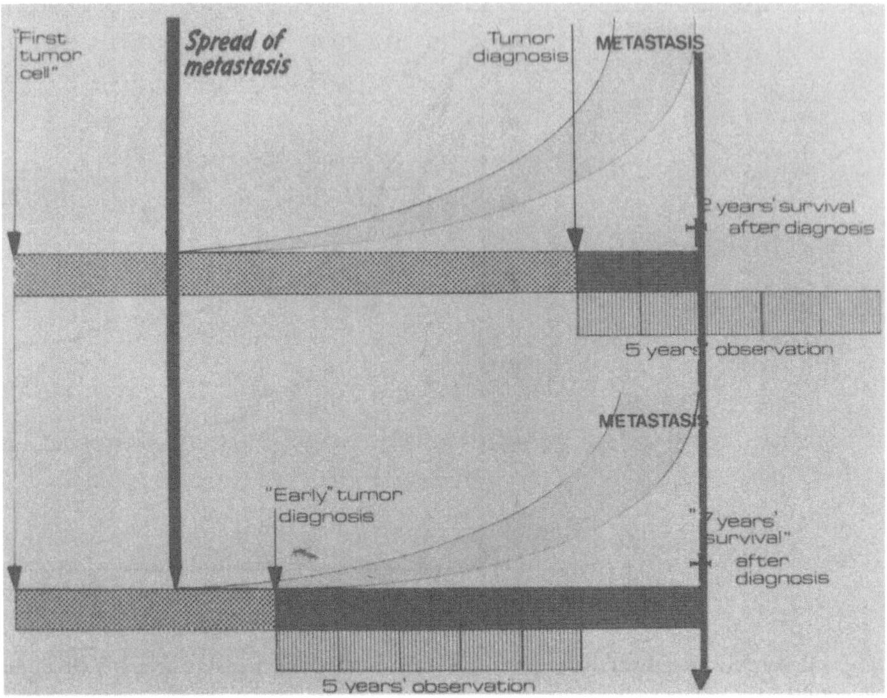

Fig. 14. The effect of so-called early diagnosis in some cases is merely that the patient knows the diagnosis 5 years earlier; there is no effect on life span when the tumor has started to metastasize before detection (lead time bias)

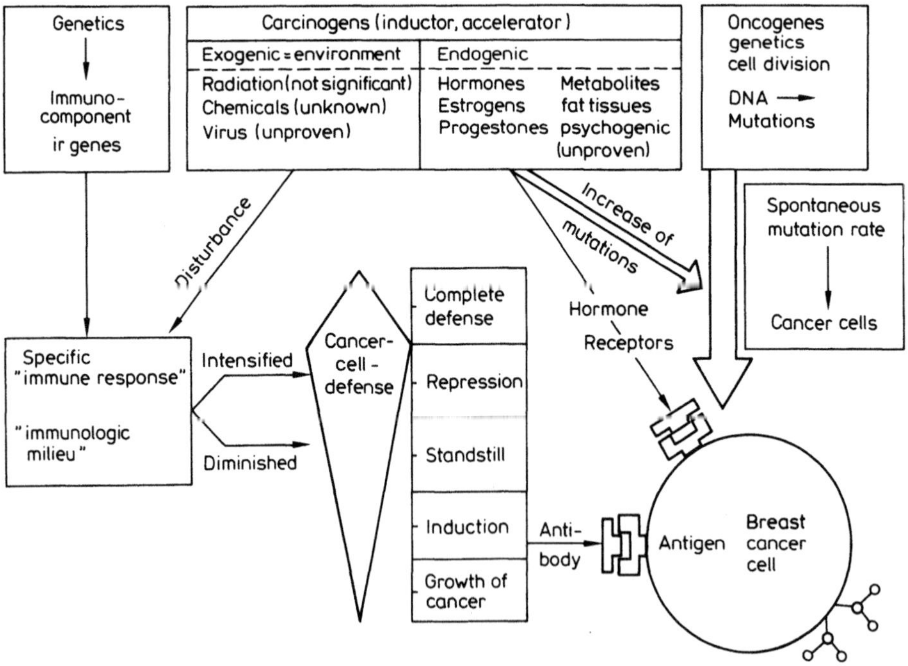

Fig. 15. Factors that can influence the growth of breast cancer (von Fournier, 1984, 1985)

the age of 30–40. The interval between screening mammographies should be 1–2 years. Examinations at intervals shorter than 6 months are usually not useful because of the growth behavior of the tumors.

Therapeutic effects, especially definitive cure rates, can be evaluated only 20 or more years later after treatment of the primary tumors. The predetermination of the life span by occult metastases gives us a rationale for the application of nonmutilating treatments in most cases. Whether systemic chemotherapy or hormonal therapies have an effect on the definitive cure rate of breast cancer can be decided only after an observation period of 10–20 years. Improved 5- or 10-year survival may mean only that the course of the disease has been slowed down somewhat.

References

1. Alvord EC Jr (1975) When do carcinomas of the breast begin to metastasize? Cited in: Spratt JS (1977) Growth kinetics in mammary cancer. In: Stoll BA (ed) Secondary spread in breast cancer. Heinemann Medical, London
2. Black MM (1975) Cell mediated response in human mammary cancer. In: Stoll BA (ed) Host defence in breast cancer. Heinemann Medical, London, p 48
3. Bloom HJG (1965) The influence of delay on the natural history and prognosis of breast cancer. Br J Cancer 19:228
4. Bloom HJG, Richardson WW, Harrier EJ (1962) Natural history of untreated breast cancer Br Med J 2:213–221
5. Bloom HJG, Richardson WW (1957) Histological grading and prognosis in breast cancer. A study of 1,409 cases of which 359 have been followed for 15 years. Br J Cancer 11:359
6. Brinkley D, Haybittle JL (1977) The curability of breast cancer. World J Surg 1:287
7. Brinkley D, Haybittle JL (1984) Long term survival of women with breast cancer. Lancet 1:1118
8. Collins VP, Loeffler RK, Tivey H (1956) Observations on growth rates of human tumours. AJR 76:988
9. Duncan W, Kerr GR (1976) The curability of breast cancer. Br Med J IV
10. Fournier vD, Kuttig H, Kubli F, Prager P, Stolpe H, Maier A, Hüter J (1976) Wachstumsgeschwindigkeit des Mammakarzinoms und röntgenologische "Frühdiagnosen". Strahlentherapie 151:318
11. Fournier vD, Weber E, Hoeffken W, Bauer M, Kubli F, Barth V (1980) Growth rate of 147 mammary carcinomas. Cancer 45:2198–2207
12. Fox MS (1979) On the diagnosis and treatment of breast cancer JAMA 241:489–494
13. Gershon-Cohen J, Berger SM, Klickstein HS (1963) Roentgenography of breast cancer moderating concept of "Biologic predeterminism". Cancer 16:961
14. Haagensen CD (1971) Diseases of the breast. Saunders, Philadelphia, p 501
15. Haagensen CD (1986) Diseases of the breast, 3rd edn. Saunders, Philadelphia
16. Henderson IC, Canellos GP (1980) Cancer of the breast: the past decade N Engl J Med 302:17–79
17. Koscielny S, Tubiana M, Le MG, et al. (1984) Breast cancer: Relationship between the size of the primary tumour and the probability of metastatic dissemination. Br J Cancer 49:709–715
18. Krokowski E (1964) Betrachtung zur Dynamik des Geschwultwachstums. Krebsforsch Krebsbekämpfung 5:189–192
19. Kusama S, Spratt JS, Donegan WL et al. (1972) The gross rates of growth of human mammary carcinoma. Cancer 30:594
20. MacDonald I (1951) Biological predeterminism in human cancer. Surg Gynecol Obstet 92443

21. Müller A, Tschahargane C, Kubli F (1988) Zum Problem der subkutanen Mastektomie. Die Bedeutung der histopathologischen Aufarbeitung des Mastektomiepräparates. Geb Fra
22. Oeser H (1974) Krebsbekämpfung: Hoffnung und Realität. Thieme, Stuttgart, pp 12–30
23. Spratt JS Jr, Kaltenbach ML, Spratt JA (1977) Cytokinetic definition of acute and chronic breast cancer. Cancer Res 37:226
24. Spratt JS, Hauser LS, Kuhns JG, Greenberg R, Polk HC (1981) Association between the actual doubling times of primary breast cancer with histopathologic characteristics and Wolf's parenchymal ammaographic patterns. Cancer 47:2265–2268
25. Tubiana M (1971) The kinetics of tumour cell proliferation. Br J Radiol 44:325
26. Tubiana M, Koscielny S (1988) Cell kinetics, growth rate and the natural history of breast cancer. The Heuson Memorial Lecture. Eur J Cancer Clin Oncol 24.1:9–14

Growth Rates and the Cytokinetic Behavior of Breast Cancer

J.S. SPRATT and J.A. SPRATT

Our purpose here is to discuss the basic cytokinetics of cancer growth, extant data on the growth rates of human breast cancer, the association of these growth rates with histopathological traits and hormone receptor levels, and the relation of growth rates to survival and screening strategies.

Cytokinetics

Breast cancer is a disorder of cellular replication, cohesion and maturation. Breast cancers arise from a single cell and the cancer cells replicate immortally, leading to successive generations of cells whose numbers are the net product of cell replication and cell death. The mutation rate inherent to each generation produces increasing heterogeneity. The interrelatedness of cell numbers, numbers of net cellular generations, gross size, actual doubling time, and potential survivorship are shown in Fig. 1.

In Fig. 2 is provided a model of the critical events in the evolution of a breast cancer. The temporal scale on this model would vary widely with breast cancer growth rates. Critical proportionalities determine the survivability of a person with cancer. An adult is composed of approximately 10^{13} cells, or $2^{40.8}$ cells. As the total body load of cancer cells approaches 10^{12} cells, or 2^{40} cells, the load is equivalent to about 10% ($10^{12}/10^{13}$) of the body's cells and death ensues beyond this point. Thus, the time required for an individual to accumulate the equivalent of 40 net generations of cancer cells approximates maximum survival from onset of the cancer. The variability of survival as a function of net actual doubling time may be appreciated in Fig. 1.

The growth rate equations best defining the progression of a human cancer are still under study. Many complex forces are at work as a cancer grows – cell replication, cell death, cell dormancy, degree of angiogenesis, diffusion of cell nutrients, rate of vasal migration of cancer cells from the focus of origin, desquamation of cells from cancers exposed to a body surface (visceral lining or skin), and inadequately understood factors controlling both cell replication (as hormones, local growth factors, prostaglandins) and cytodifferentiators. Cells in general are least cohesive at the time of mitosis. The more frequently mitosis occurs, the greater would be the prevalence of non-cohesive cells. This, coupled with any loss of natural cohesiveness in cancer cells, increases the probability of vasal shedding, particularly with angiogenesis.

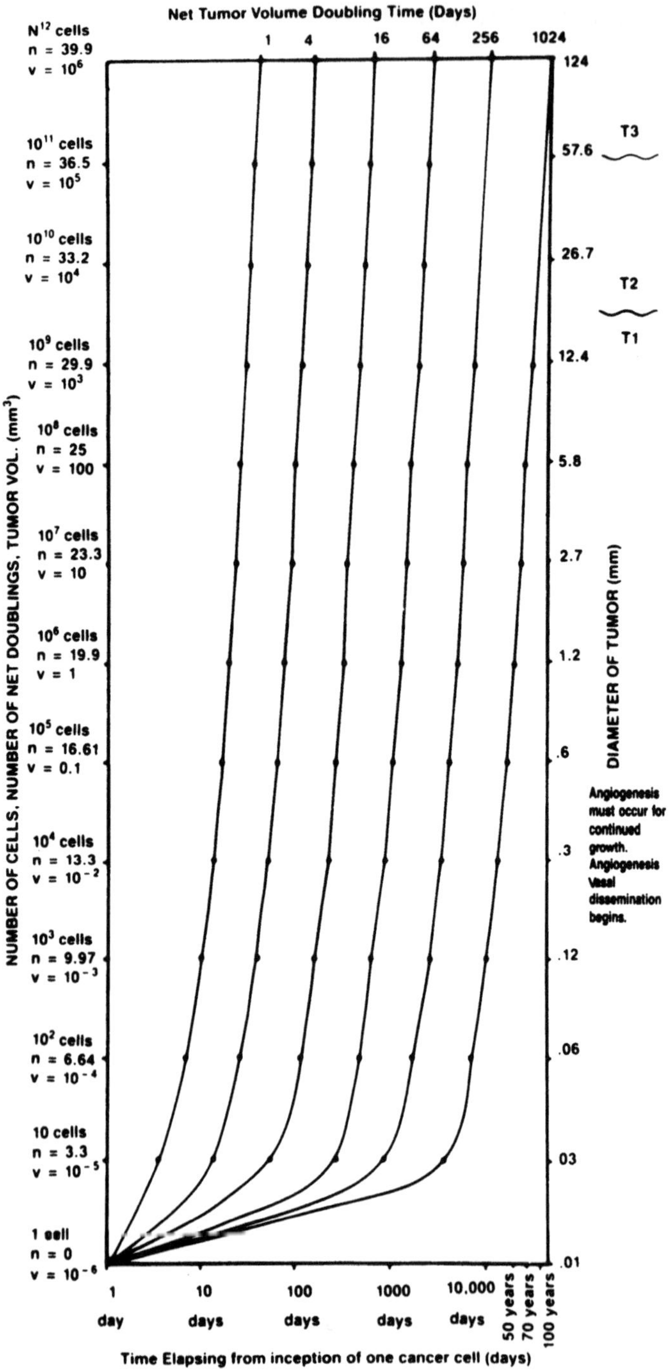

Fig. 1. The interrelationships of the number of cancer cells, cancer volume, and number of net cellular generations of cancer cells necessary to obtain the volume. The net $DT_{(act)}$ of a succession of possibilities, duration of the cancer, and the T-stage of the cancer are depicted. (Adapted from [23])

MODEL OF BREAST CANCER PROGRESSION

Asymptomatic disease of below threshold size for detection – local, locoregional, distant Normal	Asymptomatic disease above threshold size for detection	Symptomatic	End Points	
T_v Biological onset	T_w Disease now detectable if screen done	T_x Disease becomes symptomatic	T_y Death without treatment	T_z Death with treatment
	Screening takes place, can be true positive or false negative	Patient comes for diagnosis of symptomatic disease		

$T_a = T_w - T_v$:	Undetectable sojourn	T_v –	Onset
$T_b = T_x - T_w$:	Detectable asymptomatic sojourn	T_w –	Detectable but asymptomatic
$T_c = T_b - T_w$:	Delay time	T_x –	Symptomatic
$T_d = T_x - T_b$:	Lead time	T_y –	Time of death without diagnosis and treatment
$T_y - T_v =$	natural sojourn of undiagnosed, untreated disease	T_z –	Time of death with treatment
$T_z - T_v =$	natural sojourn of diagnosed disease, treated without treatment mortality	T_y, T_z	determined by lifelong follow-up to avoid truncation of results

Cancer Control Window (CCW) = time that cancer disseminates and is no longer locoregional less T_w

Fig. 2. A clinical model of breast cancer behavior adapted from Walter and Day Am J. Epid 228:865–886, 1983. The sojourn times in various intervals are dependent upon cancer growth rates, biological properties of cancers, and the sensitivity and specificity of diagnostic methods. [18]

In our studies we have used linear, exponential, and deceleratory growth equations to seek best fits for available data on the growth of human breast cancer. SKEHAN [15] fitted various data bases to a family of 18 different growth equations. He summarized these relationships by observing that cancer cell populations prevailingly follow the growth characteristics of all metazoa influenced by depletion, timekeepers, tissue sizers, and stochastic events. He affirmed that cancers have never been shown to grow faster than their tissue of origin. He extrapolated this observation to conclude that antiproliferative drugs could not be expected to cure human solid cancers.

The best fits of growth equations establish that deceleratory growth is the dominant pattern. Thus, the actual or net tumor doubling time [$DT_{(act)}$] would exhibit a progressive lengthening with increasing tumor size and the passage of time. Referring to Fig. 1, it is obvious that the clinical or observable period of human breast cancer is restricted to the end stage of the disease, when $DT_{(act)}$ would be lengthened. The tumor just visible on mammography requires a mass of 2^{22} cells about 2 mm in diameter. By 2^{30} (or 10^9) cells, a 10 mm diameter mass is produced, and symptoms do not regularly occur before a tumor of 2^{33}–2^{35} cells exists. Death will occur when cancer cell mass exceeds 2^{40} cells. Angiogenesis with a true cancer allows vasal dissemination as early as 10^4 cells ($2^{13.3}$), a cancer only 0.3 mm in diameter.

Among breast cancers, as with most other solid neoplasms, there are favorable subsets of lesions that never metastasize regardless of the size of the primary, and these tumors, as well as cancers with very long doubling times, are the ones in which favorable clinical results are obtained by locoregional treatment. These more indolent cancers also tend to accumulate favorably among cancers discovered by periodic screening as a result of length-biased sampling [17]. As early as 1905, STEINTHAL of Stuttgart [24] recognized that slow growth rate was a favorable prognostic variable for human breast cancer. The relationship of growth rate to survival is also confirmed by the consistent observation that there is no relation between the duration of symptoms before diagnosis and treatment on the one hand and survival on the other [3].

Cancer Growth and Heterogeneity

A population of cancer cells becomes more heterogeneous with each successive generation of new cells. This has been shown to be a function of the mutation rate inherent in each cycle of cellular replication. Theoretically, chemotherapy should be more effective in the less heterogeneous and therefore smaller cancers. However, this theory is frustrated by the observation that with as few as 10^9 (2^{30}) cells there is a zero probability of having nǫ cells resistant to chemotherapy [4]. A cancer of this size is barely palpable and rarely symptomatic. As SKEHAN notes, increasing cellular heterogeneity with successive generations of cells is inherent in any cellular system, associated with reduced cellular cohesiveness and possibly other feedback controls essential to promote homogeneity, and the cytodifferentiation needed to arrest the immortal replication of cancer cells. The same phenomenon is seen in replicating noncohesive bacteria that become resistant to antibiotics.

Measurements of Growth Rates of Human Breast Cancer with Clinicopathological Correlations

The accumulation of data necessary to measure the growth rates has been attempted by the senior author (JSS) since 1960. Data have come from many sources – sequential roentgen examinations of many sites harboring neoplasms, direct clinical measurements, indirect measurements of clinical duration that are dependent of growth-rate, and reports in the literature. The technology for measuring cytokinetic parameters of growth has evolved in the laboratory with tissue culture and cytometric techniques, and with radioisotopic labeling of DNA synthesis to improve the quantitation of rates of cell replication both in vitro and in vivo. A burgeoning area of research is addressing factors controlling replication at the cellular level. A comprehensive review of progress in this area is beyond our scope here. Rather, we propose to summarize actual measurements on human breast cancer and to discuss the clinical implications for screening, treatment, and prognosis.

The growth rates for any specific method or site of measurements have consistently resulted in lognormal frequency distributions [16]. These are highly skewed distributions that arise whenever there are random errors in exponential or geometric variables. The clinical expression of this phenomenon is to be found in the similarly skewed survival of persons afflicted with cancer. As a result we will report observed rates and the parameters of lognormal frequency distributions whenever the data are complete enough to permit. The distributions vary with patient age, tumor size, and histology. A selection of growth rate data available is organized by method of observation and relative tumor size.

Growth Rates in the Preclinical or Subdetectable Size Ranges

Among tumors too small to be seen on a roentgenogram or palpated, all methods of measurement are indirect. From tissue culture growth rate measurements TSENG (1986, personal communication) has estimated the average breast cancer cell doubling time to be 24–36 h. The actual cell colony growth rapidly decelerates with increasing size, generally following Gompertzian growth [5].

Cellular replication rates have also been studied by various investigators using ^{3}H-thymidine labeling of the synthesis of DNA. The ^{3}H-thymidine labeling index (TLI) obtained is a ratio (expressed in percent) of the number of labeled cells over the number of cells present as a function of the period of exposure to labeled thymidine. Using this value the potential doubling time [$DT_{(pot)}$] of a cancer can be calculated by assuming that all replicating cells survive. The relationship between $DT_{(pot)}$ and $DT_{(act)}$ is dependent upon the rate of cell loss:

$$\rho = 1 - DT_{(pot)}/DT_{(act)}$$

Cell loss ranges around 50%. Though a number of investigators have used TLI to study breast cancer cytokinetics, we will review only the work of MEYER and associates because of their sustained effort to establish correlations between TLI values and histopathological, hormone receptor levels and disease-free survival. MEYER has recently prepared a comprehensive review which we will summarize [11]. MEYER and his associates have either shown or confirmed that heterogeneity in cell cycle time for breast cancer is observable in the microenvironment. The heterogeneity in TLI values seems determined by the distance of oxygen-consuming cells from the nearest blood vessel. Avascular centers even become necrotic. The thickness of viable cells growing as spheroids is about 80 μm (0.08 mm). Growth expressed as thymidine uptake increasingly becomes restricted to perivascular cells. The complete cell cycle averages about 85 h: G_1, 58 h; S, 19 h;

G_2, 6 h or less. Mitosis (M) takes less than 30 min. The number of S phase or labeled cells will be approximately 20 times the number of M phase cells at any time.

The TLI values form lognormal frequency distributions. Among cancers with no axillary metastases, TLI values greater than 4.15% were associated with much shorter patient survivals. The same was true for cancers with positive lymph nodes. TLI values decreased in cancers with increasing host age. The higher the nuclear grade, the higher was the TLI. TLIs of $>$ 4.15% were associated with shorter survival whether the estrogen receptor levels were negative or positive. The TLI values overrode in prognostic significance all parameters of anatomical staging.

Mitotic indices determined by light microscopy parallel the prognostic significance of TLI values in spite of lower accuracy. PARL and DUPONT (1982) observed that breast cancers with high mitotic indices were associated with a standard mortality ratio (SMR) of 2.7. A combination of a high mitotic index and an absence of tubule formation produced an SMR of 2.9. Well-defined tubules and a low mitotic index were associated with an SMR of only 0.17, indicating little mortality from these indolent cancers.

Our first direct measurements of the growth of human breast cancer were of pulmonary metastases ranging in size from about 4 mm to 70 mm in greatest chordal dimension. The log mean $DT_{(act)}$ was 82 days, with 99% confidence ranging from 7 to 969 days [19]. This range is equivalent to the accumulation of from less than 1 to as many as 99 new cancer cells per 1000 existing cancer cells per day. The next data reported were for primary mammary cancers observed serially on mammograms. For the 19 cases reported, the $DT_{(act)}$ exhibited a median value of 120 days, ranging from 23 to 209 days. Were these rates constant from inception, these cancers would have required from 520 to 29 440 days (99% confidence) to produce a lethal cancer load. The diameters at the time of resection ranged from 4 to 30 mm [20].

The growth rates of breast cancers at multiple metastatic sites were reported by KUSAMA et al. [10]. Length of survival at all sites was distinctly more favorable for cancers with very long doubling times, regardless of the site. PEARLMAN and JOCHIMSON [14] addressed the relation of survival in the presence of metastatic cancer to speed of disease evolution by correlating the time interval between the appearance of the first recurrence (R_1) and the appearance of a second recurrence (R_2). Regardless of the site of recurrences, there was a direct relationship between the length of the R_1–R_2 interval and the duration of survival. The survival of patients with long R_1–R_2 intervals was unrelated to treatment when comparing local and systemic treatment. Only with visceral metastases did systemic treatment give superior results.

Our most recent studies were made possible by the Breast Cancer Detection and Demonstration Project (BCDDP) in the United States. This program, organized by the National Cancer Institute and the American Cancer Society, funded under contract 27 centers, each required to screen and provide data on 10 000 women between 35 and 70 years of age with no breast symptoms and no prior history of breast cancer. The purpose of the project was to demonstrate the feasibility of mass screening for breast cancer. Entrants underwent anamnesis and physical, mammographic, and thermographic examinations. Thermography was discontinued when found ineffective, and mammography was discontinued in women under 50.

Subjects were taught techniques for breast self-examination. All women were screened annually for 4 years. Generally, mammograms were repeated only once a year for those patients whose tumors grew measurably. This interval may result in a significant truncation of the growth rate measurements by missing very rapidly growing cancers. This truncation can be assessed by considering the frequency with which cancers are diagnosed in the interval between annual mammograms. We refer to these cancers as "interval surfacing cancers."

Though the BCDDP was not set up to test any research hypotheses, it nevertheless generated large amounts of data on a defined population of women maintained under intense surveillance with respect to the prevalence of breast cancer at first screen and the incidence at subsequent screens. In some cases cancers were observed in the breast more than once on mammograms, and some surfaced in the intervals between screens. Time between the attainment of threshold size (2 mm) and the discovery of prevalent cancers at first screen could be estimated by dividing the prevalence rates by incidence rates. The sizes of prevalent cancers were known from the mammograms, permitting the calculation of the numbers of cells in the cancers. With these data the number of generations necessary for a cancer to grow from threshold size to the size at diagnosis could be estimated. These generation numbers were then divided into the durations of time estimated to ascertain the net doubling times in this segment of the life history of a primary breast cancer. The data and conclusions from a series of studies have been published, and the original papers must be consulted for methodology and data. Here we can only summarize the major conclusions.

Interval Surfacing Cancers

PANOUSSOPOULAS et al. [12] reported the interval cancer discovery rates for the Breast Cancer Demonstration Project at the University of Kansas Medical Center. They reported that the cancers diagnosed *between* mammograms comprised 29% of all cancers diagnosed (24 of 89). In the discussion of this paper, the point was made that monitoring of the rates at which breast cancers are discovered between annual mammograms is essential for evaluating the worth of mammography and for estimating the potential truncation of the frequency distribution of mammographically measured growth rates [12,20].

As an extension of this observation, data were later provided by SPRATT et al. [22] on the "acute breast cancer." The interval surfacing cancers were classified as "fast" or "acute." They were associated significantly with a more anaplastic nuclear grade in the cancer cells, the absence of mammographic and microscopic calcifications in the cancer, occurrence in women under age 50, presence in mammographically dysplastic breasts, the lack of a family history, and a prognosis worse than with slower cancers. The slower cancers were associated with a circumscribed tumor margin and a papillary growth pattern. In this same population, the absence of calcifications and the presence of lymphatic invasion around the periphery of the primary cancer were significantly associated with the early development of metastases in the axillary lymph nodes [9].

Estimation of the $DT_{(act)}$ of Interval Surfacing Cancers

In addition to the confirmation that reported frequencies of $DT_{(act)}$ were truncated by the exclusion of interval surfacing cancers, it is possible to calculate the range of $DT_{(act)}$ excluded by the truncation. First, the lethal number of net doublings (about 40) is simply divided into 365 days: the result is 9. Any breast cancer with a net actual doubling time of less than 9 days could arise de novo and kill between annual mammograms. If this estimate is recalculated from the threshold of mammographic detection, i.e., about 2 mm or 20 net doublings, then 365 could be divided by 20 (40–20), giving 18 days. Any breast cancer that could sustain a net actual doubling time of 18 days or less could grow from the threshold of mammographic detectability to host death in less than 365 days. If the majority of breast cancers followed Gompertzian or deceleratory growth in their predetectable period, the problem of truncation would be even more serious. Not only can the accurate reporting of breast cancer development rates *between* annual mammograms help evaluate the degree of truncation, but the careful follow-up of these interval cancer cases can help confirm whether these faster-growing cancers are also more rapidly lethal. Eventually, we can even determine whether mammographic screening is having a real impact on the overall lethality of mammary cancer or whether it is simply dividing breast cancers into fast-growing and slow-growing subsets.

Definition of the Entire Spectrum of $DT_{(act)}$

The BCDDP provided an opportunity to define the entire frequency distribution of actual growth rates of primary mammary cancers because it provided growth rate data for all cancers occurring in a defined population of women over a defined span of time. This distribution falls into three subsets. The first subset consists of cancers growing too rapidly to permit measurement by annual mammography. These are the interval surfacing cancers. The second subset is composed of cancers in which two or more mammographic observations permitted a measurement of growth and a calculation of growth rates. The third subset comprises the exceedingly slow-growing cancers in which no measurable growth occurred on mammographic observations at intervals of 1 year or greater.

During the BCDDP study at Louisville [7,8], there were 115 proven cancers among the 10 180 women receiving over 30 000 mammograms. Serial measurements were possible by xeromammography in 32 cases. Doubling times for measureable cases ranged from 109 to 944 days with a median value of 324 days. The log mean doubling time was 327 days. The predominant geometric shape of small primary breast cancers observed on mammography was that of a spheroid, with the long axis following the direction of the ducts. The frequency distribution of the doubling times of the spheroids was lognormal.

Forty-three percent of these cases (49 of 115) were interval surfacing cancers, and 7.8% (9 of 115), or 28% of the cases observed by two or more mammograms (9 of 32), consisted of cancers growing too slowly to permit measurement of growth. The annual incidence of cancers increased from 0.064% to 0.239% over the first 3 years of the project and dropped to 0.144% in the 4th year when women under 50 years of age were excluded.

The conclusions were that a very large percentage of all breast cancers are exceedingly rapid in early or predetectable growth and that the annual mammogram was primarily subdividing breast cancers into fast- and slow-growing subsets. The faster-growing cancers were significantly more likely to metastasize. This is the first report of a full spectrum of growth rates in a defined population of women [7,8].

Composite Data for Considering Growth Curves Best Fit

VON FOURNIER et al. (1980) provided us with the data from his original study. These data contained measurements of tumor nucleus shadows observed on mammograms and the date of each measurement for 202 patients. To these, we added the additional 32 cases obtained from the BCDDP at Louisville. Mean Gompertz and exponential growth curves were fitted to these data.

The measurements of tumor size were made in three dimensions. Tumor volume was calculated by using the formula

$$V = 4/3\, \pi\, r_1 r_2 r_3 \tag{1}$$

Exponential doubling times were calculated by performing a linear regression between ln V and the times between the various observations. The slope of this relationship is the relative growth rate. The actual doubling time [$DT_{(act)}$] is the natural logarithm of two divided by the relative growth rate. The distribution of the doubling times was tested with the Kolmogorov-Smirnov test. The distribution was lognormal with a mean of 5.53 ± 0.81 days, corresponding to an antilog mean of 252 days.

Gompertzian Growth

The Gompertz equation is a specific deceleratory growth rate formula which is the exact solution to the following system of two differential equations:

$$dV/dt = \lambda\, V \tag{2}$$
$$d\lambda/dt = -\alpha\, \lambda \tag{3}$$

Equation 3 states that the tumor growth rate is the product of the relative growth rate and the volume. This is what is seen in exponential growth where the relative growth rate, λ, is constant. Equation 3 shows that λ is itself time-dependent. The rate of decay of λ, α, is a constant.

The Gompertz growth equation is thus:

$$V = V_o e^{(1-e^{-\alpha t})\beta/\alpha} \tag{4}$$

where α = rate of decay of relative growth rate (day^{-1}); β = relative growth rate at $\tau = 0$ (day^{-1}); $\lambda = \beta e^{-\alpha t}$ = relative growth rate at time t. The independent variables describing a given curve are therefore α and β. A plot of a Gompertz curve is shown in Fig. 3. A cancer following a Gompertzian equation grows rapidly while small but more slowly as its size increases. It approaches a horizontal asymptote determined by a size (V_{max}) that it never exceeds. The curve may seem upwardly concave initially but is actually exhibiting a steady decrease in its actual growth rate as it approaches the asymptote of V_{max}.

Since the relative growth rate is constantly decreasing, the doubling time is continuously increasing. The doubling time equation can be solved as a function of time (Eq. 5) or tumor size (Eq. 6):

$$DT_{(act)} = (-1/\alpha) \ln (1-(\alpha/\beta) \ln 2\, e^{\alpha t}), \text{ for } V < 12\, V_{max} \tag{5}$$
$$DT_{(act)} = (-1/\alpha) \ln[1-(\ln 2/\ln(V_{max}/V))], \text{ for } V < 1/2\, V_{max} \tag{6}$$

Note that doubling time has meaning only for a tumor which is less than half of its maximal size ($V < 1/2 V_{max}$).

In order to calculate Gompertz growth curves, several assumptions were made. We assumed that each cancer originated as one cell ($V_0 = 2^0$) and that the maximum size attainable was 2^{40} cells ($V_{Max} = 2^{40}$). The latter assumption follows from the observations on the usual lethal tumor mass of neoplasm. This is roughly 10^{12} cells or forty cellular generations (2^{40}).

By specifying (2^{40}) to approximate V_{max} it can be shown that

$$\alpha = \beta/(40 \ln 2) \tag{7}$$

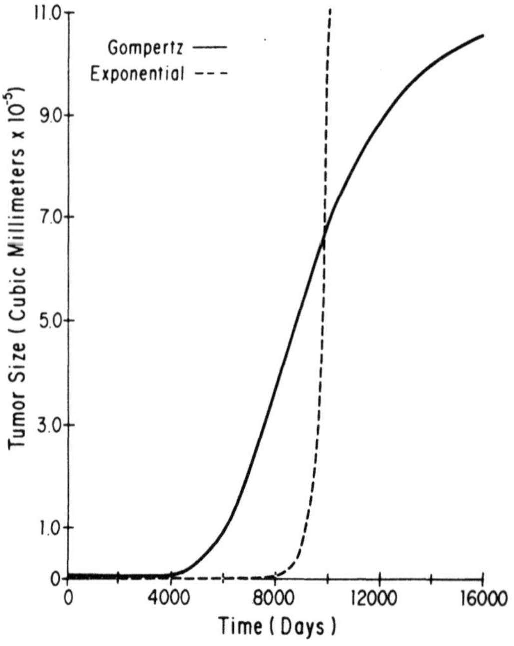

Fig. 3. Comparison of the exponential and the Gompertzian growth curves

so that the Gompertz equation then becomes

$$V = V_0 e(1\text{-}e^{\alpha t})\ 40\ \ln 2$$

Doubling time could be expressed as a function of generation number as follows:

$$DT_{(act)} = (-1/\alpha)\ \ln\,[1-(1/(40\text{-}n))] \qquad (9)$$

where n is the generation number.

The Gompertz equation can be converted into linear form by taking the logarithm of each side of the equation twice. This equation is

$$\ln \ln\,(V_{max}/V) = -\alpha t + \ln\,(\beta/\alpha) \qquad (10)$$

From our assumptions, β/α and V_{max} are known. The resulting equation is thus the relationship between tumor size and time, where $-\alpha$ is the slope of this relationship. By performing a standard regression analysis on ln ln (V_{max}/V) versus time α was calculated for each of the patients studied.

Again by using the Kolmogorov-Smirnov test, the distribution of α values was examined. This distribution was not significantly different from a lognormal distribution with mean -7.813 ± 0.844 day^{-1}. The antilog of this number, the geometric mean of α, was thus $4.034(10)^{-4}$ day^{-1}.

With Gompertzian growth, tumor doubling time is a function of time or tumor size. In order to compare sojourn time and doubling time data, assuming either Gompertzian or exponential growth, these parameters must be specified. For example, doubling times could be compared for the size at which a tumor was first detected. The mean diameter of the first mammographic tumor shadow in this study was 8.7 mm, which corresponds to a volume of 345 mm^3, the 28th net cellular generation of the tumor nucleus shadow on a mammogram. It should be emphasized that most tumors in this study were first detected at a larger size and only verified to be present at the 345 mm^3 size retrospectively.

A graph of the mean tumor growth for all patients, assuming both exponential and Gompertzian growth, is shown in Fig. 3. As can be seen, the Gompertzian growth curve begins to rise sooner but undergoes a progressively decreasing rate of growth as tumor size increases. On the other hand, the exponential growth curve shows tumor size to be very small until a sojourn time of approximately 8000 days. It then undergoes an increasingly rapid increase in size over the next 2000 days.

Doubling time is plotted as a function of sojourn time in Fig. 4. With exponential growth, mean doubling time was constant at 252 days. Assuming Gompertzian growth, however, the initial mean doubling was 62 days. Doubling time slowed to approximately 321 days at the time the tumors were discovered, then slowed even more to a mean of over 7000 days by the 38th generation.

This same effect is illustrated in Fig. 5, where doubling time is plotted as a function of generation number. Exponential doubling time is constant regardless of generation number. Gompertzian growth again begins with a net doubling time of 62 days for the first generation, but approaches infinity at the 39th generation, the last generation for which doubling time has meaning.

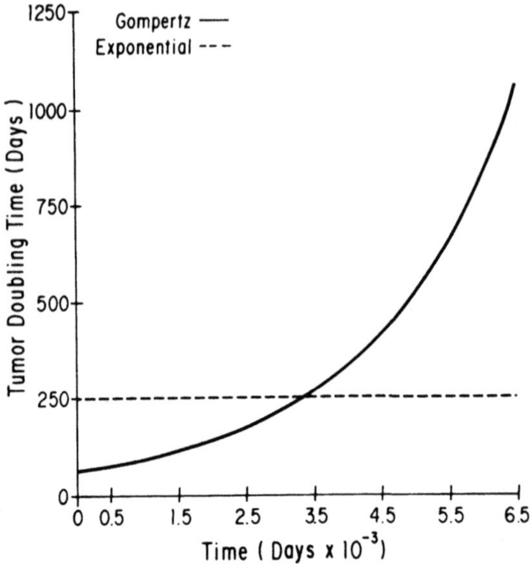

Fig. 4. Doubling time as function of cancer sojourn time, exponential growth and Gompertzian growth

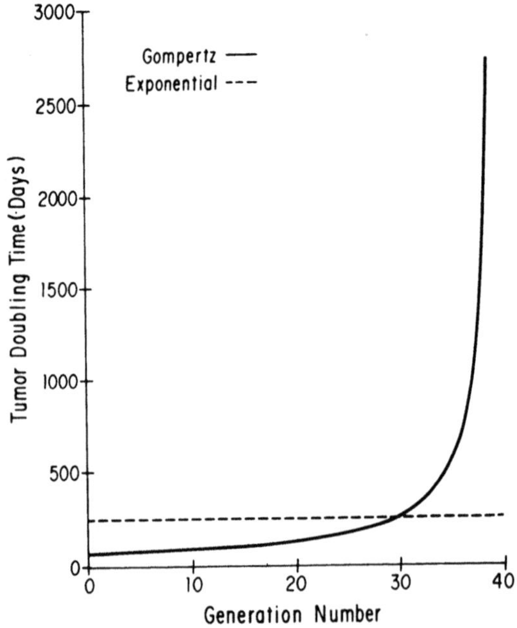

Fig. 5. Doubling time as a function of net generation number, exponential growth and Gompertzian growth

Tissue culture and thymidine labeling studies have shown that the initial doubling time of mammary cancer cells is on the order of 12–48 h. It is known from the clinical data above that tumors of approximately 1 cm^3 in size have a mean doubling time of 261 days with Gompertzian growth. Many very large tumors have been shown to have no demonstrable growth, indicating a further prolongation of the doubling time. Exponential growth curves can be accurately fitted to data in the range of clinical observation, but they clearly cannot allow for the rapid growth rates of smaller tumors. Gompertz growth equations and other deceleratory growth equations, on the other hand, can be fitted in such a way as to reflect more accurately tumor growth throughout the cancer's entire life span.

An important result from this type of analysis would be the ability to quantify the sojourn time of a tumor from one cell until it attains clinically detectable size. Assuming Gompertzian growth for the data described, the mean tumor sojourn time from one cell to 1 cm^3 was 3428 days, with 95% confidence intervals of 633–18 569 days.

Other deceleratory growth rate formulas, as suggested by SKEHAN (1986), may allow even more accurate mathematical modelling of breast cancer growth. Growth rates calculated from the measurement of tumor nucleus shadows on mammograms would be expected to be slower than the actual rate of increase in total body tumor burden if cells are being shed rapidly from small tumors to take up metastatic growth elsewhere.

Conclusions

Our conclusions from these studies are that the speed with which early breast cancers can arise and metastasize while still undetected places limits on our ability to control breast cancer by screening. Rates of growth clearly have major, often dominant, prognostic significance, overriding the significance of the cruder gross parameters of clinical stage or hormone receptors. The very rapidly growing early metastasizing cancer has to be regarded as a systemic disease and must be managed accordingly. The extremely slowly growing cancers may permit long periods of disease-free survival even in the absence of cure. Regional overtreatment of either rapid-growing, early disseminating cancers or indolent and favorable cancers by ultraradical surgery or wide-field radical radiotherapy would not be expected to enhance survival.

References

1. Bradley JV (1968) Distribution free statistical tests. Prentice-Hall, Englewood Cliffs, pp 296–303
2. Butler TP, Guillino PM (1975) Quantification of cell shedding into efferent blood of mammary adenocarcinoma. Cancer Res 35:512–516
3. Donegan WL, Spratt JS (1979) Cancer of the breast, 2nd edn. Saunders, Philadelphia
4. Goldie JH, Coldman AJ (1985) A model for tumor response to chemotherapy: an integration of the stem cell and somatic mutation hypotheses. Cancer Invest 3:553–564
5. Gompertz B (1825) On the nature of the function of the law of human mortality, and on a new mode of determining the value of life contingencies. Philos Trans R Soc Lond 114:513–583
6. Gould MN, Jirtle R, Crowley J, Clifton KH (1978) Reevaluation of the number of cells involved in the neutron induction of mammary neoplasms. Cancer Res 38:189–192
7. Heuser L, Spratt JS, Polk HC Jr, Buchanan J (1979a) Relation between mammary cancer growth kinetics and the intervals between screening. Cancer 43:857–862
8. Heuser L, Spratt JS, Polk HC Jr (1979b) Growth rates of primary mammary cancers. Cancer 43:1888–1894

9. Heuser LS, Spratt JS, Kuhns JG, Chang AF-C, Polk HC Jr, Buchanan JB (1984) The association of pathologic and mammographic characteristics of primary human breast cancer with 'slow' and 'fast' growth rates and with axillary lymph node metastases. Cancer 53:96–98
10. Kusama S, Spratt JS, Donegan WL, Watson FR, Cunningham CJ (1972) The gross rates of growth of human mammary carcinoma. Cancer 30:594–599
11. Meyer JS (1988) Cell kinetics of breast and breast tumors. In: Donegan WL, Spratt JS (eds) Cancer of the breast, 3rd edn. Saunders, Philadelphia, pp 250–269
12. Panoussopoulas D, Chang J, Humphrey LJ (1977) Screening for breast cancer. Ann Surg 186:356–862
13. Parl FP, Dupont WD (1982) A retrospective cohort study of histologic risk factors in breast cancer patients. Cancer 50:2410–2416
14. Pearlman NW, Jochimson PR (1979) Recurrent breast cancers: factors in fluency survival including treatment. J Surg Oncol 11:21–29
15. Skehan P, Friedman SJ (eds) (1984) Growth, Cancer and the Cell Cycle. Humana Press, Clifton NJ, p 323
16. Spratt JS (1969) The lognormal frequency distribution and human cancer. J Surg Res 9:151–157
17. Spratt JS (1982) The epidemiology of screening for cancer. Curr probl Cancer 5 (8)
18. Spratt JS, Spratt JA (1985) What is breast cancer doing before we can detect it? J Surg Oncol 30:156–160
19. Spratt JS, Spratt TL (1964) Rates of growth of pulmonary metastases and host survival. Ann Surg 159:161
20. Spratt JS, Kaltenbach ML, Spratt JA (1977) Cytokinetic definition of acute and chronic breast cancer. Cancer Res 37:226–330
21. Spratt JS, Heuser L, Kuhns JG, Reiman HM, Buchanan JB, Polk HC Jr, Sandoz J (1981) Association between actual doubling times of primary breast cancer with histopathologic and Wolfe's parenchymal mammographic patterson. Cancer 47:2265–2268
22. Spratt JS, Chang AF-C, Heuser LS, Kuhns JG, Buchanan JB, Polk HC Jr (1983) Acute carcinoma of the breast. Surg Gynecol Obstet 157:220–222
23. Spratt JS, Greenberg RA, Heuser LS (1986) Geometry, growth rates and duration of cancer and carcinoma in situ of the breast before detection by screening. Cancer Res 46:970–974
24. Steinthal CF (1905) Zur Dauerheilung des Brustkrebses. Beitr Klin Chir 47:226
25. Von Fournier D, Kubli F, Barth V (1980) Growth rate of 147 mammary carcinomas. Cancer 45:2198–2207

II. Diagnosis

The Value of Diagnostic Methods: Mammography, Screening and Other Imaging Techniques

M. Friedrich, D. von Fournier and W. Hoeffken

Indications for Mammography and for Supplementary Techniques

Mammography is the most effective method for the early detection of breast cancer and the discovery of occult, i.e., non-palpable, breast tumors. Two objectives of mammography should be differentiated:

- Diagnostic clarification of a finding in symptomatic patients (clinical mammography)
- Discovery of clinically occult carcinomas within a breast cancer screening program (screening mammography)

Clinical Mammography

The value of clinical mammography is hardly disputed nowadays. Numerous specialist associations unanimously recommend "achievement of a complete diagnostic clarification, including mammography, in all patients with nodes (lumps), unclear palpation findings, inversion of the skin or mamilla, discharges from the mamilla, eczematously altered mamilla (Paget's disease) or circumscribed, unilateral, cycle-independent painfulness even without palpation findings."

Clinical mammography is always performed bilaterally in two planes with dose-saving film-screen systems using the grid technique. It should always be preceded by inspection and palpation of the breast.

The informational value of mammography depends on the structure and composition of the breast: dense soft tissue tumor shadows are less easily recognizable in radiodense glandular tissue than in radiolucent fatty tissue. The assessability of microcalcifications, on the other hand, is less impaired by the tissue density.

In symptomatic patients, mammography, including pneumocystography or galactography, can yield the following *unequivocal* findings: lipoma or lipomatosis; oil cyst (post-traumatic or postoperative); calcified fibroadenoma; simple breast cyst; mammary duct ectasia.

Mammography is *relatively reliable* for indicating a carcinoma in the presence of "typical" star-shaped tissue configurations (scirrhous carcinoma) or "typical" polymorphic intraductal microcalcifications (calcified milk duct carcinoma).

Mammographic evidence is *fundamentally limited* in the presence of the following breast alterations: circumscribed tumors (noncalcified fibroadenoma, cell-rich or mucinous carcinoma); diffuse or nodular fibro-adenomatous-cystic-plastic mastopathy.

Even in cases of a clinically unequivocal carcinoma, bilateral mammography is indicated to rule out a multifocal ipsilateral or contralateral carcinoma. In all cases where the mammographic or clinical finding is doubtful, supplementary methods (ultrasound, puncture, galactography) should be employed *before* a biopsy is recommended (see below!).

Screening Mammography

The second area of application for mammography, which will expand strongly in the future, is in early breast cancer detection. The aim of screening mammography is diagnosis of clinically occult carcinomas in asymptomatic patients.

The benefit of screening mammography has been controversial, and is called in question for women under 50. It can only be proven by controlled studies in which a large patient collective is mammographed at regular intervals and compared with an age-matched and epidemiologically similar control collective that is not submitted to mammography. The final result must be the demonstration of lower breast cancer mortality in the mammographically examined collective than in the controls.

Such a result was first shown in the HIP study [Health Insurance Plan Study of Greater New York; SHAPIRO 1977]: Ten years after initiation of the study, breast cancer mortality was 32% lower in women between 50 and 59 years of age than in the controls, and 45% lower in the age group between 60 and 64. No such beneficial effect could be found in women under 50 at the time of diagnosis. This was explained by the fact that mammographic evidence is poorer in the parenchyma-rich breasts of younger women, and it was recommended that screening mammography not be performed in women under 50. However, more recent controlled screening programs using modern dose-saving soft-ray mammography in the Netherlands [20,61,83], in Sweden [4,5,39,78] and in the USA [57,58,59] unequivocally confirm the benefit of a preventive program with mammography for women under 50 as well. Thus, after an observation period of 7 years, it could be demonstrated that mammographic screening led to a 32% [78] to 50% [61] reduction in mortality for women between 40 and 75.

The increase of early tumor stages among the mammographically discovered carcinomas and the low percentage of these among tumors detectable by palpation can be regarded as supporting evidence for the effectiveness of screening mammography:

- According to PENN and HENDRIKS [61], there was a reduction of the mean tumor size from 2.8 cm to 1.3 cm with involvement of only 20% of the axillary lymph nodes as opposed to 48% among the spontaneously detected carcinomas.

- The diagnostic yield for T1 tumors in screening mammography is between 57% [20] and 75% [61].
- In all screening programs, about 50% of the detected carcinomas were impalpable [61,54].

The effectiveness of palpation as well as self-examination by women must be designated as inadequate for early diagnosis: SALTZSTEIN [67] and PHILIP et al. (1984) reported that, despite intensive instruction of the patients in a self-examination program, there was no alteration in either median or mean tumor size or lymph node involvement. In the screening program conducted in the Netherlands, 50% of the carcinomas discovered were impalpable [61].

Despite these facts, there is considerable underapplication of mammography in the USA and probably also in Europe: According to FOX et al. [31], 53%–69% of 35- to 49-year-old women performed self-examination, but mammography was accepted by only 19% and by only every fourth woman over 50. Moreover, mammography was performed for screening purposes in only 9%.

Problems of Screening Mammography

No secret is made of the problems involved in screening mammography:

- The apparent increase in survival time resulting from earlier diagnosis (lead-time bias)
- The selection of slow-growing and hence possibly biologically more benign carcinomas by screening (length-time bias)
- Discovery of very early carcinoma types and stages which would never lead to death of the host without discovery and without treatment, but which are evaluated as a success of the screening (population bias, MILLER 1983)
- The interval carcinomas discovered between the screening examinations, usually by the women themselves
- The histologically benign biopsies unnecessarily performed

The time saved by earlier diagnosis in the screening program is calculated from the difference in mean tumor size between carcinomas discovered by mammography and those detected by clinical/palpation examinations (e.g., 1.3 vs 2.8 cm in diameter, in PENN and HENDRIKS [61]) and the mean doubling time (e.g., 312 days, PENN et al. 1984) to be about 3 years (concurrent data in MOSKOWITZ [58]).

According to FEIG and coworkers [25], the alleged selection of slowly growing and hence relatively benign carcinomas by screening is not to be perceived as actually involving a different category of carcinomas. The fact is that a relatively abrupt transition from a non-invasive to an invasive state is seen in all carcinomas when they exceed a diameter of about 0.5 cm, so that the relatively large proportion of noninvasive in situ carcinomas in preventive mammography must be attributed to the extremely early tumor stages rather than to a particular carcinoma subpopulation. Even small carcinomas that appear relatively harmless pathohistologically will grow into deadly tumors if the clinical course is long enough!

A particularly disquieting phenomenon in all screening mammographic programs is the occurrence of interval carcinomas, which shakes the confidence of both the women involved and the non-medical observer of such programs in the efficiency of mammography. Advocates of high-quality, high-dose mammography have blamed this on methodological-technical shortcomings (e.g., single-plane mammography), although other causes are usually responsible. The number of interval carcinomas can range between 10% [51] and nearly 30% [33a] of all carcinomas discovered in preventive programs.

In the screening program of Nijmegen [33a], single-plane mammography, 19 of 64 interval carcinomas were simply overlooked, four of 64 were not imaged, and 41 of 64 were mammographically occult. Twenty of these 41 occult lesions were too small, and the other 21 were either masked in one plane by dense glandular tissue or displayed uncharacteristic tissue consolidation and were not recognizable as carcinoma. The following conclusion can be drawn: Two-plane mammography should be performed – even as a screening examination – in parenchyma-rich breasts, and other supplementary procedures, e.g., sonography should be employed before biopsy is recommended.

According to MARTIN et al. [51], about one-third of the interval carcinomas were not recognizable mammographically in dense glandular tissue, and about one-third were simply overlooked, though clearly recognizable. The remaining 38% could be detected only by a very experienced mammographer on the basis of discrete indirect signs, such as isolated thickening of the retromamillary duct, microcalcifications, increasing neodensity in subsequent examinations and unilateral asymmetric neodensity. Nevertheless, the percentage of carcinomas (7.6%) diagnosed in 630 interval biopsies is markedly lower than in the screening biopsies (499 carcinomas in 3271 biopsies = 15%).

The proposition that interval carcinomas are more malignant because of their – at least theoretically – more rapid growth was disproved by HOLMBURG et al. (1986), who found the same survival time with 94 interval carcinomas as with 178 screening carcinomas.

A further serious problem in all preventive mammography programs is posed by the benign biopsies unnecessarily performed. In general, a ratio of one discovered carcinoma to three benign biopsies is considered acceptable, because it is unavoidable. In some "aggressive" screening programs (e.g., MOSKOWITZ 1984), however, a ratio of just under 1:10 (i.e., nine benign biopsies to one detected carcinoma) is also tolerated.

Protocol for Screening Mammography

The temporal sequence of a breast cancer screening program can be defined rather precisely on the basis of the age-specific beneficial effect found in the controlled studies performed so far:

- A baseline mammography is usually recommended between the ages of 35 and 40 years as a basis for the later screening. MILLER [55] rightly raises the objection that, if performed too far in advance of the screening program, the baseline mammography is of limited value due to age-dependent structural changes.
- According to MOSKOWITZ [58] the screening program should start at the age of 40 and comprise annual mammography between the ages of 40 and 50, since the greatest beneficial effect is achieved in women between the ages of 45 and 49 (in contrast to the outdated statement concerning this age group in the HIP study). Two-year screening intervals are scheduled after the age of 50 years.
- The reasonable upper age limit is sometimes defined (e.g., 65 years) and sometimes left open.

The recommendations of the German Society for Senology concerning screening mammography are as follows:

1. Baseline mammography between the ages of 30 and 40 years.
2. Screening mammographies at 2-year intervals from the age of 40 onward.
3. If mammography is first performed between the ages of 40 and 50, it should subsequently be carried out at annual intervals for 3 years.
4. No upper age limit for screening mammography.
5. In high-risk patients, mammography every year or every 2 years beginning at an individually established age.

Supplementary Techniques

Techniques which can be used to supplement plain mammography comprise the following: pneumocystography (cyst insufflation); galactography (milk duct imaging with contrast media), including exfoliative cytology; breast sonography; thermography; fine-needle puncture (mammographically/stereotactically or sonographically controlled); magnetic resonance tomography.

Pneumocystography

In cases where a palpable finding is suspected to be a cyst on the basis of anamnestic, clinical and mammographic evidence, pneumocystography was already a valuable measure for the reliable diagnosis and usually also therapy of mammary cysts before the introduction of breast sonography. Moreover, insufflation of the cysts often improves the mammographic assessment of adjacent or overshadowing breast structures (e.g., microcalcifications).

Galactography

Visualization of the milk ducts with contrast media (galactography), including exfoliative cytology, is indicated in cases of a discharge from the mamilla:

- For preoperative localization of the affected milk duct
- For detection or exclusion of pathological alterations in the duct segment (filling defects, duct interruptions, extravasations)
- For detection of cytologically suspicious intraductal cellular material

KINDERMANN ([44] Table 1) was able to demonstrate a normal milk duct system or a simple mammary duct ectasia, and thus avoid an operation, in 65% of 1695 galactographies. In the other 35% biopsy was necessary, because morphological duct alterations, of whatever kind, cannot otherwise be identified as malignant or benign. Biopsy reveals papillomas or benign intraductal proliferations in about half the cases and carcinomas in only 3.3%. This shows the limited value of galactography for carcinoma diagnosis. Exfoliative cytology in cases of a discharge from the mamilla likewise has only a limited degree of accuracy (average 63.5% [45]).

Table 1. Results of galactography in cases with nipple discharge (KINDERMANN 1985)

	Number	Percentage of all cases	Percentage of all pathological findings
All cases	1694	100	
Normal findings	1105	65.1	
Pathological findings (ref. to biopsy)	589	34.9	100
Histological diagnosis			
Fibocystic mastopathy	155	9.2	26.3
Papilloma	256	15.3	43.8
Benign intraductal proliferation	89	5.3	15.2
Carcinoma in situ	18	1.0	3.0
Carcinoma	55	3.3	9.4

Sonography

Sonography is now the most efficient supplementary method to mammography. It is largely performed using manually controlled real-time sound probes in direct skin contact (with or without a water path). The *advantages* over mammography are as follows:

- Better structure imaging and assessment of mammographically dense, poorly assessable breasts

- Nearly 100% differentiation of clinically or mammographically unclear lesions as being fluid-containing or solid
- Assessability of the inner structure of solid alterations (advantage of the tomographic procedure)
- Provision of a contrast complementary to mammography between tumor tissue (usually echo-poor) and parenchyma rich in glandular and connective tissue (usually echo-rich)
- Better results in the gland- and connective tissue-rich breasts of younger women and during pregnancy
- Better assessability of breast prostheses
- Direct correlation of the palpation finding and the sonomorphological finding

Breast sonography bears, however, the following *disadvantages*:

- Inability to recognize or differentiate microcalcifications
- Poor sonographic contrast between tumorous and fatty tissue (both echo-poor; particularly disadvantageous in the fat-rich breasts of older women)
- Problematic sonographic documentation of the total organ (disadvantage of the tomographic procedure compared to mammography as a projection procedure)
- Direct examiner dependency of the method, even on primary demonstration of the findings

In the hands of an experienced examiner (!), high-resolution real-time sonography now achieves accuracy comparable to that of mammography in the diagnosis of early breast carcinomas (T1, less than 1 cm) [79]. The accuracy of sonography reaches 50% vs 53%–75% in screening mammography (see screening results above).

Of course, small in situ carcinomas only recognized mammographically because of microcalcification are not found sonographically (Rosner et al. 1980); on the other hand, sonography detects small individual carcinomas which are not visible on mammography, even retrospectively, through their identical soft-tissue density in radiodense surroundings, though they usually cannot be identified as benign or malignant.

In later tumor stages (T2), sonography is of the same value as mammography in a global sense, without considering individual cases.

On the basis of the different physical imaging properties, however, other carcinomas are sometimes detected by sonography complementary to mammography, so that the accuracy rate clearly increases with the combined and systematic application of mammography and sonography [64,19,66,41,72,47].

Largely because of methodological drawbacks (examiner dependency, incomplete documentation) and diagnostic disadvantages (no microcalcification detection), breast sonography, compared to mammography, can play only an additive role in the diagnosis and prevention of breast cancer. The relatively restrictive recommendations of the German Society for Senology on the application of breast sonography are therefore as follows:

- Breast sonography can at present be regarded only as an additive examination method to mammography. A suspicious breast finding represents an indication

for breast sonography only if it cannot be clarified unequivocally by mammography. Mammographically detected microcalcifications are not an indication for breast sonography.
- Mammography should always precede breast sonography. Breast sonography can be employed as an initial examination for detection of cysts only in patients under the age of 30 with palpation findings in the breast. In cases of confirmed macrocystic mastopathy, sonography can be employed for cyst detection between regular control mammographies if there is a new palpation finding.

Thermography

Thermography is of little significance in the early diagnosis of cancer. It is undisputed that inclusion of thermography in a screening program may lead to discovery of some clinically occult carcinomas not detectable by any other examination procedure (a category comprising just under 5% of the carcinomas). Conversely, it is equally undisputed that, within the framework of the screening, about every second occult carcinoma is overlooked if only thermography is used. Thermography is therefore the only examination method besides inspection and palpation that is *not* acceptable for breast cancer prevention [29,40,60,53].

If for no other reason, thermography is inadequate because, if the thermogram is suspicious in the absence of palpation findings, it is impossible to localize the tumor and establish an indication for biopsy. At the most, it can now play only a supplementary role alongside inspection, palpation, mammography and sonography. In this function, it can increase the accuracy by documentation of a certain risk situation on the basis of a pathological thermogram (GAUTHERIE and GROS 1980) and by a degree of prognostic classification of the primary finding on the basis of heat production. For both aspects (risk, prognostic staging), however, there are now better clinical, surgical and histological assessment parameters.

Fine-Needle Biopsy

Fine-needle biopsy is a very effective supplementary method in the hands of an experienced examiner working in close cooperation with a cytologist. It can be performed under palpatory, mammographic stereotactic or sonographic control and is indicated in the following circumstances:

- Unclear findings localized by palpation, mammography and sonography
- Impalpable uncharacteristic consolidation zones in the mammograph
- Suspicious impalpable sonographic findings not visible mammographically
- Nodes in the skin or in the scar after mastectomy
- Areas of increased consistency after excision or only irradiation of a carcinoma
- Circumscribed or diffuse "inflammatory" processes (differentiation between mastitis and inflammatory carcinomas)
- Enlarged or suspicious lymph nodes

The objective of fine-needle biopsy in the presence of mammographically or sonographically unclear or suspicious findings is non-invasive cytological characterization of the process in question without having to resort to a more aggressive operative biopsy.

According to older statistical compilations [45], the rate of false-negative findings was 13%, that of false-positive ones 1%. Of 247 histologically confirmed carcinomas, 214 (86.5%) were classified as malignant (74.9%) or suspicious (11.7%) by aspiration biopsy cytology. In a more recent statistical survey from 1977 to 1982, AUER and KRONENWETT (1985) report a false-negative rate of only 3.2% and a false-positive one of 0.04%.

While the cytologist is always responsible for false-positive findings, the numerous false-negative findings are due to inadequate material being obtained at the aspiration biopsy. In particular, cell-poor carcinomas (scirrhous) cannot be well assessed by cytological examination, and their confirmation by fine-needle biopsy is limited. This underlines the necessity for close cooperation between the cytologist and the examiner performing the biopsy.

CITOLER (1985; Table 2) reported on comparatively performed mammographic-stereotactic fine-needle or punch-needle biopsies (Tru-Cut needle) in the presence of impalpable findings. In this connection, sufficient material for unequivocal histological or cytological characterization of the lesion was provided in 67% of cases by the punch-needle biopsy and in only 46% by the fine-needle biopsy. This once again illustrates the limited value of the stereotactic fine-needle biopsy in cases of scirrhous carcinoma and fibroadenoma.

Table 2. Diagnostic accuracy of breast biopsy under stereotactic mammographic guidance of 159 impalpable lesions (CITOLER 1985)

Mammographic appearance	*n*	Percentage correct diagnosis	
		Histology (Tru-cut)	Cytology (fine-needle)
Fibrosis/scirrhosis	48	87	53
Fibroadenoma	53	70	30
Microcalcification	32	50	42
Cyst	26	33	71
Average		60	49

Finally, it remains to be said that in about 50% of cases, impalpable, mammographically unclear findings can be adequately clarified in a non-invasive manner by stereotactic fine-needle aspiration biopsy cytology. This is of great economic importance in view of the numerous biopsy recommendations that will be made in the future within the framework of screening mammography.

Magnetic Resonance Tomography of the Breast

Magnetic resonance tomography is the newest and most complex of the medical imaging techniques. It uses electromagnetic (radio-) waves in order to produce cross-sectional images of the body or individual organs from the different energy release and distribution of the stimulated hydrogen atoms in the tissue.

The hoped-for *advantages* of this procedure for breast diagnostics are:

1. High soft-tissue contrast and, in relation to mammography/sonography, complementary differentiability of benign and malignant tissue
2. Compared to mammography, better detection of the inner structure of circumscribed focal findings
3. The absence of any risk

The examination is performed with the patient in a prone position and the breast hanging into a special pot-shaped breast coil. The breast is imaged in layers in any desired plane (sagittal, transverse or coronary). The image character is decisively influenced by the relaxation times and the proton density of the tissue, as well as by the chosen measuring parameters (pulse sequences) (Fig. 1a-c).

In the so-called T1-weighted image, the signal intensity is high for fat (Fig. 1a), weak for glandular and connective tissue and for lesions with a high water and cell content (e.g., mucinous carcinomas) and poor for fluid (cysts). In the T2-weighted image, the signal intensity decreases for fat but increases relatively for cell-rich lesions and strongly for fluids. This makes tissue differentiation possible. In particular, the connective tissue fibroadenoma in older women (always of poor signal intensity, Fig. 1) can be distinguished from the mucinous or cell-rich carcinoma. Moreover, a distinction between malignant and benign tissue can currently be made only on the basis of the shape characteristics known from mammo-/sonography. Efforts are now being made to differentiate benign/malignant processes by means of paramagnetic contrast media (e.g., gadolinium-DTPA).

The present *indications* for magnetic resonance tomography of the breast are as follows:

1. Differentiation of the fiber-rich fibroadenoma in older women from the circumscribed cell-rich carcinoma
2. Differentiation of scirrhous carcinomas from star-shaped scars by means of paramagnetic contrast medium
3. Supplementation of mammo-/sonography for better assessment of the surrounding parenchyma in connection with breast prostheses/implants

The *disadvantages* of magnetic resonance tomography comprise the following:

- The inability to recognize calcium and microcalcifications
- The still long examination time
- The uncomfortable position during the examination
- The high costs
- The limited availability of the procedure

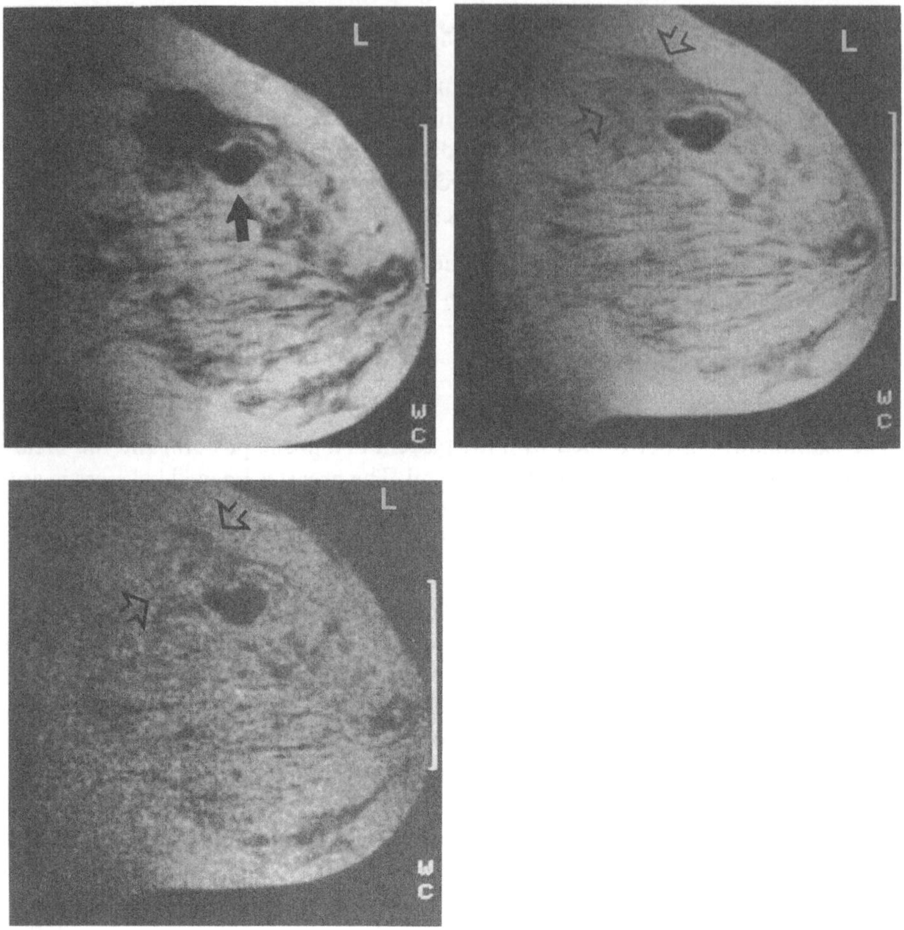

Fig. 1a-c. Tissue differentiation by magnetic resonance tomography of the breast: sagittal section. **a** T1-weighted image, spin echo mode 400/35 ms: lobular fibroma of extremely poor signal intensity (*black arrow*), above it an irregularly bordered carcinoma with weak signal intensity. **b** Proton-density image, spin echo mode 1600/35 ms: fibroma with unaltered poor signal intensity; relative signal increase in the carcinoma with a center of weak signal intensity and a fibrotic marginal border (*open arrows*). **c** T2-weighted image, spin echo mode 1600/105 ms: poor signal intensity unaltered for fibroma and identical for carcinoma and fatty tissue

Radiation Risk of Mammography

The radiation risk of mammography should be considered in two different ways:

1. For a single, clinically indicated mammography (symptomatic patient) to clarify palpation findings or other symptoms, the radiation risk is usually of no importance measured against the patient's risk of illness.
2. For screening mammography, i.e., repeated exposure of larger groups of asymptomatic women, the radiation risk must be taken into account, because

(a) many fewer women profit here by early diagnosis of a subclinical carcinoma, and (b) the cumulative radiation risk of repeated mammographies is higher than the risk from a single mammography.

In discussing the development of radiation-induced breast cancer, it is important to differentiate between a high-dose range (above 100 rad = 1 Gy) and a low-dose range (below 100 rad).

In the *high-dose range,* which is surely not reached by modern mammography, a carcinogenic effect of the radiation on the breast is indisputable. Sufficient data to this effect were obtained with adequate precision in the following study populations: (1) survivors of the atomic bombings of Hiroshima and Nagasaki: [48,74,80]; (2) fluoroscopy patients in North American tuberculosis hospitals [12]; (3) mastitis irradiation patients [71]; (4) dial painters and [1].

The essential features of high dosage can be summarized as follows:

1. There is a linear dose/effect relationship (between 100 and 400 rad).
2. The latency period from the time of exposure to the development of cancer is at least 10 years, with longer latency periods in younger women, because radiogenic carcinomas do not occur earlier than natural cancers.
3. The radiation hazard is markedly greater in younger women (under 30 years of age) than in older ones.
4. After exposure to a single radiation hazard, the risk lasts at least 40 years.
5. Radiation-induced carcinomas cannot be differentiated histologically from spontaneous cancers.

The data in the *low-dose range* are considerably more inaccurate and contradictory. The numbers of cases are usually too small and/or the dose calculations too imprecise. No increased risk of breast cancer was reported in the following study populations:

(1) fluoroscopy patients in Canadian tuberculosis hospitals [38]; (2) mastitis irradiation patients [71]; (3) atomic bomb survivors who were over 20 years of age at the time of exposure [80]; (4) radium dial painters [1]; (5) patients treated with radioiodine for hyperthyroidism [37]; (6) patients whose contralateral breast had been irradiated because of a carcinoma [34]. Other collectives (atomic bomb survivors under 20 years of age at exposure and fluoroscopy tuberculosis patients) include excess carcinomas in women with exposures below 100 rad, but the figures are not significant.

In animal experiments, radiation has been shown generally to possess a relatively lower effectiveness in the dose range of 50–100 rad than in the high-dose range [84].

In the face of these uncertainties, the National Cancer Institute of the USA gave the following *estimations on the radiation-induced breast cancer risk* for a *single exposure* [82]:

- 7.5 excess carcinomas per million women per year and rad in women under 35 years of age.
- 3.5 excess carcinomas per million women per year and rad in women over 35 years of age. This risk applies for each subsequent year, i.e., 3.5 excess carcinomas are added to the natural incidence each year.

If the radiation risk of a single mammography with an assumed mean parenchymal dose of 0.5 rad (0.005 Gy) is compared to the natural breast cancer risk for the various age groups (Table 3), it becomes apparent that the natural breast cancer risk is far higher in all age groups, even assuming this not generally accepted parenchymal dose. It also becomes evident in this connection that the cumulative radiation risk decreases with increasing age at exposure, because it can no longer express itself in view of the limited natural life expectancy. On the other hand, the natural breast cancer incidence strongly increases with age. No synergism of the radiation risk and the naturally increased breast cancer risk (familial risk or fibrocystic mastopathy) is known.

For the application of mammography in breast cancer prevention, two basic findings on radiation risk from the most recent studies are decisive:

1. In the best documented and largest collectives (atomic bomb survivors, fluoroscopy patients from Canadian tuberculosis hospitals), no increased breast cancer risk compared to nonexposed women can be found in the age groups over 40, even with doses of over 100 rad (!) [38].
2. Likewise, no increased breast cancer risk was found for atomic bomb survivors over 30 years of age with exposures below 100 rad.

These two facts *prove* that there is no radiation risk from screening mammography for women over 30 years of age.

Table 3. Radiation risk and natural breast cancer risk

Age on exposure (0.5 rad)	Radiation risk (lifelong risk per million women)	Annual incidence (per million women)
40	50	800
45	45	1400
50	35	1800
55	30	2050
60	20	2400
65	15	2700
70	10	2950

Modified according to FEIG 1983

References

1. Adams EE, Brues AM (1980) Breast cancer in female radium dial workers first employed before 1930 J Occup Med 22:583-587
2. American College of Radiology (1983) Guidelines for mammography. Am Coll Radiol Bull 38:6-7
3. American Cancer Society (1983) Mammography guidelines 1983: Background statement and update of cancer-related checkup guidelines for breast cancer detection in asymptomatic women age 40 to 49. Cancer 33:255
4. Andersson A, Andren L, Hildell J, Linell F, Ljundqvist U, Pettersson H (1979) Breast cancer screening with mammography. Radiology 132:273-276
5. Andersson I, Fagerberg G, Lundgren B, Tabar L (1980) Breast cancer screening in Sweden. Radiologe 20:608-611
6. Auer G, Kronenwett M (1985) A topical view of the reliability of fine-needle aspiration biopsy in the early detection and biological characterization of breast cancer. In: Zander J, Baltzer J (eds) Early breast cancer. Springer, Berlin Heidelberg New York
7. Bailar J (1977) Screening for early breast cancer: pros and cons Cancer 39:2783-2795
8. Baker LH (1982) Breast cancer detection demonstration project: five year summary report. Cancer 32:194-226
9. Baral E, Larson LE, Mattson B (1977) Breast cancer following irradiation of the breast. Cancer 40:2905-2910
10. Bearhs OH, Smart CR (1983) The breast cancer detection demonstration projects as viewed by the clinician. In: Feig SA, McLelland R (eds) Breast carcinoma: current diagnosis and treatment. Masson, New York, pp 307-314
11. Bekanntmachungen der Kassenärztlichen Bundesvereinigung (1980) Indikationen zur Durchführung einer Mammographie. Dtsch Artztebl 77, 914
12. Boice JD, Monson RR (1977) Breast cancer in women after repeated fluoroscopic examinations of the chest. JNCI 59:823-832
13. Boice JD Jr, Land CE, Shore RE, Norman JE, Tokunaga M (1979) Risk of breast cancer following low-dose radiation exposure. Radiology 131:589-597
14. Bolmgren J, Jacobson B, Nordenström B (1977) Stereotaxic instrument for needle biopsy of the mamma. Am J Rontgenol 129:121-125
15. Boquoi E, Kreuzer G (1974) Punktionszytologie der Mamma. Dtsch Arztebl 45:3229
16. Breslow L, Thomas LB, Upton AC (1977) Final reports of the National Cancer Institute ad hoc working groups on mammography in screening for breast cancer and summary report of their joint findings and recommendations. JNCI 59:467-541
17. Brezina K (1975) Ergebnisse der Mammographie mit gezielter Nadelbiopsie. Klin Wochenschr 87:666-670
18. Citoler P (1985) Histology and cytology following stereotactic needle biopsy. In: Zander J, Baltzer J (eds) Early breast cancer. Springer, Berlin Heidelberg New York
19. Cole-Beuglet C, Goldberg BB, Kurtz AB, Rubin CS, Patchefsky AS, Shaber GS (1981) Ultrasound mammography: a comparison with radiographic mammography. Radiology 139:693-698
20. Collete HJA, Day NE, Rombach JJ, de Waard F (1984) Evaluation of screening for breast cancer in a non-randomised study (the Dom project) by means of a case-control study. Lancet: 1224-1226
21. Dixon JM, Anderson TJ, Lamb J, Nixon SJ, Forrest APM (1984) Fine needle aspiration cytology in relationship to clinical examination and mammography in the diagnosis of a solid breast mass. Br J Surg 71:593-596
22. El Yousef SJ, Connell DMO, Duchesneau RH, Smith MJ, Hubay CA, Guyton SP (1985) Benign and malignant breast disease: magnetic resonance and radiofrequency pulse sequences. Am J Rontgenol 145:1-8
23. Feig SA (1982) Die Kontroll-Intervall bei mammographischen Reihenuntersuchungen. In: Frischbier H-J (ed) Die Erkrankungen der weiblichen Brustdrüse. Thieme, Stuttgart
24. Feig SA (1984) Radiation risk from mammography: is it clinically significant? Am J Rontgenol 143:469-475

25. Feig SA, Schwartz GF, Nerlinger R, Édeicken J (1979) Prognostic factors of breast neoplasms detected on screening by mammography and physical examination. Radiology 133:577–582
26. Friedrich M (1982) Was leistet die Mamma-Sonographie? Gynakol Prax 6:393–414
27. Friedrich M (1985) Recent progress in the ultrasonic detection of breast cancer. In: Zander J, Baltzer J (eds) Early breast cancer. Springer, Berlin Heidelberg New York
28. Friedrich M, Semmler W (1987) MR-Tomographie der Brust – Zusatzinformationen in ausgewählten Fällen. Radiologe 27:
29. Frischbier HJ, Lohbeck HU (1977) Frühdiagnostik des Mammacarcinoms. Thieme, Stuttgart
30. Frischbier HJ (1985) Empfehlungen zum Einsatz der Mammasonographie. Dtsch Artztebl 82,44 (1985) 44
31. Fox S, Baum JK, Klos DS, Tsou CV (1985) Breast cancer screening: the underuse of mammography. Radiology 156:607–611
32. Gisvold JJ, Martin JK (1984) Prebiopsy localization of nonpalpable breast lesions. Am J Rontgenol 143:477–481
33. Hall FM, Frank HA (1979) Preoperative localization of nonpalpable breast lesions. Am J Rontgenol 132:101–105
33a. Holland RM, Mravunac M, Hendriks JHCL, Bekker BV (1982) So-called interval cancers of the breast. Cancer 49:2527–2533
34. Hankey BF, Curtis RE, Naughton MD, Boice JE Jr, Flannery JT (1983) A retrospective cohort analysis of second breast cancer risk for primary breast cancer patients with an assessment of the effect of radiation therapy. JNCI 70:797–804
35. Heywang SH, Frenzl G, Edmaier M, Eiermann W, Bassermann R, Krischke I (1985) Kernspintomographie in der Mammadiagnostik Fortschr Rontgenstr 143:207–212
36. Heywang SH, Hahn D, Schmidt H, Krischke I, Eirmann W, Bassermann R, Lissner J (1986) MR imaging of the breast using gadolinium-DTPA. J Comput Assist Tomogr 10:199–204
37. Hoffman DA, McConahey WM (1983) Breast cancer following iodine 131 therapy for hyperthyroidism. JNCI 70:63–67
38. Howe GR (1984) Epidemiology of Radiogenic breast cancer. In: Boice JD Jr, Fraumeni JF Jr (eds) Radiation carcinogenesis: epidemiology and biological significance. Raven, New York
39. Holmberg LH, Adami HO, Tabar L, Bergström R (1986) Survival in breast cancer diagnosed between mammographic screening examinations. Lancet:27–30
40. Hüppe JR (1976) Mammographie und Thermographie in der Früherkennung des Mammakarzinoms. Med Welt 27:1017–1023
41. Kessler M, Igl W, Krauss B, Bassermann R, Bohmert DH, Eiermann W, Lohe KJ, Lissner J (1983) Vergleich von Mammographie und automatisierter Sonographie an 700 Patientinnen. Fortschr Rontgenstr 138:331–339
42. Kaiser W, Zeitler E (1986) Die Kernspintomographie der Mamma – Diagnose, Differentialdiagnose, Probleme und Lösungsmöglichkeiten Teil I: Untersuchungsverfahren. Fortschr Rontgenstr 144:459–465
43. Kaiser W, Zeitler E (1986) Die Kernspintomographie der Mamma – Diagnose, Differentialdiagnose, Probleme und Lösungsmöglichkeiten Teil II: Diagnostik. Fortschr Rontgenstr 144:572–579
44. Kindermann G (1985) Diagnostic value of galactography in the detection of breast cancer. In: Zander J, Baltzer J (eds) Early breast cancer. Springer, Berlin Heidelberg New York
45. Kreuzer G (1977) Zytologische Diagnostik. In: Frischbier HJ, Lohbeck HH (eds) Frühdiagnostik des Mammakarzinoms. Thieme, Stuttgart
46. Land CE, Boice JD Jr, Shore RE, Norman JE, Tokunaga M (1980) Breast cancer risk from low-dose exposure to ionizing radiation: results of parallel analysis of three exposed populations of women. JNCI 65:353–376
47. Lauth G, Duda V, Hackelöer B-J (1984) Ultrasound mammography: possibilities and limitations in the detection of early breast cancer. In: Zander J, Baltzer J (eds) Early breast cancer. Springer, Berlin Heidelberg New York

48. Loewe WE, Mendelsohn E (1981) Revised dose estimates at hiroshima and nagasaki. Health Phys 41:663-666
49. Lundgren B (1979) Efficiency of single-view mammography: Rate of interval cancer cases. JNCI 62:799-803
50. Lundgren B, Jakobsson S (1979) Single-view mammography screening. Radiology 130:109-112
51. Martin JE, Moskowitz M, Milbrath JR (1979) Breast cancer missed by mammography. Am J Rontgenol 132:737-739
52. Meyer JE, Kopans DB, Stomper PC, Lindfors KK (1984) Occult breast abnormalities: percutaneous preoperative needle localization. Radiology 150:335-337
53. Milbrath JR (1977) Does thermography aid in breast cancer detection? In: Logan WW (ed) Breast carcinoma. Wiley, New York, pp 255-258
54. Miller AB (1978) Risk benefit in mass screening programs for breast cancer. Semin Oncol 5:351-359
55. Miller AB (1983) Controversies in screening for breast cancer. In: Margolese RG (ed) Breast cancer. Churchill Livingstone, New York, pp 1-22
56. Moskowitz M (1982) Reihenuntersuchungen zur Diagnostik des Mammakarzinoms: Wie wirksam sind unsere Untersuchungsmethoden? Ein kritischer Überblick. In: Frischbier H-J (ed) Die Erkrankungen der wieblichen Brustdrüse. Thieme, Stuttgart
57. Moskowitz M (1984) Mammography to screen asymptomatic women for breast cancer. Am J Rontgenol 143:457-459
58. Moskowitz M (1986) Breast Cancer: Age-Specific Growth Rates and Screening Strategies Radiology 161 (1986) 37-41
59. Moskowitz M, Gartside PS (1982) Evidence of breast cancer mortality reduction: aggressive screening in women under age 50. Am J Rontgenol 138:911-916
60. Moskowitz M, Milbrath J, Gartside P, Zermeno A, Mandel D (1976) Lack of efficacy of thermography as a screening for minimal and stage I breast cancer. New Engl J Med 295:249-252
61. Penn W, Hendriks JHCL (1984) Die Bedeutung von breit angelegten Vorsorgeuntersuchungen für die Prognose des Mammacacinoms. Chirurg 55:211-217
62. Peyster RG, Kalisher L (1979) Needle localization of nonpalpable lesions of the breast. Surg Gynecol Obstet 148:703-706
63. Philip J, Harris WG, Flaherty C, Joslin CAF, Rustage JH, Wijesinghe DP (1984) Breast self-examination: clinical results from a palpulation-based prospective study. Br J Cancer 50:7-12
64. Pluygers E, Rombeau M (1980) Ultrasonic diagnosis of breast diseases. Tumor Diagn 4:187-194
65. Pochin EE (1978) Why be quantitative about radiation risk estimates? In: The Lauriston S. Taylor lecture series in radiation protection and measurements: National Council on Radiation Protection and Measurements, Washington, D.C. (Lecture 2)
66. Rosner D, Weiss L, Norman M (1980) Ultrasonography in the diagnosis of breast disease. J Surg Oncol 14:83-96
67. Saltzstein SL (1984) Potential limits of physical examination and breast self-examination in detecting small cancers of the breast. Cancer 54:1443 1446
68. Schöndorf H (1977) Die Aspirationszytologie der Brustdrüse. Schattauer, Stuttgart
69. Schwartz FW, Robra BP (1982) Zur Frage der unteren Altersgrenze beim gesetzlichen Screening auf Brustkrebs. Geburtshilte Frauenheilkd 42:137
70. Shapiro S, Venet W, Strax P, Venet L, Roeser R (1982) Ten-to-fourteen-year effect of screening on breast cancer mortality. JNCI 69:349-355
71. Shore RE, Hempelmann LH, Kowaluk E, Mansur PS, Pasternack BS, Albert RE, Haughie GE (1977) Breast neoplasms in women treated with X-rays for acute postpartum mastitis. JNCI 59:813-822
72. Sickles EA, Filly RA, Callen PW (1983) Breast cancer detection with sonography and mammography: comparison using state-of-the-art equipment. Am J Rontgenol 140:843-845
73. Stosiek U, Breitbach GP, Lindner R (1983) Kombinierte präoperative Diagnostik von Mammatumoren. Tumordiagnostik Ther 4:175-178

74. Straume T, Dobson RL (1981) Implications of new Hiroshima and Nagasaki dose estimates: cancer risks and neutron RBE. Health Phys 41:666–671
75. Tabar L, Dean PB (1979) Interventional radiologic procedures in the investigation of lesions of the breast. Radiol Clin North Am 27:607–621
76. Tabar L, Dean PB (1984) Risks and benefits of mammography in population screening for breast cancer. In: Bonadonna G (ed) Breast cancer: diagnosis and management. Wiley, New York
77. Tabar L, Gad A, Akerlund E, Holmberg L (1983) Screening for breast cancer in Sweden. In: Feig SA, McLelland R (eds) Breast carcinoma: current diagnosis and treatment. Masson, New York, pp 315–326
78. Tabar L, Gad A, Holmberg LH, Ljundquist U, Fagerberg CJG, Baldertorp L, Gröntoft O, Lundström B, Manson JC, Eklund G, Day NE, Pettersson F (1985) Reduction in mortality from breast cancer after mass screening with mammography. Lancet:829–832
79. Teubner J, van Kaick G, Junkermann H, Pickenhan L, Wesch H, Eggert W, Kruse W, Müller A, Tschahargane C, von Fournier D, Kubli F (1985) 5 MHz Realtime-Sonographie der Brustdrüse Teil 2: Untersuchungstecnik und diagnostische Wertigkeit. Radiologe 25:457–467
80. Tokunaga M, Land CE, Yamamoto T, Asano M, Tokuoka S, Ezaki H, Nishimori I, Fujikura T (1984) Breast cancer among atomic bomb survivors. In: Boice JC Jr, Fraumeni JF Jr (eds) Radiation carcinogenesis: epidemiology and biological significance. Raven, New York
81. United Nations Scientific Committee on the Effect of Atomic Radiation (1972) Ionizing radiation: levels and effects, vol 2. New York, United Nations
82. Upton AC, Beebe GW, Brown JM, Quimby EH, Shellabarger C (1977) Report of the NCI ad hoc working group on the risks associated with mammography in mass screening for detection of breast cancer. JNCI 59:481–493
83. Verbeek ALM, Holland R, Sturmans F, Hendriks JHCL, Mravunac M, Day NE (1984) Reduction of breast cancer mortality through mass screening with modern mammography. Lancet: 1222–1224
84. Webster EW (1981) On the question of cancer induction by small X-ray doses. Am J Rontgenol 137:647–666
85. Zajicek J (1977) Fine-needle aspiration biopsy of palpable breast lesions. In: Westinghouse Logan W (ed) Breast carcinoma – the radiologists expanded role. Wiley, New York

Standards in the Technique of Mammography

M. SÄBEL and H. AICHINGER

Considerable advances have been achieved in recent years in the field of mammography in terms of improvement in image quality and reduction of radiation exposure. These improvements in mammography must be taken into consideration when installing a new mammography unit. The following text describes in brief the technical specifications which now can (and indeed must) be met by this kind of radiographic equipment, in order to produce mammograms with good image quality.

Standard Technique

Because of the higher radiation yield of the X-ray tube and lower radiation exposure of the organ examined, the high-voltage generator must be at least a six-pulse device. The X-ray tube can be either a molybdenum anode tube (with a minimum additional filtration of 30 μm molybdenum) or a tungsten anode tube with K-edge filters [5,6]. The tungsten anode tube thereby offers the facility, through choice of tube voltage and filter material, of matching the energy distribution of the image-producing X-rays to the tissue condition and thickness of the breast, and thus of achieving a certain degree of optimization with respect to radiation exposure and image quality (Figs. 1, 2). A tungsten anode tube (at least at greater thicknesses of the compressed breast) yields mammograms with the same diagnostic information and about half the radiation exposure of a molybdenum anode tube (Fig. 3).

Since the sharpness of the image of structures located distant from the film is materially affected by focal spot size, this should be as small as possible. However, the tube power also decreases as the focal spot becomes smaller. In order to avoid exposure times of several seconds, there must be a compromise.

Clinical experience has shown that a focal spot of nominal value 0.4 (IEC) is adequate for conventional radiography (with and without antiscatter grid) at focus-film distances of about 60 cm.

The mammography unit must have a compression device, in which both the breast thickness under compression and the position of the radiation detector of the automatic exposure timer must be indicated.

An antiscatter grid at greater thicknesses of the breast ($\geqq$ 5 cm) makes an important contribution to reducing scattered radiation, and thus to improving radiation contrast [3]; however, it also increases radiation exposure by a factor of

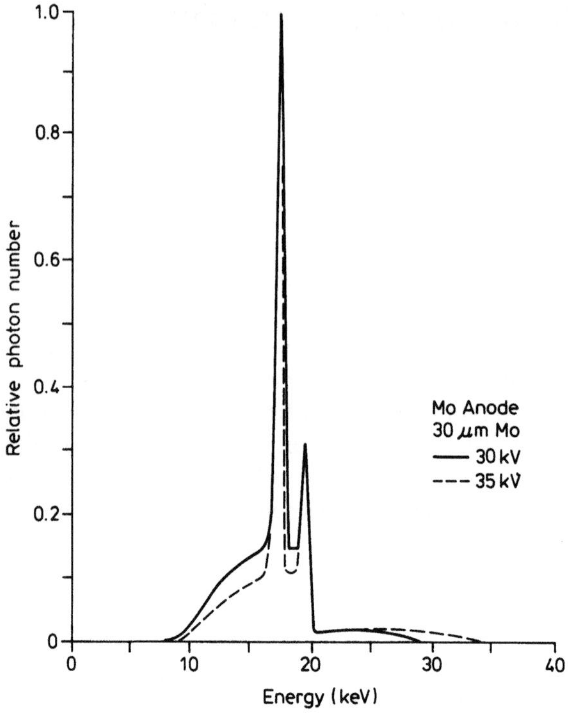

Fig. 1. X-ray spectra filtered by molybdenum generated by a molybdenum anode at 30 kV and 35 kV

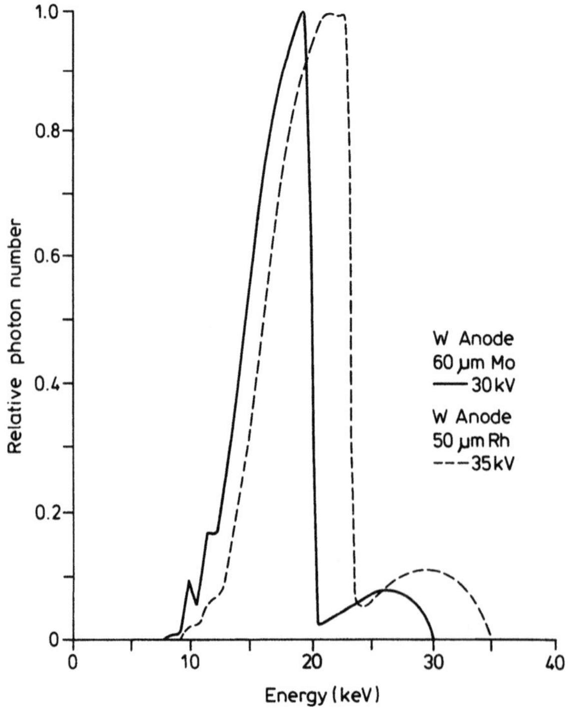

Fig. 2. X-ray spectra filtered by molybdenum or rhodium generated by a tungsten anode at 30 kV or 35 kV

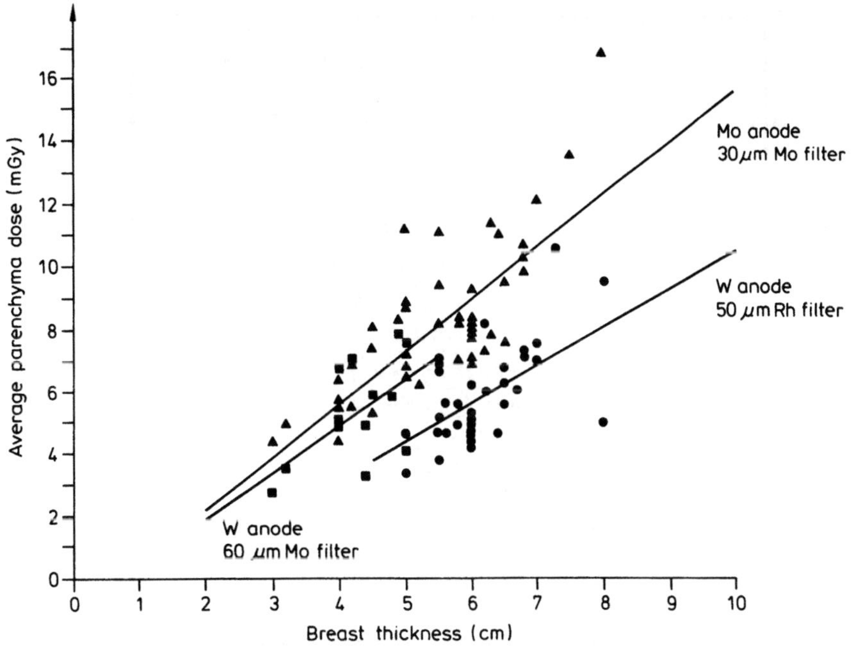

Fig. 3. Radiation exposure in mammography with a molybdenum and a tungsten anode

about 2–3. The facility should therefore also be provided for working without a grid in the case of small breasts.

Automatic exposure timing must be provided, as only by this means is it possible to compensate for the influences of thickness and tissue composition of the breast (Fig. 4) and to achieve a constant mean optical density ("blackening") of the mammogram. When – as is usual – the detector of the automatic exposure timer is located behind the image receptor, there must be a facility for correcting the dependence of the exposure on the tube voltage and breast thickness caused by the variable transmission of the image receptor [7].

The image receptor to be used in film mammography must be a screen-film system developed for this field of application. The use of non-screen film is no longer justified, because of the associated high radiation exposure (Tables 1, 2). There is now a whole series of suitable screen-film systems, and Table 2 gives a selection [8]. The more sensitive systems produce more blurring and noise, but their widespread use in clinical practice indicates that the image quality is satisfactory.

In xeromammography, the reduction in dosage compared with non-screen film (Table 1) has so far been achieved mainly through the use of higher tube voltages (up to 50 kV) and thicker additional filters (up to 3 mm aluminum) [9]. This is due to the characteristics ("edge enhancement effect") of the xeroradiographic development process, which also allows an antiscatter grid to be omitted. Xeromammograms should also be produced using automatic exposure timing. Because

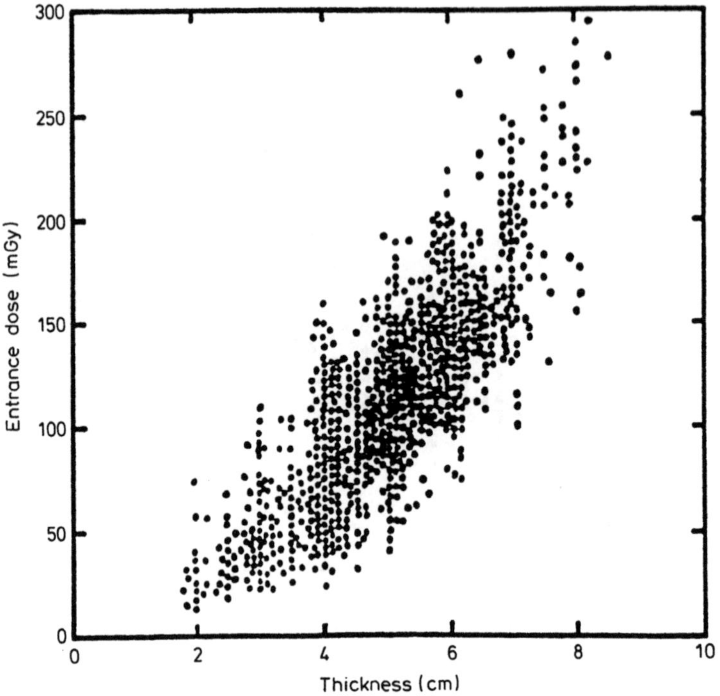

Fig. 4. Entrance doses in film mammography in relation to thickness of the compressed breast. Molybdenum anode tube with 30-μm molybdenum filter; tube voltage 28–35 kV; image receptor Kodak Definix Medical (non-screen film); exit dose 3 mGy; number of patients 1593. Average values for this batch: entrance dose 105 mGy; parenchyma dose 20 mGy; thickness of the compressed breast 4.8 cm; age of patients 49 years

Table 1. Average parenchyma dose per radiograph (1D) for various mammographic procedures. Average breast with 5 cm thickness, molybdenum anode tube

	D (mGy)
Non-screen film	20
Screen-film system	1– 4
Grid technique	2–10
Xeromammography	5–20

From [8]

Table 2. Approximate values for relative dose requirement of some screen-film systems

Film	Screen	Relative dose requirement (%)
Dupont NDT 70	Agfa MR 50	20
Dupont LD+	Kodak Min-R	13
Dupont Lo Dose	Dupont Lo Dose	13
3M Trimax M	3M Trimax Alpha 2M	11
Dupont Lo Dose	Dupont Lo Dose/2	8
Kodak Min-R MR-1	Kodak Min-R	7
Dupont LD+	Agfa MR 50	6
Agfa Mamoray M3	Agfa MR 50	6
Kodak Ortho-MA	Kodak Min-R	5
3M Trimax MS	3M Trimax Alpha 2M	3

The values stated are based on an average optical density (including fog) of 1.5 and on the dose requirement of a non-screen film (Kodak Definix Medical or Agfa T3), which (with an average optical density of 2.0) has been set equal to 100%

of the low transmission of the Xerox cassette, the ("shadow-free") measuring chamber of the automatic exposure control should be placed in front of the image receptor [10].

Magnification Technique

The standard grid technique is suitable for high-quality routine diagnosis. The additional use of the magnification technique will therefore remain restricted to the clarification of suspected microcalcifications and finest tissue structures. The reasons for this are the difficult patient positioning, the larger film size required to display the entire breast and the radiation exposure, which increases with the square of the magnification factor M.

For the magnified image to provide more diagnostic information than a Bucky mammogram viewed with a magnifying glass, tumor masses must also be reproduced with equally good image quality. Achievement of the same limiting resolution as when using the grid technique, a focus-film distance of 60 cm and a magnification factor of 2, for instances, requires a focal spot size of 0.15 (IEC), as can be proved by calculation of the modulation transfer function of the entire imaging system. The magnification technique will then also successfully display microcalcifications with diameters of the order of 200 μm, which is necessary from a medical point of view [11]. Taking into account the chemical composition of the microcalcifications and the physiological parameters governing visualization, the limit of perceptibility may be around 100 μm [4].

The scattered radiation component in the film plane when using magnification is, in any case, less than with a contact radiograph, because of the large object-film distance. This, coupled with the increase in radiation exposure and exposure time, means that use of a antiscatter grid is prohibited here. For the X-ray system, this in turn means that on changing from grid technique to magnification technique, there must be a simple method of removing the grid from the radiation beam.

In order to obtain contrast comparable with a Bucky mammogram for a particular tube voltage, the scattered radiation component in the film plane must not be very much higher. Table 3 shows the scattered radiation component and contrast improvement factor for exposures with and without grid, as well as for magnification factors 1.4 and 2.2. It can be seen that an object-film distance of around 30 cm is needed to achieve the required goal.

Table 3. Scatter fraction in the film plane for grid and magnification technique in mammography

	Air gap	Scatter fraction[a]	Contrast improvement factor[b]
Without grid	OFD 1.1 cm	45%	1
Grid	OFD 1.1 cm	19%	1.47
Magnification 1.4	15 cm	30%	1.27
Magnification 2.2	30.7 cm	22%	1.42

OFD, object-film distance
[a]Measured at 30 kV employing a tungsten anode/molybdenum filter combination. Phantom dimensions 20 cm × 20 cm × 4 cm
[b]Primary fraction with grid divided by primary fraction without grid

An advantage of magnification is the fact that the influence of noise on image quality decreases with the square of the magnification factor M [2]. This opens up the possibility of the use of more sensitive systems for the magnification technique and avoidance of the increase in radiation exposure. If a screen-film system with about twice the sensitivity is used for the magnification technique with a magnification factor $M=2$, approximately the same radiation exposure results as for the grid technique.

One way of checking the statements regarding the image quality of grid versus magnification techniques is the method of Receiver Operating Characteristic (ROC) analysis. Figure 5 shows the result of an investigation of this kind to clarify the discernibility of microcalcifications. A special test phantom [13] is used which consists of individual small blocks that can be interchanged with one another. These blocks contain granules with decreasing diameter as a model for microcalcifications. The imaging system improves the closer the ROC curve moves toward the top left corner of the graph. This method shows that a magnification factor of $M \geqq 1.7$ must be used for the Min R/Ortho MA system, if the magnification technique is to provide additional diagnostic information.

Summarizing, it can be stated that the magnification technique should be used to supplement the grid technique only when no clear diagnosis is possible with the latter alone. But then only sectional radiographs should be taken in order to reduce radiation exposure and film costs, i.e., the equipment must provide the necessary collimation facilities.

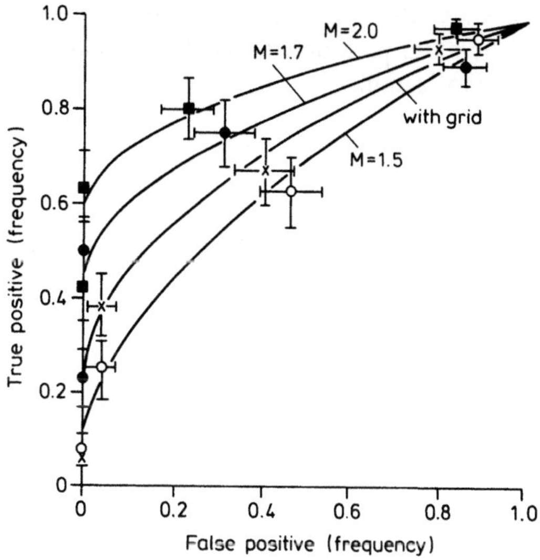

Fig. 5. Detail perceptibility (ROC method) of test granules in mammography

Quality Control

X-ray examinations of the female breast must be accompanied by technical quality control. The legislators of the Federal Republic of Germany have now insisted on this in the amended X-ray law (§ 16 of the *Röntgenverordnung*). Based on WHO guidelines [12], three types of test are thereby used with increasing complexity (and reducing frequency): testing for constancy, condition and acceptance testing (Table 4). The regularly repeated constancy testing is carried out by the user himself. For the particularly important check of the film processing (best carried out each

Table 4. Parameters to be checked for technical quality control in mammography

	Test		
	Acceptance	Condition	Constancy
Tube voltage	×	×	
Radiation quality	×	×	×
Filtration	×		
Dose	×	×	×
Radiation yield	×	×	
Focal spot size	×	×	
Radiation field limitation	×		
Antiscatter grid	×	×	
mAs product	×	×	
Automatic exposure timer	×	×	×
Image receptor	×	×	×
Film processing	×	×	×

After [12]

workday), there is already a proven method of testing [1]. The methods of checking of the other parameters (see Table 4) are, on the other hand, still the subject of standardization.

References

1. DIN 6868 (1985) Teil 2: Sicherung der Bildqualität in röntgendiagnostischen Betrieben. Filmverarbeitung: Konstanzprüfung der visuellen optischen Dichte. Beuth, Berlin
2. Doi K, Imhof H (1977) Noise reduction by radiographic magnification. Radiology 122:479–487
3. Friedrich M (1978) Neuere Entwicklungstendenzen der Mammographietechnik: die Rastermammographie. Fortschr Geb Rōntgenstr 128:207–222
4. Klein J (1979) Zur filmmammographischen Nachweisbarkeitsgrenze von Mikroverkalkungen. Fortschr Rōntgenstr 131:205–210
5. Säbel M, Aichinger H, Dierker J, Willgeroth F (1985) Strahlenexposition und Bildgüte bei der Mammographie mit einer Wolfram-Anodenröhre in Verbindung mit Kantenfiltern. In: Poretti G (ed) Medizinische Physik. Deutsche Gesellschaft für Medizinische Physik Bern, pp 280–285
6. Säbel M, Willgeroth F, Aichinger H, Dierker J (1986) Röntgenspektren und Bildqualität in der Mammographie. Electromedica 54:158–165
7. Säbel M, Paterok EM, Weishaar J, Aichinger H (1979) Belichtungsmessung bei der Mammographie mit Film-Folien-Systemen. Electromedica, Heft 3:127–136
8. Säbel M, Willgeroth F, Aichinger H (1987) Strahlenschutz bei der Mammographie: Möglichkeiten der Dosisreduktion. Rōntgenpraxis 40:65–71
9. Säbel M (1982) Strahlenexposition und Bildgüte bei der Xeromammographie. Rōntgenpraxis 35:463–468
10. Säbel M, Weishaar J, Aichinger H (1977) Die Belichtungsmessung bei der Xeromammographie. Electromedica, Heft 5:150–157
11. Stender H-S (1985) Bildqualität in physiologischer und diagnostischer Sicht. In: Stender H-S, Stiere FE (eds) Qualitätssicherung in der Rōntgendiagnostik. Thieme, Stuttgart, pp 76–84
12. World Health Organisation (1982) Quality assurance in diagnostic radiology. WHO, Geneva
13. Wurm J, Säbel M, Weishaar J (1982) Anwendung der ROC-Methode auf Probleme der Bildgute und Qualitätskontrolle in der Mammographie. Fortschr Rōntgenstr 137:201–211

Current Status of Ultrasound Mammography

W. LEUCHT and DAGMAR RABE

Introduction and Methods

The value of ultrasound as an adjunct to mammography is beginning to be recognized. Although most of the initial studies on breast sonography were carried out by WILD and REID [11, 12] during the early 1950s, it is essentially only during the past few years that its efficacy as a tool for breast diagnosis has been seriously considered by many physicians. Sonography of the breast can be performed either with a hand-held, high-resolution contact transducer or with whole-breast waterbath units capable of displaying the entire breast in multiple thin sections. One of the advantages of hand-held real-time sonography is the fact that many of the users of ultrasound – gynecologists and radiologists – are prepared to extend their existing equipment with a high-resolution contact transducer for ultrasound mammography. In accordance with the recommendation on the application of ultrasound mammography adopted by a joint commission of the German Society of Senology and the German Society for Ultrasound in Medicine in 1983, a real-time linear array should have an operating frequency of at least 5 MHz with a minimal width and depth of the visual area of 5 cm and electronically induced focusing over a depth of 0.5–5 cm with direct skin contact of the ultrasound probe.

Diagnostic Value

Most investigators have pointed out that the domain of ultrasound mammography is the possibility of differentiating between cystic and solid masses. Another well-known fact is the superiority of ultrasound compared with radiography in recognizing masses in radiologically dense breasts. A number of recent articles is concerned with the comparison of ultrasound and radiographic mammography in diagnosing breast tumors. A review of the international trends in rates of diagnostic accuracy found an average of 86% for carcinomas and 82% for benign lesions [1]. The accuracy rates of X-ray mammography were 76% for carcinomas and 60% for benign lesions. We found accuracy rates in palpable masses of 91% for carcinomas and 74% for benign masses. The relatively low rate of 74% is due to the exclusion of cystic masses [3]. In agreement with PLUYGERS et al. [9], we found ultrasound sufficiently reliable in 86% of small breast cancers (T1). In subclinical cases below

1 cm in diameter, the accuracy rate is less. The main indication for ultrasound mammography is the presence of a palpable mass.

The reliability of ultrasound in dense breasts is better than that of X-ray mammography, which is the better diagnostic tool in fatty breasts. That means the most advantage from ultrasound is to be gained by younger women, especially those suffering from fibrocystic disease [2]. The breast which has been therapeutically irradiated after conservative surgery is another reason for using ultrasound mammography [7]. In cases with inconclusive X-ray mammograms, a correct diagnosis can be made before biopsy in 70% using ultrasound; 23% remain doubtful; 7% of the ultrasound diagnoses are wrong [4].

Needle aspiration with ultrasound guidance additionally allows us to drain cysts for diagnostic and therapeutic purposes. Ultrasound guidance makes needle-aspiration biopsies of solid masses more certain of success. In a prospective study, we are trying to mark areas of clustered microcalcification preoperatively; the position of the needle must then be proved by X-ray mammography [5].

Another application of ultrasound mammography is in follow-up of patients after mastectomy to detect local recurrence in the chest wall or axilla. A correct diagnosis of a palpable mass in these areas is made in 94%, and by palpation in only 47% [10]. In postoperative follow-up it is possible to detect seromas and hematomas. There is also no problem in checking prostheses.

The indications for ultrasound mammography are:

1. Palpable masses
2. Young women
3. Radiologically dense breasts (as in fibrocystic disease or following irradiation)
4. Inconclusive mammograms
5. Pregnant and breastfeeding women
6. Ultrasound-guided needle aspiration of cysts, aspiration biopsies, and prebiopsy localization
7. Local recurrence of carcinoma
8. Postoperative follow-up of seromas, hematomas, and prostheses

Our experience is based on about 4000 investigations with about 1300 biopsy-proved findings. For this reason, it is unquestionable that comparable results cannot be expected from every user. It is important in particular to know the interpretative criteria used for sonographic appraisal and their different diagnostic implications, and to reexamine diagnoses continuously, for the development of histologic precision in ultrasound mammography. Although areas of overlap between benign and malignant conditions are found when interpreting sonographic abnormalities, we believe that the differentiation is better than with X-ray mammography [6]. Examples of sonograms are presented in Figs. 1-6.

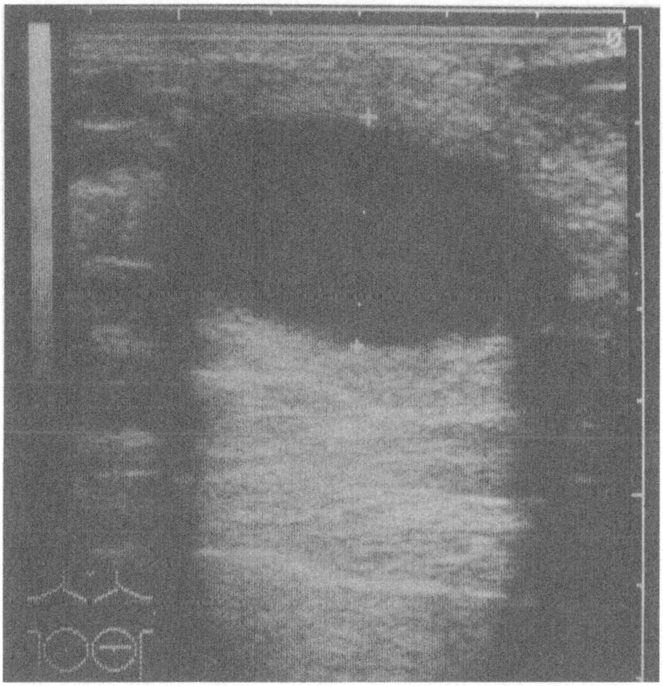

Fig. 1. Typical cyst, showing posterior echo enhancement with lateral shadows

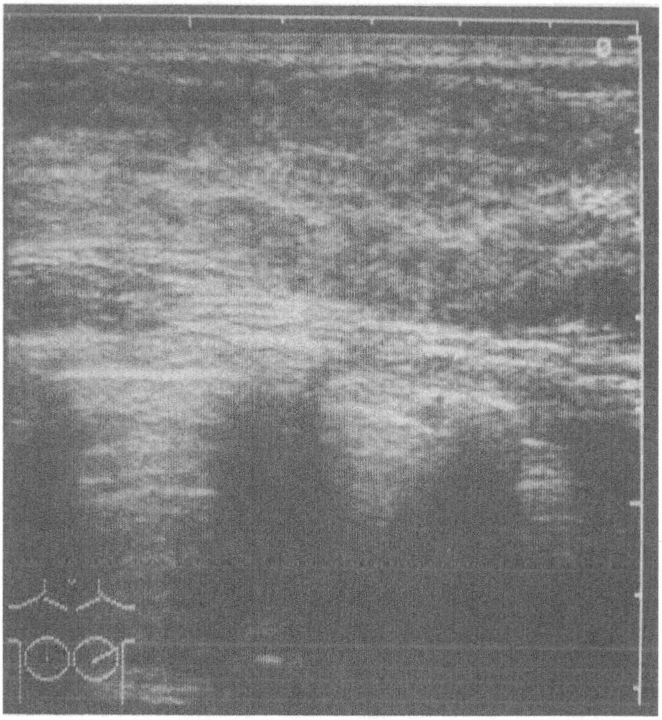

Fig. 2. Fibrocystic disease

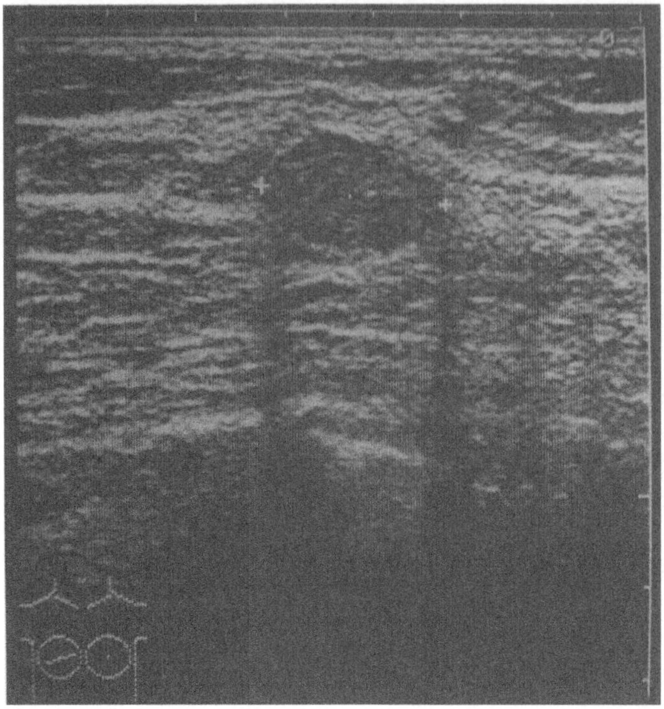

Fig. 3. Typical fibroadenoma, showing homogeneous internal echo-structure with lateral shadows

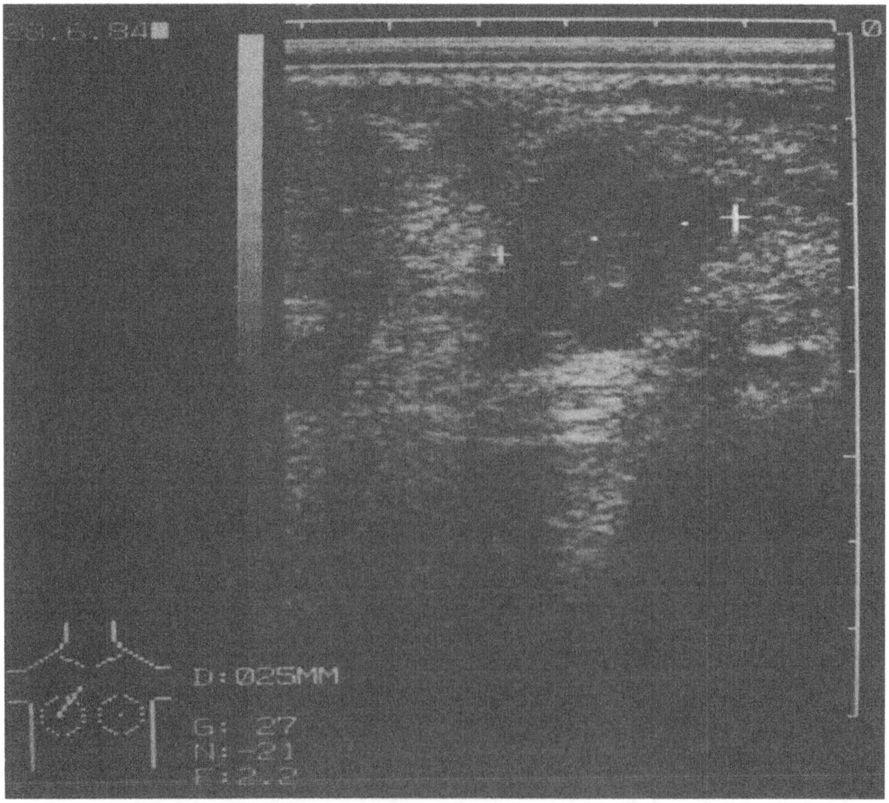

Fig. 4. Medullary carcinoma, showing heterogeneous internal echo-structure, minimal posterior echo enhancement, and irregular boundary

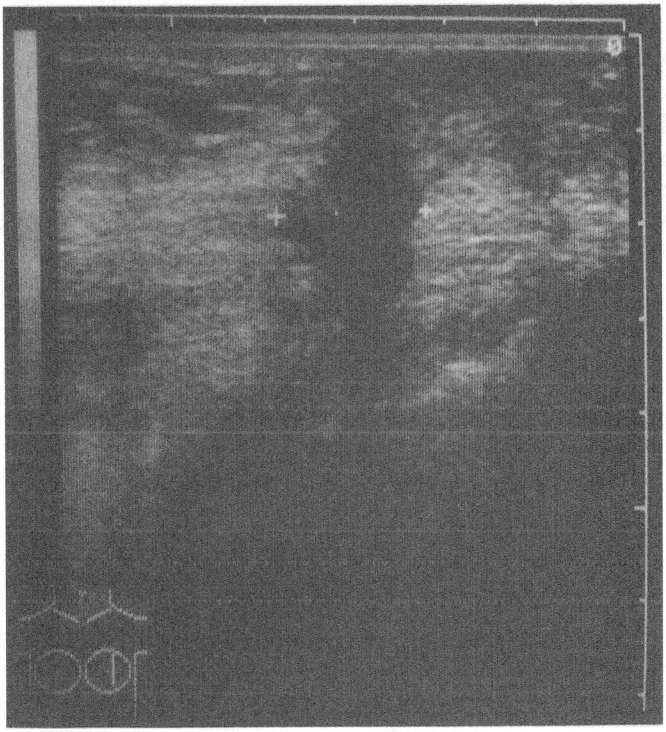

Fig. 5. Scirrhous carcinoma, a nearly anechogenic tumor with distinct posterior middle shadowing

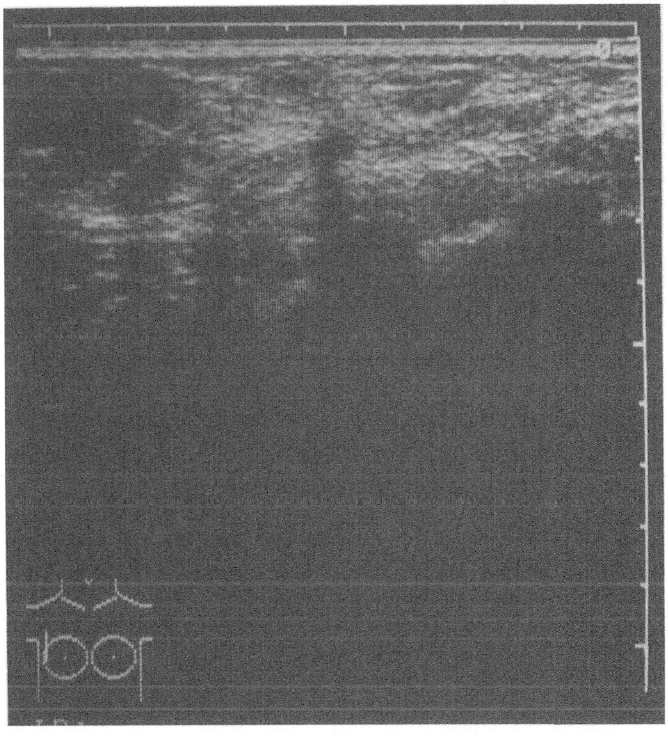

Fig. 6. Small carcinoma of 6 mm diameter, a nearly anechogenic tumor with intermediate posterior shadowing

Conclusion

Despite the promising good results, it should become standard to use ultrasound mammography chiefly as an adjunct to X-ray mammography. Present knowledge and technical possibilities do not yet allow the use of sonography as a screening method. In particular, one must warn against considering sonography as a general substitute for mammography. Currently, there is an increased willingness to recognize the benefits of ultrasound as an adjunctive technique to X-ray mammography and as a sole examination modality under certain specific circumstances.

References

1. Hackelöer BJ, Duda V, Lauth G (1986) Ultraschallmammographie. Springer, Berlin Heidelberg New York
2. Leucht W, Schmidt W, Humbert KD, Rabe D, Kubli F (1984) Real-time Echomammographie bei benignen Prozessen der Mamma. In: Lutz H, Reichel L (eds) Ultraschalldiagnostik 83, Thieme Stuttgart
3. Leucht W, Rabe D, Müller A, von Fournier D, Humbert KD, Schmidt W (1985a) Verbesserung der präoperativen Abklärung von palpablen nicht-zystischen Prozessen der Mamma durch die Echomammographie. Ultraschall 6:15-25
4. Leucht W, Rabe D, Boos R, von Fournier D, Schmidt W (1985b) Stellenwert der real-time Echomammographie bei röntgenmammographisch unklaren Befunden. In: Judmaier G, Frommhold H, Kratochwil A (eds) Ultraschalldiagnostik 84, Thieme Stuttgart
5. Leucht W, von Fournier D, Rabe D, Humbert KD, Kühn W, Schmidt W (1987) Mikrokalk in der Mammasonographie Darstellung und Bewertung. Ultraschall Klin Prax 2:195-204
6. Leucht W, Rabe D, Schmidt W (1988a) Beurteilungskriterien für die Mammasonographie. Geburtsch u Frauenheilk 48:78-91
7. Leucht W, Rabe D (1988b) Sonographic findings following conservative surgery and irradiation for breast carcinoma. Ultrasound Med & Biol 14: 27-41
8. Leucht W (1989) Lehratlas der Mammasonographie. Thieme Stuttgart (in press)
9. Pluygers E, Rombaut M, Dormal C (1983) The accuracy of ultrasonics in the diagnosis of small and subclinical breast cancer. In: Jellins J, Kobayashi T (eds) Ultrasonic examination of the breast. Wiley and Sons, New York
10. Rabe D, Leucht W, Schmid H, Leppien G, Schmidt W (1986) Stellenwert der Real-time Sonographie bei der Entdeckung von loco-regionären Rezidiven nach Mamma-Carcinom. In: Otto R Ch, Schnaars P (eds) Ultraschalldiagnostik 85, Thieme Stuttgart
11. Wild JJ, Reid JM (1952) Further pilot echographic studies on the histologic structure of tumors of the living intact human breast. Am J Pathol 28:839-861
12. Wild JJ, Reid JM (1954) Echographic visualization of lesions of the living intact human breast. Cancer Res 14:277-283

Cytologic Diagnosis of Breast Cancer

W. KÜBLER, W. KÜHN, and H.H. RUMMEL

Introduction

With the increasing differentiation of therapy for breast carcinoma, the cytology of malignant breast tumors is becoming more and more important in the context of an expanded range of breast diagnostic techniques. Progress in grid mammography and the innovation of breast sonography have helped to define the significance of abnormal breast findings with a high degree of accuracy. Following clinical examination, breast cytology meets the need for preoperative morphologic diagnosis. A trend toward performing preoperative cytology has already been mentioned by VERHAEGHE et al. (1969) and GROS et al. (1972). More formerly necessary tissue biopsies can be avoided by employing all these new diagnostic procedures [13].

Extraction of Specimen and Cytologic Examination

Puncture Cytology

This is the most frequently used method. Cells are obtained using a syringe and a thin needle (gauge 12). Usually, a puncture handle of the CAMECO (STORNBY) or FRANZEN type is used (Fig. 1). Cells of the lesion are forced out of the tissue by negative pressure or separated by the cutting effect of the needle and aspirated into it. Aspiration of blood is unpleasant, but cannot always be avoided. Cellular material that flows from the needle into the syringe is useless for cytologic examination. For fine-needle aspiration we use the pistol-handle type of CAMECO needle with a 10-ml disposable syringe and disposable needles. Before transcutaneous puncture of the breast, the overlying skin must be cleaned and disinfected. Anesthesia is not necessary. By stretching the skin between two palpating fingers, the puncture can be made nearly painless (Fig. 2). The suspicious area is held with two fingers of one hand while the other hand controls the syringe. Once the needle has passed through the subcutaneous fat and the glandular tissue and has penetrated the lesion, the piston of the syringe is retracted with a jerk. In fibrous tumors, definite resistance is felt on penetrating the lesion. While maintaining the negative pressure within the lesion, the needle is pushed rapidly forward and retracted with a fanlike movement. This is repeated four or five times. After the aspiration, the piston of the syringe is returned to its original position with the needle still in the

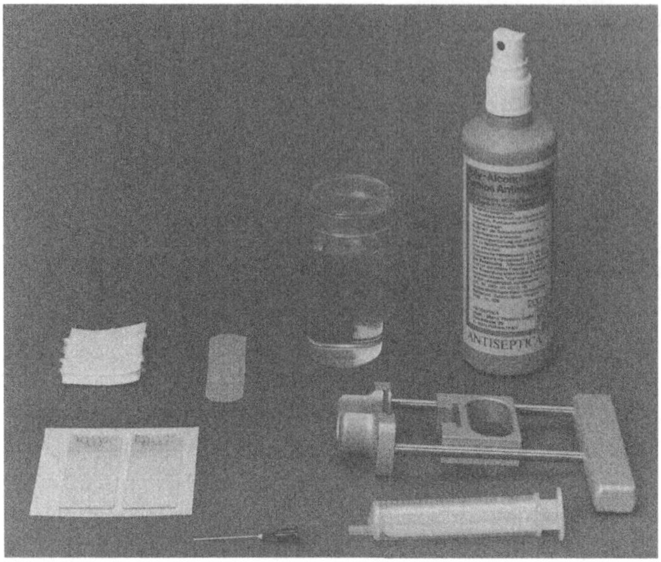

Fig. 1. Fine-needle biopsy kit consisting of a puncture handle (Cameco), a 10-ml syringe with a fine needle (gauge 12), two glass slides, alcohol and swab for disinfection of the skin, fixation medium (95% alcohol), and a dressing (photo by Liedtke)

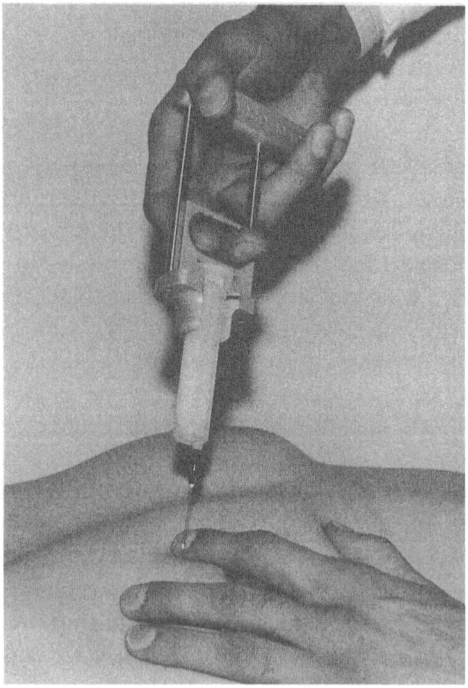

Fig. 2. Puncture position, showing the palpable mass held between two fingers of the left hand. Lesions deep in the gland must be punctured tangentially to avoid causing a pneumothorax (photo by Liedtke)

lesion, the negative pressure thus being removed. The needle is then pulled out of the punctured lesion. Retraction of the needle before equalizing the pressure should be avoided, as there is danger of drawing biopsy material into the syringe and additionally of aspirating inadequate and unrepresentative tissue from the area around the lesion. Metastases in the puncture channel have been histologically proven in cases of inadequate aspiration techniques [1]. At the end of the puncturing process the needle is removed from the syringe, and air is drawn into the latter. The needle is replaced and the cells from within its lumen are extruded onto the microscope slide. This process can be repeated once or twice. The aspirated material is spread by placing a second slide over the specimen and pulling the slide back rapidly while applying slight pressure. The usual result is two equally thin smears of cells. Both slides must be immediately transferred into an appropriate medium (95% alcohol). If the specimens are to be stained according to the Pappenheim method [MAY-GRÜNWALD-GIEMSA], the smears are air-dried.

Cytology of Fine-Needle Aspirate

In fine-needle aspiration material from the breast, the following elements can be found:

1. Glandular epithelium
2. Duct epithelium
3. Lobular epithelium
4. Myoepithelial cells and/or bipolar nuclei
5. Foam cells and/or histiocytes
6. Apocrine epithelial metaplasia
7. Fibroblasts and fibrocytes
8. Additional cells such as granulocytes, lymphocytes, plasma cells, erythrocytes, and squamous epithelial cells of the skin
9. Tumor cells

Cyst Punctures

Aspiration of fluid from a mammary structure that offers resistance confirms that a cyst has been punctured. The cyst should always be completely emptied and pneumocystography performed. Fluid from all cysts should be examined if several cysts are punctured. The color of the fluid varies from chocolate-brown to green, yellow, or a watery clear color. The following components can be found in fluid from a benign breast cyst:

1. Glandular epithelium
2. Apocrine metaplasia of epithelium
3. Foam cells

4. Histiocytes
5. Erythrocytes
6. Lymphocytes
7. Granulocytes
8. Bluish blobs (cell detritus)

Intracystic carcinomas can seldom be demonstrated cytologically. Proof of papillomas can be obtained more often.

Breast Secretions

A pathologic discharge from the nipple should be cytologically examined on principle. Pathologic nipple secretions are spontaneous, usually unilateral, secretions of the breast occurring outside pregnancy or lactation. The fluid is usually serous, sanguinous or watery, varying in color from red-brown to green or yellowish. The specimen is taken by smoothly pressing the nipple with the thumb and second finger. The secretion is smeared onto a slide, directly from the nipple. It is advisable to compress the breast slightly first, accompanied by pressure in the direction of the nipple, If there is too much cell material, the specimen can be spread onto two slides according to the method described above. Cytologic interpretation can be rendered more difficult by increased degeneration of the desquamated cells, caused by prolonged stasis of secretion in the mammary ducts.

Exfoliative Cytology of the Nipple and Areola

Specimens are taken from clinically suspicious regions by scraping with either a scalpel or the edge of a slide. With ulcerated or discharging lesions, the slide is pressed directly onto the suspicious area (*klatsch* preparation). The following cell elements are found in smears of the nipple and areola:

1. Denucleated plaques (keratinized epidermal cells)
2. Cell groups representing ductal epithelium (in benign adenomas)
3. Tumor cells
4. Paget's cells
5. Round cells (signifying inflammation)

Indications

All palpable breast abnormalities should be investigated by fine-needle puncture. In theory sonographically conspicuous but nonpalpable nodes can be biopsied under sonographic guidance. Further indications are suspected recurrence of carcinoma, and clinically and paraclinically suspicious tissue alterations after previous surgery for breast carcinoma, especially in an irradiated area. Suspicious supraclavicular lymph nodes can also be punctured if surgery poses an increased risk. This method is convenient for patients who decline surgical diagnosis or therapy. Puncture is the alternative to sonography if cysts must be differentiated from solid masses.

The nature of any spontaneous discharge from the nipple, pathologic or sanguinous secretion of the lactiferous ducts, or eczematous, discharging, nodular, or ulcerated skin lesion in the nipple and areola area should be clarified cytologically. This is simplified by easy accessibility; however, the presence of keratinized squamous epithelium makes it difficult to obtain representative cells. A good result can be expected in all cases of skin infiltration, e.g., Paget's disease, carcinoma of the nipple, and benign adenoma. Cytologic examination is less suitable for diagnosing inflammatory alterations of the nipple.

Cytology of Breast Cancer

No single cytologic criterion is sufficient to indicate the significance of a lesion. An exact diagnosis is only possible if several criteria of malignancy are found, the following nuclear alterations being of greatest importance (Fig. 3):

1. Hyperchromasia
2. Enlargement

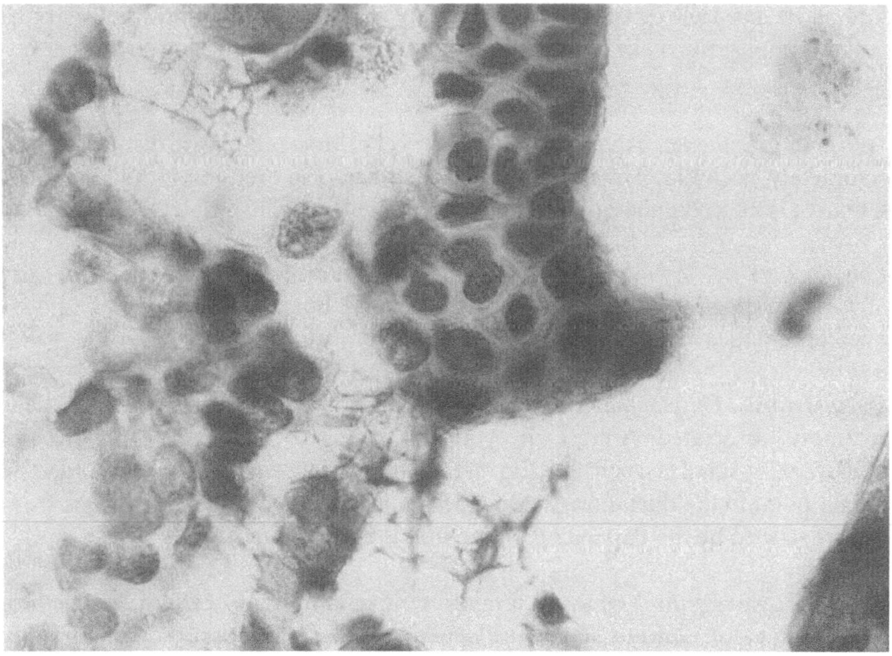

Fig. 3. Criteria of malignancy seen in a ductal invasive carcinoma showing hyperchromasia, enlargement, and polymorphism of nuclei, irregular chromatin pattern, and macronucleoli. (Papanicolaou stain) X 630

3. Polymorphism
4. Irregular chromatin clumping (salt-and-pepper pattern)
5. Macronucleoli
6. Multiple nuclei
7. Mitoses and atypical mitotic figures

Cytoplasmic criteria of malignancy, e.g., alterations in size, form, or nucleus-cytoplasm ratio, are of secondary importance. So-called indirect criteria of malignancy, helpful when scanning the specimen under low magnification are:

1. Dissociation of cancer cells due to loss of intercellular cohesion
2. Abundance of nuclei in specimens containing malignant alterations

Exceptions are puncture biopsies of scirrhous carcinomas, i.e., tumors rich in fibrous tissue. Differentiation, grading, size, and degree of polymorphism of tumor cells can often be assessed nearly as well cytologically as by histology. However, fine-needle puncture does not clarify the histogenesis of a tumor.

Mucinous Carcinoma. Blue - violet mucus is easy to recognize in smears stained by the Papanicolaou method. The cancer cells are isolated or in typical round clusters surrounded by mucus. Signet-ring cells are occasionally seen.

Medullary Carcinoma. These contain a high density of cancer cells, and therefore slides are rich in cells, with extremely dissociated tumor cells. Enlarged, polymorphous and naked tumor nuclei with prominent nucleoli are predominant.

Scirrhous Carcinoma. Almost all cell types occur. Most tumors are distinctly, even completely, acellular. The more marked the fibrosis in the tumor, the less representative is the cell material obtained.

Lobular Invasive Carcinoma. Cytologic diagnosis is difficult because of the density of cancer cells. The tumor cells are dissociated but are uniform and seldom hyperchromatic (Fig. 4).

Ductal Invasive Carcinoma. In smears from undifferentiated forms, the tumor cells are more dissociated. Almost all cytologic criteria of malignancy are present. Occasionally, small cell clusters (Fig. 5) that appear to form lumina surrounded by intima point to the ductal origin (Fig. 6). In these cases cytologic diagnosis from smears stained by the Papanicolaou method is more difficult.

Paget's Disease of the Nipple. In a mixture of squamous epithelium, leukocytes, and inflammatory detritus, Paget's cells stand out clearly because of their markedly enlarged nuclei with coarse-grained chromatin (Fig. 7). Cytologically these tumor cells resemble atypical squamous epithelium, whereas their morphology resembles that of adeno-carcinoma.

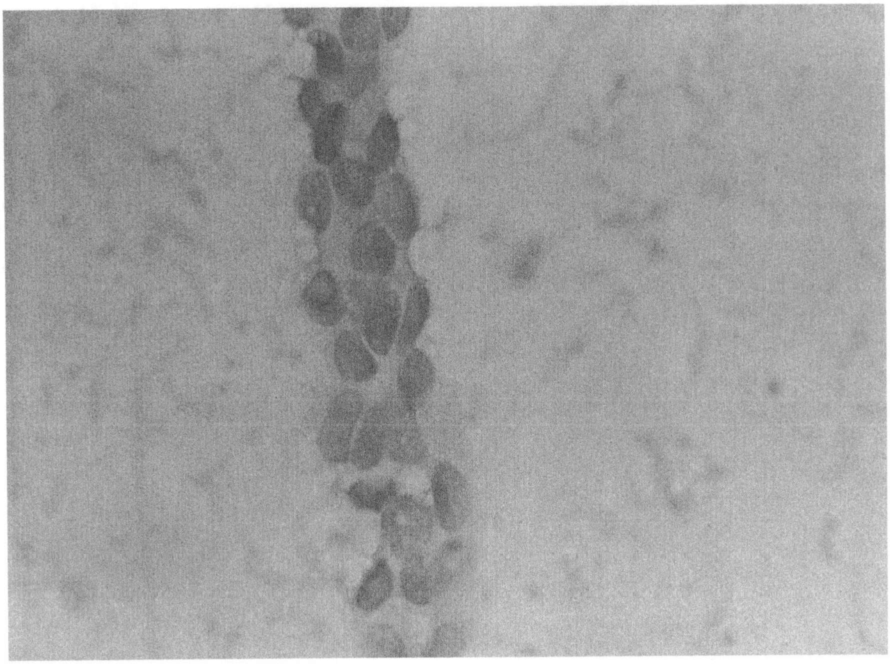

Fig. 4. Uniform normochromatic tumor cells in a tubular arrangement within a lobular invasive carcinoma (Papanicolaou stain) X 630

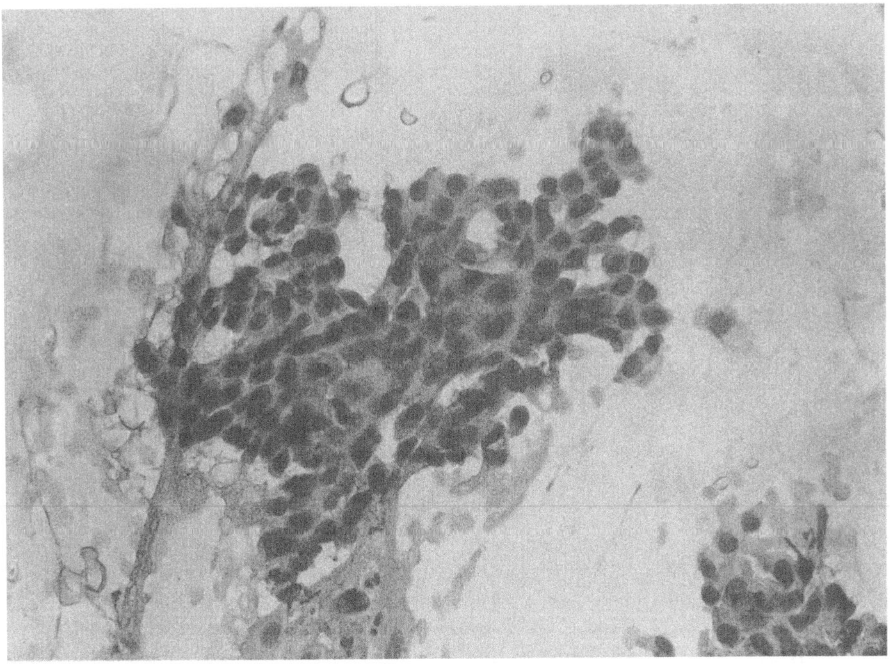

Fig. 5. Cell cluster seen in a poorly differentiated ductal invasive carcinoma (Papanicolaou stain) X 252

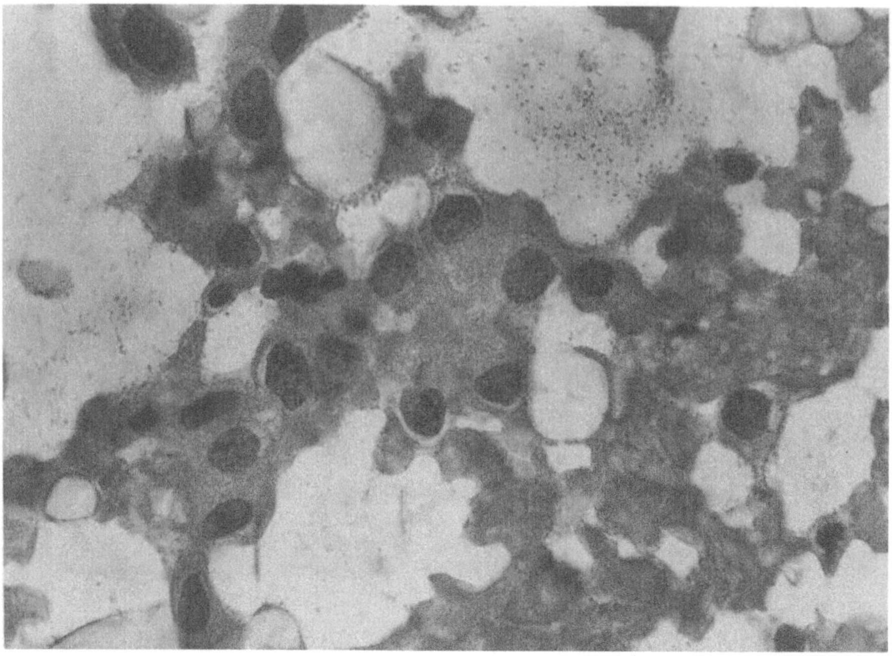

Fig. 6. Ductal invasive carcinoma, showing glandular arrangement of tumor cells in the *center* (Papanicolaou stain) X 630

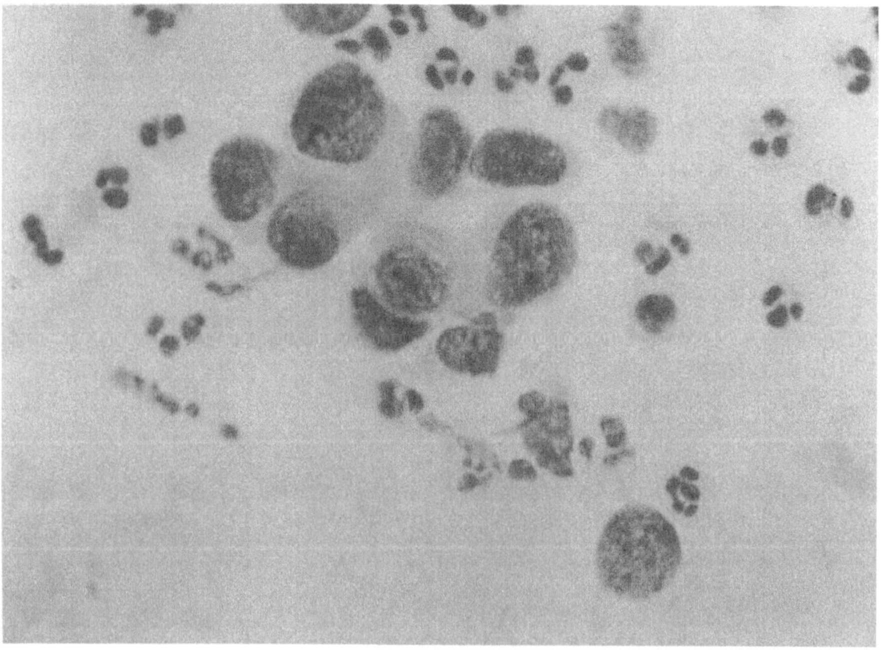

Fig. 7. Paget's disease of the nipple, showing tumor cells with coarse-grained chromatin and prominent nucleoli, surrounded by leukocytes and cell detritus (Papanicolaou stain) X 1050

Intracystic Carcinoma. This diagnosis is made when tumor cells occur together with the usual cell components in fluid obtained by puncture of a cyst. Identification of intracystic malignancies is seldom possible. HOFFKEN [9] discovered only 4 carcinomas in 2100 cytologically examined aspirated specimens, BARTH [2] found 1 carcinoma in 1500 aspirates and KREUZER and BOQUOI [11], 2 in more than 2000 punctured cysts. In our own patient group we found 1 carcinoma in 292 cysts punctured in 1986.

Breast Cancer with Secretion. These are discovered by cytology in about two-thirds of cases [12]. Only 5%–10% of all breast diseases and only 4% of all breast carcinomas are accompanied by pathologic secretions, a fact which influences cytologic results considerably. Cytologic examination of pathologic nipple secretions yields a diagnosis of carcinoma in 2.5% [11]. Summarizing the data from the literature, we found the incidence of carcinoma to be 0%–32%. The probability that a discharge from the nipple is caused by a carcinoma increases with the age of the patient [15]. As a rule, breast cancers are not the cause of pathologic secretions as often as benign breast diseases are, carcinoma being associated in 0.44%–11%, and benign alterations in 6.2%–42% of cases with nipple discharge [7].

Breast Cancer Diagnosed by Exfoliative Cytology. The scanty information available concerning the diagnostic accuracy achieved with exfoliative cytology of the nipple shows relatively frequent cytologic verification of existent carcinomas. Cytologic diagnosis is rather difficult, but because the nipple is so accessible and cell extraction unproblematic, lesions of the skin in the nipple region should be clarified routinely by cytology.

Results

In 1986 about 870 breast punctures were performed and the aspirates, including fluid from cyst punctures, examined cytologically. 239 were examined histologically as well. The patient group comprised 118 with malignancies and 121 with benign alterations of the breast (Table 1). In 58% of the tumors classified as malignant by histology, cytology had been correctly interpreted. In a further 22%,

Table 1. Relationship between histologic and cytologic findings in 239 breast lesions

Cytologic diagnosis	*n*	Histologic diagnosis	
		Malignant	Benign
	239	118 (100%)	121 (100%)
Malignant	68	68 (58%)	0
Suspicious	53	26 (22%)	27 (22.3%)
Benign	118	24 (20%)	94 (77.7%)

n, no. of cases

Table 2. Cytologic results reported by other authors

Author	n	Histo-logically malignant n(%)		Cytologic diagnosis False-positive n(%)		False-negative n(%)	
Bothmann (1974)	114	58	(50.8)	19	(16.6)	5	(8.6)
Eisenberg (1986)	993	665	(67)	0		–	
Furnival (1975)	178	51	(28.6)	5	(4)	2	(4)
Geier (1975)	338	179	(53)	15	(8.4)	15	(9.4)
Kreuzer and Boquoi (1976)	602	247	(41)	4	(1.1)	33	(13.4)
Rummel (1975)	191	116	(60.4)	8	(8.9)	7	(6.0
Schöndorf (1977)	532	333	(62.6)	10	(3.0)	6	(3.0)
Zaijcek (1970)	2077	1068	(51.4)	1	(0.1)	106	(10.5)
Mean			(51.8%)		(5.2%)		(7.8%)

cytology had indicated that the lesion was suspicious. Another 20% of punctures yielded a false-negative result. Cytologic diagnoses reported by other authors are shown in Table 2.

False-positive diagnoses are usually the result of cytologic misinterpretation. This mainly occurs in the following conditions:

1. Proliferative mastopathy
2. Fat necrosis
3. Pregnancy and lactation
4. Papilloma
5. Fibroadenoma

Insufficient material and misinterpretation of malignant cells are the usual causes of false-negative diagnosis. Highly differentiated or small-cell carcinomas are generally involved.

Role of Cytology Breast Diagnosis

Cytology of the breast, especially puncture cytology now occupies a prominent position in breast diagnosis. Together with clinical examination and mammography, it forms the so-called triple diagnostic. Mammography records some of the macroscopic alterations present in malignancy, cytology some of the microscopic ones. Mammography is more accurate in fibrous carcinomas, whereas puncture cytology is more accurate in diagnosing cancers with little fibrosis, medullary carcinomas, and mucous carcinomas. Finally, mammography seldom results in false-negative findings, whereas cytology very rarely yields a false-positive diagnosis.

The practical implications of this are that:

1. Having positive results from all three methods (clinical examination) mammography, and cytology) makes obtaining cryostatic intraoperative section unnecessary, so that surgery can be planned more exactly. In "small therapy" the incision can be marked preoperatively, according to the location of the tumor. Better cosmetic results can be expected.
2. Use of all three diagnostic methods makes many formerly unavoidable biopsies, which impede subsequent radiologic diagnosis, superfluous. However, good results from puncture cytology are only possible if the puncture is performed by well-trained examiners. According to experience, an increasing puncture frequency results in greater accuracy. Cytologic technique and experience play important parts as well.

References

1. Ad hoc Kommission des wissenschaftlichen Beirates der Bundesärztekammer (1980) Metastasenförderung durch diagnostische Gewebsentnahme (Biopsie)? Dtsch Arztebl 22:1460–1467
2. Barth V (1979) Brustdrüse. In: Frommhold W (ed) Röntgen, wie? wann? Thieme, Stuttgart
3. Bothmann G, Rummel HH, Kubli F (1974) Stellung der Aspirationscytologie bei der Frühdiagnose des Mammacarcinoms. Geburtshilfe Frauenheilk 34:287–293
4. Eisenberg AJ, Hajdu SI, Wilhelmus J, et al. (1986) Preoperative aspiration cytology of breast tumours. Acta Cytol Baltimore 30:135–146
5. Furnival CM, Hughes HE, Hocking MA, Reid MMW, Blumgart LH (1975) Aspiration cytology in breast cancer, its relevance to diagnosis. Lancet II: 446–449
6. Geier G, Schuhmann R, Kraus H (1975) Mammapunktionscytologie. Beitr Pathol 156:223–225
7. Gregl A (1979) Farbatlas der Galaktographie: Klinische, radiologische Symptomatik und Therapie der sezernierenden Brust. Schattauer, Stuttgart
8. Gros C, Gautherie M, Bourjat P, Girardie J (1972) Necessity of complementary investigation methods for early diagnosis of breast cancer. Arch Geschwulstforsch 39:304–314
9. Höffken W (1978) Diagnostik und Therapie isolierter Cysten in der Mamma. Gynakol Prax 2:427–438
10. Kreuzer G, Boquoi E (1976) Aspiration biopsy cytology, mammography and clinical exploration: A modern set up in diagnosis of tumors of the breast. Acta Cytol Baltimore 20:319–324
11. Kreuzer G, Boquoi E (1981) Cytologie der weiblichen Brustdrüse. Thieme, Stuttgart
12. Ries P (1976) Cytodiagnostik der weiblichen Brustdrüse. In: Soost H-J (ed) Lehrbuch der klinischen Cytodiagnostik. Thieme, Stuttgart
13. Rummel HH, Bothmann G, Kubli F (1975) Die Stellung der Aspirationscytologie bei der Frühdiagnose des Mammacarcinoms. Dtsch Arztebl 72:2532–2534
14. Schöndorf H (1977) Die Aspirationscytologie der Brustdrüse. Schattauer, Stuttgart
15. Seltzer MH, Perloff LJ, Kelley RI (1970) The significance of age in patients with nipple discharge. Surg Gynecol Obstet 131:519–521
16. Verhaeghe M, Cornillot M, Herbeau J, Wurtz A, Verhaeghe G (1959) Le triple diagnostic cyto-radio-clinique dans les tumeurs du sein. Mem Acad Chir 95:48–61
17. Zaijcek J, Caspersson T, Jakobsson P, et al. (1979) Cytologic diagnosis of mammary tumors from aspiration biopsy smears. I. Comparison of cytologic and histologic findings in 2111 lesions and use of cytophotometry. Acta Cytol Baltimore 14:370–382

III. Primary Treatment

Growth Behavior and Implications for Staging and Therapy

D. VON FOURNIER

Breast Cancer as a Primarily Loco-regional Disease

In accordance with the concept of breast cancer as a primarily loco-regional disease, a type of therapy was developed that quickly became linked with the names of HALSTED (1894), STEINTHAL (1905) and, in the German-speaking countries, ROTTER (1896), and was accepted throughout the world for many years.

From the middle of the nineteenth century onward, the vast majority of surgeons saw breast cancer as a disease that first spread locally and then formed metastases step by step throughout the body, spreading initially by way of the lymph nodes and later via the lymph vessels and blood vessels. For this reason, it seemed essential to use the most radical techniques possible in the performance of corrective surgery.

Therefore the Halsted-Rotter operation, as it is called in the German-speaking countries, was the surgical technique most frequently applied in the treatment of breast cancer throughout the world for more than 80 years, from 1890 (HALSTED 1894) until about 1970. HALSTED published his treatment strategy after a trip to Europe, where he found that some aspects of his technique of loco-regional surgery had already been developed by various Central European surgeons who were practicing it in different forms. DE MOULIN (1983) noted that the Halsted-Rotter principle represented a synthesis of the knowledge current among leading Central European and North American authors between 1850 and 1894 (Table 1).

Only 10 days after the appearance of HALSTED's publication, MEYER [28,29] a German born surgeon in New York, published an almost identical operative technique, which makes it obvious that the HALSTED-ROTTER strategy was rooted in the international medical thinking of that time. We are indebted to Halsted for integrating the empirical observations recorded by the leading surgeons of the day to yield a therapeutic concept that was logical in its context. At the same time, he proved that this concept represented a step forward: in his patient population he achieved the highest rate of freedom from loco-regional recurrence and also the seemingly highest survival rate which was not reconfirmed later on [Table 1] among all contemporary authors (see Table 1).

The clinical classification system devised by STEINTHAL (Stuttgart, 1905) also shows that even then a clear and logical dependence of the prognosis on the size of the tumor, the lymph node involvement and the speed of growth had been recognized. This classification was widely used, especially in German-speaking countries, until about 1970. In many countries, especially in the United States of America, the Columbia Clinical Classification was introduced increasingly and

Table 1. The historical development of radical mastectomy and the 3-year cure rates achieved. (After DE MOULIN 1983)

Type of operation	Author	Year	No. of cases	Three-year cure rate (%)
Partial or complete mastectomy with or without removal of pectoral fascia and axillary nodes	Winiwarter (Billroth)	1867–1875	143	4.7
Complete mastectomy and axillary dissection in most cases	Oldekop (Esmarch, Kiel)	1850–1878	220	11.7
	Dietrich (Lücke, Strasbourg)	1872–1890	148	16.2
	Horner (Krönlein, Zürich)	1881–1893	144	19.4
	Poulsen (Copenhagen)	1870–1888	110	19.4
	Banks (Liverpool)	1877	46	20
	Schmid (Küster, Berlin)	1871–1885	228	21.5
			Average:	18.1
Complete mastectomy, axillary dissection, removal of pectoral facia and varying amount of pectoral muscle	Sprengel (Volkmann, Halle)	1874–1878	200	11
	Schmidt (Czerny, Heidelberg)	1877–1886	112	18.8
	Rotter (Bergmann, Berlin)		30	20
	Mahler (Czerny, Heidelberg)	1887–1897	150	21
	Joerss (Helferich, Greifswald)	1885–1893	98	28.5
			Average:	19.9
Modern radical mastectomy	Halsted	1889–1894	76	45[1)]
	Halsted	1907	232	38.3
	Meyer	1894		
	Rotter	1896		

[1)] For comments on the relevance of this result see W.L. DONEGAN and J.S. SPRATT (1988) Cancer of the Breast, Saunders: pp 4–10.

with modifications (Cooley) from 1943 onward [17,18]. In 1961, the International Union Against Cancer (UICC) started publishing the TNM staging system for breast cancer, influenced by Denoix of Paris more than anyone else. This classification system has been subject to continuous improvement and updating ever since, and is now accepted by most therapists. Even the TNM system, albeit more detailed, ultimately reflects Steinthal's realization that the prognosis of the tumor is closely correlated with the loco-regional extension and metastasis. It is a more precise system for description of tumor spread, but does not take account of tumor biology.

Leading experts in breast oncology are now tending to the opinion that it is the biological properties of the breast cancer cells that dictate the clinical course in the individual case. It must be borne in mind that the TNM stage at diagnosis is largely a consequence of the tumor biology; the pattern of loco-regional spread and occult metastasis has been determined for some years, before the initial diagnosis is made.

Breast Cancer as a Primarily Disseminated Disease

The concept of breast cancer as a primarily disseminated disease has been strongly influenced by B. FISHER et al. [13], NISSEN-MEYER et al. [32] and BONADONNA et al. [3,4], among many others. In a review entitled "What Is 'Early Breast Cancer'?", E. FISHER [14] stated: "... operable breast cancer in a large proportion of instances is already a systemic disease".

These authors are becoming more and more convinced that breast cancer is usually already a systemic disease at the time of first diagnosis and that consequently the survival rate can hardly be influenced by loco-regional treatment variations. This opinion is supported by a retrospective comparison of untreated patients from the Middlesex Hospital (1805–1933) with those figuring in Halsted's original report [21,24]. As shown in Fig. 1, the survival curves for the two patient groups are similar, so Halsted's radical surgery apparently did not lead to any impressive increase in survival rates. It should be noted that the primary tumors were in advanced stages before surgery. Compared with untreated patients, Halsted achieved only a limited improvement in survival, but an impressive improvement in local control (LEWIS and REINHOFF 1932). Evidently, this improved local control led to the widespread acceptance of the Halsted operation.

The new concept of breast cancer as a primarily systemic disease has also derived support from a study comparing radical mastectomy with and without radiotherapy. The loco-regional recurrence rates differed according to local treatment, while overall survival (OAS) was the same 10 years later [13].

The proportion of lymph nodes that are positive in unscreened women with breast cancer is now over 50% on average. This reflects cell dissemination as well as indicating a host-tumor relationship that permits the growth of metastasized tumor cells.

BRINKLEY and HAYBITTLE [5,6] estimated on the basis of long-term studies that only about 18% of all breast cancer patients, and only about 30% of those with stage I or II disease, are still alive after more than 25 years of follow up. This supports the concept of breast cancer as a primarily disseminated disease, at least in advanced stages, over this observation period (Fig. 2). It is interesting to compare the following breast cancer survival curves: (1) untreated cases from 1805–1933 [$n=250$; BLOOM et al. 1962] (Fig. 1a); (2) treated cases from 1947–1950 ($n=704$; BRINKLEY et al. [6]) (see Fig. 1b); (3) treated cases with tumor sizes of 1 cm, 2 cm and 3 cm at time of first treatment [11] (Fig. 13, page 91). It can be assumed that:

I. Local treatment of breast cancer seems to lead to better survival than no treatment.

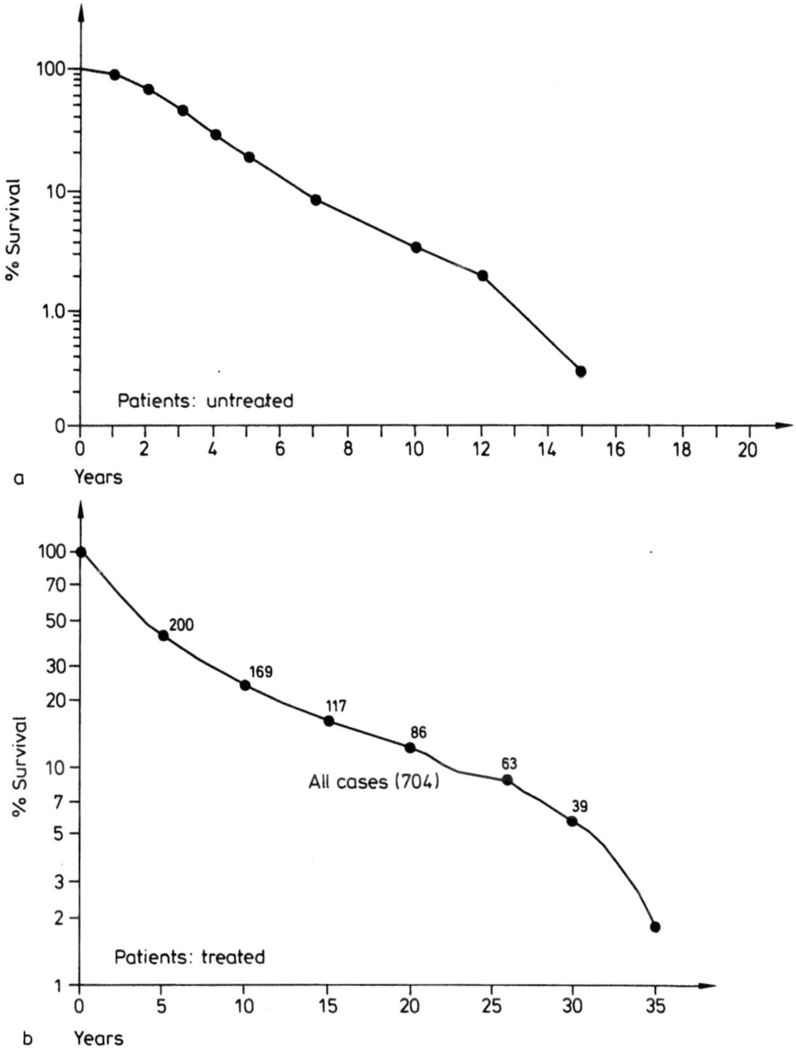

Fig. 1a,b. Survival curves of patients with breast cancer. **a** Untreated patients ($n=250$), Middlesex Hospital, 1805–1933 (BLOOM et al. 1962); **b** Treated patients ($n=704$), Cambridge, 1947–1950 (BRINKLEY and HAYBITTLE 1984). Source J.R. HARRIS et al. (1987), Breast Diseases, Lippincott, pp 234–235

II. The smaller the tumor at therapy, the better the long-term survival, with the following exceptions: In some cases "early detection" may not influence survival (lead time bias). Screening will tend to detect the slower growing rather than the faster growing tumors (length-time bias) and so to separate patients with a more favorable prognosis from those with a less favorable prognosis.

If the modern concept of the presence of predominantly systemic tumor spread at the time of primary therapy is correct, an adequate systemic therapy adminis-

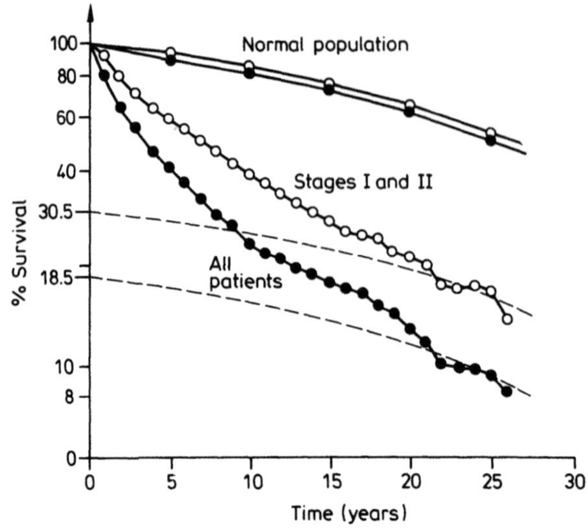

Fig. 2. Survival for breast cancer patients compared with normal population of same age distribution. [5]

tered at the same time as the primary therapy might be expected to lead to an increase in the complete cure rate. The concept of systemic therapy in the form of hormonal therapy (oophorectomy or ovarian irradiation) was in fact the subject of a randomized study at the Christie Hospital in Manchester initiated in 1948 [8], and there have been other randomized trials on this since. After 5–15 years of follow-up, the survival rate was 5% better. Significant improvements in OAS were observed only in premenopausal women and only in a few studies (Toronto trial with 7.5 mg prednisone; MEAKIN et al. 1983). It is important to realize that in one study (Saskatchewan trial; BRYANT and WEIR 1981), the 10-year survival rate was 11% higher ($p < 0.05$) in patients who had undergone oophorectomy than in controls. Thus, the improvement in survival rate was comparable to that achieved by NISSEN-MEYER et al. [32] and NISSEN-MEYER and KJELLGREN [30] with adjuvant chemotherapy.

That the elimination of ovarian function in premenopausal women prevents the growth of breast cancer has recently been confirmed by an international study on women who had had radiotherapy for cervical carcinoma (BOICE et al. 1988), this volume. If we assume that breast cancer starts developing in women at the age of 35 years on average [15], there were two possible effects of radiologic castration: either the formation of cancer was prevented, or the growth of occult early stages into clinically detectable tumors was reduced. Figure 3 shows the improvement in survival with oophorectomy compared with controls [7].

The following prospective studies on adjuvant chemotherapy were of special importance for the concept of breast cancer as a primarily disseminated disease: B. FISHER et al. [12] treated patients with thio-TEPA between 1958 and 1961; NISSEN-MEYER et al. [32] prescribed cyclophosphamide for 6 days perioperatively between 1965 and 1975; BONADONNA et al. [3] administered CMF over 12 months between 1973 and 1975. All of these and other studies showed a significant

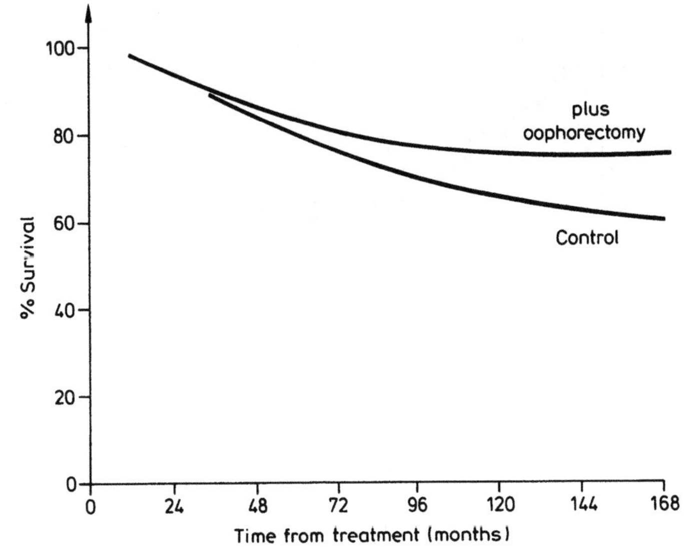

Fig. 3. Survival rate after mastectomy plus oophorectomy ($n = 182$) compared with mastectomy alone (*control;* $n = 177$). (From BRYANT and WEIR 1981) Source J.R. HARRIS et al. (1987), Breast Diseases, Lippincott, p 326

improvement in disease-free survival (DFS) and OAS, especially in subgroups of premenopausal women. The constancy of results reported by NISSEN-MEYER et al. [32] is quite impressive: significant differences in OAS after 15 years and after 20 years, with about 10% more survivors (Fig. 4).

Thus the concept of early dissemination was indirectly proved by the therapeutic success in a limited number of patients. On the whole, however, the results of systemic cytotoxic adjuvant therapy, seen in relation to its side effects, have been disappointing, except in premenopausal women with one to three positive lymph nodes.

The limited nature of the effect of any adjuvant therapy may be due to the following facts:

1. In premenopausal women chemotherapy seems to work partly by the castration effect, which is still to be proved in prospective trials.
2. The tumor burden seems to be so large in the majority of patients treated (patients with many positive lymph nodes) that, in the long term, survival cannot be further improved by chemotherapy.
3. The majority of tumors display long-term resistance to all chemotherapeutic combinations used so far. For this reason, in the situation of first metastatic relapse (large tumor burden), no increase in 7-year-survival by chemotherapy has been definitely proved so far. POWLES (1988) (23) showed that 7-year-survival curves after the first relapse are very similar with no chemotherapy (pre-1974 in Fig. 5), a mild form of chemotherapy (1974–1979 in Fig. 5) or a more aggressive form of multidrug chemotherapy (1980- in Fig. 5). From this it becomes clear that even in the adjuvant phase (smaller tumor burden), chemotherapy is rarely able to improve long-term survival.

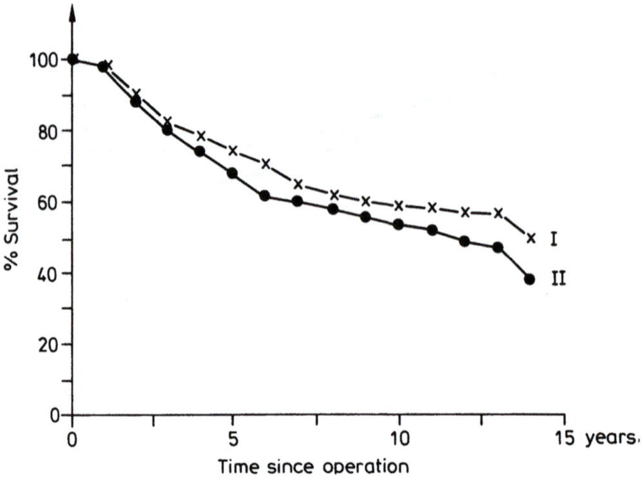

Fig. 4. Fifteen-year survival rate in patients with perioperative adjuvant chemotherapy (Cytoxan, 6 days). *II* Control group without chemotherapy. The 15-year survival (and also the 20-year survival) was significantly better in patients with chemotherapy in the Scandinavian trial. (From NISSEN-MEYER et al. 1984, 1986) Source J.R. HARRIS et al. (1987), Breast Diseases, Lippincott, p 329

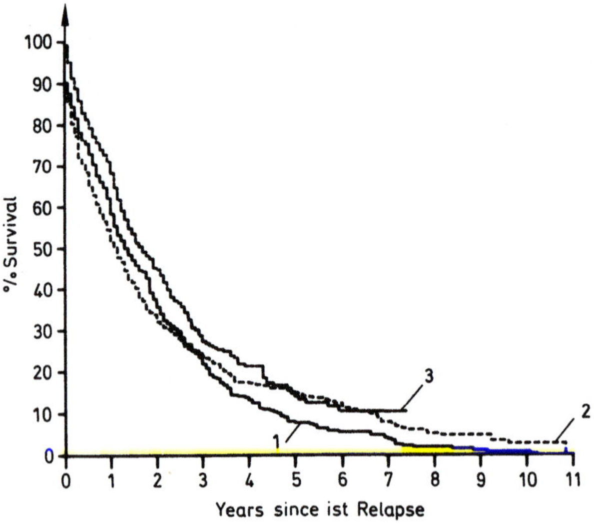

Fig. 5. Survival curves (probability of survival) in breast cancer patients with first relapse followed by *1* no chemotherapy (before 1974); *2* chemotherapy with low toxicity (1974–1979); *3* multiple-drug chemotherapy (1980 onward). The survival curves for 10 years observation time apparently do not differ. (From POWLES 1988)

"Biologic Predeterminism" in Relation to the Growth Behavior of Individual Breast Cancers

Important papers on the concept of biologic predeterminism in relation to breast cancer growth have been appearing for some decades [9,16,33,39,41]. Studies on prognostic factors lend continuously more credence to this concept. Significant studies by authors subscribing to concepts 1 and 2 also lend support to the idea of biological predeterminism, however, as their results can be better explained in this light. This concept is still developing piece by piece as our knowledge of the clinical behavior of breast cancer increases.

In summary, the basic tenets of this concept so far are as follows. It is not rare for carcinoma of the breast to develop polycentrically or bilaterally. With a few exceptions (perhaps inflammatory carcinoma) the disease first goes through the phase of carcinoma in situ and then through the early invasive phase. Even in the early invasive phase, mammary carcinoma is initially localized and grows without metastasizing, so that it can theoretically still be cured by local radical treatment. Metastatic dissemination does not start until a certain tumor size is reached, and depends on individual tumor cell biology. The "malignant potential" for metastatic dissemination is reflected in the various prognostic factors known so far, all of which are different forms of expression of the same tumor characteristic (potential for metastasis). Thus, all factors that correlate closely with the prognosis must naturally also correlate with each other.

Some factors with a high prognostic value are histological grading, number of positive axillary lymph nodes, mitosis rate and S-phase fraction, receptor content, growth rate, ploidy, proliferation rate and labeling index (LI), and oncogene expression and/or amplification. These factors can be classified as markers of *metastatic potential* or markers of *tumor response* (Table 2).

The (measurable) natural speed of growth is by far the most unequivocal parameter of malignancy, because it makes the tumor's malignant potency directly apparent on clinical examination (palpable tumor) or directly visible in X-ray pictures. The natural speed of growth observed allows predictions concerning the later clinical course of each individual tumor (within the margins of error). If these predictions later prove accurate this lends further credence to the concept of biological predeterminism of the individual breast carcinoma. Evidence of disease (EOD), growth rate and death are unequivocal signs of malignant potency (Fig. 6).

According to this concept, fast-growing tumors metastasize while quite small (diameter 1–5 mm, for example), whereas with more slowly growing tumors metastatic dissemination does not begin until they are quite large on average (range of diameter: 1–3 cm). This means that every invasive carcinoma has a metastasis-free early phase in which early diagnosis could theoretically mean the possibility of cure.

The concept of biological predeterminism involves the statement that the long-term survival rate is improved more effectively by early diagnosis than by any other means known so far, despite the possibilities of length-time and lead-time bias. In keeping with this, DUNCAN and KERR [11] found that after 20 years of

Table 2. Factors influencing outcome in breast cancer and their prognostic relevance

FACTOR				**Prognostic relevance**
Oncogene amplification	Not amplified	In between	Amplified	
Growth factor receptors	Negative	Fairly low	Positive	As yet undetermined
Nuclear grade	Good	Fairly good	Poor	Low
Histological findings	No invasion of blood/lymphatic vessels	–	Invasion of bloody/lymphatic vessels	
Ploidy	Diploid		Polyploid	
Histological grading	Well differentiated	Fairly well differentiated	Poorly differentiated	
Hormone receptor content	ER and PR very high ($\geq$ 300 fmol)	ER and PR fairly high ($\geq$ 100 fmol)	ER and PR low/negative ($\leq$ 10 fmol)	
LI	Low	Fairly low	High	High
S-phase rate (mitotic rate)	Low ($<$ 2%)	2–9%	$>$ 10%	
Lymph nodes	Negative	One to nine positive	Ten or more positive	
Doubling time (growth rate)	$>$ 500 days	51–499 days	$\leq$ 50 days	
Size	$\leq$ 0.5 (minimal cancer)	0.6–3.5 cm	T4	
Cure	Probable	Questionable	Unlikely	

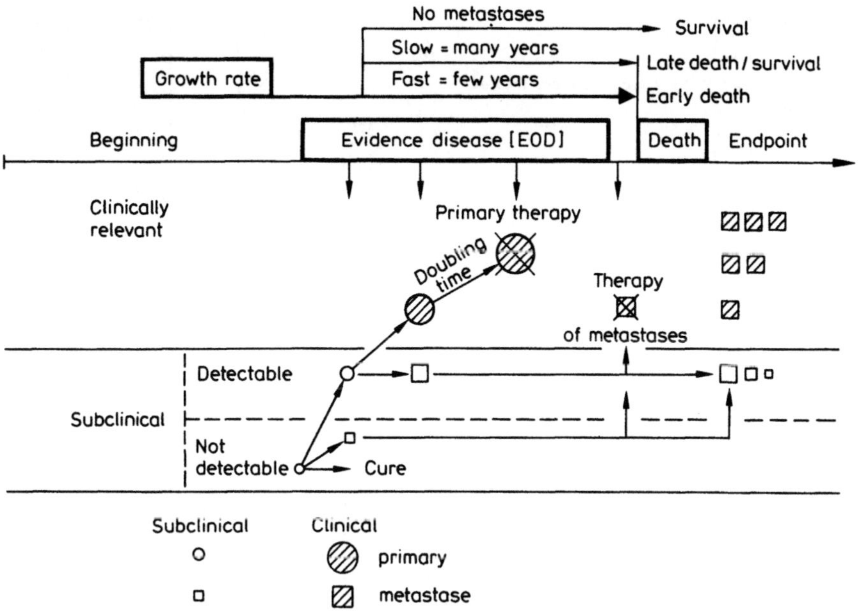

Fig. 6. Unequivocal signs of malignant potency: evidence of disease, growth rate and death

follow-up patients with tumors 1 cm in diameter had survived in a distinctly greater proportion of cases than patients with tumors 2 cm in diameter at the time of therapy. The concept demands the safest possible loco-regional care, since even in the presence of some quite large (i.e., slowly growing) tumors metastasis will not have started in some cases. Since the speed of growth of the metastases and that of the primary tumor correlate with each other, it is possible to forecast the duration of survival to be expected on the basis of the observed speed of growth (within the margins of error): with fast-growing tumors the remaining life expectancy will be short, with slowly growing tumors, long. Life expectancy can be extended in the case of tumors that are susceptible to chemotherapy or hormone therapy, primarily because such therapy slows down the growth rate. Cure may be achieved in a few case (see Fig. 6).

Since chemotherapy has hardly and influence on survival once distant metastases have arisen (POWLES 1988), the concept of biological predeterminism also explains the rather small effect of adjuvant chemotherapy on long-term survival. It also makes it clear why patients die of breast cancer even after an interval of 15–20 years. Most patients in earlier follow-up studies already had advanced tumors, and therefore distant metastases, at the time of the primary operation. The slow growth in many patients explains the long survival times despite the presence of metastases (N pos.). Patients in whom tumor growth was monitored by serial mammographies were on average 58 years old when their tumors were 2 cm in diameter. They had been an average of 35 years old at the beginning of breast cancer growth [15] (Fig. 8), which makes it obvious that different degrees of radicality and different adjuvant regimens had led to similar survival rates.

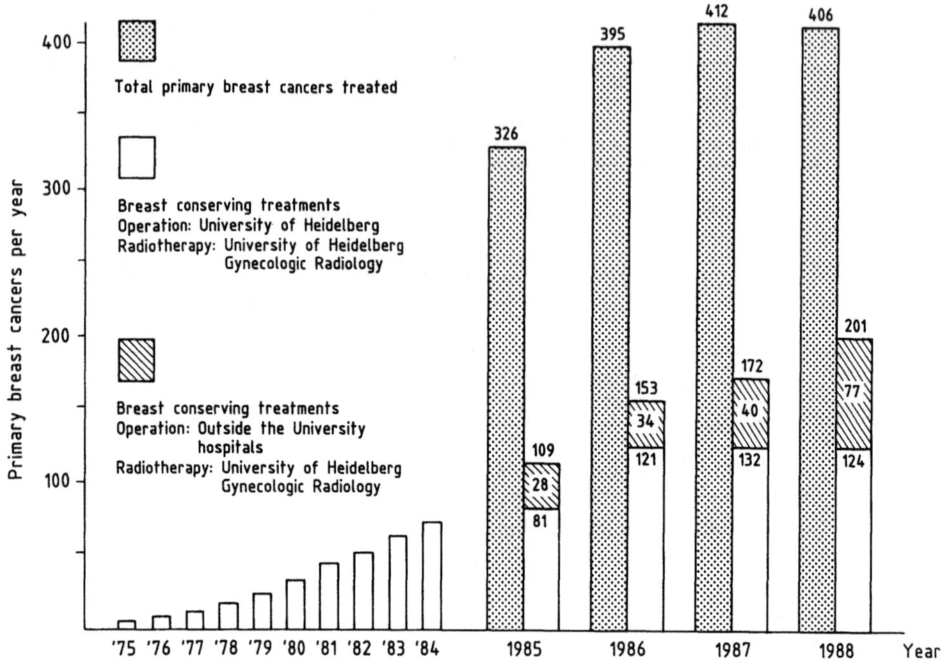

Fig. 7. Increase of Breast Conserving Therapy (BCT) between 1974 and 1988 of the University of Heidelberg

It is implicit to this concept that only limited improvement in long-term cure rates will be possible as long as no effective form of therapy has been established for metastases. The facts of the growth behavior of breast carcinoma explain why the concept of a primarily systemic disease has met with general acceptance. The acceptance of "biologic predeterminism" has led to a rapid increase in breast-conserving therapies, see Fig. 7.

The concept of biological predeterminism, however, suggests that mass screening might now allow survival and definitive cure following detection of some types of tumor, mainly those with primarily slow growth. Screening will hardly influence the survival rate in fast-growing tumors, which can potentially spread metastases even at the smallest detectable size.

Furthermore, this concept explains why, particularly in the more slowly growing tumors, loco-regional cure is imperative to prevent the persistence of residual tumor or multicentric tumors ("second primaries") which could potentially metastasize later on. This explains how insufficient loco-regional radicality in breast-conserving therapy may result in a reduction in survival, as has for instance been observed following inadequate irradiation [20].

This concept intimates that, owing to the wide range of speed of growth, there must be a large number of extremely slowly growing occult preinvasive and invasive breast cancers that do not reach a clinically detectable size during the host's lifetime. Screening for early diagnosis is revealing such early cancers – referred to as "academic cancers" – with increasing frequency. Important confirmation was

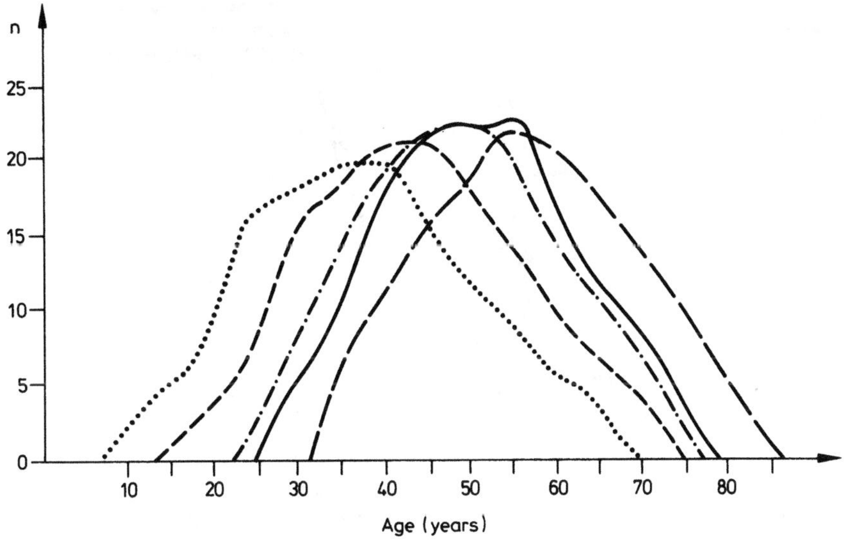

Fig. 8. Frequency distribution of estimated ages at tumor diameters of 0.01 mm (....), 0.1 mm (----), 1 mm (-.-.-), 2 mm (———) and 20 mm (— — —) (From VON FOURNIER et al. 1985)

provided by ANDERSEN et al. [1] who found invasive or in situ carcinoma of the breast in 21 (25.4%) of the 83 autopsies performed on women in 1 year in the Danish county of Ribe. The lifelong cumulated incidence of invasive breast cancer in this county was 9.4%. Thus, it is estimated that two thirds of occult breast cancers never develop to a clinically detectable size.

Finally, the concept explains the increase in breast carcinoma incidence with increasing age (Fig. 9): slowly growing tumors appear clinically at a rate which increases exponentially with age in older patients while the period in which the tumor originates probably covers a much shorter period of life. This leads to the conclusion that there are only differences of degree between premenopausal and postmenopausal breast cancers: Premenopausal carcinomas grow under the influence of cyclic estrogenic and progestogenic stimulation, while postmenopausal carcinomas "emerge" clinically when the hormonal stimulus is lacking. The latter, therefore, can be influenced more frequently by hormonal therapy, e.g., with anti-estrogens. According to this concept, postmenopausal primary carcinomas might be expected to grow more slowly with increasing age. Nevertheless, the average time between first diagnosis and death from the tumor in older patients can be even shorter than in premenopausal women: in slowly growing primary tumors, the metastases have also had long periods of growth up to the date of diagnosis. The growth behavior of the metastases is generally similar to that of the primary tumor; in the course of time, however, growth accelerates increasingly because of the selection of faster-growing metastatic cells.

As far as the consequences for the patients are concerned, the concept of biological predeterminism differs only slightly from the concept of breast cancer as a primarily disseminated disease. However, it explains empirical phenomena of

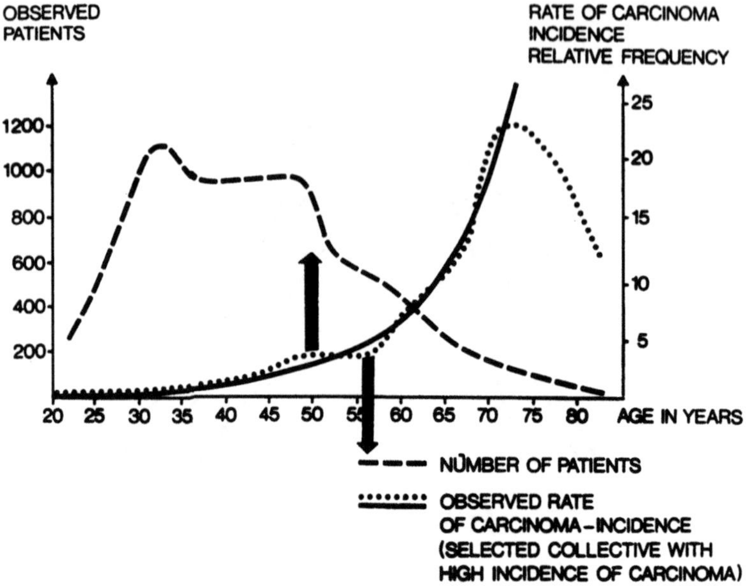

Fig. 9. Age-related incidence of breast cancer in a selection of patients at very high risk of breast cancer. The incidence displays a strictly exponential increase with increasing age. Note the slight increase before and decrease after the menopause (*arrows*). — — —, number of patients; ......, incidence of breast cancer

breast carcinoma more precisely and provides a rational basis for more individualized treatment depending on the biological behavior of the particular tumor. The most important implication is the necessity for early detection by screening.

Data Underlying the Concept of Biologic Predeterminism Based on Variable Speed of Growth

The work of a few authors who have influenced the still developing concept of biological predeterminism will be discussed briefly at this point:

1. STEINTHAL [41] included in stage I the tumors which were "slowly growing", in addition to having other qualities of a small, unextended tumor with clinically free lymph nodes.
2. COLLINS et al. [9] presumed an exponential model for tumor growth and observed lung metastases of breast carcinomas in 24 patients in serial chest X-rays. They noted great heterogeneity of individual tumors, with doubling times ranging from 28 to 164 days (median 78 days). For a rather fast growing primary tumor with a doubling time of 100 days, they estimated that the time required for growth from the first malignant cell to the clinically detectable size of 1 cm would be more than 8 years.

3. GERSHON-COHEN et al. [16] were the first to observe the growth of primary breast cancer on serial mammograms, in 18 patients. They noted a very wide variation in the speed of growth of the primaries, with doubling times ranging from 23 to 209 days. They, too, formulated the concept of biologic predeterminism in breast carcinoma.
4. SPRATT and SPRATT [38,40] summarized the data relating to growth of the primary tumor and its metastases and established exponential growth in breast carcinoma on the basis of comprehensive data in the literature. They were the first to describe the speed of growth of breast cancer as the most important prognostic factor, exerting more influence on the course of the disease than any therapeutic procedure.
5. PEARLMAN [34] estimated the doubling time on the basis of scar recurrence after mastectomy. Patients whose recurrent tumor had a doubling time of less than 25 days (53%) had a 5-year survival rate of 5%, whereas in the case of slowly growing relapses with a doubling time of over 75 days (15%) the 5-year survival rate was 100%.
6. TUBIANA and MALAISE [43] and TUBIANA and KOSCIELNY (1988) found a cell cycle in breast cancer of around 2 days, a growth fraction of 5% and "cell loss factor" in the range of 75%. Slow tumor growth over many years becomes understandable when it is known that the majority of cancer cells are not involved in cell division (resting cells) and that a high percentage of new cells perish daily.
7. KOSCIELNY et al. [22] examined the relation between the size of the primary tumor at operation and the probability of later metastatic spread, with a follow-up of 10 to over 25 years. They found a linear correlation (log normal distribution), with a median tumor diameter of 3.6 cm. At this size, 50% of the tumors had not metastasized during the follow-up period. Accordingly, clinically relevant metastatic spread in 50% of patients does not begin until the tumor reaches a palpable size, contradicting the concept of breast cancer as a primarily system disease.
8. FOURNIER et al. [15] found that the volume doubling time shows a log normal distribution in clinically relevant primary tumors, with 27% of carcinomas growing fast (doubling time less than 150 days), 39% exhibiting medium-fast growth (doubling time 150–300 days) and 33% displaying slow growth (doubling time more than 300 days). He showed correlations between growth rate, S-phase rate, mitotic rate, ploidy, grading and, especially, frequency of metastatic spread. See page 76–94, this volume.
9. Following mass screening by mammography, LUNDGREN [25] found 5-year survival rates of 14% for very fast-growing tumors (doubling time less than 30 days); 60% for tumors with doubling times between 30 and 90 days and 100% for tumors with doubling times of more than 90 days.

TUBIANA [42,44] found a threshold volume (in experimental tumors) at which the first metastasis is initiated for every single type of tumor. As mentioned above the prognostic factors correlate well between each other: For instance, the thymidine labelling index (LI) correlates significantly with the histopathological grading

(Kusama, 1972; Meyer, 1986). Patients with a low LI showed a 6-year relapse-free survival of 80% and patients with a high LI of 60% (Silvestrini, 1985).

TUBIANA [42] found that the low incidence of relapse in low LI subgroups cannot be explained merely by different rates of growth, but also partly by differences in the metastasizing probability of the cancer cells.

Staging of Breast Cancer in Correlation to Prognostic Factors

The staging of breast cancer has two main aims:

1. The stage of anatomical extension of the tumor should be described because it directly determines the possibilities and limits of an operative technique. If local surgery is no longer possible, alternative procedures of treatment as a first step must be considered: primary radiotherapy or chemotherapy for example.
2. Preoperative staging is today routinely supplemented by a postoperative staging mostly with the TNM classification. Postoperative staging indicates the actual histological tumor extension, particularly in the area of the axillary lymph nodes. Further therapy, e.g. adjuvant chemotherapy, adjuvant hormonal therapy, adjuvant radiotherapy, currently depends on tumor size, involvement of lymph nodes as well as further established prognostic factors.

Apart from the classic factors, in the meanwhile further prognostic factors are established (see Kaufmann, this volume). So it seems useful for the future to integrate these factors in a postoperative tumor classification which combines the old patho-anatomical findings with the new biological expression of the tumor. Not all prognostic factors known today can be used for staging yet.

Some prognostic factors (e.g. growth rate) can often not be directly obtained by serial mammographies. The indirect estimation of the growth rate using the LI-assay is a limited method because it does not reflect the host factor. An extension of staging with prognostic factors is only useful if it has new consequences for the therapeutical procedure compared with the staging systems (TNM) used so far. At present, the following parameters can give substantial information for a useful staging:

1st group: Good prognosis, definite cure possible

Anatomic extension, prognostic criteria	*Therapeutic consequences*
– small tumor – very slowly growing tumor (doubling time over 300 days)	– every type of standard operation leads to local cure in most cases
– histologically not affected lymph nodes	– breast-conserving therapy is possible with low risk
– diploid – grading I	– local radicality and adjuvant therapies have little impact on survival

- low LI
- receptor content: high

- cure through early detection possible

Percentage of these patients: small (less than 20%) in historical collectives

2nd group: uncertain prognosis, on average relatively long, relapse free survival

Prognostic criteria
- small, fast-growing tumors *or*
- slowly growing or very slowly growing medium-sized and large tumors
- not affected or only few affected lymph nodes
- grading II
- Medium to high LI
- medium to high S-phase-fraction [4%–8%]
- aneuploid DNA-index
- frequently prevailing occult metastases

Therapeutical consequences
- loco-regional radicality is necessary
- possible cure of a small part of tumors by local eradication and adjuvant therapy
- insufficient local radicality in some tumors shortens survival
- receptor status and age dependent adjuvant therapies improve relapse free interval and to some extent also survival
- breast-conserving therapy possible
- no long-term cure in the majority of the cases because of occult metastases

Percentage of these patients: high. The prognosis depends strongly on the tumor size

3rd group: poor prognosis, no curative therapy

Prognostic criteria
- large, inoperable tumors
- very fast-growing tumors (doubling time less than 50 days)
- locally inoperable or inflammatory carcinoma
- subtotally or totally affected lymph nodes
- receptor content: low
- DNA-index: aneuploid
- grading III
- S-phase fraction more than 8%
- high LI-index

Therapeutic consequences
- no operative or other primary treatment technique cures.
- every therapy is palliativc
- a prolongation of survival by additional therapies is limited
- occult or apparent metastases in each case
- predominant are quality of life and control of the tumor at the chest wall
- screening for early detection is not possible

References

1. Andersen JA, Nielsen M, Jensen J (1985) Essential histological findings in the female breast at autopsy. In: Zander J, Baltzer J (eds) Early breast cancer. Springer, Berlin Heidelberg New York, pp 52–63
2. Boice J et al. (1988) Radiation dose and second cancer risk in patients treated for cancer of the cervix. JNCI : -
3. Bonadonna D, Valagussa P, Rossi A (1985a) Ten-year experience with CMF-based adjuvant chemotherapy in resectable breast cancer. Breast Cancer Res Treat 5:95–115
4. Bonadonna G, Rossi A, Valagussa P (1985b) Adjuvant CMF chemotherapy in operable breast cancer. Ten years later. World J Surg 9:707–713
5. Brinkley D, Haybittle JL (1977) The curability of breast cancer. World J Surg 1:287
6. Brinkley D, Haybittle JL (1984) Long-term survival of women with breast cancer. Lancet 1:1118
7. Bryant AJ, Weir JA (1981) Prophylactic oophorectomy in operable instances of carcinoma of the breast. Surg Gynecol Obstet 153:660–664
8. Cole MP (1975) A clinical trial of an artificial menopause in carcinoma of the breast. Inserm 55:143–150
9. Collins V, Loeffler RK, Tivey H (1956) Observations on growth rates of human tumors. Am J Roentgenol 76:988–1000
10. De Moulin D (1983) A short history of breast cancer. Martinus Nijhoff, Boston, p 86
11. Duncan W, Kerr GR (1976) The curability of breast cancer. Br Med J IV:781
12. Fisher B, Slack N, Katrych D (1975) Ten year follow-up results of patients with carcinoma of the breast in a co-operative clinical trial evaluating surgical adjuvant chemotherapy. Surg Gynecol Obstet 140:528–534
13. Fisher B, Redmond C, Fisher ER (1985) Ten-year results of a randomized clinical trial comparing radical mastectomy and total mastectomy with or without radiation. N Engl J Med 312:674
14. Fisher E (1985) What is early breast cancer? In: Zander J, Baltzer J (eds) Early breast cancer. Springer, Berlin Heidelberg New York, pp 1–13
15. Fournier D von, Hoeffken W, Junkermann H, Bauer M, Kühn W (1985) Growth rate of primary mammary carcinoma and its metastases: consequences for early detection and therapy. In: Zander J, Baltzer J (eds) Early breast cancer. Springer, Berlin Heidelberg New York, pp 73–86
16. Gershon-Cohen J, Berger SM, Klickstein HS (1963) Roentgenography of breast cancer moderating concept of "biological predeterminism." Cancer 16:961–964
17. Haagensen CD (1971) Diseases of the breast. Saunders, Philadelphia
18. Haagensen CD (1986) Diseases of the breast, 3rd edn. Saunders, Philadelphia
19. Halsted WS (1907) The results of radical operations for the cure of cancer of the breast. Ann Surg 46:1–19
20. Hayward JL (1985) Trials of wide excision and radiation therapy at the Breast Unit, Guy's Hospital, London. In: Zander J, Baltzer J (eds) Early breast cancer. Springer, Berlin Heidelberg New York, pp 253–263
21. Henderson IC, Canellos G (1980) Cancer of the breast: the past decade. N Engl J Med 302:17,79
22. Koscielny S, Tubiana M, Le MG (1984) Breast cancer: relationship between the size of the primary tumour and the probability of metastatic dissemination. Br J Cancer 49:709–715
23. Kusama S, Spratt JS, Donegan WL (1972) The gross rates of growth of human mammary carcinoma. Cancer 30:594–599
24. Lewis D, Rienhoff WF (1932) A study of results – John Hopkins Hospital 1889-1931. Ann Surg 25:336
25. Lundgren B (1983) The growth rate of breast cancer as a dynamic indicator of prognosis. Australas Radiol 27:178–180
26. Meakin JW, Allt WEC, Beale FA (1983) Ovarian irradiation and prednisone following surgery and radiotherapy for carcinoma of the breast. Breast Cancer Res Treat [Suppl] 3:45–48

27. Meyer JS, Prey MU, Babcock DS, McDivitt RW (1986) Breast carcinoma cell kinetics, morphology, stage and host characteristics: a thymidine labeling study. Lab Invest 54:41–51
28. Meyer W (1894) An improved method of the radical operation for carcinoma of the breast. Med Red 46:745
29. Meyer W (1905) Carcinoma of the breast: 10-year experience with my method of radical operation. JAMA 45:297
30. Nissen-Meyer R, Kjellgren K (1986) Perioperative adjuvant chemotherapy of breast cancer: the Scandinavian experience. Recent Results Cancer Res 00:00–00
31. Nissen-Meyer R, Kjellgren K, Manssen R (1982) Adjuvant chemotherapy in breast cancer. Recent Results Cancer Res 80:142–148
32. Nissen-Meyer R, Host H, Kjellgren K (1984) Scandinavian trials with one single post-operative course vs 12 courses. Recent Results Cancer Res 96:48–54
33. Oeser H (1974) Krebsbekämpfung: Hoffnung und Realität. Thieme, Stuttgart, pp 12–39
34. Pearlman AW (1976) Breast cancer – influence of growth rate on prognosis and treatment evaluation. A study based on mastectomy scar recurrences. Cancer 38:1826
35. Powles TJ (1988) Advanced breast cancer – new approaches to treatment. A review. Eur J Cancer Clin Oncol
36. Rotter J (1896) Günstigere Dauererfolge durch ein verbessertes Operationsverfahren der Mammakarzinome. Berl Klin Wochenschr 33:69–99
37. Silvestrini R, Diadone MG, Gasparini G (1985) Cell kinetics as a persistent prognostic marker in node-negative breast cancer. Cancer 56:1982–1987
38. Spratt JS, Spratt JA (1979) Growth rates. In: Donegan WL, Spratt JS (1979) Cancer of the breast. Saunders, Philadelphia, pp 197–221
39. Spratt JS, Kaltenbach ML, Spratt JA (1977) Cytokinetic definition of acute and chronic breast cancer. Cancer Res 37:226
40. Spratt SS, Spratt JA (1985) What is breast cancer before we can detect it? J Surg Oncol 30:156–160
41. Steinthal CF (1905) Zur Dauerheilung des Brustkrebses. Beitr Klin Chir 47:226
42. Tubiana M, Koscielny S (1988) Cell kinetics, growth rate and the natural history of breast cancer. The Heuson Memorial Lecture. Eur J Cancer Clin Oncol 24:9–14
43. Tubiana M, Malaise EP (1976) Comparison of cell proliferation kinetics in human and experimental tumors: response to irradiation. Cancer Treat Rep 60:1887–1895
44. Tubiana M, Malaise EP (1984) Growth rate and cell kinetics in human tumors. In: Symington T, Carter RL (eds) On scientific functions of oncology. Year Book Medical, Chicago, pp 126–136
45. Tubiana M, Pejovic MH, Chavaudra N et al. (1984) The long term prognostic significance of the thymidine labeling index in breast cancer. Int J Cancer 33:441–445

Rationale for the Choice of Treatment

D. VON FOURNIER and F. KUBLI

General Points

The treatment of breast cancer is currently based on the following ideas:

1. In the majority of cases the tumor has already reached the stage of dissemination at the time of the primary treatment. This can be inferred from the mortality among patients with locally completely cured breast cancer, especially against the backdrop of what we know about the comparatively slight influence of the radicality of locoregional treatment on survival rates. In 60%–80% of cases distant metastases are the first indication of tumor recurrence [38]. The concept of adjuvant systemic cytotoxic therapy is derived from these facts.
2. The prognosis is dependent primarily on how aggressive the tumor is and on its growth behavior. Indications of the aggressiveness of the cancer can be obtained from a number of morphological and biochemical characteristics of the tumor. These are currently used to allocate patients to particular risk groups and thus to tailor the therapy to suit the level of risk in individual patients.
3. The prognosis is obviously also dependent on the immune status of the affected organism, though the degree of this dependence cannot be quantitatively estimated. According to DONEGAN and SPRATT (1979, 1988) and FISHER et al. (1980), involvement of the axillary lymph nodes by carcinoma is an indicator of the tumor-host relationship and should alert us to the likelihood that the tumor is also attacking the organism at other locations. Attempts to influence the immunological defense situation have so far not been successful or are still experimental [29,41]. An effect of psychic factors has not been rejected [22] but has not been unequivocally demonstrated, and the extent of their importance is completely undefined.
4. There is still no consensus on the bearing of the radicality of the locoregional treatment of the tumor on the survival rates. ATKINS et al. [2] have shown that inadequate clearance of quite large tumor masses (breast-conserving treatment without axillary lymph node dissection and with inadequately dosed radiotherapy) reduces the chances of survival significantly: their follow-up period is now 15 years [see HAYWARD, this volume]. Local control of disease is an essential part of conservation treatments, especially in small (T1) tumors with negative nodes, in which cure can be achieved.

On the other hand, the large-scale prospective studies reported in the Anglo-Saxon literature – protocol 04 of the NSABP [15], the Manchester study [31], and the

King's Cambridge trial [9] – indicate that incomplete clearance of the axillary lymph nodes in clinical stage I does not have effects on the overall survival rate. Histologically demonstrable lymph node metastases must be expected in about 40% of cases in this stage. Performance of more radical surgery including the parasternal lymph drainage area also has no influence on the cure rates [VERONESI et al. 1981].

The same is true, finally, for the radicality of the treatment of the chest wall following mastectomy: the survival rates are identical regardless of whether the chest wall is irradiated or not [16,31,9].

It must therefore now be assumed that neither the persistence of small tumor masses in the axilla and at the chest wall nor the failure to remove affected parasternal lymph nodes exerts any statistically significant influence on the final cure rates. According to BELLER [3], the stepwise changes in operative radicality during the last 100 years reflect this experience (Fig. 1).

In contrast, it has been shown in several studies and is unanimously agreed that the frequency of locoregional recurrence bears a direct relationship to the radicality of the clearance in the locoregional sector – whether this is accomplished by surgery or by radiotherapy – and that the frequency of locoregional recurrence rises with declining radicality.

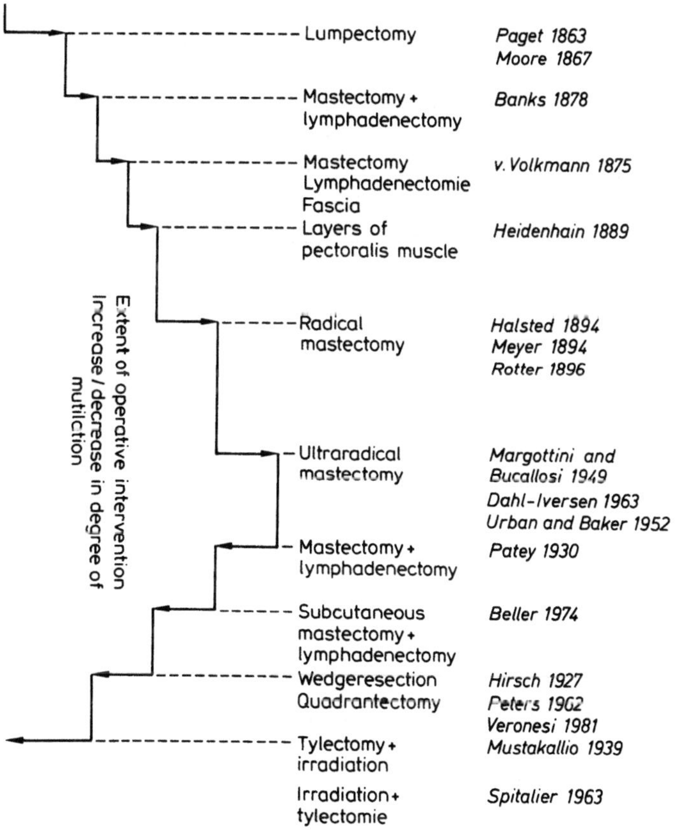

Fig. 1. The last 100 years of breast surgery: increasing radicality of surgical procedures and associated deterioration in the quality of life, followed by a reversal of this trend. (From BELLER 1985)

Factors in Prognosis

In addition to the histological type of the tumor – medullary, colloidal, tubular and papillary carcinomas have a relatively good prognosis compared with invasive ductal carcinoma, which is the most frequently occurring type – the following tumor characteristics are relevant to the prognosis to varying degrees: tumor size, lymph node involvement, hormone receptor status, growth rate/cell kinetics (S-phase rate or labeling index), degree of differentiation of tumor and presence or absence of lymph vessel invasion.

There are other factors whose clinical significance has been established but which are still of lesser importance today ([26,40,43] see also 3 VON FOURNIER and KAUFMANN et al. in this volume).

Locoregional Therapy

One aim of therapy in every case is the avoidance of locoregional recurrence. This is particularly so when the quality of life and the possibility of breast-conserving therapy and reconstruction are also borne in mind. Every local recurrence means a reduction in the patient's quality of life. Local failure following primary breast-conserving therapy is in some cases associated with ultimate loss of the breast, and following mastectomy it makes any planned reconstruction difficult.

There is therefore general agreement that the first objective of any locoregional treatment must be complete control of the tumor progress in the locoregional sector, but this influences the chances of survival only within relatively narrow limits [21]. Numerous studies (summarized by HARRIS and HELLMAN 1987; DONOGEN and SPRATT 1979) have shown the identical survival rates after Halsted's operation, modified mastectomy and breast conservation. Halsted's operation is now therefore generally not performed except in the cases where the pectoral muscles are largely affected by the tumor.

The three sectors – breast and chest wall, axillary lymph drainage areas and parasternal lymph drainage areas – can be considered separately.

Breast and Chest Wall

The procedures considered are modified radical mastectomy (with or without postoperative irradiation of the chest wall) breast-conserving therapy with subsequent irradiation of the breast and, finally, subtotal resection of the breast with no irradiation.

Modified Radical Mastectomy

Modified radical mastectomy is almost universally accepted as the standard procedure and the treatment of choice for mobile tumors of any size that still permit excision with sufficient tumor-free margins. Local recurrences in the chest wall arise in about 10%–20% of cases, depending on the one hand on tumor size and the aggressiveness of the tumor and on the other on the radicality of the surgery performed. Their frequency can be lowered by postoperative irradiation to the chest wall. Even so, irradiation seems to be omitted more and more frequently [30]. In the case of small tumors with a good prognosis, irradiation seems unnecessary in view of the relative rarity of recurrences in the scars and the good prospects for their successful treatment. Irradiation makes the basic position less favorable for any planned reconstruction. In the case of tumors with a worse prognosis, rapid initiation of an aggressive systemic adjuvant therapy currently appears to be the first priority. Irradiation of the chest wall is easier to incorporate into the primary treatment schedule with less radical surgical intervention and increasing size and aggressiveness of the tumor.

Technically, there is obviously a wide variation in the understanding of radicality, even in the definition of modified radical mastectomy. In our opinion, it is most advantageous for the surgical procedure to be designed in such a way that it is possible with a good conscience to omit irradiation from the primary treatment. This means that the space between the resection line and the primary tumor must be at least 4 cm, since with intervals smaller than 3 cm the frequency of local treatment failure rises significantly [13] (see Fig. 2). In young women especially, the breast inserts in the chest wall over a large area, and in the peripheral areas very extensive dissection of the body of the gland from the remaining skin/subcutis is frequently necessary.

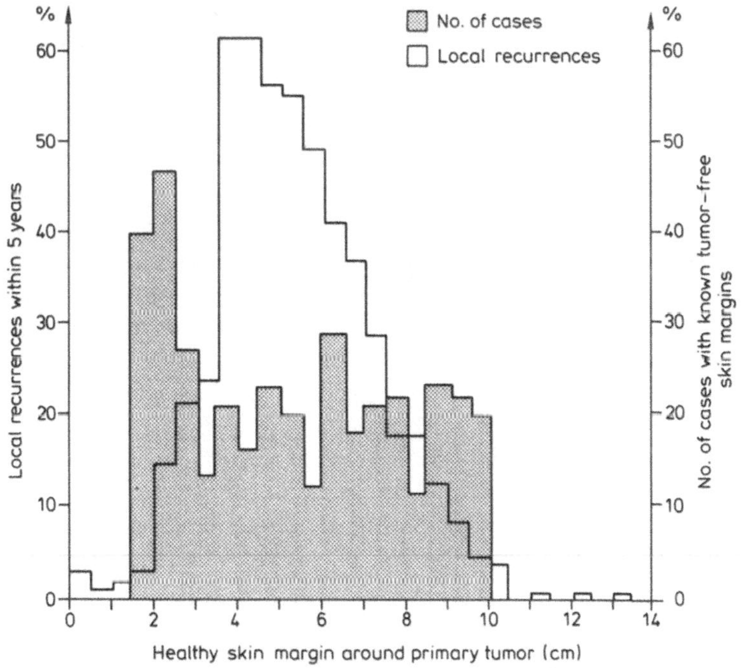

Fig. 2. Relationship between tumor-free skin margins in operative specimen and local recurrence within 5 years. Significant elevation of recurrence with tumor resection margins < 3 cm. [13]

Breast-Conserving Surgery with Subsequent Irradiation

The classical concept of therapy with total ablation of the breast whenever possible is based on knowledge of the frequency of multifocal disease or micrometastatic foci even in the quadrants not initially affected by cancer, which ranges up to 50% (see MÜLLER this volume). The frequency of multifocal microscopic tumor foci rises with increasing size of primary tumor.

The experience of breast irradiation in individual French and Scandinavian treatment centers in particular, however, has shown that modern irradiation techniques have made it possible to give doses of radiation adequate for tumor destruction with relatively good cosmetic results [1,6,21,35,36].

Primary therapy consisting exclusively of irradiation is certainly followed by local recurrence and secondary amputation of the breast in a great many cases, especially in the case of quite large primary tumors [6,7,36]. The probability that a given irradiation dose will prove to have a genuinely curative effect is inversely related to the size of the tumor. Thus, the situation in which the prospects of successful radiotherapy are best is that in which the primary tumor has been surgically removed and only microscopic carcinomatous foci are present.

So far, however, the results of two prospective controlled studies have been published in which the number of patients has been high enough and the follow-up period at all adequate: that by ATKINS and HAYWARD (this volume) and the later one by VERONESI et al. [44,45]. In both these studies, the therapy consisted basically in wide excision or quadrantectomy combined with irradiation. It must be remarked that the dosages of radiotherapy were too low according to present-day standards as described in the first Guy's Hospital study. Even in these circumstances, the duration of survival after a 15-year follow-up period is comparable to radical mastectomy for stage I tumors, though with a decisively higher frequency of relapse, while the survival rates were significantly lower following breast-conserving therapy of stage II tumors. In the more recent study by VERONESI et al. the follow-up periods amount to 15 years, the irradiation technique is in keeping with present-day ideas and only patients with clinical stage T1, N0 disease were admitted to the study. Survival rates, frequency of distant metastases and frequency of locoregional recurrences are the same so far for breast-conserving therapy and for radical mastectomy according to Halsted.

In the case of relatively small tumors (T1), there are now unequivocal indications that quadrantectomy or wide excision with subsequent radiotherapy can be a reasonable alternative to modified radical mastectomy if adequate local control is achieved.

The cosmetic results of simple lumpectomy and subsequent irradiation are even better. There are reports of very good cure rates with this procedure in individual centers, in some cases with long follow-up periods.

The question as to whether the breast-conserving forms of therapy briefly described above should now be widely used outside controlled studies is generally greeted with some hesitation and a rather negative attitude. This is connected with the fact that in the Milan study, in which the radiotherapy administered is in keeping with modern ideas, the follow-up periods are still relatively short compared with the time that mammary carcinoma takes to metastasize and with the fact that the overall number of prospective controlled studies published is limited. There is still agreement on the fact that breast-conserving forms of therapy are substantially more difficult, technically, than modified radical mastectomy. After all, adequate radiotherapy is no simple matter, especially when the forms of interstitial radiotherapy [35,36] are considered.

Axillary Lymph Nodes

The following rules can now be considered as widely accepted for the therapeutic management of the axillary lymph nodes:

1. At least in clinical stage I, the survival rates are the same whether the axillary lymph drainage areas are treated or not. However, local recurrences are definitely more frequent without treatment of the axillary area [2,16,20].
2. The result of surgical clearance of the axilla is superior to that of radiological clearance [20].
3. Histological examination of the lymph nodes following surgical dissection yields information that is of high significance for determination of the individual prognosis. This appears to be particularly reliable if more than 10 lymph nodes have been removed and examined.
4. Adequate surgical clearance of the axilla does not necessary involve removal of both pectoral muscles.

Our procedure of choice is therefore as thorough a clearance of the axilla as possible, regardless of what therapy is performed for treatment of the primary.

It is of advantage for both diagnostic and therapeutic purposes if clearance of the axilla includes at least groups I and II (Fig. 3) in the case of smaller tumor and apparently uninvolved lymph nodes. This is generally possible with both the surgical techniques mentioned. The diagnostic and therapeutic usefulness of clearance of group III of the axilla is probably low.

We remove or divide the pectoralis minor muscle when we find during surgery that the axilla is indubitably affected. The mean number of lymph nodes removed gives an indication of how radical the surgical technique is (see ENGEL, this volume). Also crucial of course, is the amount of care devoted to the histological preparation. With optimal preparation and a fairly radical surgical procedure the number of lymph nodes removed varies between 10 and more than 30, the mean being around 20 or more with our technique.

When surgery is sufficiently radical, postoperative irradiation of the axilla is not indicated even if lymph nodes are affected, in view of the low rate of local relapse. For the axillary region it is also true that the therapy must, as far as possible, be directed at complete locoregional control of the tumor, regardless of the influence of the treatment on the survival rate. If for any reason surgical clearance of the axilla is not carried out, or is restricted to subradical lymphadenectomy, radiotherapy to the axilla will usually be administered as a matter of policy: there is nothing to recommend the alternative approach of waiting for a relapse and then treating it.

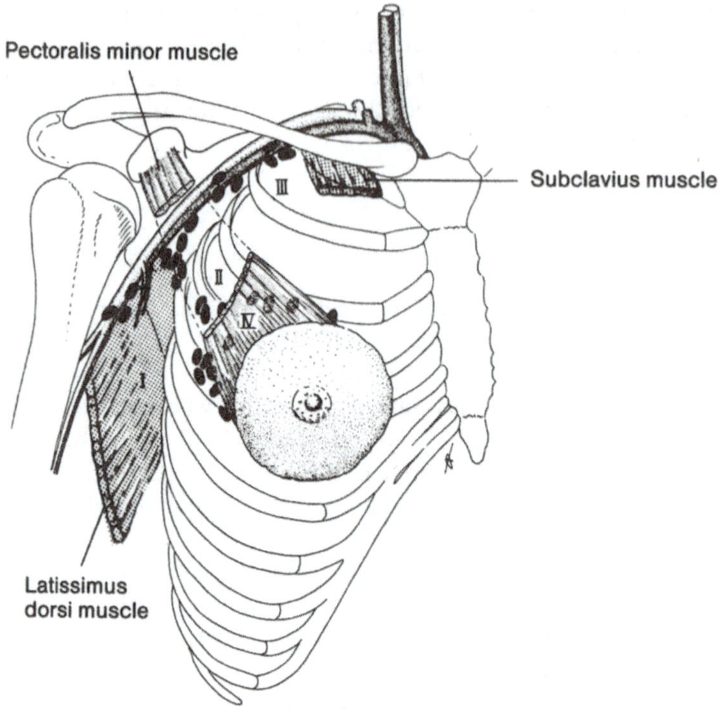

Fig. 3. Group I, II and III lymph nodes in the axilla. IV, interpectoral lymph nodes

Parasternal Lymph Nodes

There is still no agreement on the treatment of the parasternal drainage areas.

Medially situated tumors metastasize to parasternal areas in about 10% of cases when the axillary lymph nodes are negative and in 30% when the axillary lymph nodes are positive [44]. Surgical therapy directed at the lymph nodes has not brought about any improvement of the cure rates [44], and neither has irradiation to the parasternal region in several large-scale prospective Anglosaxon studies [9,16,31[. The prospective randomized studies currently in progress include one, the Stockholm study, in which radiotherapy is linked with a significantly improved survival rate in the subgroup of patients with medially situated tumors [46,47].

While supraradical mastectomy with surgical clearance of the parasternal lymph drainage areas has been largely abandoned, irradiation of the parasternal lymph drainage areas in the case of medial tumors is supported by some workers and rejected by others, both sides citing the results of prospective studies with relatively long follow-up periods in support of their views.

Adjuvant Systemic Therapy

Adjuvant Chemotherapy

Results are now available which were recorded over relatively long periods in studies that are significant in terms of patient numbers and study design (Scandinavian trial, NSABP projects 05 and 07, Milan study), as are a large body of results of studies still in progress (see HENDERSON, this volume). The results vary in some of the details, but the general trend and the broad features are the same:

1. The relapse-free survival rates are significantly increased in premenopausal patients when adjuvant chemotherapy is given.
2. In postmenopausal patients this effect is less pronounced in some studies.
3. Differences from the control populations in terms of overall survival are less pronounced. In some studies early significant differences have disappeared (temporarily?) in the course of the follow-up period, while in others such differences still exist for the total population but not for subgroups, or vice versa. This effect is also much more clearly seen in premenopausal patients.
4. The relapse-free survival rates are on the order of 10% to over 30% higher than in control populations, with corresponding figures for overall survival of around 10% or more.
5. The castration effect of adjuvant chemotherapy is the probable main effect in premenopausal women. For this reason it is necessary in studies to compare adjuvant chemotherapy with castration (LHRH analogs, ovariectomy, irradiation of the ovaries; see HENDERSON, this volume; KAUFMANN, this volume).

The long-term results in the Scandinavian study [33], which has yielded a significant improvement of 10% in the overall survival rates after short-term preoperative chemotherapy with a follow-up period of 20 years, suggest that the time at which chemotherapy is started may be of importance. There is a trend to shorten the duration of treatment, which apart from the aforementioned sequential administration of different combinations of drugs generally no longer exceeds 6 months.

While the beneficial effect of adjuvant chemotherapy is now beyond all doubt [37], the initially enthusiastic overall assessment has rather given way to sober scepticism. In particular, it remains obscure whether the declared aim of adjuvant chemotherapy – a significant increase in the long-term cure rate is really achieved – "Disease-free survival will be prolonged for many, but few will be cured." In this situation the benefits of adjuvant chemotherapy must be balanced against their disadvantages: short-term and long-term toxicity and subjective side effects. Serious complications attributable to the short-term toxicity are surprisingly rare. A higher frequency of secondary carcinomas has not so far been observed following adjuvant chemotherapy, in contrast to the experience with palliative chemotherapy, where secondary carcinomas occur with long-term administration and high total doses.

The subjective tolerance of aggressive adjuvant chemotherapy, however, is mostly poor. The negative psychological impact of this form of therapy is considerable, and greater significance will doubtless be imputed to this in future. Therefore regimes with less severe side effects are now being tested in prospective trials. Another problem for the future is the further improvement of the selection of patients suitable for treatment, since at present many patients show no appreciable benefit compared with untreated control populations and are suffering severe side effects.

Despite all potential reservations, adjuvant chemotherapy currently represents the only chance of improving the prognosis, especially for those premenopausal patients in high-risk groups, i.e., with axillary lymph node metastases, in particular when the tumor is receptor negative. Premenopausal patients with negative lymph nodes but whose other tumor characteristics have an unfavorable influence on the prognosis are also certainly candidates for adjuvant chemotherapy. Adjuvant chemotherapy will generally also be administered in postmenopausal women in the presence of a high degree of risk, but according to CARTER [11], for example, control arms without chemotherapy are quite permissible and even desirable.

Adjuvant chemotherapy is best administered as part of a controlled study. Where this is not possible it will be necessary to make a particularly careful review of the pros and cons in each case, and it seems to us essential that the following conditions be fulfilled:

- Unequivocal determination of the individual risk, based on consideration of the parameters of prognosis
- Adequate experience with cytotoxic drugs on the part of those administering the therapy
- Guaranteed availability of regular monitoring for recognition and avoidance or treatment of toxic side effects
- Guaranteed availability of a long-term documentation method valid for all these factors

Adjuvant Endocrine Therapy

The idea of *castration* as a form of adjuvant therapy continues to be the subject of controversy. It should be mentioned that there are indications of a positive long-term effect of this form of therapy in terms of survival rates [5,32].

Greater interest, however, is focused on the antiestrogens, in particular on tamoxifen (Nolvadex). A fairly large number of prospective studies are in progress. The preliminary results of the relevant NSABP study, with significantly higher recurrence-free survival rates for the combination with adjuvant chemotherapy, have attracted particular attention [18,19]. The relapse-free survival was directly dependent on the estrogen and progesterone receptor content [19]. In addition, the results recorded so far suggest that an effect of antiestrogen therapy can be expected mainly in postmenopausal patients. For premenopausal patients the discussion is still centered on castration. This can be attained by oophorectomy, by irradiation with 16 Gy or by a subcutaneous depot injection of LHRH analog (Zoladex) every 4 weeks (reversible castration). There is general agreement, however, that the as yet relatively short observation periods do not allow any definite conclusions as to in which subgroups of premenopausal patients castration is superior to adjuvant chemotherapy.

In practice, the minimal side effects of antiestrogen therapy compared with chemotherapy means that adjuvant administration of antiestrogens (20–30 mg tamoxifen/day) will probably be widely used nonetheless in postmenopausal patients with receptor-positive tumors, both now and in the near future.

Reconstruction Following Amputation of the Breast

Especially in the case of younger patients, the possibility of surgical reconstruction following amputation should be taken account of in the primary treatment plan. It is, however, wrong to perform an insufficiently radical operation in such cases – with regard to the resection margin on the skin, for example – because this leads to a higher frequency of local recurrence.

The operative manipulation necessary in surgical reconstruction, and the introduction of foreign material into an area that may at least theoretically, still be harboring cancer cells, obviously do not have a negative influence on the prognosis. In those of our patients in whom reconstruction was performed, the survival rate and the frequency of distant metastases and locoregional recurrences over follow-up periods of 5 to 10 years were comparable with the results in a control group of patients who did not have reconstructions and were paired for the most important variables known to influence the prognosis (see ENGELS, this volume). Reconstruction obviously helps the patients come to terms with the psychological trauma involved in amputation of the breast; relevant results collected in prospective controlled studies have been published by the Edinburgh group (DEAN 1983).

Viewed objectively, the results are not considered good, mainly because the Silastic implant frequently leads to capsular contraction beneath the skin. It should be borne in mind, however, that less than ideal results can still also help a patient considerably in her daily life.

From the technical viewpoint numerous modifications have been described (for survey see BOHMERT 1982). In general, at least two more than minor operations are necessary, though in some cases it is possible to perform the first of these at the same time as the primary treatment. The prospects of good long-term cosmetic results are best if the Silastic implant has a submuscular localization, generally below the pectoralis major. If this muscle is not present a latissimus dorsi island graft is now the treatment of choice. The possibility of reconstruction by means of endogenous material, e.g., rectus abdominis muscle-skin flaps, is attracting increasing interest. The timing of a reconstruction procedure is dependent on the individual prognosis. In the case of tumors with a favorable prognosis, for example $T1\ N_0$, reconstruction can be performed soon after the primary surgical treatment. Sometimes reconstruction can even be started at the time of the primary operation, but in any case it can be done after primary wound healing is complete.

In the case of tumors with a less favorable prognosis, reconstruction is generally not performed until 2–3 years after the primary treatment. The main reason for this is that local recurrences or distant metastases are observed within this period in a considerable proportion of such cases. We are, however, increasingly of the opinion that if a patient urgently desires reconstruction her request should not be refused.

The possibility of surgical reconstruction should be discussed, as a matter of policy, with every patient whose prognosis is not too unfavorable. In our experience, only a minority of the patients considered suitable – about 10%–30% – accept, predominantly younger women. Reconstructions are relatively difficult plastic operations, and the long-term results are not always fully satisfactory. It would probably be best to leave them to centers where the surgeons have had adequate experience.

Locally Advanced Carcinomas

Locally advanced carcinomas in stages T3 and T4 with lymph node involvement are generally no longer curable, and occult or even manifest dissemination is the rule. Locoregional recurrences also have to be expected with great regularity if only surgical treatment is given. Even though cure is not possible, it seems important to control the tumor locoregionally for reasons connected with the quality of life (avoidance of cancer en cuirasse). The procedure must be decided on individually for each patient. If the pectoralis major muscle is involved, its partial or total resection is generally indicated. As a rule, the surgical treatment is combined with radiotherapy delivered to the locoregional area and with systemic therapy. If tolerance is adequate, combined systemic chemotherapy is recommended.

Guidelines and Recommendations

There is no authority at present that can give universally binding guidelines and recommendations for the treatment of breast carcinoma.

As described by KINNE and ROBBINS [27] at the moment the selection of therapeutic procedures for women with carcinoma of the breast is a challenge for potential patients, their families, and the doctors concerned. This situation is not attributable solely to rapid progress in research, but just as much, or even more, to an incredible number of prematurely published partial results, which are then reproduced manifold in the lay press. It really should be borne in mind that for breast cancer, the results after 5 years are relatively short-term results, and that studies from different centers on the same topic, even if their design is beyond reproach, frequently yield divergent results (e.g., effect of adjuvant castration in premenopausal women).

It therefore seems necessary to differentiate between the therapeutic procedures whose value and range of application have been confirmed by many studies of the same kind with adequate follow-up periods and those treatment modalities for which this is not true even though theoretical considerations, experience at individual centers and isolated prospective studies point in their favor. The latter group of modalities should be employed with caution and the necessary degree of skepsis, preferably under controlled conditions. This group includes the procedures used for primary breast-conserving therapy and, strictly speaking, adjuvant chemotherapy too. There are specific risks of overtreatment and undertreatment, which must be avoided as far as possible.

Areas of Certainty in Therapeutic Action

For mobile tumors that can be excised with adequate margins – basically tumor stages T1 and T2 – the therapy that has been confirmed in its effect and is recognized throughout the world as suitable is modified radical mastectomy with axillary lymphadenectomy of nodes in groups I, II and III (Fig. 3). This is true regardless of the lymph node status. If the tumor can no longer be moved against pectoralis major part or all of the muscle must be removed with the tumor. If the operation is sufficiently radical and an adequate surgical technique is used, irradiation of the axillary lymph node areas is not indicated and neither is additional radiotherapy of the chest wall, unless the risk of local recurrence is very high because of the tumor biology. We consider this treatment to be most logical and rational.

Variants of the therapy that can be justified and are also accepted throughout the world consist in restriction of the surgical radicality (especially concerning group III nodes in the axillary region) and the use of compensatory radiotherapy.

Postoperative irradiation of the parasternal lymph node area when the tumor is medially situated may have some advantage, but this has not been confirmed. For locally advanced tumors (T3 and T4), surgical treatment alone is not sufficient as a rule; it must be combined with postoperative – and possibly also preoperative – radiotherapy and/or chemotherapy.

Areas of Therapeutic Action That Are Currently Largely Accepted Though Not Unequivocally Confirmed

Although the effectiveness of adjuvant chemotherapy is not proved beyond all doubt, this form of therapy is currently recognized as an integral part of the treatment in premenstrual high-risk patients, i.e., those with axillary lymph node involvement. For postmenopausal high-risk patients the effect is even less clear, but adjuvant cytotoxic therapy is still carried out in subgroups.

Surgical reconstruction can presumably now also be included among the areas of therapeutic action that are largely accepted, although studies on the effect of reconstruction on the prognosis are extremely sparse.

Forms of Therapy That Have Not Been Definitely Confirmed and are Currently Largely Categorized as Experimental

This category currently includes all forms of primary breast-conserving therapy; these should therefore be carried out only under controlled conditions (see HAYWARD, this volume).

Overtreatment

It has now been proved that the side effects and/or the cost of a number of therapies are out of all proportion to the benefit they confer. These include Halsted's modified radical operation in the case of small mobile tumors without involvement of pectoralis major, postoperative irradiation of the axilla and the chest wall after Halsted's mastectomy and postoperative irradiation of axillary lymph drainage areas and chest wall when the histological staging reveals a tumor *falling* in the category T1 N0, especially when the tumor is highly differentiated, even after a modified radical operation. Aggressive adjuvant chemotherapy administered over a long period to patients with no lymph node involvement and no specific risk factors should now also be classed as overtreatment.

Areas in which Undertreatment is Possible

The burst of publicity and popular appeal surrounding breast-conserving forms of therapy carries with it the potential risk of undertreatment if these forms of therapy do not remain confined to centers with a great deal of experience and are employed outside the protective framework of controlled studies and possibly with inadequate technical expertise and equipment. It is not yet known whether this danger is real or how serious it is. Nonetheless, it should be borne in mind. The power of the media to influence the course of science has been fundamentally discussed by HAAGENSEN (1986): see C.D. HAAGENSEN (1986), Diseases of the Breast, Saunders, pp 933–937.

References

1. Amalric R, Santamaria F, Robert F, Seigle J et al. (1981) Curative radiotherapy for operable breast cancer: 5- and 10-year results. In: Lewison EF, Montague ACW (eds) Diagnosis and treatment of breast cancer. Williams & Wilkins, Baltimore, p 185
2. Atkins H, Hayward JL, Klugnar DJ, Wayle AB (1972) Treatment of early breast cancer. A report after ten years of a clinical trial. Br Med J II: 423
3. Beller FK (1985) Atlas der Mammachirurgie. Schattauer, Stuttgart
4. Bohmert H (1982) Brustkrebs und Brustrekonstruktion. Thieme, Stuttgart
5. Bryant AJS, Weir JA (1981) Prophylactic oophorectomy in operable instances of carcinoma of the breast. Surg Gynecol Obstet 153:660
6. Calle R, Pilleron JP, Schlienger P, Vilcoq JR (1978) Conservative management of operable breast cancer. Ten years experience at the Foundation Curie. Cancer 42:2045
7. Calle R, Vilcoq JR, Pilleron JP et al. (1983) Conservative treatment of operable breast carcinoma by irradiation with or without limited surgery – ten-year results. In: Harris JR, Hellman S, Silen W (eds) Conservative management of breast cancer. Lippincott, Philadelphia, pp 3–9
8. Campbell FC, Blamey RW, Elston CW, Morris AH et al. (1981) Quantitative oestradiol receptor values in primary breast cancer and response of metastases to endocrine therapy. Lancet 2:1317
9. Cancer Research Campaign Working Party (1980) Cancer Research Campaign (King's Cambridge) trial of early breast cancer. Lancet 2:55

10. Carter SK (1981a) Predictors of response and their clinical evaluation. Cancer Chemother Pharmacol 7:1
11. Carter SK (1981b) Adjuvant chemotherapy of breast cancer. N Engl J Med 304:45
12. Croton R, Cooke T, Holt S, George WP, Nicolson R, Griffitts K (1981) Oestrogen receptors and survival in early breast cancer. Br Med J 283:1289
13. Donegan WL, Spratt JS (ed) (1979) Cancer of the breast. Saunders, Philadelphia
14. Duncan W, Kerr GR (1976) The curability of breast cancer. Br Med J IV:781
15. Fisher B (1980) Laboratory and clinical research in breast cancer – a personal adventure. The David A. Karnofsky Memorial Lecture. Cancer Res 40:3863
16. Fisher B, Redmond C, Fisher ER, participating NSABP investigators (1980) The contribution of recent NSABP clinical trial of primary breast cancer therapy to an understanding of tumor biology – an overview of findings. Cancer 46:1009
17. Fisher B, Wolmark N, Redmond E, Deutsch M et al. (1981a) Findings from NSABP protocol NB-OH: comparison of radical mastectomy with alternative treatments. II. The clinical and biological significance of medial-central breast cancers. Cancer 48:1863
18. Fisher B, Redmond C, Brown A et al. (1981b) Treatment of primary breast cancer with chemotherapy and tamoxifen. N Engl J Med 305:1
19. Fisher B, Redmond C et al. (1983) Tumors estrogen and progesterone receptor levels on the response to tamoxifen and chemotherapy in primary breast cancer. J Clin Oncol 1:227
20. Fisher B, Redmond C, Fisher ER et al. (1985) Ten-year results of a randomized clinical trial comparing radical mastectomy and total mastectomy with or without radiation. N Engl J Med 312:674
21. Fournier D von, zum Winkel K, Kuttig H, Kubli F (1986) Strahlentherapie als adjuvante Maßnahme beim Mammakarzinom. In: Kadach U, Kaufmann M, Kubli F (eds) Hormone Antihormone Zytostatika zur adjuvanten Therapie des Mammakarzinoms. Zuckschwerdt, München, pp 82–97
22. Greer S, Morris T, Pettingale KW (1979) Psychological response to breast cancer. Effect on outcome. Lancet 2:785
23. Harris JR, Hellmann S (1987) Conservative surgery and radiotherapy. In: Harris JR, Hellman S, Henderson IC, Kinne DW (eds) Breast diseases. Lippincott, Philadelphia, pp 299–323
24. Harris JR, Hellman S (1987) Adjuvant radiotherapy. In: Harris JR, Hellman S, Henderson IC, Kinne DW (eds) Breast diseases. JB Lippincott, Philadelphia, pp 284–299
25. Kaufmann M (1982) Prognostische Behandlung des Mammakarzinoms. Habilitationsschrift, Heidelberg
26. Kaufmann M, Klinga K, Runnebaum B, Kubli F (1982) Steroid-Rezeptor und Prognose beim primären Mammakarzinom. In: Frischbier HJ (ed) Die Erkrankungen der weiblichen Brustdrüse. Thieme, Stuttgart
27. Kinne D, Robbins GF (1981) The dilemma of carcinoma of the breast. Surg Gynecol Obstet 153:577
28. Knight WA, Livingstone RB, Gregory EJ, McGuire WL (1977) Estrogen receptor as an independent prognostic factor for early recurrence in breast cancer. Cancer Res 37:4669
29. Lacour J, Lacour F, Spira A, Michelson M et al. (1980) Adjuvant treatment with polyadenylic-polyuridylic acid (Poly A, Poly U) in operable breast cancer. Lancet 2:161
30. Lipsett MB (1981) Postoperative radiation for women with cancer of the breast and positive axillary lymph nodes. Should it continue? N Engl J Med 304:112
31. Lithgoe JP, Leck J, Swindell R (1978) Manchester Regional Breast Study: preliminary results. Lancet 1:744
32. Meakin JW, Allt WEC, Beale RA et al. (1977) Ovarian irradiation and prednisone following surgery for carcinoma of the breast. In: Salmor SE (ed) Adjuvant therapy of cancer. North Holland, New York
33. Nissen-Meyer R, Host H, Kjellgren K (1984) Scandinavian trials with one single postoperative course vs 12 courses of Chemotherapy. Recent Results Cancer Res 96:48–54

34. Ober KG (1984) Alternative Behandlungsmethoden des frühen Mammakarzinoms. In: Kubli F, Fournier D von (eds) Neue Konzepte der Diagnostik und Therapie des Mammakarzinoms. Springer, Berlin Heidelberg New York, pp 128–133
35. Pierquin B, LeBourgeois JP, Brun B, Mazeron JJ, Huart J (1981) Radiotherapy as primary treatment of operable breast cancer. In: Lewison EF, Montague ACW (eds) Diagnosis and treatment of breast cancer. Williams & Wilkins, Baltimore, p 175
36. Pierquin B, Otmetzquine Y, Lobo PA (1985) Conservative management of breast carcinoma. In: Zander J, Balzer J (eds) Early breast cancer. Springer, Berlin Heidelberg New York, pp 276–284
37. Rossi A, Bonadonna G, Valagussa P, Veronesi U (1981) Multimodal treatment in operable breast cancer: five year results of the CMF programme. Br Med J 282:1427
38. Senn HJ (1981) Adjuvante Chemotherapie beim Mammakarzinom. Dtsch Med Wochensehr 106:1626
39. Silvestrini R, Diadone MG, Gasparini G (1985) Cell kinetics as a persistent prognostic marker in node-negative breast cancer. Cancer 56:1982–1987
40. Sulkes A, Livingstone RB, Murphy WK (1979) Tritriated thymidine labeling index and response in human breast cancer. Cancer 62:513
41. Terman DS, Young JV, Shearer WT et al. (1981) Preliminary observations of the effects on breast adenocarcinoma of plasma perfused over immobilized protein A. New Engl J Med 305:1195
42. Tubiana M, Koscielny S (1988) Cell kinetics, growth rate and the natural history of breast cancer: The Heuson Memorial Lecture. Eur J Cancer Clin Oncol 24:9–14
43. Tubiana M, Pejovic A, Renand G et al. (1981) Kinetic parameters and the course of the disease in breast cancer. Cancer 47:937
44. Veronesi U, Saccozzi R, Del Vacchino M et al. (1981) Comparing radical mastectomy with quadrantectomy, axillary dissection and radiotherapy in patients with small cancers of the breast. N Engl J Med 305:6
45. Veronesi U, Zucali R, Luini A, Belle F, Crispino S, Merson M (1985) Conservative treatment of breast cancer with the "Qu.A.RT" technique. In: Zander J, Baltzer J (eds) Early breast cancer. Springer, Berlin Heidelberg New York, pp 264–270
46. Wallgren A et al. (1980) The value of preoperative radiotherapy in operable mammary carcinoma. Int J Radiat Oncol Biol Phys 6:287
47. Wallgren A, Arner O, Bergstrom J et al. (1988) Radiation therapy in operable breast cancer – results from the Stockholm trial in adjuvant radiotherapy. Int J Radiat Oncol Biol Phys

Perioperative Clarification of Diagnosis

D. von Fournier, F. Kubli and E. Krapfl

Preoperative Procedures

Even when preoperative diagnostic procedures have been reliably carried out in another clinic, before the operation the surgeon still needs to familiarize himself or herself personally with the findings in the particular patient; the surgeon's own impression can lead to a change in the intended treatment plan.

In a tumor clinic, it is advisable for all examinations that have to be carried out before the operation be checked over again, if possible with reference to existing records (X-ray films, cytological and histological preparations etc.) It is not uncommon for the preoperative assessment of the tumor to be changed.

We carry out the following preoperative examinations in all cases:

- Clinical examination
- Evaluation of the mammography films available
- Puncture of any nodes palpated (if not already done elsewhere) if a cyst seems possible
- Ultrasound examination when solid or cystic masses are present

Thermography (electronic thermography) can sometimes yield valuable supplementary information, but is basically of secondary importance.

Procedure for Exclusion of Cyst

If clinical, radiological or sonographic examination gives rise to the suspicion of a cyst, or if the findings are inconclusive and do not allow definite exclusion of a cyst, a puncture is carried out. Following disinfection of the skin a no. 1 disposable cannula is used for the puncture, and the complete contents of the cyst, if possible, are aspirated under pressure. The needle is left in place, and a second disposable syringe is used to introduce a volume of air equal to the volume of fluid removed. The patient must then compress the puncture site for at least 5 min to prevent the formation of a hematoma along the path of the cannula.

Pneumocystography of the breast is then carried out in two planes (Fig. 1). The contents of the cyst are subjected to cytological examination. If cells suggestive of malignancy are found (this is rare), or if the radiological appearance of the wall of the cyst gives rise to the suspicion of malignancy, the whole of the cyst must be

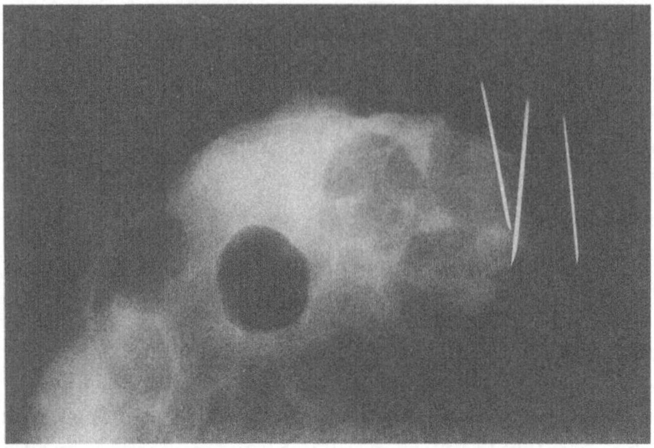

Fig. 1. Pneumocystography. Following aspiration of the cyst content the "shell" of the cyst is filled with the same volume of air. Pneumocystography is performed to find out whether there are any changes in the cyst wall suggestive of malignancy or requiring excision for other reasons

removed. If the contents of the cyst are found on puncture to be solid, a puncture specimen is taken for cytological examination.

If the cyst fluid and the cyst wall are unremarkable there is no need for a surgical operation. In this case a clinical examination is performed 3 months later to check whether the cyst has disappeared or refilled. When cysts recur frequently we tend to remove them surgically.

Solid Nodes

All solid palpable nodes should be surgically removed, even if they appear to be benign. This rule should be adhered to except in exceptional cases, and certain precautions must be observed even then. These include very careful monitoring and morphological checks at least by means of cytological examination of a puncture specimen. It must be noted that false-negative results have to be reckoned with in 10% of cases even when puncture cytology is carried out by experienced staff. Punch biopsy or drill biopsy may give greater certainty, since these admit of histological examination.

Indications for and Implementation of Preoperative Punch and Drill Biopsies

When a *punch biopsy* is to be taken the skin is first disinfected and local anesthesia of the skin and the projected route of puncture is accomplished with 1% Scandicaine. The punch biopsy needle is then advanced with a trocar up to the surface

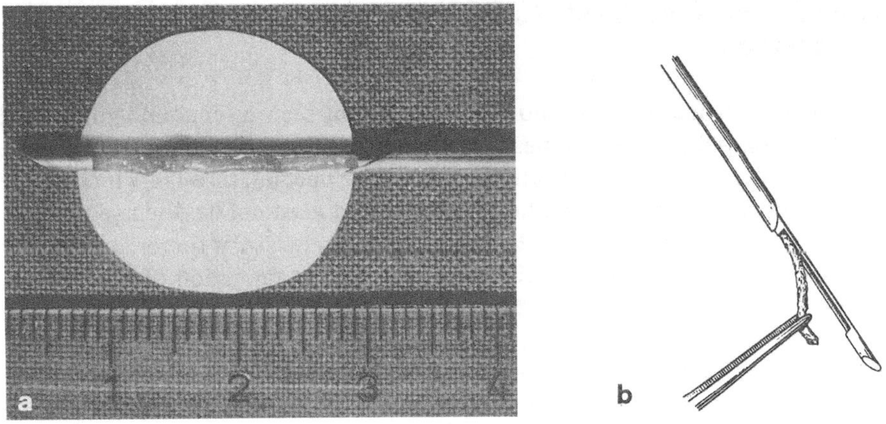

Fig. 2a,b. Punch biopsy: Representation of punch needle and removal of tissue **a**. A cylinder of tissue is punched out. **b**. Cylinder of tissue is taken out through gap in needle

of the tumor, pushed right into the tumor and the cutter sleeve advanced over the needle so that a cylinder is punched out. Once the cutter sleeve with the needle inside has been withdrawn, the cylinder of tissue can be pulled out through the gap in the needle (Fig. 2).

There are various advantages to *drill biopsy*. The high speed of rotation makes it possible for the instrument to be advanced into the tissue precisely and with no difficulty even in the case of really tough fibrotic tumors, while a considerable amount of force has to be applied when a punch biopsy is taken in such circumstances, and this is painful. Preparation is the same as for a punch biopsy, and a 3-mm incision is then made with a scalpel. A drill needle less than 3-mm in diameter is pushed forward or drilled as far as the tumor with a mandrin in place. The mandrin is then removed and the hollow needle is advanced through the tumor by means of the drill motor at 1000–22 000 rpm. The needle is removed by hand after release of the drill chuck, or else removed by moving the drill, and the cylinder of tissue is pushed out by means of saline solution from syringe.

The path of the puncture is compressed firmly by the patient for 10 min and an elastic pressure dressing is then applied for 24 h.

When the patient is examined subsequently it must be borne in mind that this method is also prone to false-negative results, albeit seldom.

General Preoperative Examinations

All patients should undergo examination by an internist to determine the level of risk involved in surgery. If clinical examination has given rise to the suspicion that distant metastases are already present, bone scintigraphy and the necessary X-ray and blood investigations should be carried out before surgery, so that any surgical procedure planned can be corrected if appropriate.

Resection of Nonpalpable Changes Revealed Only by X-ray Examination

For the localization of occult, nonpalpable lesions seen on mammography, the instruments supplied as accessories to modern mammography equipment are used. These instruments allow localization by means of needles, through which a wire with a hook is inserted. The method is precise and need not be discussed further here. If the lesion is not a microcalcification but an occult solid tumor, we monitor the localization by ultrasound. Modern ultrasound examination of the mamma allows definite localization of solid foci of as little as 2 mm in diameter, depending on the size of the breast. It must be pointed out that in breasts with a high fat content, solid foci and even cysts up to 1 cm in size can sometimes not be definitely visualized.

As many clinics do not have the instrumentation needed for mammographic localization, just one method is described here that almost always shows up the occult focus with an adequate degree of certainty even in large breasts. Our procedure is as follows: Mammography in two planes with the patient seated allows an approximate estimate of the location of the lesion in the breast. Three no. 18 cannules are then advanced toward the lesion in such a way that the points of their insertion make a triangle on the skin (Fig. 3). In the control mammography in two planes one of these needles is almost always in a relatively good position close to or even directly in the focus of disease they were all aimed at. The position of the nearest needle is corrected, if necessary, and the other two are removed. A sketch is prepared by hand for the surgeon. A sterile wire with a 3-mm hook-shaped end is inserted through the needle (no. 1.2 diameter = size of the needle) after careful positioning. The wire left protruding at the skin is cropped to 4 cm and fixed sterilely to the skin. Mammography is performed in two planes to check how close the tip of the needle is to the occult disease focus; the distance from the focus in millimeters is recorded for the surgeon's information. The hook is generally inserted on the day before the operation. Patients who are not inpatients in the hospital where surgery is to be performed can have the hook in the breast for up to a week, though they must then wear a well-fitting brassiere. The patients do not have any symptoms when the

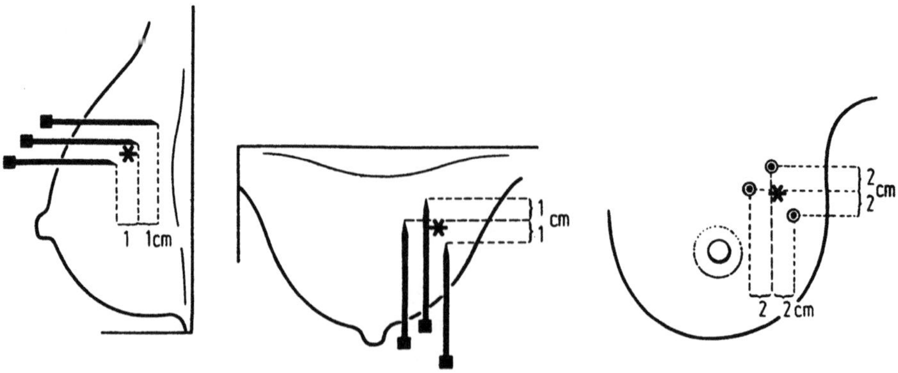

Fig. 3. Marking of findings seen on mammography with needles: Needles are inserted vertically – 2 cm apart in each plane – with depths of points differing by 1 cm

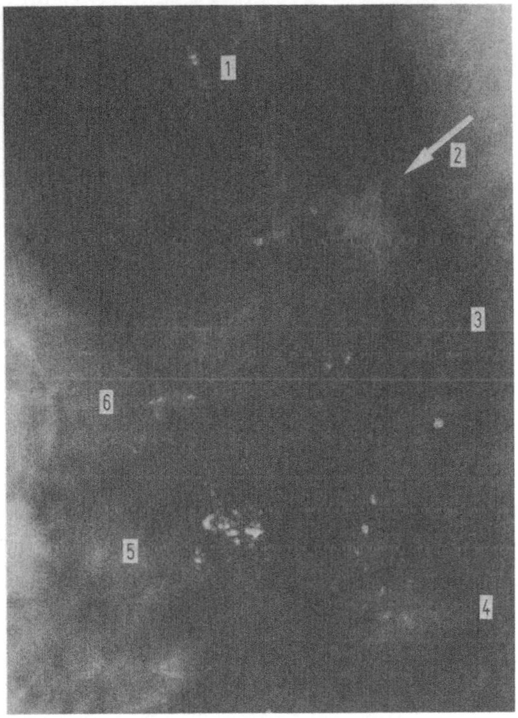

Fig. 4. Multiple areas of carcinoma in situ (*1–6*) seen on a magnified mammogram, at one point (*arrow*) giving way to a 2-mm invasive carcinoma. The nonpalpable lesions can be extirpated only following marking at the correct point

hook is in place, and after over 2000 localization procedures we have not seen any infections. During the operation the surgeon can use the scalpel to check along the length of the wire to the end of the hook for the occult lesion. The hooked wire is removed together with the lesion and the whole is sent for section radiography before being prepared for pathohistological examination.

In all cases, before the wound is closed the specimen must be X-rayed, and this must show that the entire lesion has really been removed. Figure 4 shows multiple carcinoma in situ with incipient invasive carcinoma 2 mm in diameter, which can be revealed by marking.

Procedure in the Presence of Pathologic Alterations to the Milk Ducts

If gaps or breaks are seen on galactography, the pathological alterations seen on the galactogram and also the adjacent duct system must be removed in toto in a single operation. The difficulty for the surgeon is to determine the extent of resection. It is possible to inject indigo blue into the duct at the beginning of the operation. We

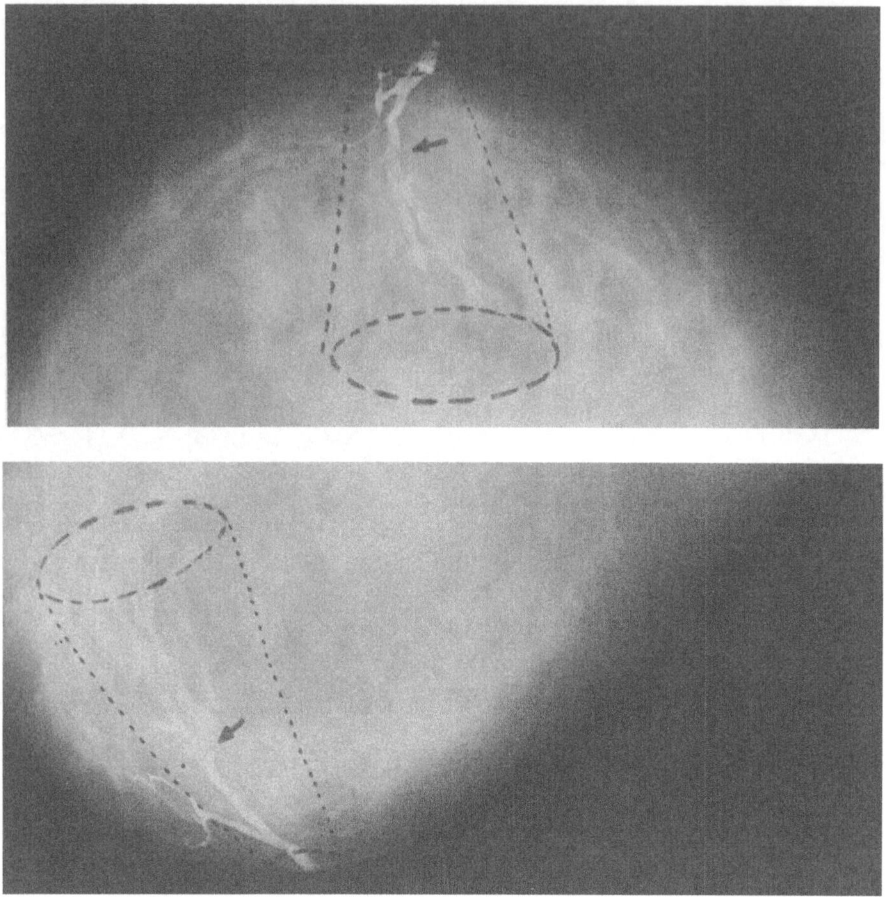

Fig. 5. Galactography. In this case, the milk duct had an appearance suggestive of malignancy and gaps in its course. It was extirpated with generous margins, the *broken lines* indicating the tissue excised. Histological examination revealed noninvasive ductal carcinoma that had arisen from papillomatosis

have found it worthwhile for the radiologist to mark the segment on the mammography in two planes (Fig. 5).

In the event of a mamillary duct alteration, a corresponding blunt-cone-shaped segment can be resected through a curved perimamillary incision (Fig. 6). If the defect is extensive and localized more peripherally, the necessary reconstruction can be accomplished more easily via a radial incision. The tissue to be removed is marked with a thread near the mamilla, the milk duct is opened up, and areas with a macroscopic appearance suggestive of malignancy are marked with threads. The tissue is spread out on a cork base and subjected to further work-up for histological examination.

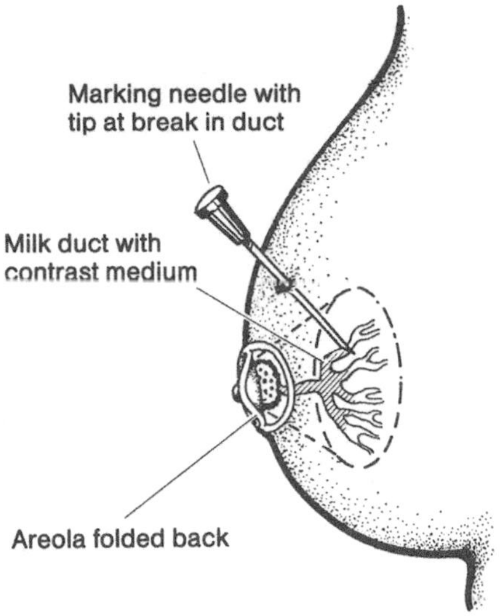

Fig. 6. Schematic representation of incision following a curved line around the areola. The milk duct system to be removed is cut out in the form of a truncated cone. The suspect gaps in the milk duct are marked with indigo blue injected through a marking needle

Excision of Tissue Samples

First a check is carried out to see whether the palpated node fits in with the suggestive findings in the X-ray picture. It is not rare for cysts to be palpated when radiography reveals a small breast carcinoma at another site. Among 1000 cases of carcinoma in the 3 years from 1984 to 1987, we saw 232 patients in whom there were nonpalpable changes requiring explanation in either the same breast or the contralateral breast in addition to the lesions palpated previously and given as the reason for referral. In 34 cases these changes were found to result from invasive carcinomas and in a further 32, from carcinoma in situ or atypical epithelial proliferation.

Selection of Incision

The incision selected depends on the situation of the tumor and the patient's ideas of what constitutes an acceptable cosmetic result. The best cosmetic results are obtained with the curved periareolar incision and the Bardenheuer incision in the skin fold (Fig. 7). Lesions located further laterally or cranially can be reached by way of an incision along the free edge of the pectoralis major muscle. Most lesions, however, are situated in segments of the mammary gland in which the incision should run directly over the lesion along the skin cleavage lines (Langer's lines, Fig. 8). In this way the shortest distance to the lesion is selected, and the healthy tissue is not unnecessarily destroyed by the cutting of a tunnel as shown in Fig. 10.

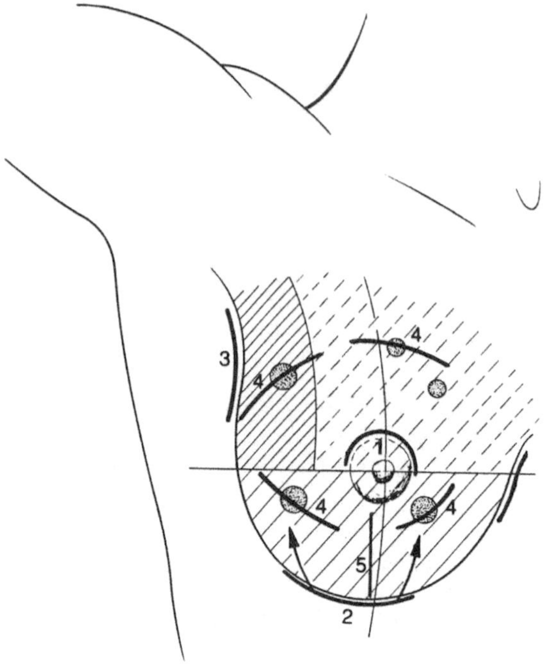

Fig. 7. Choice of skin incision in the case of different tumor sites. *1*, Not recommended; *2*, recommended for tumors in very caudal locations; *3*, recommended only for laterocranial tumors; *4*, recommended: incision over tumor; *5*, radial incision: recommended only for large caudally located tumors

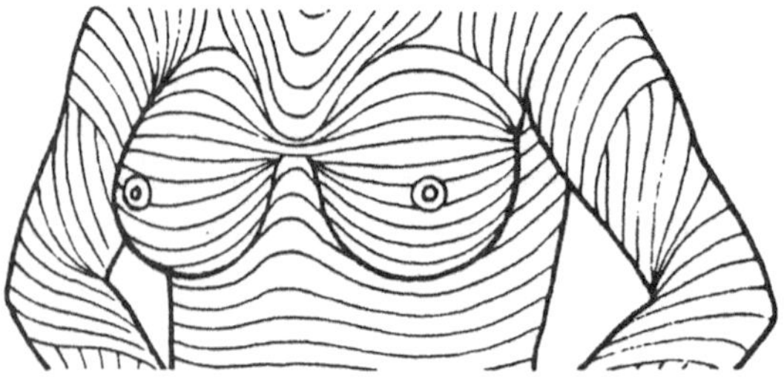

Fig. 8. Course of Langer's lines of the skin. [1]

The volume defect is best concealed by an incision of this kind, and usually no approximation sutures are needed, only subcutaneous suturing of the fascia and an intracutaneous suture.

Volume of Tissue To Be Removed, Excisional Biopsy

If it seems possible that a nodule is malignant, the following points must be borne in mind when selecting the incision:

1. The course of the incision should be suitable for performance of a segmentectomy with a good cosmetic result; this means it should follow the cleavage lines of the skin (Fig. 8).
2. The tissue must be removed in the first instance with a safety margin of at least 1–2 cm.
3. In the case of larger tumors, when organ conservation is planned, a spindle-shaped piece of skin about 2 cm wide is also removed, so that following the removal of a relatively large volume of tissue not too much skin will be left which would fall in wrinkles. If the tumor is located in one of the upper quadrants, the nipple is usually shifted upward, which the patient quite often sees as positive from the cosmetic aspect.
4. When a radical incision is made in the case of tumors sited below the nipple close to the transmamillary line this prevents the nipple from being pulled downward; this can have a negative cosmetic result if a curved incision is made and a spindle-shaped piece of skin is removed (Fig. 9).
5. If the lesion is more than 3 cm below the skin, a 1-cm-thick layer of subcutaneous fat can be left in place, which improves the cosmetic result.
6. Such operations must always be performed exclusively with a scalpel, to ensure clean sharp edges to the incision. This also makes it easier to keep relatively accurately to the recommended safety margin of 1–2 cm from the suspect disease focus. Hemostasis must be accomplished by precise damping of the blood vessels during cutting; coagulation of large areas is not permissible.
7. The tissue should not be removed in a rush; bleeding vessels must be coagulated step by step. This makes it possible to achieve the correct safety margin from the surface of the tumor at the first operation and to avoid unnecessary further resections if wide excision has to be performed.
8. If the tumor is sited peripherally, which can make excision problematic, and if the patient is not excessively concerned about cosmetically ideal results, the incision is made over the tumor. A semicircular course following the natural lines of the skin is beneficial.
9. We generally excise the specimens of tissue with the patient under general anesthesia. This seems necessary particularly when the tumor is sited some distance away from an incision designed for an optimum cosmetic result. Local anesthesia is used only at the express request of the patient, when changes are known to be sited relatively superficially, and when the general medical risk involved in general anesthesia is high.

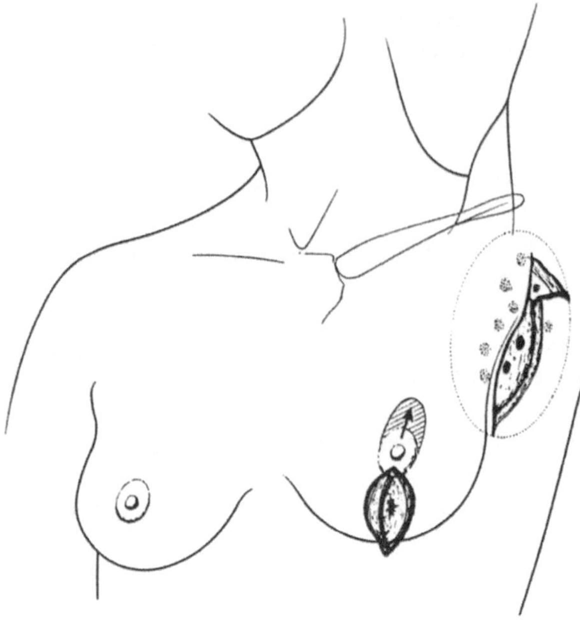

Fig. 9. Schematic representation of a wide excision with axillary lymphadenectomy. Dotted line: volume of resected tissue from beneath the skin

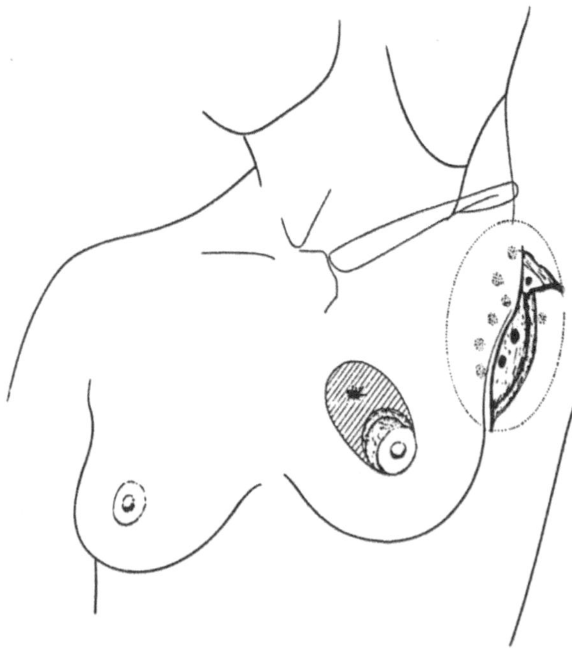

Fig. 10. Schematic representation of a tumorectomy with axillary lymphadenectomy. This type of tumorectomy from a perimamillary incision is *not* recommended by us

Intraoperative Processing of Excised Tissue

When tissue is removed for testing, the tumor palpated or the area with a suggestive radiological appearance must always be removed in toto. The surgeon cuts up the tissue immediately after removal and measures the solid parts in three dimensions.

Fixation of the Tissue: The tissue segment, with the tumor located centrally, is marked at two points: we mark the cranial incision line with green and the medial incision line with blue stitches. If it is suspected that the tumor is a carcinoma, the following are removed at once:

a) A tissue sample about the size of a pea (without any fat) for hormone receptor determination
b) A tissue sample at least the size of a lentil for immediate histological examination if indicated
c) A tissue sample about the size of a pea for determination of ploidy, proportion of cells in S-phase or other parameters
d) A tissue sample for determination of the labeling index

Care and Closure of the Wound

Careful hemostasis is important, and when large vessels are spurting blood we use electrocautery for this purpose. Large areas of tissue are not electrocauterized, because re-excision has to be performed if the tumor is found to have reached the edge of the tissue excised, either invasively or as carcinoma in situ, and electrocautery may cause damage. An aspiration drain is normally used. We prefer soft drains in this situation, the size depending on the size of the wound (Fig. 11). The drain is removed when less than 20 ml fluid per day is draining away, usually on the 3rd day after surgery. Approximation of the deep tissue of the breast by suturing is not worthwhile in most cases; after intracutaneous or subcutaneous alignment the tissue settles to give an optimal cosmetic result. A compression dressing is applied to the entire breast for 24 h after surgery to prevent seepage. In the same way, when surgery has been performed in the axilla (see below) a pressure dressing is applied for a few days to prevent later seepage of serum and the formation of serum pockets. Occasionally the glandular adipose tissue surrounding the defect needs to be mobilized to a varying extent from the adjacent skin, so that the filling of the defect does not lead to the skin being pulled in. The subcutis is adapted relatively close to the skin with resorbable single button sutures. Intracutaneous suturing is performed for closure of all other incisions. The breast is immobilized with a firm brassiere for about 2 weeks.

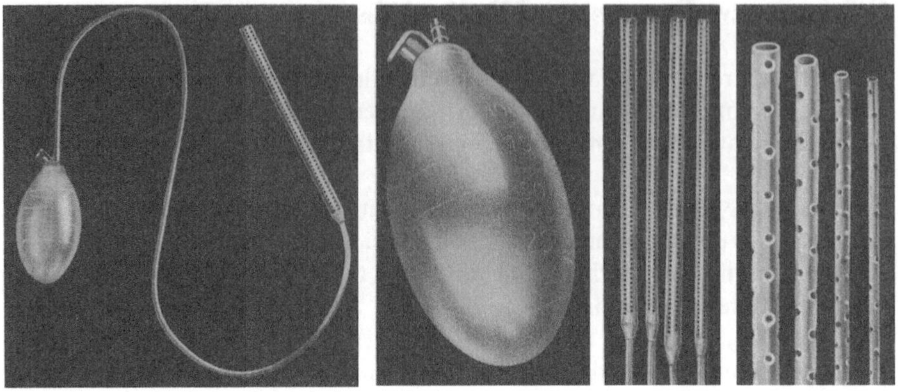

Fig. 11. Examples of round and flat soft drains provided with a decompression reservoir

The Problem of Frozen Section Examination

As a basic rule, the interval between removal of the biopsy and initiation of the treatment ultimately decided upon should be kept as short as possible. Contrary to frequently expressed opinion, however, it is not essential for tumor biological reasons that biopsy and final surgery be performed in the same operative session. On the other hand, it is better to perform both procedures in a single session in the case of aged patients and those whose poor general medical condition restricts their ability to withstand surgery. In these situations the patient must be given full information beforehand and the expected diagnosis must be confirmed by immediate frozen section.

There is also a relative indication for immediate frozen section examination when a patient in whom a carcinoma has been clearly revealed by radiological and clinical examination, and who has been fully informed beforehand, with an unhurried discussion of the treatment plan, has asked for the operation ultimately decided on to be performed in the same session.

If the diagnosis of carcinoma is not clear before surgery, for psychological reasons we prefer the two-step procedure. If the tumor turns out to be benign, this spares the patient the trauma of having to consent to a mastectomy on the previous evening. The two-step procedure can also be of advantage in the case of an obviously malignant tumor when alternative therapeutic procedures, e.g., amputation and breast-conserving treatment, are being discussed. Definite information on tumor type, intraoperative and histological extension and degree of differentiation make the decision easier.

Reference

1. Beller FK (1985) Atlas der Mammographie. Schattauer, Stuttgart, p 10

Surgical Treatment[1]

D. von Fournier and F. Kubli

Modified Radical Operation

The modified radical operation, consisting of total mastectomy with clearance of the axilla while one (Patey) or both (Auchincloss-Madden) of the pectoralis muscles is left in place is now regarded as the standard operation for operable carcinoma of the breast and has been described several times in the literature [1,3,5,7,9,11]. Therefore only a few points are dealt with here.

Positioning of Patient

The proximal upper arm and shoulder and the whole of the breast to be operated on must be sterile and completely exposed for the operation – medially up to the vertical transmamillary line on the contralateral side, caudally to 20 cm below the fold line, laterally up to 10 cm behind the posterior line of the axilla and cranially to above the clavicle. Surgical drapes should be attached with adhesive film at these borders. The arm should be draped free so that it can later be moved in a cranial direction.

Surgical Technique

The incision of the skin should be at least 4 cm from the tumor. The incision should be elliptical in form, encompassing the tumor and the nipple and areola. As a whole the incision should have a slightly oblique course, being higher at the lateral end, and everything should be done to ensure that tension-free closure of the skin will be possible. If these two requirements cannot both be realized we leave a narrower margin and, if it seems appropriate, administer postoperative irradiation to the chest wall. This is rarely necessary, since adaptation of the typical transverse oval incision to the individual position of the tumor generally makes it possible to ensure both adequate resection margins and tension-free closure.

---

[1]This topic was presented by F. Kubli as a lecture. It has been written by the co-author in accordance on the basis of the joint publication: F. Kubli and D. von Fournier (Eds), Neue Konzepte der Diagnostik und Therapie des Mammakarcinoms, Springer (1984) [8].

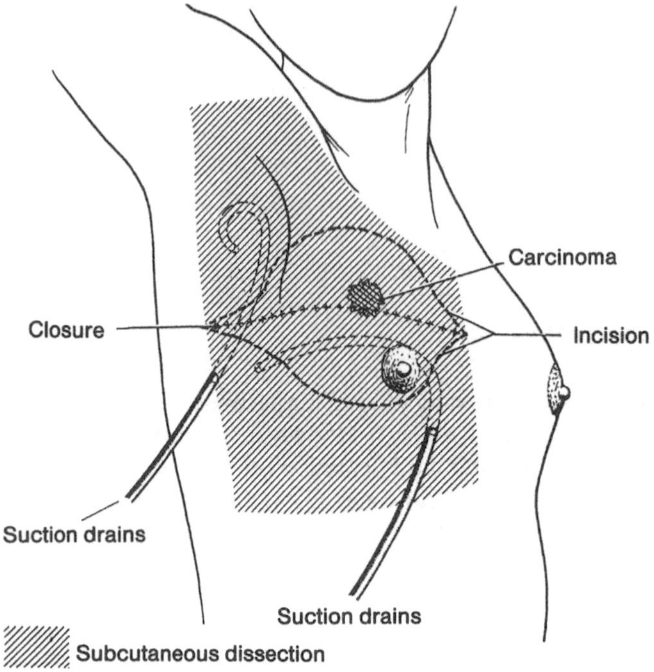

Fig. 1. Modified radical mastectomy: type of incision, extension of subcutaneous dissection, drainage and closure of the wound

As long as the tumor is not sited in the medial quadrant, for cosmetic reasons it is better to restrict the skin incision in the medial direction and terminate it clearly before the edge of the sternum.

In contrast, dissection of the body of the gland away from the cutis must be as near complete as possible; especially in young women a large area of skin, extending to the sternum in the medial direction, almost to the clavicle in the cranial direction and as far as the insertion of the right abdominal muscle in the caudal direction, must be undermined (Fig. 1). During this process the gland is dissected away from the pectoralis muscle from mediocaudal laterocranial. If the tumor is 2 cm or less from the pectoral fascia the part of the muscle underlying the tumor is also removed.

The mammary gland is generally removed with the pectoral fascia of the pectoralis major muscle. We make exceptions to this in the case of small tumors, especially when primary or secondary reconstruction is planned.

Preparation of the axilla begins with undermining of the skin up to the edge of the latissimus dorsi muscle and, cranially, approximately as far as the axillary vein. We prepare the axilla en bloc, and the lymphatic adipose tissue in the axilla remains connected with the body of the gland after it has been rolled away in the lateral direction. The two large nerves (long thoracic nerve, thoracodorsal nerve) and the thoracodorsal vascular bundle are spared. Conservation of the latter has attained some importance in connection with use of the latissimus dorsi islet flap for reconstruction. It is recommended that the medial and lateral thoracic nerve extending to the lateral edge of the pectoralis major muscle also be spared to avoid later atrophy of the laterocaudal parts of the pectoralis major muscle [4].

The lymphatic adipose tissue between the two pectoral muscles is examined digitally. We have hardly ever found carcinomatous involvement of interpectoral lymph nodes. For complete removal of Rotter's lymph nodes it is essential to remove the pectoralis minor muscle. It might be mentioned at this point that Rotter's lymph nodes are found in only 73% of cases, and in one study they were affected in only 8% patients in whom the axilla was positive and only 0.5% of these with negative axillary nodes (CODY et al. 1984). The arm must be mobilized with caution for clearance of the axilla, in order to prevent the medial pectoral nerve from being either cut through or ruptured. Axillary node dissection at level III – medial to the pectoralis minor muscle and lateral to the subclavius muscle – is performed with conservation of pectoralis minor by carefully retracting this muscle [1]. Level III, II and I dissection is best performed as an en bloc resection. The borders between levels I and II and levels II and III are marked with clips or sutures for the pathologist on the operative specimen. Our own standard procedure is to make a transverse cut through pectoralis minor, reuniting the ends at the end of the operation. If there is extensive invasion of the group II nodes pectoralis minor is completely excised. If the clinical tumor status is favorable (T1 N0) and the group I and II axillary lymph nodes are found at surgery to be free of disease, we do not cut through pectoralis minor. The apex of the axilla is marked with a clip in every case, because if postoperative irradiation is necessary, only radiotherapy delivered cranial to the axilla is of any use. If the operation is sufficiently radical no additional radiotherapy should be administered caudal to the clip, i.e., in the operative field.

If possible, the lateral pectoral nerve, which supplies the caudal third of the pectoralis major muscle, should also be spared. This prevents stiffness in the shoulder and atrophy of the caudal part of the pectoralis muscle. In 62% of cases this nerve passes through the belly of pectoralis minor and in the remaining 38% sweeps around its lateral border [10].

Radicality of Axillary Lymph Node Dissection

The radicality of axillary dissection varies in degree, this being reflected in the terms used for the different procedures.

Axillary Sampling

Axillary sampling involves removal of only a few axillary nodes, mostly of group I, with no exact description of the anatomical extent. The procedure is absolutely lacking in precision: it yields no accurate information that might be helpful to the doctor, and there is no therapeutic benefit to the patient. Axillary sampling thus cannot be recommended.

Dissection of the Low Axilla

This involves clearance of group I nodes in the axilla within the following limits: cranial, axillary vein; medial, edge of pectoralis minor muscle; lateral, edge of latissimus dorsi muscle. The apex and medial edge should be marked with clips if the region of groups II and III is to be irradiated in the case of lymph node invasion. This form of dissection can only be recommended in exceptional cases in the following situations: advanced age of patient and low risk; very low risk of axillary invasion, e.g., in the case of minimal cancer (< 5 mm) or noninvasive intraductal carcinoma extending over no more than 2 cm.

Dissection of Group I and II Nodes

This dissection involves the lymph nodes within the following limits: medial, medial edge of the pectoralis minor muscle; cranial, axillary vein; lateral, latissimus dorsi. Pectoralis minor is lifted for this procedure, and pectoralis major is relaxed by raising the arm. The apex of level II should be marked with a clip. This form of dissection can be recommended for patients with small tumors, especially any classified as T1 N0, when the nodes of groups I and II have also been found on intraoperative examination to be histologically negative. So-called skip metastases in group III occur in only 1% of patients in whom groups I and II are histologically negative [12].

Full Dissection of Axilla with Removal of Group I, II and III Nodes

The medial limit of full axillary dissection is the subclavius muscle, and the apex of the axilla should be marked with a clip. If group III nodes are affected radiotherapy can be delivered cranial to the clip. This type of dissection is advisable whenever intraoperative examination suggests that group I or II nodes are affected. The area of the wound is drained by means of an axillary and prepectoral suction drain. Intracutaneous sutures are used to close the skin in the medial two-thirds of the wound and individual button sutures in the lateral third.

Radical Mastectomy According to Rotter and Halsted

Classical radical mastectomy is now rarely carried out, the most common indication being extensive involvement of the pectoralis major muscle. Radical mastectomy is rather easier than the modified radical operation, and like the latter has been described by KASER et al. [7].

Breast-Conserving Operations

The following classification of operation technique has become accepted.

Tumorectomy

In tumorectomy (synonym: lumpectomy) the line of resection directly follows the surface of the tumor. This procedure obviously gives the best cosmetic results and is carried out in some trials. We abandoned tumorectomy some years ago because histological examination frequently shows that invasive or noninvasive tumor in situ extends beyond the line of resection. In this case re-excision is essential, because the local recurrence rate is directly dependent on the mass of invasive and noninvasive tumor cells left behind (see also A. MÜLLER, this volume).

Wide Excision

In wide excision (synonyms: partial mastectomy, limited resection) the tumor is removed with a wide margin of grossly normal tissue. Wide excision, described below, is now our standard technique.

Quadrantectomy

In quadrantectomy the tumor is excised together with the healthy tissue immediately surrounding it within one quadrant. The fascia of the pectoralis major muscle and the overlying skin are also removed. This technique has been described in detail by VERONESI et al. [13] and is so far the one that is followed by the lowest rate of local recurrences. The cosmetic results are not so pleasing as those attained with tumorectomy and wide excision.

Indications for Breast-Conserving Therapy

We carry out breast-conserving therapy within the context of a prospective controlled trial. The following conditions favor such treatment: small tumor; peripheral location (i.e., far distant from the mamilla); patient's desire for breast conservation. We perform breast-conserving surgery routinely when tumors are not more than 3 cm in size according to measurements from X-ray images; in the case of a very large breast this size limit is extended to 4 cm.

Patients to whom any of the following apply should *not* be selected for breast-conserving treatment: multifocal cancer; extensive noninvasive intraductal carcinoma, either demonstrated histologically or indicated by the microcalcifications typical for carcinoma on mammography; central location of the tumor behind the nipple; Paget's disease; pregnancy (no irradiation would be possible). When histological examination after wide excision shows that invasive or extensive noninvasive tumor has persisted, re-excision can still be performed as breast-conserving therapy.

One disadvantage of wide excision is the impossibility of keeping to a standard operation technique. A positive feature of it is the relatively good cosmetic result: it is seldom necessary to relocate the nipple or any healthy glandular tissue. The difference in volume between the treated and the untreated breast is usually so small that no cosmetic approximation of the healthy breast is necessary.

Reduction Mammoplasty

Large breasts with a high proportion of adipose tissue can be unsuitable for wide excision and, in particular, for radiotherapy. In such cases we carry out wide excision in combination with reduction mammoplasty. The course of the incision is selected with reference to the site of the tumor in each case. The contralateral breast must be reduced to achieve a good cosmetic result with breasts of approximately the same size. The advantage of this operation in patients with large breasts is that the line of resection is generally a long way into the healthy tissue, so that the volume of breast tissue remaining is sufficiently small to give favorable conditions for the radiotherapy.

Course of Incision for Wide Excision

We make the excision as described above for the modified radical operation. This means that we almost always make a curvilinear incision directly over the tumor, removing a spindle-shaped area of skin the size of which depends on the volume of tissue to be excised. If no skin is removed, wrinkles result if a large amount of tissue is excised, see Figs. 7, 8, 9 and 10 (pages 196, 198).

We do not generally make an incision running around the areola, because this requires a tunnel to the tumor, which is otherwise unnecessary. In exceptional cases, when the tumor is large and is sited caudal to the nipple we make a radial incision. In these cases a curvilinear incision and removal of a wide spindle-shaped area of skin would lead to caudal retraction of the mamilla.

Line of Excision

The tumor must be excised with grossly normal margins of 1–2 cm. Even then it is not uncommon to find residual invasive and noninvasive tumor at the margins. In such cases re-excision is performed if this is still possible from the cosmetic point of view. If the distance between tumor and pectoralis major muscle is 2 cm or less the underlying part of the muscle is also resected. Electrocautery should be avoided whenever possible in order to allow accurate histological assessment following re-excision. We perform careful cauterization of the visible blood vessels only.

The cranial and medial edges of the tissue removed are marked with different-colored sutures, and in addition the surface of the tissue is marked with a blue dye. The pathologist can then make a precise reconstruction of the cutting lines.

Examination of Tumor

The tumor is completely opened up and measured in three dimensions. The surgeon takes tissue for determination of hormone receptors, proportion of cells in S-phase, labeling index and ploidy. The tissue excised is weighed before and after removal of the tissue specimens. This allows the pathologist to estimate the total volume of the tumor, which is especially important in the case of very small tumors. Following removal of tissue specimens the segment is closed again with a continuous suture.

Wound Closure

Deep sutures for approximation of the wound cavity are avoided, and closure is accomplished by means of a fascial suture and subcuticular approximation. This usually gives an optimum form. A suction drain is inserted and left in place until less than 20 ml fluid per day is draining away. A pressure dressing is applied for 24 h, and the breast is supported with a firm brassiere for 2 weeks.

Stepwise Approach

As a rule we use the two-step procedure. Only wide excision is performed at the first operation. If the pathologist confirms that the margins are clear, axillary dissection is carried out in the second step. If the histological examination shows that multifocal invasive or noninvasive malignant disease has been left behind, re-excision is performed if still cosmetically possible. If necessary, mastectomy is carried out, and in this case axillary lymph node resection is also performed during this second step. If we explain this procedure to the patient and stress how safe it is, she is usually ready to accept the two-step approach and the necessity for general anesthesia.

If interstitial implantation is necessary for boost irradiation we do this 10 or more days later.

Axillary Dissection

The axillary dissection is performed as described above, for the modified radical operation. We make a transverse incision below the skin folds, extending it in the craniocaudal direction. If the disease status is relatively good (TI N0) the nodes of groups I and II are dissected, and if the lymph nodes are affected group III is dissected in addition, see Fig. 9.

Initiation of Radiotherapy

Postoperative irradiation of the remaining breast tissue is performed routinely 3 weeks after the operation. If interstitial boost radiation is necessary this is carried out first, the external teletherapy subsequently.

References

1. Auchincloss H (1963) Significance of location and number of axillary metastases in carcinoma of the breast, a justification for a conservative operation. Ann Surg 158:37
2. Cody HS III, Egeli RA, Urban JA (1984) Rotter's node metastases. Therapeutic and prognostic considerations in early breast carcinoma. Ann Surg 199:266
3. Donegan WL, Spratt JS (1979) Cancer of the breast. Saunders, Philadelphia
4. Gant TD, Vasconez LD (eds) (1981) Postmastectomy reconstruction. Williams and Wilkins, Baltimore
5. Handley R, Thackray A (1969) Conservative radical mastectomy (Patey's operation). Surgery 170:880
6. Harris JR, Hellmann S, Kinne DW (1985) Limited surgery and radiotherapy for early breast cancer. N Engl J Med 313:1365
7. Käser O, Iklé FA, Hirsch HA (1983) Atlas der Gynäkologischen Operationen, 4th edn. Thieme, Stuttgart
8. Kubli F und von Fournier D Eds (1984) Neue Konzepte der Diagnostik und Therapie des Mammakarzinoms. Springer, Berlin Heidelberg New York
9. Madden JL, Kandalaff S, Bourque R (1956) Modified radical mastectomy. Ann Surg 175:624
10. Moosman DA (1980) Anatomy of the pectoral nerves and their preservation in modified mastectomy. Am J Surg 139:883
11. Patey DH, Dyson WH (1948) The prognosis of carcinoma of the breast in relation to the type of operation performed. Br J Cancer 2:7
12. Rosen PP, Lesser MT, Kinne DW (1983) Discontinuous or "skip" metastases in breast carcinoma. Analysis of 128 axillary dissections. Ann Surg 197:276
13. Veronesi U, Saccozzi R, Del Vecchio M et al (1981) Comparing radical mastectomy with quadrantectomy, axillary dissection and radiotherapy in patients with small cancers of the breast. N Engl J Med 305:6

Breast-Conserving Therapy or Amputation with Reconstruction: The Patient's View

K. Engel, D. von Fournier, F. Kubli and M. Kaufmann

Summary

By means of a retrospective study, we compared the subjective appreciation of cosmetic results, complaints, and psychosocial problems of patients who underwent either breast amputation with reconstruction or breast-conserving therapy at the University Women's Clinic, Heidelberg, between 1983 and 1986. Questionnaires completed by two groups of 50 patients were evaluated, taking into consideration the match criteria – absence of recurrence, menopausal status, and time elapsed since therapy was completed. The more-positive attitude toward cosmetic results, tolerance of therapy, acceptance of physical appearance, unchanged sensation of shame and self-consciousness, partner relationship, professional situation, and fear of recurrence – showed that patients who had undergone breast-conserving therapy were significantly more often satisfied with their treatment. Comparison with the group of patients who had amputation with reconstruction showed no significant differences in patients' complaints. From an oncologic point of view, amputation with reconstruction and breast conservation are equivalent therapies, if we consider indications and limitations. From the patient's point of view, breast conservation is clearly to be preferred.

Introduction

The historical change in the conception of breast carcinoma as a systemic disease has radically changed the therapy of locally operable carcinoma in recent years. Radical operations have been increasingly replaced by organ-conserving procedures which combine local control of tumors with concern for cosmetic results and a maximal chance of cure. Comparative studies have shown that amputation of the breast, a mutilating intervention, is not oncologically superior to local excision (tumorectomy, wide rejection, quadrantectomy or tumor-adapted partial mastectomy) with subsequent irradiation of the residual breast [8]. Less favorable results of breast-conserving therapy [1] can essentially be traced back to inadequate local tumor control. Nevertheless, because of these experiences breast conservation is not yet generally accepted as an alternative to breast amputation and has by no means replaced it. In these cases breast reconstruction after amputation is essential for the patient's positive acceptance of her cancer, stabilizing her self-confidence and psychic condition.

Breast-conserving therapy is a more differentiated and complex procedure than amputation with reconstruction. It is very exacting for the patient and requires close cooperation between surgeon, pathologist, radiotherapist, and oncologist. In judging whether both procedures are equivalent not only from both the oncologic and the patient's points of view, purely objective examination of cosmetic results and complaints is not sufficient. These factors are often judged very differently by patient and physician. When establishing indications it seems useful to consider patients' appraisal of cosmetic results, complaints, and psychosocial problems. We directly compared two patient groups, one receiving breast-conserving therapy, the other amputation with primary reconstruction.

Material and Methods

Between May 1983 and June 1986, 116 patients underwent breast amputation at the University Women's Clinic in Heidelberg. After amputation, the breast was reconstructed by insertion of a subpectoral tissue expander [5]. In 62 patients phase II or III of reconstruction was completed (Table 1). Patients were matched with respect to absence of recurrence, menopausal status, and time elapsed since conclusion of therapy, so that 50 of the patients treated with amputation-reconstruction surgery could be compared with 50 patients treated with breast-conserving therapy (Table 2). Each patient's opinion of the cosmetic results, postoperative complaints, and psychosocial problems was determined of both groups by means of a specially designed questionnaire completed by the patients.

Table 1. Steps in amputation-reconstruction treatment

Step	Management
1	Modified radical mastectomy Radical axillary lymph-node dissection (levels I–III) Phase-I reconstruction (subpectoral expansion prosthesis)
2	Phase-II reconstruction (final gel prosthesis, creation of submammary fold)
3	Phase-III reconstruction (nipple and areola)
4	N+, adjuvant chemotherapy, 6× CMF (FEC) before phase II

N+, patients with lymph-node involvement; CMF, FEC

Table 2. Steps in breast-conserving therapy

Step	Management
1	Tumorectomy, wide resection, quadrantectomy or partial mastectomy with or without contralateral adjustment Radical axillary lymph-node dissection (levels I–III)
2	Irradiation – Homogeneous (residual breast) 45–55 (60) Gy "Boost" (tumor bed) 5–10 (15) Gy
3	N+, combination adjuvant chemotherapy/irradiation ("sandwich" technique) 3× CMF (FEC) // 3× CMF (FEC)

Table 3. Comparison of premenopausal ($n=41$) and postmenopausal ($n=9$) patient groups

	Premenopausal		Postmenopausal	
	Amputation with reconstruction	Breast-conserving therapy	Amputation with reconstruction	Breast-conserving therapy
Age (in years)				
Mean	41.6	42.8	53.4	56.1
Min.	30	27	51	50
Max.	47	54	58	61
Tumor stage (in number of patients)				
T1	21	29	4	6
T2	20	12	5	3
N+	12	7	4	4

Comparison of the groups showed that in the group treated with organ-conserving measures, smaller, nodal-negative tumors were overrepresented (Table 3). For certain questions the patients of both groups were rematched according to tumor stage, thus taking into account the predominance of less favorable tumors in the amputation-reconstruction group.

Results

Cosmetic Results

When evaluating cosmetic results (Table 4), patients who had undergone breast-conserving therapy more rarely reported an unpleasant or awkward difference in shape or size between the two breasts. Moreover, scars following irradiation looked better than those which followed breast reconstruction, which more often resulted in rather ugly scars, due to stretching of the skin.

Table 4. Patients' opinion of cosmetic results after amputation ($n=50$) and breast-conserving therapy ($n=50$)

Cosmetic results	Amputation with reconstruction (%)	Breast-conserving therapy (%)
Unsatisfactory shape or size difference	30	10
Unsatisfactory scars	26	14
Evaluation		
Excellent	16	44
Good	44	40
Fair	32	16
Poor	8	0

Postoperative Complaints (Table 5)

Patients of both groups generally complained of the same type of postoperative symptoms. They referred to chronic pain, sensory disturbances, shoulder stiffness, and lymphedema of the arms – all of variable severity. The patients' evaluation of these disturbances, albeit subjective, is of special importance. The severity of symptoms described, reported degree of functional impairment, and subjective estimation of disability were the same in both groups.

Psychosocial Problems

Impairment by Therapy (Table 6). Despite the necessary irradiation, patients who had breast-conserving therapy generally coped better with the treatment they had to undergo. This also remained valid if we compared only those patients of both groups who, because of a positive nodal finding, had to undergo adjuvant chemotherapy. Generally more patients found reconstruction caused impairment, as it required several surgical interventions and thus hospitalizations.

Table 5. Postoperative complaints after amputation ($n = 50$) and breast-conserving therapy ($n = 50$)

Complaints	Amputation with reconstruction (%)	Breast-conserving therapy (%)
None or few symptoms, no disability	44	50
Few symptoms, occasional disability	36	32
Definite symptoms with disability	16	18
Severe symptoms, marked disability	4	0

Table 6. Psychosocial impairment as a result of amputation ($n = 50$) and breast-conserving therapy ($n = 50$)

Reported impairment due to therapy	Amputation with reconstruction (%)	Breast-conserving therapy (%)
Well tolerated, practically no adverse effects	22	40
Hardly any impairment, relatively well tolerated	48	46
Great impairment, badly tolerated	26	14
Hardly bearable	4	0

Acceptance of Physical Appearance (Table 7). Acceptance of physical appearance was significantly better in patients who had breast-conserving therapy. In this group, even patients who regarded the cosmetic results as unfavorable could still fully regard the breast as part of themselves. After reconstruction, most patients – even if the cosmetic results were satisfactory – merely "put up with" the prosthesis. However, even in patients who described a "foreign-body" sensation, there was a close correlation with unsatisfactory cosmetic results. This difference in patient attitude between the two groups was also noted in their evaluation of self-confidence and sensation of shame.

Partnership and Marriage (Table 8). Breast-conserving therapy had comparatively less effect on the patients relationship with her partner(s). These patients more rarely described the relationship with a partner as having "cooled down" emotionally and sexually or were threatened by loss of the partner, but the number of patients was too small to allow a definite conclusion. Surely other factors, e.g., the partner's attitude, were also responsible for the fact that in the reconstruction group a closer relationship was somewhat more often described.

Table 7. Patients' acceptance of physical appearance after amputation ($n = 50$) and breast-conserving therapy ($n = 50$)

	Amputation with reconstruction (%)	Breast-conserving therapy (%)
"This is my breast"	16	80
"I have put up with it"	68	20
"The breast is foreign to me"	14	0
"The breast does not belong to me"	2	0
Loss of self confidence	36	8
Changed sense of shame	40	16

Table 8. Effect of amputation ($n = 50$) and breast-conserving therapy ($n = 50$) on partnership/marriage

Reported effect	Amputation with reconstruction (%)	Breast-conserving therapy (%)
No change	56	74
"Cooled down" emotionally	5	2
"Cooled down" sexually	10	7
Loss or change of partner	4	0
Closer relationship	25	17

Professional Situation (Table 9). Questions relating to professional situation also showed a tendency toward more positive responses by patients who had breast-conserving therapy. Reintegration at work was considerably more difficult in the breast-reconstruction group, as data referring to disability and changes in employment show. However, the greater frequency of unfavorable tumor stages also played an important part in this.

Fear of Recurrence (Table 10). Patients who underwent reconstruction more often reported fear of tumor recurrence. When comparing patients of the two groups on the basis of tumor stage, we also found that there was less potential for fear after breast-conserving therapy. To this corresponds the fact that this group of patients more rarely had doubts as to the right choice of therapy.

Table 9. Effect of amputation ($n = 50$) and breast-conserving therapy ($n = 50$) on professional situation

Reported Effect	Amputation with reconstruction (%)	Breast-conserving therapy (%)
No change	52	72
Activity made more difficult by handicap	32	20
Different activity	0	4
Loss of employment/ incapable of working or earning a living	16	4

Table 10. Postoperative anxieties reported by patients after amputation ($n = 50$) and breast-conserving therapy ($n = 50$)

	Amputation with reconstruction (%)	Breast-conserving therapy (%)
Fear of recurrence		
Often	32	22
Sometimes	54	44
Rarely	12	26
Never	2	8
Doubts as to the right choice of therapy		
Often	12	4
Sometimes	22	10
Rarely	14	12
Never	52	74

Final Evaluation (Table 11). The final evaluation once more confirmed the better quality of life in patients who had breast-conserving therapy. However, one must certainly also note that, despite the generally less favorable cosmetic results in the reconstruction group, only 12% of all the patients of this group were definitely not satisfied with the choice of therapy. This fact may suggest that the importance of cosmetic results to the patient's basic attitude is minor relative to other factors.

Table 11. Final evaluation

	Amputation with reconstruction (%)	Breast-conserving therapy (%)
"If you could choose, would it be the same therapy?"		
Certainly	58	96
Possibly	30	4
Probably not/certainly not	12	0
"Would you recommend the therapy you underwent?"		
Certainly	64	94
Possibly	24	6
Probably not/certainly not	12	0

Discussion

In the critical evaluation of our comparison between patients who underwent amputation with reconstruction and those, with breast-conserving therapy, the basic difficulties of a retrospective study cannot be neglected. In reality, prospective studies, like that of the German Federal Ministry of Research and Technology (BMFT; see [6]), encounter considerable difficulties, especially in the randomization of patients. In total, the patients' answers to our questions clearly showed that breast conservation is preferred to reconstruction with a prosthesis. At the University Women's Clinic in Heidelberg, indications for breast-conserving therapy are, besides the patient's urgent desire for organ conservation, a series of oncologic factors: tumor size less than 3 cm, more than eight extirpated lymph nodes, tumor without excessive intraductal growth and completely removed [4]. Patients with larger tumors or mainly central localization of the tumor generally do not receive breast-conserving therapy. In determining indications, the relationship between size of the breast and tumor size is also of importance, as in the case of an unfavorable relationship, e.g., a very small breast with a large tumor, an acceptable cosmetic result can hardly be obtained. Thus from the beginning a series of patients must be excluded, to whom only breast amputation with primary reconstruction can be offered as an alternative. This decision made by the physician, irrespective of the patient's attitude towards breast conservation, is certainly relevant to further developments, as amputation is for many patients equivalent, on the basis of personal experiences derived from their surroundings, to a less-favorable prognosis, while breast conservation promises a prognostically better first stage. Apparently, fear of recurrence in the conserved breast is secondary to the certainty that amputation was not yet necessary. Evidently in most cases not even breast reconstruction can affect this basically pessimistic evaluation of amputation. A comparison with the reconstruction group shows for different comparable tumor stages a positive evaluation by patients after breast-conserving therapy, even among those with positive axillary lymph nodes who required chemotherapy.

The patient's evaluation of cosmetic results is often very different from the physician's. Various factors play an important role in the patient's evaluation: acceptance of personal physical appearance prior to the illness, individual appreciation of the prognosis, reaction to the reality of cancer, social integration, etc. At the same time, patients' complaints can only partially be made objective by the physician. At the same time, there was a positive correlation between a cosmetic result appreciated as unfavorable and a "foreign-body" response in the reconstruction group. In these cases a good cosmetic result was essential for toleration of the prosthesis and even for its acceptance as the patient's own breast. The possibilities of breast reconstruction by means of a temporary tissue expander not only depend on operative techniques, but also on factors that cannot or can only with difficulty be influenced, e.g., subpectoral capsule formation; variable atrophy of the pectoralis major muscle; movement of the prosthesis (due to muscle contraction, prosthesis dislocation, or defects); unfavorable scar formation; and omitted adjustment of the contralateral breast. It is interesting to note that after breast-conserving therapy many patients find the operated breast more pleasant than the healthy one, as a favorable relationship between tumor size and breast size often results in a "lifting" effect, especially of ptotic breasts, due to radiogenic fibrosis of the mammary gland.

Our results concerning patients' evaluation of amputation with reconstruction enlarge the studies of BULMAN et al. (1986) and VAN DONGEN (1986), ascertaining that the degree of psychic morbidity in patients after breast-conserving therapy is less than in patients after simple amputation without reconstruction. BRODERICK et al. (1986) conducted a pilot study of 41 patients who had breast-conserving therapy and found no correlation between cosmetic results and depressive or anxiety states. These states, however, occurred significantly more often when there were accompanying severe functional disturbances such as lymphedema of the arm or shoulder stiffness. Besides taking into account oncologic and cosmetic factors, this correlation seems to make it necessary, when planning therapy, to consider post therapeutic complaints and functional disturbances more thoroughly, as well as to recognize and treat existing disturbances early by systematic postoperative follow-up.

References

1. Atkins H, Hayward JL, Klugman DJ, et al. (1972) Treatment of early breast cancer: a report after ten years of clinical trial. Br J Breast Cancer Res Treat 1:27–32
2. Broderick MM, Evans JE, Yarnold JR, Maguire P (1986) Cosmetic results and psychological morbidity in women treated for early stage breast cancer by local excision and high dose radiotherapy. Seminar on Conservative Treatments in Breast Cancer of the European School of Oncology, Milano
3. Bulman S, Gomez J, Phillips RH, Ellis H (1986) Anxiety and depression in breast cancer patients treated by local tumor excision and radical radiotheraphy. Seminar on Conservative Treatments in Breast Cancer of the European School of Oncology, Milano
4. Kubli F, von Fournier D (1986) Brusterhaltende Therapie des Mammacarcinoms. In: Melchert H, Beck L, Hepp H, Knappstein PG, Kreienberg R (eds) Aktuelle Geburtshilfe und Gynäkologie. Springer, Berlin Heidelberg New York
5. Radovan C (1982) Breast reconstruction after mastectomy using temporary expander. Plast Reconstr Surg 69(2):195–205
6. Rauschecker H, Sauer R, Schauer A, Scheurlen H, Peiper HJ (1985) Our experience in setting up the BMFT multicer trial: therapy of small breast cancer. In: Zander J, Baltzer J (eds) Early breast cancer. Springer, Berlin Heidelberg New York
7. Van Dongen J (1986) Parameters for the evaluation of the results, including the quality of life, in breast conserving therapy. International Workshop on Conservative Treatment of Breast Cancer, Oct 3–5, Heidelberg
8. Veronesi U, Succosi R, et al. (1981) Comparing radical mastectomy with quadrantectomy, axillary dissection, and radiotherapy in patients with small cancer of the breast. N Engl Med J 305:6

Surgical Techniques of Breast Preservation for Early Breast Cancer

D. W. KINNE

Increased use of conservative surgery combined with radiotherapy as primary treatment for women with early breast cancer has given rise to a set of guidelines to be used in these cases. Published reports from retrospective and prospective randomized studies have indicated that local tumor control and cosmetic results have been satisfactory and that the overall disease-free survival, so far, has been comparable to that of mastectomy. Other prospective studies are underway, and will generate more data in the future. The purpose of this paper is not to review these results in comparison to mastectomy; instead, it addresses how best to select surgical approaches to the breast primary and the axilla in patients undergoing breast preservation.

The actual details of surgical treatment have yet to be standardized. The extent of the excision in the breast and the approach to the axillary nodes varies considerably. Accordingly, a workshop was held in June, 1985 in New York City, sponsored jointly by the Memorial Sloan-Kettering Cancer Center and The Joint Center for Radiation Therapy (Harvard) to improve the definition of terms and to select which approaches seem most appropriate. The results of this conference, and our present techniques at Memorial Hospital, will be discussed.

Definition of Terms

The terms currently used in describing the resection of a primary breast tumor are as follows:

1. Local excision (excisional biopsy, tumorectomy) implies simple gross excision of the tumor without regard to the microscopic margins of resection. "Lumpectomy" is an imprecise term, but probably is in this category.
2. Wide (local) excision (limited resection, partial mastectomy, segmental mastectomy) implies resection of the tumor, with 1–2 cm adjacent breast tissue, designed to provide clear margins of resection.
3. Quadrantectomy implies resection of the tumor, along with the involved quadrant of the breast, including the overlying skin.

Axillary dissection is described as follows:

1. Lateral (level 1) – dissection of the axillary contents, extending from the tail of the breast inferiorly, the latissimus dorsi muscle laterally, the axillary vein superiorly, and the lateral border of the pectoralis minor muscle medially.
2. Levels I and II – a procedure similar to that described above, but also including removal of axillary tissue beneath the pectoralis minor. This dissection is typically facilitated by retraction of the muscle and manipulation of the arm position during the operation.
3. Full – complete dissection of all three levels of the axilla, with or without resection of the pectoralis minor muscle.

The term "axillary sampling" is not used by us, as it does not denote a precise surgical procedure.

Patient Selection

Adequate resection of the breast tumor without major cosmetic deformity is the major goal of this type of treatment. Poor surgical candidates, or those with relative contraindications for breast preservation, include patients with the following characteristics:

1. Radiographically or clinically evident, widely separated tumors in the same breast
2. Clustered microcalcification in multiple quadrants, even without histologic evidence of malignancy (high-quality mammographic studies are therefore necessary)
3. Unfavorable size of the tumor in relation to the size of the breast (no absolute upper limit of size is defined, but adequate excision without resultant breast deformity is the objective)
4. Certain histologic types (the presence of intraductal cancer within and outside of the primary tumor, or microscopically involved margins, indicate the need for reexcision)
5. Unfavorable location of the tumor. This applies primarily to central tumors requiring excision of the nipple-areola complex. (This procedure can be done, nevertheless, and after irradiation of the breast mound, nipple-areola reconstruction can be considered)

Other relative contraindications are psychological problems, pregnancy, very large and/or pendulous breasts, extreme age or youth, a clinically positive axilla and, on biopsy, the presence of in situ ductal carcinoma only. It must be emphasized that these clinical settings do not represent absolute contraindications to breast preservation, but indicate the need for cooperation and joint consultation between radiation and surgical oncologists to decide the appropriate treatment.

Pathologic Review

For evaluation of the resected specimen by the pathologist, sutures are placed in the specimen for orientation. The specimen is sent intact to the pathology laboratory, where the exterior surface is inked to facilitate microscopic assessment of the resection margins for tumor involvement. This assessment is most accurate using paraffin, not frozen, sections. Gross description should include measurement of tumor dimensions, and shortest distance from periphery to margin of resection. Tissue samples for measurement of estrogen- and progesterone-receptors should be obtained with minimal interference during evaluation of the margin. It is important to determine the presence of microscopic tumor involvement in the resection margins. Microscopic tumor features should be recorded, as they may influence the need for further resection, particularly, as noted above, the presence of intraductal carcinoma in the primary tumor and in grossly normal adjacent tissue. Negative margins are the goal of surgery; if the histology indicates it, further resection should be done before starting radiotherapy. If local resection is not feasible or would not achieve the cosmetic goal, then mastectomy would reasonably be considered.

Surgery

In most cases, breast excision and the incision for axillary dissection should be separate, as this improves the cosmetic result. However, primary tumors located in the axillary tail of the breast may be resected with the axillary contents, as the sites are close to each other. The incision should be placed directly over the primary tumor to minimize the possibility of contamination by tumor cells through a tunnel, and to indicate to the radiologist the exact site of the tumor for planning a boost dose. Circumareolar incisions are therefore avoided. In the upper part of the breast, curvilinear incisions are best. In the lower half of the breast, the type of incision is adapted to the extent of reapproximation required. Radial incisions are often best for major reapproximation, and curvilinear for minimal reapproximation.

Axillary dissection is performed to determine the presence of positive lymph nodes in that site. Patients with positive nodes are at greater risk of distant relapse than those with negative nodes, and are currently considered candidates for adjuvant systemic therapy or hormonal therapy. Complete axillary dissection is indicated in all patients with clinically suspicious axillary nodes.

The dissection should be extensive enough to

1. Allow a reasonable certainty of detecting axillary metastases if present (staging)
2. Provide local tumor control in itself
3. Be easily integrated with subsequent radiotherapy to the breast.
4. Not pose a major risk that complications of cosmetic deformity will occur

The optimal incision for axillary dissection is horizontal, extending from just posterior to the pectoralis major muscle to the border of the latissimus dorsi muscle.

This allows good exposure and gives a good cosmetic result. An alternative incision is vertical, in the anterior axilla, just posterior to the lateral border of pectoralis major. A vertical incision carried too high in the axilla can be associated with an adverse "bowstringing" effect and should be avoided.

In patients with clinically negative nodes at the time of dissection, it is advisable to spare the thoracodorsal vessels and nerve. The long thoracic nerve (innervating the serratus anterior) is always identified and protected throughout the dissection. The medial nerve to pectoralis major, coursing around the lateral border of pectoralis minor, is also preserved. The intercostobrachial nerve(s) innervating the skin of the medial upper arm can be spared in cases with negative axillary nodes, but this may compromise the dissection. This usually results in division of these nerves to achieve adequate axillary clearance.

In summary, the ideal excision of a breast primary is a wide excision (or limited resection) with pathological confirmation of clear margins. Quadrantectomy is considered potentially deforming for many patients, and simple local excision without attention to margins may lead to a high rate of local recurrence. The ideal axillary dissection for patients with a clinically negative axilla is a level I – II dissection. For patients with involved nodes, complete axillary dissection is preferred. Coordination between surgeons and radiotherapists is critical in these approaches.

References

1. Bluming AZ, Dosik G, Lowitz B, et al. (1986) Treatment of primary breast cancer without mastectomy: the Los Angeles community experience and review of the literature. Ann Surg 204:136–147
2. Carter D (1986) Margins of "lumpectomy" for breast cancer. Hum Pathol 17:330–332
3. Harris JR, Hellman S, Kinne DW (1985) Limited surgery and radiotherapy for early breast cancer. N Engl J Med 313:1365–1368
4. Levitt S, Potish RA, Boen JR, et al. (1986) The effect of definitive irradiation on local control and disease free survival in breast cancer. Int J Radiat Oncol Biol Phys 12:673–679
5. Solin LJ, Fowble B, Martz K, et al. (1986) Results of re-excisional biopsy of the primary tumor in preparation for definitive irradiation of patients with early stage breast cancer. Int J Radiat Oncol Biol Phys 12:721–725

Conservation Trials in Early Breast Cancer

J. Hayward

The first controlled trial on conservation treatment in the management of early breast cancer was carried out at Guy's Hospital in London between 1961 and 1975. It was conducted in two series; entry to the first was between 1961 and 1971 and to the second between 1971 and 1975. The difference between the two series was that the first included all patients aged 50 years or over with operable breast cancer, irrespective of the axillary-node status. In the second series, patients under 50 years of age were also included, but only those who did not have clinically involved lymph nodes. The patients were randomly assigned one of two treatment options. The first option was modified radical mastectomy, in which the whole breast was removed with all the axillary contents and that part of the pectoralis major muscle lying behind the tumour. The second option was wide local excision, in which the tumour was removed together with 3 cm of normal breast tissue surrounding it. All patients were subsequently treated by radiation therapy to the lymphatic drainage fields, and those treated by wide excision were also given radiation therapy to the retained breast. Precise details of the treatment and the doses of radiation have been described elsewhere [2].

These patients have now been observed for up to 25 years, and it seems unlikely that the results will change. The principal finding is that patients who had only wide excision had a significantly higher incidence of loco-regional recurrence – principally in the axilla. In the first series, those who had clinically involved axillary lymph nodes also had a higher incidence of distant recurrence and diminished survival. In those who had no clinically involved nodes, the distant recurrence rate and survival were the same for both options. In the second series, which included only patients with no clinically involved axillary nodes, there was again a higher incidence of loco-regional recurrence in the wide-excision group, and furthermore the wide-excision patients also had a higher incidence of distant recurrence and significantly diminished survival. Again, life tables detailing the results of these two series have been published elsewhere [2].

The assumption from the results of this trial is that, because the dose of radiation to the axilla was inadequate by today's standards, there was a high incidence of recurrence in the axilla and this in turn was responsible for the increased incidence of distant metastases and diminished survival. What has been difficult to explain has been that the high incidence of distant recurrence and diminished survival was not demonstrated in patients who had clinically uninvolved axillary lymph nodes in the first series, but was clearly demonstrated in the second series. This difference appeared to occur because the results of radical mastectomy in the second series were significantly better than in the first, whereas the results in patients having a wide excision were unchanged. Recent analysis has demonstrated a probable cause for this. In the second series there were twice as many patients with T1 tumours as in the first, and it was in this group that those who had a radical mastectomy did better. This operation achieved local control, whereas wide excision with inadequate radiation treatment of the axilla, did not. This can be interpreted as showing that achieving local control of disease is particularly important when dealing with patients who have small tumours. In patients with larger tumours, local control probably does not significantly affect life expectancy. Most patients with large tumours already have occult metastases before they present to the clinic, and the management of the local disease has little effect on their ultimate fate.

Local Control of Disease

The early studies from Guy's Hospital indicate that local control is important, particularly in those with small tumours, but it has been difficult to find confirmation elsewhere. Nevertheless, a recent trial by the National Surgical Adjuvant Breast Project in the USA, seems to support this suggestion. In this study [1], a randomised clinical trial was carried out comparing total mastectomy and segmental mastectomy with or without radiation therapy in the treatment of early breast cancer. All patients had axillary dissection, and consequently the nodal status was known. Patients who had positive nodes were given adjuvant chemotherapy. Life-table estimates based on data from 1843 women suggest that treatment by segmental mastectomy with or without breast irradiation results in disease-free, distant disease-free and overall survival at 5 years that is no worse than after total breast removal. Nevertheless, in the comparison of segmental mastectomy with segmental mastectomy plus radiation therapy, it was shown that patients who received segmental mastectomy alone and had negative nodes had significantly poorer disease-free survival than those who also had negative nodes and received radiotherapy as well as segmental mastectomy. Moreover, distant disease-free survival was also significantly worse in those who did not receive radiation therapy. At present there is no significant difference in survival rate between these two groups, but if distant disease-free survival is significantly worse in those not receiving radiation therapy, it would be reasonable to suppose that survival itself will eventually be affected. This finding again strongly suggests that because local control of disease was not achieved in those patients who received neither local radiation therapy nor adjuvant chemotherapy, the incidence of distant metastases was significantly increased, which will probably affect survival.

Logically, local control of disease must be an essential part of the design of future conservative treatments. Indeed, if local control of disease was not important, there would be no purpose in encouraging early diagnosis. If diagnosing breast cancer early had no effect on survival, the whole purpose of screening would be lost. The results of many studies indicate that the opposite has occurred. Through the use of mammography and clinical examination, breast cancer can be diagnosed at an earlier stage, and mortality from the disease has subsequently been reduced. This can result only from the fact that, by early treatment, permanent local control of the disease is achieved in more cases and this has its effect on the patients' ultimate fate. It is probably true to say that this effect can be shown only in patients with small tumours, but this in no way suggests that small tumours require minimal treatment. If anything, it indicates the opposite. If treated properly, patients with small tumours have a real chance of permanent cure. The principal problem now is to determine how such tumours can be treated effectively whilst giving the best cosmetic result. Essentially two policies of management are now being debated. In one, surgery is principally used to achieve local control of disease, with radiation therapy as a supporting measure. In the second, minimal surgery is employed and radiotherapy is given the major role in eradicating local disease.

The Case for Wide Local Surgery

There seems little doubt that, with small tumours, the use of wide local surgery plus subsequent radiation therapy to the breast can achieve local control as effectively as radical mastectomy. It is interesting that in both the major trials in which this procedure has been undertaken, complete axillary dissection was also included as part of the primary treatment. This procedure not only gives full information about axillary-node status, which is important in the management of the patient by adjuvant therapy, but also effectively treats the axilla, so that radiation therapy to the area is not necessary. The earliest trial using a procedure of this nature was that carried out in Milan [3] in which patients with tumours under 2 cm in diameter were subjected to "quadrantectomy" plus total axillary dissection. Subsequently each patient underwent radiation therapy to the retained breast, and those with involved axillary nodes were treated with adjuvant CMF. Patients in the control group underwent radical mastectomy. Follow-up in this study now exceeds 10 years, and there is no discernible difference in the incidence of local or distant recurrence, or in survival

Similarly, in the United States, the trial by FISHER et al. [1] compared total mastectomy and segmental mastectomy with or without radiation therapy. In this particular study, segmental mastectomy was carried out when the margins of the resected specimen were pathologically clear of tumour. In approximately 10% of patients, this could not be achieved; these were treated by total mastectomy. Patients with tumours up to 4 cm in diameter were included, and again all patients underwent total axillary dissection. Those with axillary nodes were given adjuvant therapy by melphalan and 5-fluorouracil. The follow-up of this series is much shorter but, up to 5 years, there appears to be no difference in disease-free, distant disease-free or overall survival between total mastectomy and segmental mastectomy plus radiation therapy. As has been explained earlier, the third group in this trial, in which the patients were treated by segmental mastectomy without subsequent radiation therapy, appeared to fare worse if they had no involved nodes and hence received no adjuvant chemotherapy.

In summary, it would seem that wide local excision – as variously defined – followed by adequate radiation therapy, axillary dissection and, where indicated, adjuvant chemotherapy appears to pose no additional hazard to patients with small tumours when compared with radical mastectomy. The principal problem with wide excision as a conservative surgical procedure is the cosmetic defect that often occurs in the retained breast. In patients with large breasts, this defect is probably not great, but in those with small breasts, particularly those in which the tumour lies behind the nipple, the cosmetic result may be poor. It is because of this that other techniques, in which the surgical procedure is less extensive, have been investigated.

The Use of Minimal Local Surgery with Boost Radiation Therapy

Most of the pioneer work on these techniques was carried out in France and in the United States. The aim is local excision of the tumour – with no attempt to obtain a pathologically clear margin – with boost radiation treatment to treat any residual tumour cells. This boost radiation treatment can be given in a number of ways, but those principally undertaken are the use of implants of iridium 192 or the external application of electrons. Noncontrolled studies have suggested that the cosmetic results of such procedures are excellent, and there appears to be no penalty in terms of increased loco-regional recurrence or diminished survival. To try to determine the precise value of this technique, a new trial was commenced at Guy's Hospital in 1981. In this trial, patients were randomly allocated to two groups. One group of patients received a modified radical mastectomy, and the other group had the tumour alone excised, together with complete axillary dissection. In this second group, at the same time as the tumour was excised, plastic tubes were inserted through the tumour bed. Radioactive iridium 192 was inserted into the tubes 2 days later. These patients thus received a boost dose of iridium to the tumour bed within 48 h after removal of the lesion. The dose of iridium given by this technique was 2000 cGy. Subsequently, all patients were given external radiation therapy, receiving a further 5000 cGy, in 200-cGy fractions each day for 5 days per week. Patients who had positive axillary nodes in each group were randomly allocated to receive 12 courses of adjuvant CMF or no adjuvant treatment. This trial at Guy's Hospital is being undertaken in combination with a European Organization for Research and Treatment of Cancer (EORTC) study but, in the EORTC cases, the boost dose of iridium is not given until after the external radiation treatment to the breast.

Intake to this trial has now been completed, but it is too early to give results in terms of loco-regional recurrence, distant recurrence or survival. The advantage of the method is that the cosmetic result is excellent in almost every case. There is minimal disturbance to the breast, and very little residual radiation reaction. The cosmetic results from this technique will almost certainly be better than those from wider surgical procedures. What is not known is whether loco-regional recurrence will occur at an excessive rate, or whether, when it occurs, it can adequately and safely be treated by salvage mastectomy.

The Future

It now seems almost certain that some form of breast-conserving technique can be included amongst orthodox therapies for patients with early breast cancer. It is not yet known which technique will prove to be the best; indeed, it is unlikely that the same procedure will be of value in all cases. Quite possibly, minimal local surgery with boost radiation treatment will be more suitable for patients with small-to-medium breasts, whereas wider local excision may be more feasible in patients with larger breasts. Similarly, it is not known whether the size of the tumour may affect the type of treatment, nor whether different histological types of tumour will demand different approaches. We certainly know that a few breast tumours are radio-insensitive, but we do not yet know how these can be detected.

The whole concept of conservative treatment for breast cancer is still in its infancy, and much work still needs to be done to determine the best treatment for the individual patient. Almost certainly, mastectomy will continue to be needed for some types of tumour. What can be stated with absolute certainty is that conservative treatment of the breast is not the simple option. It involves the use of sophisticated techniques and must be carried out by people who are skilled in using them. Similarly, it is not an easy treatment for the patient to undergo. It often requires long periods of radiation treatment, demanding considerable patience and forbearance. There is no place for trivial methods of treatment in this disease, and if they are undertaken, their effect will be mirrored by trivial results.

References

1. Fisher B, Bauer M, Margolese R, et al. (1985) Five-year results of a randomised clinical trial comparing total mastectomy and segmental mastectomy with or without radiation in the treatment of breast cancer. N Engl J Med 312:665–673
2. Hayward JL (1983) The Guy's Hospital trials on breast conservation. In: Harris JR, Hellman S, Silen W (eds) Conservative management of breast cancer. Lippincott, Philadelphia, pp 77–90
3. Veronesi U, del Vecchio M, Greco M, et al. (1983) Results of quadrantectomy, axillary dissection and radiotherapy (QUART) in T1No patients. In: Harris JR, Hellman S, Silen W (eds) Conservative management of breast cancer. Lippincott, Philadelphia, pp 91–99

Surgical Complications After Conservative Treatment of Breast Cancer

F. Harder, N. Lüscher, U. Laffer, R. Hünig, E. Walther,
A. Almendral, and J. Torhorst

The complications following treatment of breast cancer are related to surgery, radiotherapy, chemotherapy, and, in a broader sense, regional and local recurrence. The surgical complications of conservative treatment for breast cancer are the same as after the various forms of mastectomy, i.e., hematoma, seroma, wound infection, and lymphedema of the arm.

Hematomas requiring surgical evacuation or needle aspiration are relatively rare complications. Among our own patients at the General Surgical Clinic of the University of Basel, they occur in 5%. After tumorectomy, large tumors are associated with a slightly higher rate of hematoma formation. The development of a hematoma is, however, predominantly a consequence of the surgical approach, technique, and drainage. The incision chosen for tumorectomy must allow meticulous preparation under direct vision using the shortest distance from the skin to the tumor. This implies that the incision should be situated directly on top of the tumor. When we started our study of conservative treatment for breast cancer in 1977, we first used incisions in natural folds and skin creases in order to optimize the cosmetic result. These incisions were behind the pectoral fold, around the areola, and in the submammary fold. Depending on the tumor location, incisions of this type then required a relatively long, tunnelled approach to the tumor. The surgeon does not have the best view of the tumor to be excised. The chance of cutting frankly into the cancer itself is not negligible. Judgment of the margins becomes more difficult. Spilling of tumor cells deep in the hidden operative field may easily occur. Control of hemostasis may be inadequate and hematoma formation will occur more easily. Incisions are best positioned directly on top of the tumor, curvilinear, and concentric to the nipple (Fig. 1). Access to the axilla is through a longitudinal incision between the pectoral fold and that of the latissimus dorsi into the hair-covered part of the axilla. This incision, which does not need to be extended very far distally, is mostly invisible and allows easy dissection of the axilla en bloc with access to the level-I and -II lymph nodes. If the arm is positioned in order to be freely movable, elevation of the arm will move the pectoralis major and minor muscles away from the anterolateral chest wall and open up the axilla, giving access to the space posterior to the insertion of pectoralis minor. The inferior aspect of the axillary vein can thus be easily followed and cleared without totally denuding the vessel. The thoracodorsal neurovascular bundle, and the long thoracic nerve, are separated from surrounding tissue but left intact.

The tumor bed is marked with a metal clip to facilitate the aiming of an electron-beam boost and is provided with suction drainage. The production of a

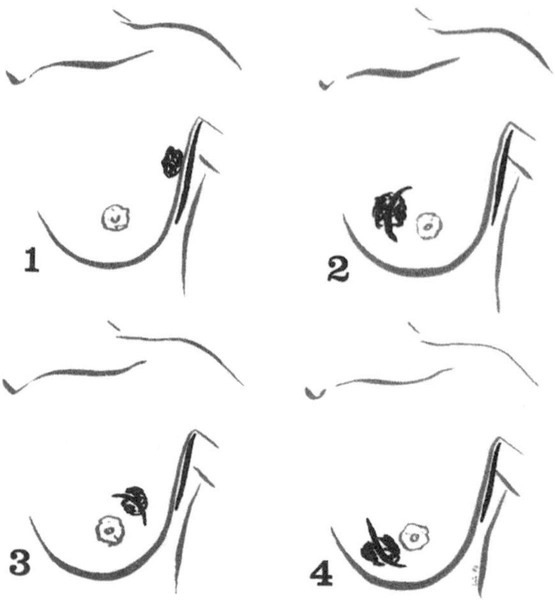

Fig. 1. Recommended curvilinear incisions and access to the axilla depending on the tumor location; incisions should always be placed directly above the palpable or suspected mass. Exception may be made in the case of a tumor placed very laterally in the axillary tail [1]

skin depression in the area of the defect created by tumor resection is avoided by mobilization of the adjacent gland and closure of the defect. Care must be taken not to thereby induce tension of the skin and increase deformation. Before closing the skin, the breast should be moved about and checked for any distortion. Some authors [3,4] recommend against trying to adapt the defect created by tumor resection or applying drainage. They argue that suction will inevitably create deformity; if no drain is installed, subcutaneous cavities will be filled by hematoma, and guarantee good cosmesis. In our experience, however, hematoma formation reduces tolerance of postoperative high-dose irradiation and may even cause skin necrosis associated with irradiation. For this reason we continue with careful adaptation of gland tissue and suction drainage.

After breast surgery, axillary seroma is more common than hematoma [4,6,8]. Seromas are observed in up to 35% of patients after mastectomy. In our own patients we observed accumulation of fluid requiring evacuation by puncture in 16% of patients after tumorectomy of lesions measuring up to 2 cm, and in 20% when the lesions were more than 2 cm in diameter. Seroma formation is correlated to breast size, age of the patient, presence of hypertension, the time at which physiotherapy for mobilization of the shoulder was started, and whether perioperative and postoperative prophylaxis against thromboembolism was applied [7]. Within the time during which 91 patients of our surgical clinic have been treated conservatively for breast cancer, our routine perioperative prophylaxis of thromboembolism with

Table 1. Frequency of hematomas and seromas requiring needle puncture or surgical evacuation; relationship to prophylaxis of thromboembolism in 91 patients at the Surgical Clinic of the University of Basel

Type of prophylactic treatment	Patients with hematoma/seroma *n*	%
Dextran	12/63	19
Heparin-DHE	5/15	33
None	1/13	8
	18/91	21

dextran has been temporarily replaced by the use of heparin and dihydroergotamine. The frequency of seroma formation is shown in Table 1. The low numbers indicate only a trend. It seems that after we ceased prophylaxis against thromboembolism in connection with any surgery for breast cancer, the observed frequency of seroma formation declined to 8%.

Wound infection rarely follows breast surgery. Only 1 of 91 patients who had conservative breast surgery developed such a complication. Tejler and Aspegren [8] observed a rate of 3.6% among 385 patients treated by either mastectomy or tumorectomy. Other authors found this complication to have a slightly higher frequency [1]. It is demonstrated in Table 2 that diagnostic procedures penetrating the skin, performed before definitive breast surgery, did influence wound infection. Among 294 patients who had mastectomy, wound infection was observed in 3.2% after a preceding fine-needle biopsy, in 5.3% when intraoperative frozen section had been performed, and in 12.4% when a surgical biopsy had been done less than 4 days before mastectomy. If this surgical biopsy was performed 4–7 days before the mastectomy, the wound-infection rate reached 23%. This strikingly high infection rate was not observed in our own series. We used fine-needle biopsy very liberally in the outpatient clinic and preoperatively, and very frequently avoided in-

Table 2. Frequency of wound infection after mastectomy correlated to preoperative fine-needle aspiration cytology (FNP), intraoperative frozen section (FS), and surgical biopsy less than 4 days before mastectomy (Δ T < 4) or surgical biopsy between 4–7 days mastectomy (Δ T=4–7) [8]

No. of LK lymph nodes	No. of patients	Percentage with edema
1–4	22	0
5–10	70	3
11–20	86	5
> 20	23	13
	201	4.5

traoperative frozen section to prove the presence of breast cancer. Any palpable lesion in which breast cancer is suspected should be analyzed by fine-needle-aspiration cytology. A positive result will allow meaningful and usually definitive preoperative discussion of treatment alternatives with the patient and relatives.

Probably the most troublesome complication after surgery for breast cancer is arm lymphedema. The correlation of arm lymphedema with the extent of axillary lymph-node dissection, postoperative radiotherapy to the draining nodes, wound infection, and locoregional recurrence is well known. If we analyze all the patients conservatively treated up to December 31, 1984, and irradiated in a single institution (the Radiotherapy Unit of the University of Basel) we find that a difference of more than 3 cm between the upperarm circumference of the treated side and that of the untreated one was correlated with the number of axillary lymph-nodes removed (Table 3).These 201 patients were equally distributed between surgical and gynecologic clinics, and local institutions outside the University. The difference in upper arm circumference between the treated and the untreated side was most pronounced in patients who had more than 20 lymph-nodes removed from the axilla. All these patients had postoperative radiotherapy of the lateral lymph-node areas. This irradiation was discontinued in January 1985, which is why these patients were not included in our analysis. Prior to that date, all patients had irradiation of the breast as well as of the draining lymph-node areas, whether there was nodal involvement or not. On average, 11.5 lymph-nodes per patient were found in the axillary specimen removed. Today, since we have abandoned radiotherapy to the lateral lymph-node area, the number of lymph-nodes removed has been deliberately increased.

Clearly, unsatisfactory cosmetic results should also be regarded as complications of conservative breast-cancer treatment. In fact, the aim of this treatment is to achieve a late cosmetic result that at least matches those of amputation with

Table 3. Frequency of arm lymphedema with a difference in upper-arm circumference of more than 3 cm as a function of the number of lymph nodes counted in the axillary specimen removed en bloc; all 201 patients (from our surgical clinic, gynecologic institutions, and smaller local institutions) received irradiation of the lateral lymph-node areas. This component of radiotherapy was abandoned at the end of 1984

FNP + mastectomy	3.2%
FS + mastectomy	5.3%
Biopsy + mastectomy Δ T < 4 days	12.4%
Biopsy + mastectomy Δ T 4–7 days	23 %

[a]Wound infection occurred in 8.2% of 294 patients

reconstruction. Unsatisfactory cosmetic results from: selection of patients with excessive tumor size or an unfavorable ratio of tumor size to breast size (e.g., a relatively large tumor in a small breast); a poor choice of skin incision; and (to a large extent) poor technique and tolerance of radiotherapy and possible supplementary chemotherapy.

The least-visible scars are found if incisions are parallel to Langer's lines, curvilinear, and concentric to the areola. Although it is tempting to place such an incision in a cosmetically favorable position (the periareolar area, submammary fold, or lateral mammary fold behind the pectoral muscle; Fig. 2), these incisions are not to be recommended in tumor surgery. The shortest route to the tumor is the best (Fig. 1). The single exception to this rule is a tumor in the uppermost axillary tail of the mammary gland, where a common incision for the axilla and the tumor itself may be selected (Fig. 1, insert). Radial incisions generally result in more visible, broader scars. This is especially true if the incision reaches into the presternal area. Here, there is a pronounced tendency to form keloid (Fig. 3).

A curvilinear incision over the tumor does not necessarily mean that excision of the tumor itself has to be carried out in the same direction. After diligent skin mobilisation, and pulling out the diseased part of the gland, with stay sutures placed outside the tumor itself, tumorectomy can be performed using a radial excision (Fig. 4). This will facilitate adaptation of the gland to bridge the defect by carefully suturing the two resection lines, if this suture is at all necessary. Figure 1 shows the longitudinal skin incision used for access to the lymph-nodes of levels 1 and 2. This incision, which should be oriented toward, but not reach, the top of the axilla, is not

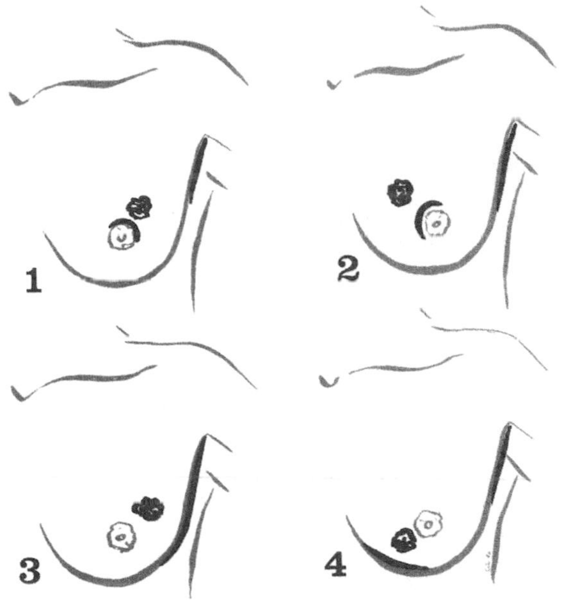

Fig. 2. Although cosmetically tempting, subcutaneous tunnelling to the tumor from a cosmetically hidden incision is not to be recommended. Tumor-cell spilling and hematoma formation may result

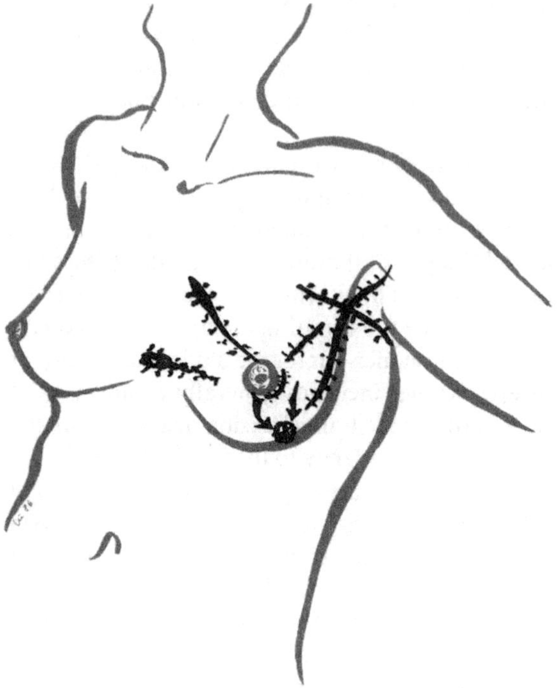

Fig. 3. Radial incisions are not to be recommended

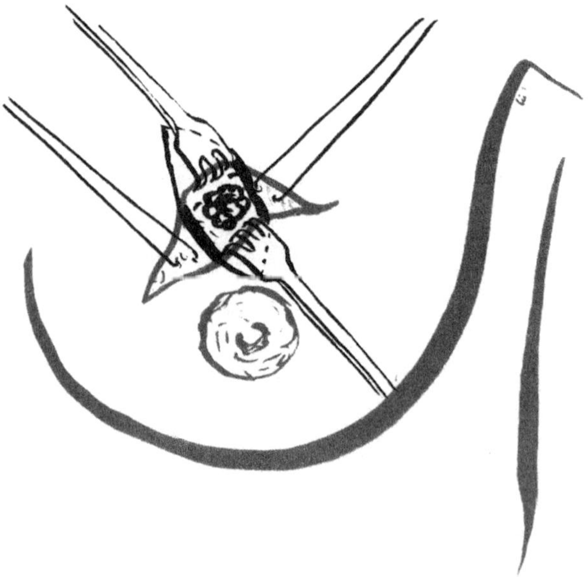

Fig. 4. Curvilinear incision in the upper-inner quadrant; stay sutures and exteriorization of the tumor-bearing part of the gland; radial excision of the specimen, allowing optimal readaptation of breast tissue

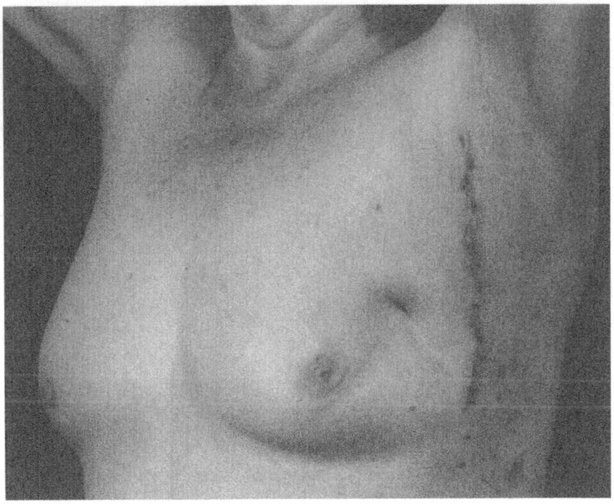

Fig. 5. Vertical access to the axilla has been placed too far ventrally here, causing a defect of lateral breast tissue

infrequently placed too far ventrally (Fig. 5). This may later form an ugly cord of scar tissue which may even be functionally inconvenient.

At times, it may be difficult to remove tumors of the upper-inner quadrant in such a way that neither an ugly scar, nor a defect with skin depression at the original tumor location will remain. This area is also difficult to hide in the décollettage. It is exactly here that radial incisions are especially unpleasant. They run vertical to the usual garments (bra, swimsuit, blouse, etc.), and the medial end tends to form keloid (Fig. 6). If possible, curvilinear incisions and radial excision of the specimen may be advantageously combined (Figs. 7 and 8).

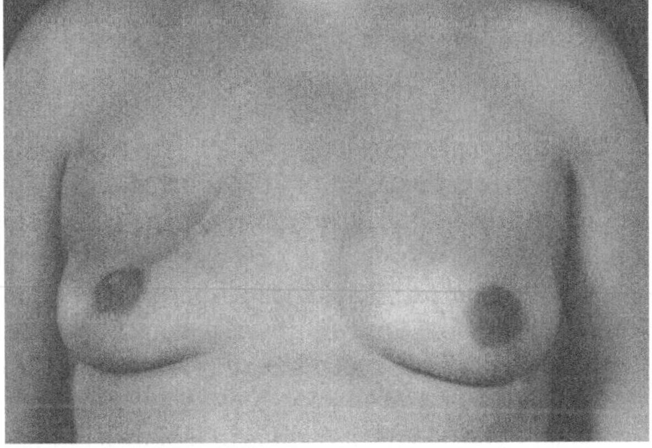

Fig. 6. Radial incision in the inner-upper quadrant, running vertical to Langer's lines and clearly visible in the décolletage. The scar tends to form keloid in the presternal area

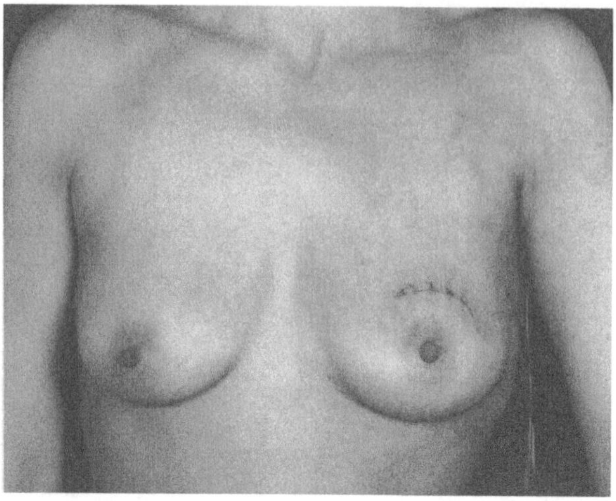

Fig. 7. Early postoperative appearance of a curvilinear incision in the upper-inner quadrant

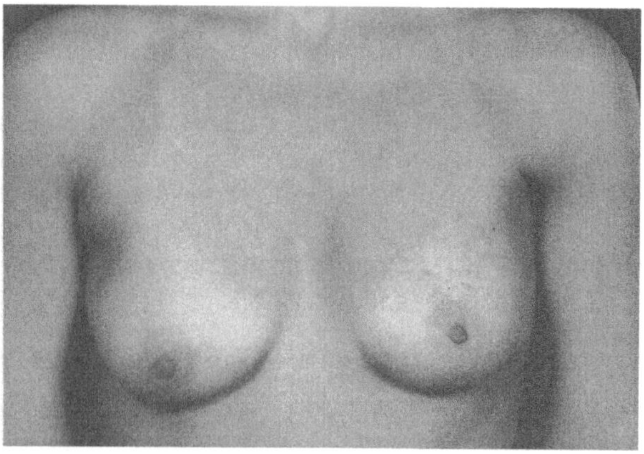

Fig. 8. Same patient as in Fig. 7, showing the result after 2 years

In the patient shown in Fig. 9, a relatively large tumor was removed from the region between the two lower quadrants. Mobilization of breast tissue, which could easily have been done from lateral to medial in order to bridge the defect, was omitted. The deformity was already distinctly visible in the early postoperative period. It is unrealistic to expect spontaneous amelioration with time. On the contrary, radiotherapy will, by inducing fibrous-tissue formation, induce progressive slight retraction and thereby accentuate the defect (Fig. 10).

Very large and pendulous breasts are usually less suitable for conservative treatment. The body-conscious actress shown in Fig. 11 had developed symmetric synchronous breast cancers in the upper-outer quadrants of both breasts. A simple bilateral tumorectomy with axillary resection and postoperative radiotherapy

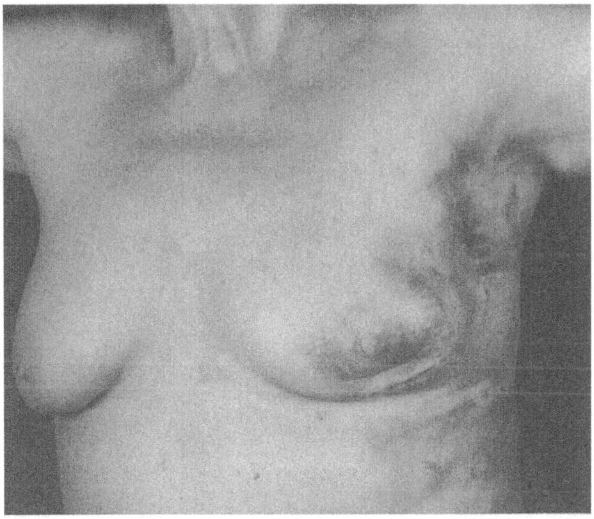

Fig. 9. Tissue defect of the inferior quadrants in the early postoperative period, due to insufficient mobilization of lateral breast tissue and omission of adaptation after tumorectomy

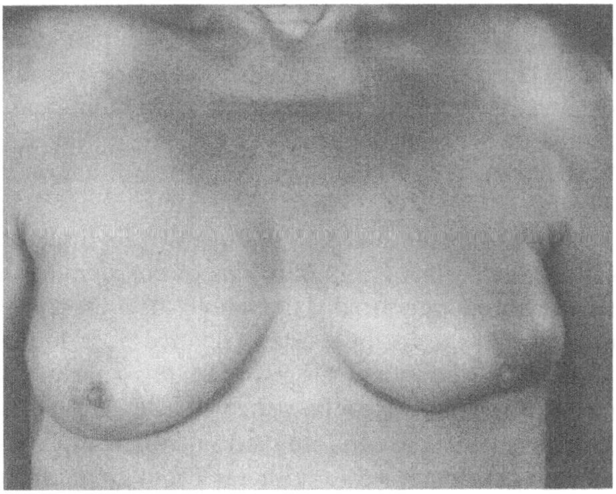

Fig. 10. Same patient as in Fig. 9: the tissue defect will not be filled later. Slight scarring of tissue as a consequence of radiotherapy may accentuate the deformity in time

would have been very likely to induce retraction of the breast due to scarring, with elevation and unpredictable asymmetry. Therefore, and because the patient had a longstanding desire for reduction mammoplasty anyway, bilateral tumorectomy and axillary clearance was performed as a first step, with strict regard for our protocols of surgical conservative treatment. This was followed during the same period of anesthesia, by bilateral autologous reconstruction with a pedicled fat-

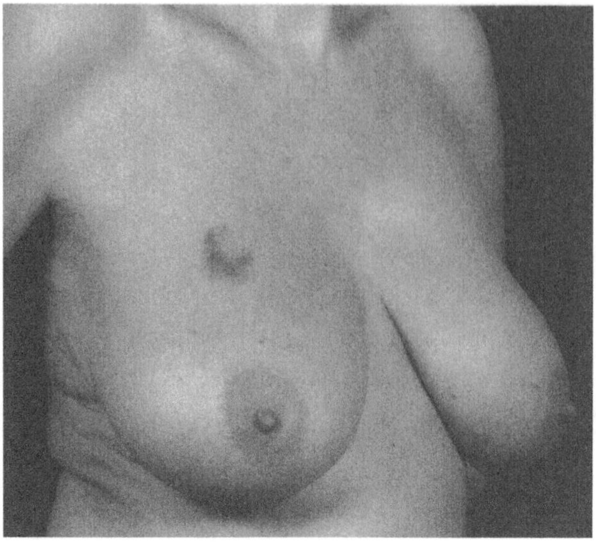

Fig. 11. Synchronous, symmetrical, bilateral breast cancer in the outer-upper quadrants of large, pendulous fatty breasts, represents difficult conditions for obtaining an excellent cosmetic result after simple tumorectomy followed by radiotherapy (because of fibrosis and asymetric retraction)

dermis flap and free transposition of the nipple-areola complex [5]. The wound healed uneventfully, and the usual postoperative irradiation of both breasts, but not the area of lymphatic drainage followed. In another patient, in whom the same procedure had been applied 3 years earlier, the late result is shown in Fig. 12. Both breasts are soft and symmetric. A nearly normal silhouette was achieved without prosthesis.

Apart from the classical postoperative complications of surgery for breast cancer, the cosmetic complications of conservative treatment for breast cancer should not go unnoticed. They play a decisive role. Conservative breast-cancer treatment has to follow a clearly defined plan, thoroughly discussed among the participating disciplines. Disregard for this principle, and furthermore omission of frequent and thorough follow-up, will lead to results such as the one shown in Fig. 13. This patient had to endure every possible complication: extended necrosis of the breast after combined radiotherapy and chemotherapy, local recurrence with extensive carcinomatous lymphangitis, and breast lymphedema with regional lymph-node metastasis.

Radiotherapy must be based on excellent surgical conditions. With the recommended incisions and bridging of the defect (very frequently superfluous, especially in larger breasts), tumor resection is usually possible without noticeable deformity of the breast. Of course, the tumor-to-breast ratio plays a role. Level-1 and level-2 nodes may be removed en bloc, especially when the arm can be moved about. The cosmetic and functional result should at least correspond to that of breast amputation with reconstruction. If not, this interdisciplinary breast-conserving procedure should be reevaluated and improved.

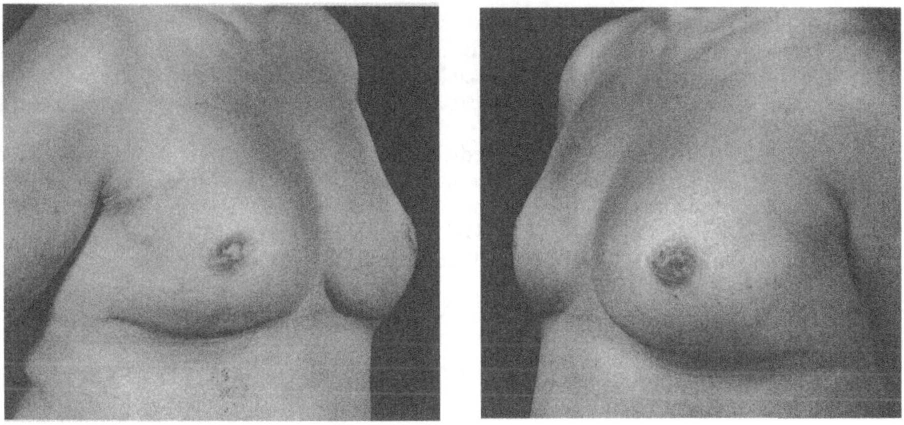

Fig. 12. Under the conditions outlined in Fig. 11, this picture is from a different patient, 2 years after tumor excision, subcutaneous mastectomy, and autologous reconstruction with a pedicled, deepithelialized fat-dermis flap originating from the inferior quadrants of the breast. Free transposition of the nipple-areola complex was carried out

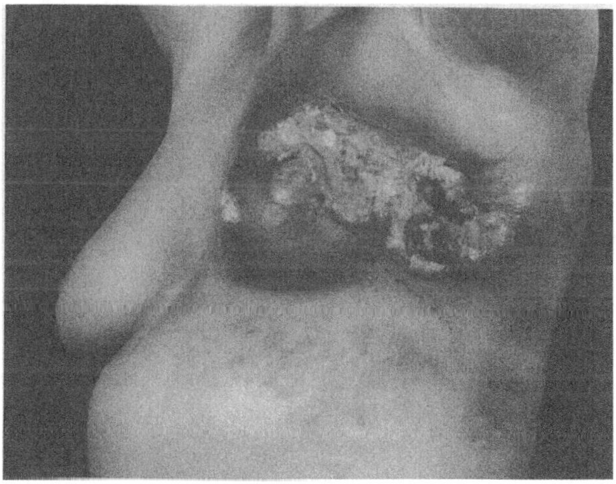

Fig. 13. Dreadful complication after attempted conservative treatment of breast cancer by surgery, radiotherapy, and chemotherapy, resulting in partial necrosis of the breast, hyperpigmentation in the irradiated area, carcinomatous lymphangitis, local and regional recurrence, and arm lymphedema

References

1. Beatty JD, Robinson GV, Zaia JA, Benfield JR, Kemeny MM, Meguid MM, Riihimaki DU, Terz JJ, Lemmelin ME (1983) A prospective analysis of nosocomial wound infection after mastectomy. Arch Surg 118:1421–1424
2. Corneillie P, Gruwez JA, Lerut T, van Elst F (1984) Early and late postoperative sequelae after surgery for carcinoma of the breast. Acta Chir Belg 84:227–231

3. Fisher B, Montague E, Redmond C, et al. (1977) Comparison of radical mastectomy with alternative treatments for primary breast cancer. Cancer 39:2827–2839
4. Fisher B, Wolmark N, Fisher ER, Deutsch M (1985) Lumpectomy and axillary dissection for breast cancer: Surgical, pathological and radiation considerations. World J Surg 9:676–681
5. Longacre JJ (1953) The use of local pedicle flaps for reconstruction of the breast after subtotal or total extirbation of the mammary gland and for the correction of distortion and atrophy of the breast due to excessive scar. Plast Reconstr Surg 11:380–403
6. McCarthy PM, Martin JK Jr, Wells DC, Welch JS, Ilstrup DM (1986) An aborted, prospective, randomized trial of sclerotherapy for prolonged drainage after mastectomy. Surg Gynecol Obstet 162:418–420
7. Salmon RJ, Cody HS, Vedrenne JB, Asselain B, Durand JC, Pilleron JP (1985) Prevention of postoperative lymphocele after breast amputation. Presse Med 14:27–29
8. Tejler G, Aspegren K (1985) Complications and hospital stay after surgery for breast cancer: a prospective study of 385 patients. Br J Surg 72:542–544

IV. Radiology

Status of Radiotherapy after Ablative and Breast-Preserving Treatment of Breast Cancer

D. VON FOURNIER, A. MÜLLER, H. JUNKERMANN and W. SCHLEGEL

Postoperative Irradiation

Radiotherapy was first used for the treatment of breast cancer by H. GOCHT [11] in 1896. One year after the discovery of röntgen rays. Improved survival rates after postoperative radiotherapy were first described by PFAHLER and PARRY [20] from studies carried out between 1902 and 1928, and a breast radium implant was first used in 1908 by FINZI [6].

The following are the currently significant uses of radiotherapy in treatment of breast cancer:

1. Adjuvant irradiation after modified radical operations
2. Primary irradiation of the remaining breast tissue in breast-preserving treatment
3. Irradiation of locoregional recurrences
4. Primary sole treatment of inoperable advanced breast cancers
5. Preoperative irradiation
6. Irradiation of metastases

Only the first two uses of radiotherapy will be discussed here, as its value in the other cases is only little disputed.

Response of Breast Cancer to Radiotherapy

The response to radiotherapy can be measured in short-term follow-up observations by complete degeneration (complete response) of irradiated and clinically detectable cancer tissue. Decisive, however, is ultimate destruction of the tumor tissue, shown by long-term observation of the irradiated region. The rate of local recurrences with and without postoperative radiotherapy also gives information about the efficacy of irradiation, particular for clinically undetectable locoregional microscopic tumor cell seeding (e.g., in the thoracic wall and regional lymph nodes).

According to retrospective studies in Manchester and New York reported by FLETCHER [9], the incidence of later supraclavicular lymph node metastases was about 20%–26% in patients with positive lymph nodes if no postoperative radiotherapy was given. The incidence of lymph node metastases was reduced to 7% when 30–35 Gy was given, to 3% with 40 Gy, and to 1.5% with 50–55 Gy.

With postoperative irradiation of the thoracic wall FLETCHER found a similar but less strong dependence of the destruction of subclinical metastases on dose of irradiation. After radical mastectomy in patients with positive lymph nodes, the 5-year thoracic wall recurrence rate was 10%, instead of the estimated probability in this series of 30% without irradiation.

This result was confirmed in the 10-year results of the NSABP study B-04 [FISHER et al. [7,8]. Axillary recurrences occurred after total mastectomy in 21% of patients with clinically negative lymph nodes (N0) without irradiation or surgical treatment of the axilla. If the axilla was irradiated at 50 Gy and no lymphadenectomy was carried out, recurrences occurred in 3% only. It is estimated that 50 Gy irradiation decreases the risk of axillary recurrence in diseased women by 86% [HARRIS 1985].

Value of Adjuvant Radiotherapy after Mastectomy

Historically, the standard treatment of breast cancer was ablation followed by irradiation of the thoracic wall and the regional lymph nodes. The first reason for prophylactic locoregional irradiation was that residual microscopic tumor cell seeds lead later to local recurrences, which are known to increase in frequency in correlation with unfavorable tumor parameters. According to the literature, local recurrences can only be treated effectively at the time of their appearance in about 50% of patients who have not previously undergone radiotherapy.

The second reason was the assumption that postoperative irradiation could improve the survival rate. If a local recurrence is the only manifestation of recurrence, new distant metastases can spread from it.

Various forms of mastectomy (radical, modified radical, total) with and without postoperative irradiation have been compared in randomized studies.

In the Manchester trial, the thoracic wall and axilla were irradiated with 32 Gy in the first series, but only the axilla in the second series (1953–1955). The rate of locoregional recurrence within 10 years was approximately halved, and the survival rates after 30 years were the same (Fig. 1).

The Stockholm trial [29] compared, between 1971 and 1976, irradiation (45 Gy, cobalt 60) of the lymph nodes and the thoracic wall with no irradiation in patients who had had radical mastectomy. In the first arm irradiation was preoperative, in the second arm it was postoperative, and in the third arm no radiotherapy was given. The rate of locoregional recurrences was reduced from 26% to 7% by irradiation, and rates of distant metastases were the same with and without irradiation (30% and 34%; see Table 1), as were the 10-year survival rates (Table 2). There was no difference between preoperative and postoperative irradiation. However, radiotherapy led to a decrease of about 7% in the rate of deaths from breast cancer in the subgroup of patients with positive lymph nodes ($p = 0.09$ not significantly).

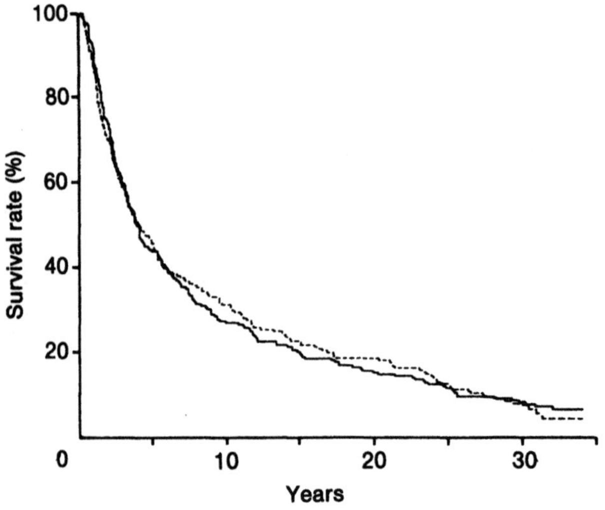

Fig. 1. Survival rates in the Manchester trial. Radical mastectomy with (*interrupted line*, $n=222$) and without irradiation (*continuous line*, $n=251$) in patients with positive lymph nodes ($p=0.9$). (PALMER and RIBEIRO 1985)

Table 1. Local recurrences and distant metastases after surgery with and without radiotherapy (Wallgren et al. 1986) Frequency and sites of recurrence within 8 years in 639 patients treated by radiotherapy and in 321 controls

	Radiotherapy		No radiotherapy	
Sites	No.	%	No.	%
All chest wall	33	5.2	62	19.3
All nodes	19	3.0	42	13.1
All distant	191	29.9	110	34.3
All with recurrence	199	31.1	135	42.1

Table 2. Observed (O) and "Expected" (E) number of deaths, if there were no differences in the three treatment groups

Treatment group	No. of patients	Observed no. dead	Expected no. dead	O/E
Preop. radiotherapy	316	121	125.3	0.97
Postop. radiotherapy	321	119	125.7	0.95
No. radiotherapy	321	132	121.6	1.09
All	960	372	372.0	1.00

Effect of Radiotherapy on Thoracic Wall Recurrences

The modified radical mastectomy that is usual now is associated with a higher rate of recurrences in the thoracic wall than radical mastectomy [HALSTED]. Naturally, the local recurrence rate increases with unfavorable tumor stages and with observation time. HØST and BRENNHOVD [16] and HØST et al. [17] found thoracic wall recurrences in 8.7% of patients in whom the lymph nodes were involved and no radiotherapy was given. We have observed local recurrences after 5 years in 40% of patients with the histologically unfavorable stages T3/T4 N+ when no radiotherapy was given [FOURNIER et al. 1986].

These recurrences were largely indications of generalization of tumors at advanced stages. On these grounds, we do not consider routine prophylactic irradiation of the thoracic wall justifiable for early stages. In the unfavorable stages T3/T4 N+ the probability of local recurrence is so high that in our view postoperative irradiation at 50–60 Gy is indicated. The survival rate is unchanged, but the patient may be spared the psychological and physical stress of a visible, local thoracic wall recurrence. Also, patients with these advanced stages are often being treated at this point anyway for distant metastases. Moreover, with these stages and without pretreatment local eradication of a thoracic wall recurrence at the time of its appearance can only be expected in 50% of cases, and so immediate postoperative local eradication using a sufficiently high dose of irradiation is more promising and should be aimed for. Even then, despite the previous radiotherapy, local thoracic wall recurrences are still to be expected long term (up to 10 years), in about one-third of cases. Anyway, within this time period the vast majority of patients with these unfavorable tumor stages either die or are ill because of metastases.

FLETCHER et al. [9] found that even in patients with four involved lymph nodes the rate of thoracic wall recurrences after radical mastectomy was 20%, and that this decreased to 11% with postoperative irradiation.

Value of Axillary Irradiation

FISHER et al. [7,8] showed in the NSABP study B-04 that in patients with clinically positive axillary lymph nodes (N+) surgery is superior to irradiation of the axilla. After 10 years, axillary recurrences were observed in 1% of patients who had had surgery (this figure is low in comparison with the rest of the literature) but in 11.9% after axillary irradiation alone. Hence it follows that suitable axillary lymphadenectomy (levels I and II; with involvement of level II, also level III) is the method of choice. The low rates of axillary recurrences after suitable surgery (local elimination is probable) do not usually justify adjuvant radiotherapy, as the combined trauma leads to too high a rate of lymphedema. FISHER et al.]7,8] found no difference in disease-free survival rates in patients with or without positive lymph nodes when (a) radical mastectomy, (b) total mastectomy with axillary irradiation, and (c) total mastectomy without treatment of the axilla were compared.

Only with subtotal involvement of the axilla or with extensive infiltration of the axillary fatty tissue can additional postoperative irradiation of the surgically treated axilla be indicated, namely when remaining tumor masses make axillary recurrences likely. Given that up to 80% of patients with axillary lymph node involvement also have occult distant metastases, the effect of axillary irradiation on survival is really minimal.

Value of Irradiation of the Supra- and Infraclavicular Lymph Nodes

As mentioned above, when there is axillary lymph node involvement, supraclavicular lymph node metastases appear in 20%–15% patients, but only in 1.5% with 50 Gy irradiation [9]. The rate of supraclavicular recurrences increases with the number of involved lymph nodes, and with total involvement is already over 40% within 5 years [10]. Thus it should be weighed up whether, with involvement of more than ten axillary lymph nodes, the supra- and the (unoperated) retro- and infraclavicular regions (clip to mark the cranial limit of surgery) should subsequently be irradiated with at least 50 Gy. No influence of this on survival has been proven.

Irradiation of the Sternal Lymph Vessels

CALLE [3] and CALLE et al. [4] showed that within 5 years retrosternal recurrences occurred in 4%–7% of patients who had not received radiotherapy and in 0–1% of those who had. WALLGREEN et al. (1988) showed that for medially located tumors postoperative (and also preoperative) irradiation of the sternal lymph nodes significantly improved the survival rate. This is *not* explicable given the low recurrence rates found in CALLE's survey.

Of interest for radiotherapy is the subgroup of patients with medially located tumors and axillary lymph node involvement, in 40%–50% of whom this also indicates retrosternal lymph node involvement. In these cases we recommend irradiation of the retrosternal lymph nodes with 50 Gy (e.g., cobalt – 60 photons combined with "fast electrons"), for the following reasons:

1. The side effects are minimal and the treatment is well tolerated
2. Retrosternal recurrences are fewer
3. An effect on survival is, according to WALLGREEN et al. (1988), at least possible in N^+ patients

Summary of the Value of Postoperative Irradiation

The thoracic wall, the supraclavicular lymph nodes cranial to the limit of surgery, and the sternal lymph nodes should be irradiated postoperatively if statistically there is a high risk (e.g., above 30% or 40%) of local recurrence within 5 years. It must be remembered that radiotherapy is also effective at the time of recurrence, and that as many patients who have a low risk of recurrence as possible should be spared postoperative irradiation. It has not been proven that this locoregional irradiation significantly improves survival. However, the appearance of a visible local recurrence is an extraordinary psychological strain on a patient, and so if the risk of this is sufficiently high postoperative radiotherapy is completely justified. Locoregional eradication by the most effective possible means is indispensible in the primary treatment of breast cancer.

Irradiation of the axilla after sufficiently radical surgery should remain reserved for the exceptional cases where it is suspected that there is residual tumor and a higher probability of recurrence. For megavolt irradiation (accelerator photons, cobalt-60 X-rays) the dose to the lymph node regions should be 50 Gy over 5 weeks, and to the thoracic wall, 60 Gy. For electrons the dose to the thoracic wall should be 45–50 Gy, daily doses not exceeding 2 Gy and the weekly dose 10 Gy.

Combination of Postoperative Radiotherapy with Adjuvant Chemotherapy

Combining radiotherapy with simultaneous adjuvant hormone therapy is possible without particularly increasing complications. In many centers adjuvant chemotherapy is given simultaneously with radiotherapy. An increase in side effects must be expected with both simultaneous and consecutive administration (sandwich technique). Therefore, in normal cases we first give two (or three) cycles of standard adjuvant chemotherapy (CMF, i.e., cyclophosphamide, methotrexate, 5-flourouracil), followed after a 10-day interval by radiotherapy and after a further 10-day interval by the remaining cycles (to make a total of six) of adjuvant chemotherapy.

As regards lengthening the patients' recurrence-free survival adjuvant chemotherapy is particularly effective in premenopausal women with one to three positive lymph nodes [1,2]. Therefore, at present this therapy should not be neglected even when radiotherapy is indicated. However, in retrospective studies prophylactic elimination of ovarian function (ovarectomy, irradiation of the ovaries) has been just as effective. In future studies adjuvant chemotherapy will be compared with medical ovarectomy using luteinizing hormone releasing hormone analogues like Zoladex. With Zoladex postoperative radiotherapy is easily possible.

For postmenopausal women who are receptor positive, adjuvant hormone therapy using antiestrogens (e.g., tamoxifen) or gestagens (e.g., medroxyprogesterone) seems to be more effective than adjuvant chemotherapy and so results in no delay in postoperative radiotherapy.

Adjuvant chemotherapy on its own hardly ever led to a significant decrease in locoregional recurrences. In the Milan study the 10-year recurrence-free survival rate was 43% with CMF in contrast to 31% in controls ($p = 0.01$). In contrast to the survival rate, the rate of locoregional recurrences after 10 years was not improved by chemotherapy: the rate was 11.6% with CMF, and 14.5% in controls (no significant difference; BONADONNA et al. 1985a,b).

Similar results were found by RAO et al. from the Dana Farber Institute (1985). After adjuvant chemotherapy was completed, patients were randomly assigned to receiving either postoperative radiotherapy or no further treatment. After a median follow-up period of 44 months, a high rate of local recurrences was found in patients with four or more positive lymph nodes (25%). The rate in patients who also received radiotherapy was significantly lower (7%). In patients with one to three involved lymph nodes no difference was seen (6% locoregional recurrences in each case).

Thus, locoregional recurrences are also clearly reduced by postoperative radiotherapy combined with adjuvant chemotherapy, which by itself does not significantly reduce locoregional recurrences. Radiotherapy is thus superior to adjuvant chemotherapy in reducing locoregional recurrences.

MARCIAL et al. [18] came to similar conclusions. The locoregional recurrence rates in patients with four or more positive lymph nodes were the same after six and 12 cycles of CMF (10% and 11%). With additional radiotherapy the recurrence rate was lower (4%), although the difference was not statistically significant because of the small number of cases.

In summary, postoperative radiotherapy should be given, independently of adjuvant chemotherapy, when the indications mentioned above are present.

Radiotherapy in Breast-Conserving Therapy

Radiotherapy in the treatment of breast cancer underwent a renaissance with the strategy of breast-preserving treatment; the irradiation techniques most frequently used now have been and are still being determined in some retrospective and prospective studies.

Retrospective Studies

CALLE et al. [4] showed that the 10-year cure rate for tumors of up to 3 cm in diameter was as good with tumorectomy and radiotherapy as with radical mastectomy in a comparison group in New York. Treatment failure (locoregional recurrences in the breast or axilla) occurred in 14% of patients within 10 years. In tumors larger than 3 cm confirmed histologically by means of needle biopsy, breast irradiation (up to 60 Gy) and a boost dose to the tumor (cobalt 60 or electrons, 20 Gy) alone did not lead to adequate local control. Tumor persisted in 163 (35%) of 463 patients who received radiotherapy, so in these cases irradiation was broken off after up to 50 Gy and a mastectomy carried out. Of patients who responded initially to radiotherapy alone (up to 80 Gy in the boost region), 28% showed locoregional failure within 10 years; of these, 75% occurred in the first 5 years and 25% between the 5th and 10th years. Thus, radiotherapy alone (without tumorectomy) resulted in locoregional failure within 10 years in a total of 247 out of 463 patients (53.3%) with tumors that were over 3 cm in diameter. Although the survival rate (54% with no evidence of disease) was just as good as in the control group, only 35% survived 10 years and retained the breast. CALLE et al. concluded from these results that removal of macroscopic tumors (tumorectomy or extensive local resection) is helpful in breast-preserving treatment.

PIERQUIN [21] and PIERQUIN et al. [22] demonstrated that boost therapy using the interstitial irradiation method (iridium 192) leads to better local control of residual tumor than external irradiation alone. After tumorectomy, external irradiation of the remaining breast tissue (45 Gy), irradiation of the lymph vessels, and an interstitial boost dose of 15–25 Gy, the locoregional recurrence rate after 10 years was only 8% in patients with T1 tumors.

In patients with T2 or T3 tumors, before therapy the tumors were only confirmed histologically by needle biopsy and left in situ. Here too the recurrence rates were low: only 9% for T2 and 15% for T3, which are clearly better than without interstitial therapy.

Prospective Randomized Studies of Breast-Preserving Therapy

A few prospective randomized studies have influenced decisively the present strategy of radiotherapy in breast-preserving treatment: the Guy's Hospital study [14,15], the Milan study [24,25], and the NSABP trial B-06 [7,8]. These studies are discussed elsewhere in this volume (see HAYWARD, this volume; MARGOLESE, this volume; HENDERSON, this volume).

Present Value of Irradiation in Primary Treatment of Breast Cancer

After no clear improvement in survival rates had been obtained with adjuvant radiotherapy and after hopes that adjuvant chemotherapy would clearly improve survival rates were damped, the use of radiotherapy in the primary treatment of breast cancer underwent a renaissance in two areas:

1. Postoperative irradiation of the thoracic wall and the regional lymph vessels that have not been treated surgically is being employed again when known unfavorable prognostic factors indicate a risk of 40% or more of recurrences in these regions.
2. The radicality of the breast operation apparently does not affect the survival rate. To improve the quality of life, increasingly the tumor is removed (quadrantectomy, segment resection, tumorectomy) and any tumor cells (or other focuses in multifocal disease) that may remain are treated using radiotherapy.

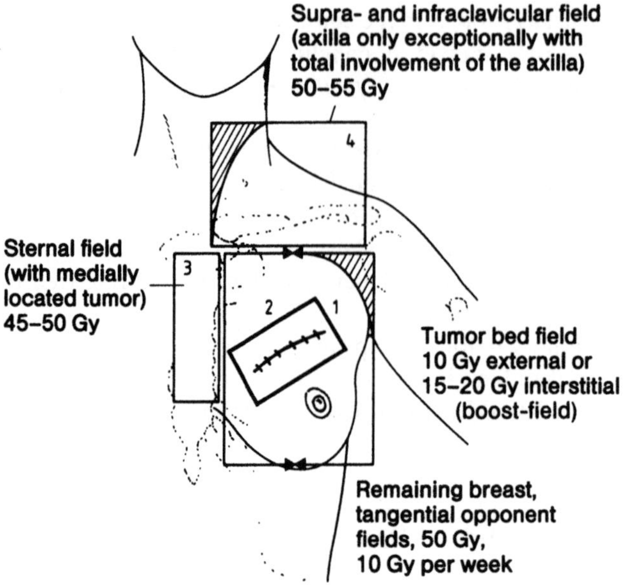

Fig. 2. Arrangement of fields for radiotherapy after surgical treatment of breast cancer. *1*, Irradiation of the remaining breast tissue (or thoracic wall) with opponent fields. *2*, Tumor bed field (with breast preservation). *3*, Sternal field. *4*, Supra- and infraclavicular lymph node field, if level III axillary lymph nodes are involved. *Shaded areas*, shielding of organs that should be protected

Techniques used at the University Women's Hospital, Heidelberg

Irradiation of the Breast

In 1988 the proportion of breast-conserving treatments (tumor size 3 cm or less) to radical treatments increased to 194 from a total of 412 primary cases, which is approximately 50%, see Fig. 1 in our clinic..

In breast-conserving therapy, irradiation of the breast is used instead of surgical removal of breast tissue. The radiotherapy aims at sterilizing tumor remnants that are left in tissue adjacent to the excision site and multicentric subclinical lesions. This means that the target volume comprises the breast from about the second intercostal space (there is great anatomic variability) to the intramammary fold. The medial boundary is the sternal edge, while the lateral boundary is the median axillary line. The thoracic wall and the pectoral muscle are *not* included in the target volume, except when the margin of the resection was not sufficiently far from these structures (2 cm or more). These structures do, however, usually receive the full dose because of the curvature of the thoracic wall.

Homogeneous irradiation. Small and medium-sized breasts are irradiated using cobalt 60 (Fig. 3). Photons from an accelerator (4–6 MeV) can be used with normal sized and moderately large breasts but are only slightly more effective (Figs. 4,5).

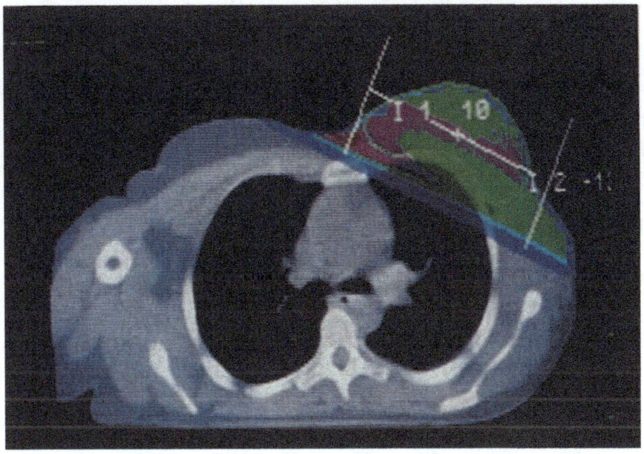

Fig. 3. Axial CT section of three-dimensional treatment of a woman with normal-sized breasts, target volume 443 cm^3. Irradiation with Cobalt 60 using 30° wedges. *Dark blue*, 50%–90% of reference dose; *pale blue*, 90%–95%; *green*, 95%–100%; *violet*, 100%–105%; *red*, 105%–110%

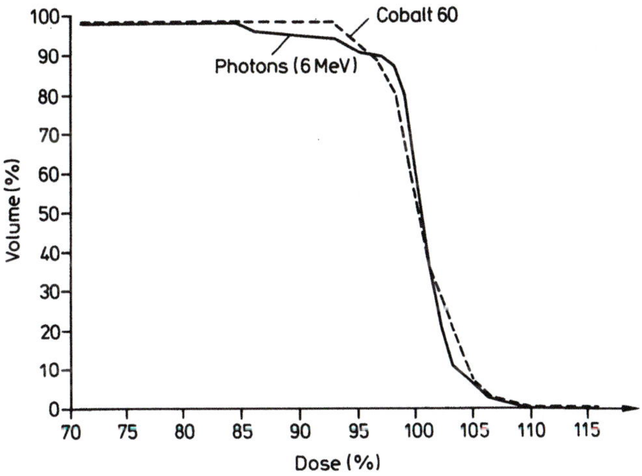

Fig. 4. Dose–volume curve for the three-dimensional treatment illustrated in Fig. 3. Comparison of Cobalt 60 and 6-MeV photons, both with 30° wedges. The curve is slightly steeper in the central region but the subcutaneous tissue receives a lower dose with 6-MV photons

Very large breasts with a wide field separation are better irradiated with 8-MeV photons. However, the subcutaneous tissue then does not receive a sufficiently high dose. Compensating by using bolus material or an increased boost dose compromises cosmetic results. We therefore prefer to do a reduction mammoplasty in patients with very large breasts.

Wedges are used if the tumor is located near the thoracic wall as this makes raising the dose at the base of the breast advisable. The dose of homogeneous

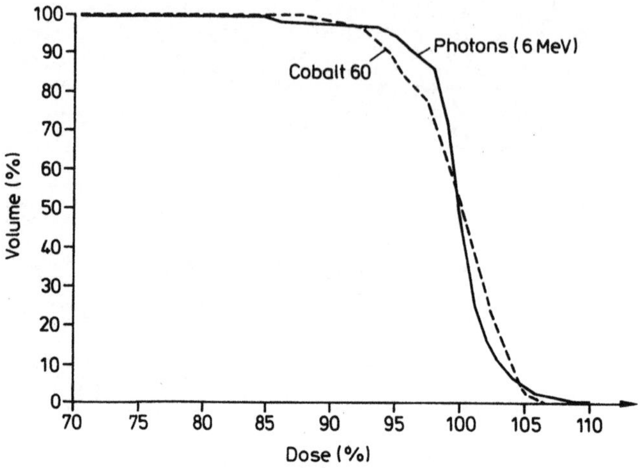

Fig. 5. Dose-volume curve for a women with a large breast (target volume 1150 cm^3). Comparison of Cobalt 60 and 6-MeV photons, both with 30° wedges. The curve is considerably steeper in the central region but the subcutaneous region receives a lower dose with 6-MV photons

irradiation is calculated for a point 2 cm below the breast, and is normally 5×2 Gy per week for 5 weeks.

Boost Irradiation. Recurrences can either develop from multicentric carcinomas or from tumor remnants. Tumor remnants have, on average, a higher volume than multicentric tumors (MÜLLER et al., this volume). As the tumor-sterilizing dose depends on tumor volume we feel it is appropriate to give a boost dose to the tumor bed if there is a high probability of tumor remnants. The boost dose is calculated for the region of the tumor bed. For the boost dose, small field photons or interstitial iridium are used. For boosts of up to 10 Gy we prefer small field photons; higher doses are best given by interstitial iridium using an remote-controlled machine (Selectron; Fig. 6).

We give a boost dose of 10 Gy to 20 Gy in the region of the tumor bed in the following situations, some of which, according to CONNOLLY et al. (1983), also indicate a significantly increased risk of local recurrence:

1. Insufficiently wide surgical excision or locally too extensive tumor
2. Intraductal carcinoma in the tumor
3. Carcinoma in situ at the border of the tumor extending to the margin of the resection
4. Invasive tumor almost reaching the margin of the resection line
5. High degree of polyploidy
6. High mitotic index
7. Extensive lymphangiosis carcinomatosa

With us, situations 1, 3, and 4 call in all cases for boost irradiation but the others only lead to boost irradiation in combination. In situations 1, 3, and 4 we give an

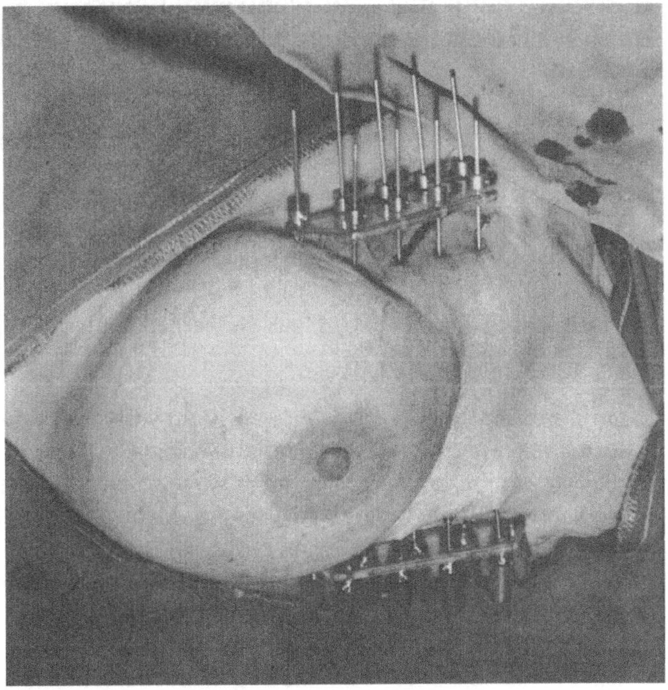

Fig. 6. Interstitial needles placed in the breast of a woman with extensive intraductal carcinoma, ready for loading using the remote-controlled afterloading (Selectron)

interstitial boost dose of 15 Gy at a high dose rate (HDR) or 20 Gy at a low dose rate (LDR), and in the others a 10-Gy external boost. Whilst the NSABP trial considered boost irradiation unnecessary, the majority of centers worldwide give boost irradiation either in all cases or if there is an increased risk of local recurrence. It is unclear, however, when boost irradiation is best given using electrons, photons, or interstitially. The efficacy of external breast irradiation and the interstitial irradiation must be further clarified in prospective studies. (For our results see Table 3).

Table 3. Overall survival (OAS), recurrence free survival (RFS), rate of local failure, death from tumor, death without tumor in the University Women's Hospital, Heidelberg 1974-April 1987, N = 665, (% follow-up = 91,3%)

5-year observation	N = 160	100%
OAS		86,9%
death without tumor included		7%
RFS		84,4%
Local failure		6,9%
Distant metastases		19 %
Local or distant failure		21 %

Residual Tumor and Multicentricity Following Wide Excision as a Basis for Determining Irradiation Dose (by A. Müller and D. von Fournier)

Of the various kinds of operation for breast-conserving therapy, wide excision has now become established at most centers (for a review of the methods, see FOURNIER, this volume). Since we hence have performed quadrant resection of the Veronesi type (see VERONESI, this volume) at the University Women's Hospital, Heidelberg since 1974, wide excision has also become established almost exclusively here in the meantime.

The investigations discussed here concerned unanswered questions about wide excision and the risk of local failure:

1. How frequently does invasive and noninvasive residual tumor remain after segmental resection in the immediate vicinity of the resection margin in patients selected for breast-conserving therapy (see below for selection criteria)?
2. How frequently are multiple focuses present in other quadrants of the remaining breast after segmental resection?
3. What volume of residual invasive and noninvasive carcinoma is left behind in the quadrant of the wide excision in comparison to the tumor volume of multicentric carcinoma in the remaining breast?
4. Up to what distance from the segmental resection margin are the residual carcinomas associated with the primary tumor be followed histologically?

Since 70% of local failures occurred in the same quadrant in the Heidelberg patients (see A. MÜLLER, this volume), this being comparable with the results of the NSABP study (FISHER et al. 1985), the hypothesis was investigated of whether larger volumes of residual tumor remaining in the quadrant of the primary tumor lead to an increased rate of recurrence. If this hypothesis is correct, two consequences regarding prevention of local failure arise:

1. Local radicality should be increased
2. A higher radiation dose (boost irradiation) should be given when there is a high risk of residual tumor.

The latter is in contrast to the policy advocated by the NSABP study (FISHER et al. 1985), according to which an upper limit for total dose to the remaining breast is 50–55 Gy.

Materials and Methods

Patient Selection

Modified radical operations (ablation, axillary lymphadenectomy, modification according to Patey) were carried out for invasive carcinomas in 695 patients at the University Women's Hospital, Heidelberg between 1978 and 1981. Of these patients, 131 which fulfilled our criteria for breast-conserving therapy were selected. These criteria were:

- Tumor size, preoperative (X-ray, clinical examination) and intraoperative (macroscopic, palpable) ≤ 3 cm
- Distance between the tumor and mamilla ≥ 2 cm
- No preoperative indication of multicentric growth (X-ray, clinical examination, ultrasound)
- No contralateral carcinoma known

In this study, a workup technique which allowed complete histological investigation of the ablated breast was used for the first time. This was based on the technique of plastination developed by VON HAGENS [28].

The glandular bodies were cut into 2.5-mm-thick sagittal slices after formalin fixation. These slices were stained with hemalum in accordance with the procedure of WELLINGS et al. [30]. With this technique, only the cell nuclei are stained. Afterwards, the 2.5-mm-thick tissue slices were impregnated with a plastic which can be polymerized in the tissue. By choosing a suitable refractive index of this plastic, these tissue slices could be made completely transparent (Fig. 7). After hardening of the lamellae (degree of hardness of lamellae could be freely chosen), microscopic examination at a magnification of up to at least 100× was possible. Pathological alterations could be followed through the entire lamellar thickness of 2.5 mm by focusing the microscope. A three-dimensional picture of all relevant

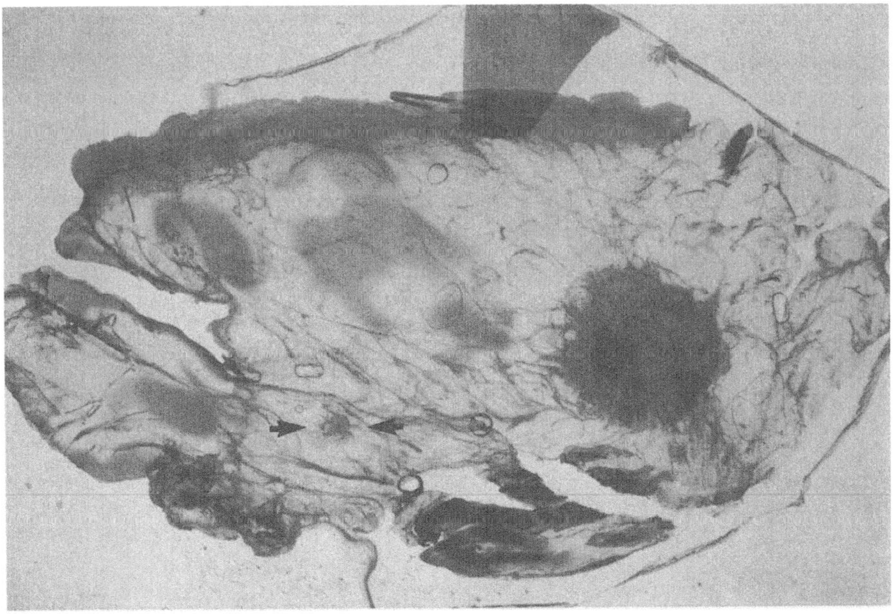

Fig. 7. Plastinated 2.5-mm-thick breast slice. An invasive carcinoma with a maximum diameter of 2.7 cm is situated in the glandular tissue. In the area marked with *arrows*, a second invasive focus was found

morphological alterations of the total breast was obtained by joining together the lamellae (see Fig. 10).

After microscopic investigation of the 2.5-mm-thick slices, the method allowed preparation of histological sections of any desired thickness from initially unclear tissue regions (5 μm in our case) and retrospective staining of these sections with hematoxylin-eosin (HE). Figure 8 is a photomicrograph of an epithelial proliferation which was unclear even when magnified in the transparent lamella. Figure 9 shows a 5-μm-thick section of the same tissue region which permits a final diagnosis of noninvasive ductal carcinoma after HE staining. A comprehensive histological examination of the entire breast, including the tiniest morphological alterations, was thus possible.

The carcinomas found in the entire breast were documented in topographic charts. Figure 10 shows a chart recording a primary tumor, the invasive and noninvasive tumor residuals, and a simulated wide excision. Our guideline that the margin of the section for a wide excision should be at least 2 cm away from the macroscopic surface of the primary tumor was observed.

Measurement of the Volume of the Carcinoma

All noninvasive and invasive carcinomas which were found in the breast remaining after simulated segmental resection were measured by means of a point counting method. Figure 11 shows the segmental resection margins, residual tumor in the remaining breast, and a tissue lamella with a grid projected onto areas containing microscopic and invasive residual tumor.

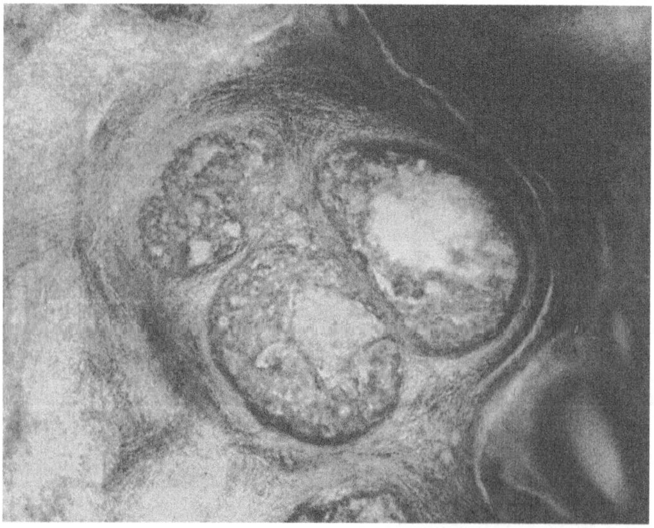

Fig. 8. Photomicrograph of a 2.5-mm-thick plastinated tissue slice. The diagnosis is unclear; proliferative mastopathy with epithelial atypia or noninvasive ductal carcinoma. ×63

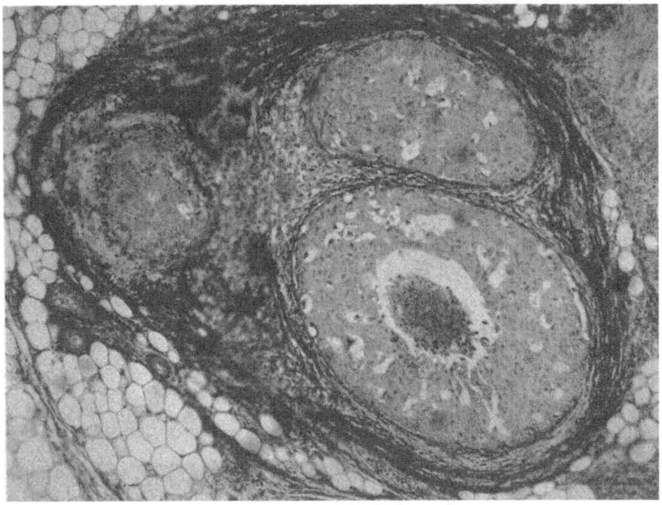

Fig. 9. Histological appearance of the glandular region in Fig. 8 after preparation of a 5-μm-thick section stained with hematoxylin-eosin. Diagnosis: ductal carcinoma in situ. ×100

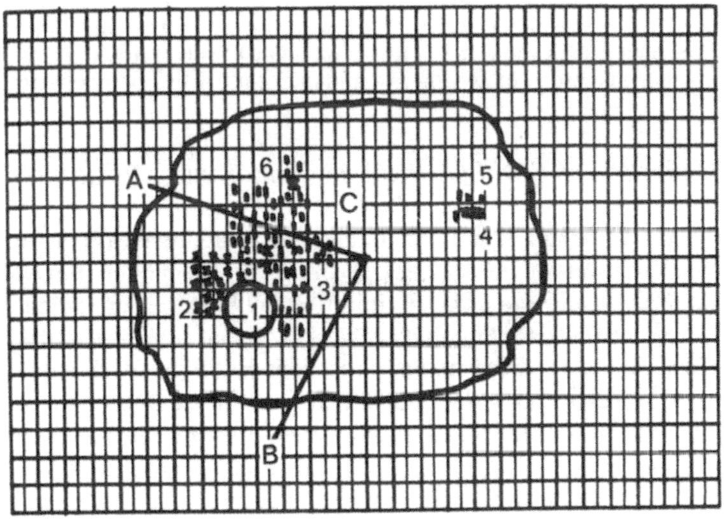

Fig. 10. Topographic chart of a preparation. Vertical lines are 0.5 cm apart and horizontal lines 1.0 cm. After simulated segment resection, residual primary tumor remains in the breast at the resection margin. Multicentric tumor focuses with multicentric invasive growth also remain. *Crosses*, invasive carcinoma; *lines*, noninvasive ductal carcinoma. *A,B*, lines of simulated wide excision; *C*, remaining breast after wide excision. *1*, Primary tumor. *2*, Invasive focus of the primary tumor, detected by this technique only. *3*, Noninvasive focus of the primary tumor. Both *2* and *3* are between the lines of resection. *4*, *5*, Invasive (*4*) and noninvasive (*5*) microscopically detected tumor. These tumors are "true multicentric foci" in the remaining breast. *6*, Primary tumor residuals in the breast remaining after wide excision

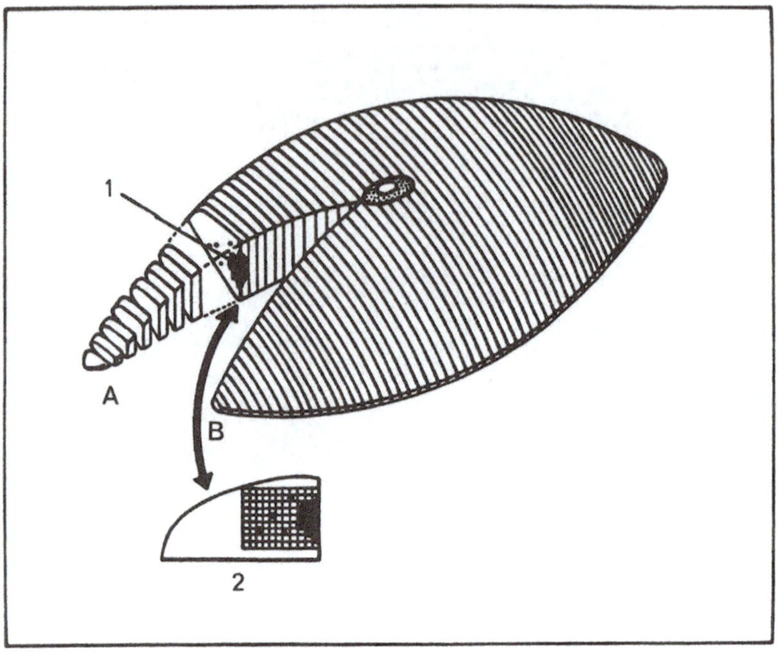

Fig. 11. Schematic representation of the volume measurement of the residual tumor after simulated segmental resection. *Black area*, invasive carcinoma; *black dots*, intraductal carcinoma ramification. *A,B,* lines of simulated wide excision; *1*, residual tumor in the remaining breast; *2*, projection of a grid onto parts with microscopic residual tumor

Definition of Residual Primary Tumor and Multicentric Tumor

Residual primary tumor was defined as a carcinoma (invasive or noninvasive) which was outside the segment, according to this method, but which had a spatial connection with the primary tumor. A multicentric carcinoma was defined as a carcinoma (invasive or noninvasive) situated outside the simulated segment in the remaining breast, but with no spatial connection (no carcinomatous tissue bridge) to the primary tumor. A tumor which was situated outside the segment but in the same quadrant as the primary tumor and not connected with the primary tumor via a tissue bridge was a multicentric carcinoma according to this definition. This definition has the logical consequence that carcinomas which remain in the breast when the resection margin is histologically free of tumor are multicentric, irrespective of their location.

Results

Residual Primary Tumor

After simulated segmental resection, we found residual tumor outside the segment that had histological connections with the primary tumor in 19.1% of the patients

(25/131). Of the 25/131 residual tumors, 15 (11%) displayed invasive growth and 10 (8%) showed no invasive growth.

Multicentric Carcinomas

In 24.4% of the cases (32/131), multicentric focuses were found in the breast remaining after simulated segmental resection with no connection to the primary tumor. Of these 32/131 multicentric carcinomas, 15 (11%) had invasive growth and 17 (13%) showed noninvasive growth.

Volumes of Residual Tumors and Multicentric Carcinomas after Segment Resection

The volumes of the residual tumors (invasive and noninvasive) were compared with the volumes of multicentric carcinomas (invasive and noninvasive). The average volume of the residual tumors was 670.2 mm³ and that of the multicentric carcinomas was 209.6 mm³. The size difference was statistically significant ($P = 0.0004$; Wilcoxon rank). Tumor volume of the residuals was more than 1400 mm³ in 4.5% of all patients, but in none with multicentric carcinoma (Fig. 12).

This shows that the total volume of the tumor focuses was markedly greater in residual tumors than in multicentric carcinoma. It must be taken into consideration that with this technique only carcinoma tissue was measured, and not the sur-

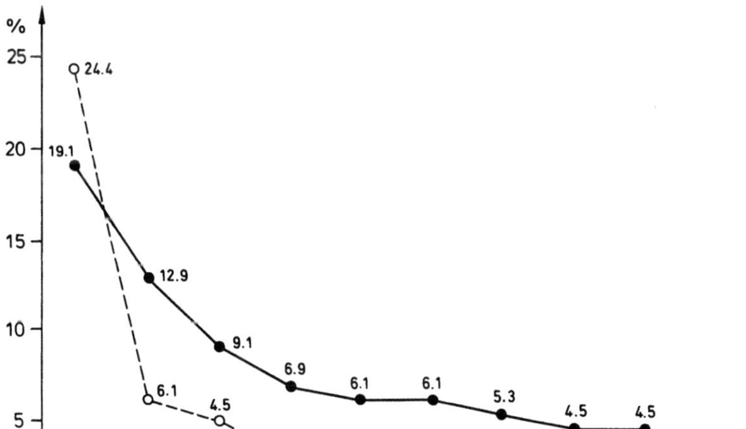

Fig. 12. Representation of the volumes of residual tumor and multicentric carcinoma remaining in the breast after simulated wide excision. The figures on the curves and on the ordinate are the percentage of the overall study population of 131 patients. *Continuous line*, volume of residual primary tumor; *dotted line*, volume of remaining multicentric carcinoma

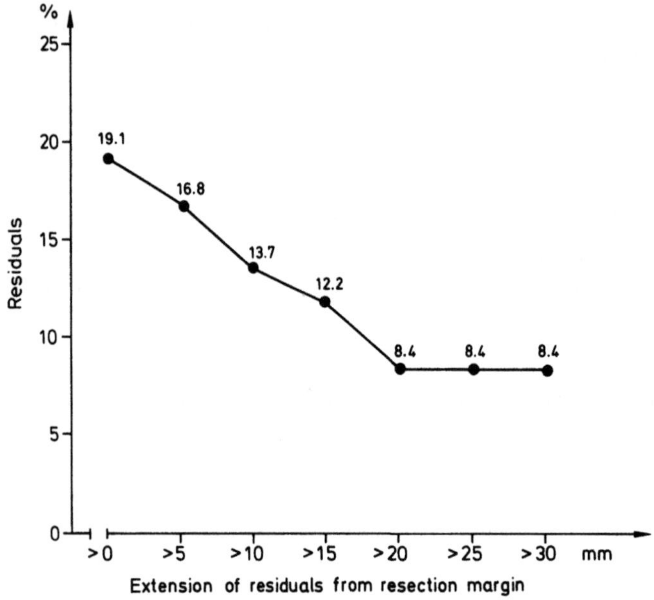

Fig. 13. Extension of residual tumor beyond the resection margin of a simulated wide excision. The *figures* on the curve and on the ordinate are the percentage of the overall study population of 131 patients

rounding connective tissue. A volume of 1400 mm^3 thus corresponds roughly to a sphere 1.4 cm in diameter consisting exclusively of tumor cells. Since the tumors contained large proportions of interstitial connective tissue, the actual sizes of both the residual tumors and the multicentric carcinomas were very much greater than the volume measured here.

Distance of Residual Tumors from the Resection Margin after Wide Excision

Measurements were made of how far the residual tumor extended from the resection margin of a wide excision (simulated segmental resection). Figure 13 shows the frequency distributions. Residual tumors were present in 19.1% of the patients studied; in 13.7% the residual tumors extended more than 1 cm and in 8.4% more than 3 cm beyond the resection margin.

Discussion

The study provided the following results relevant to breast-conserving therapy: in patients selected for breast-conserving therapy (tumor size up to 3 cm, macroscopic distance of the resection margin from the primary tumor: 2cm), residual tumor was found in one in five patients (19.1%) and multicentric focuses were found in the remaining breast in one in four patients (24.4%). The volume of the residual tumors was clearly larger than the total volume of the multicentric carcinomas.

In addition, from a radiobiological point of view, the residual tumors are situated relatively close together in the vicinity of the primary tumor. Consequently, a relatively large interconnected tumor mass arises. The multicentric carcinomas were distributed over the entire remaining breast and, as well as having a smaller total volume, the individual focuses were very much smaller. It is known [9] that breast cancer can be more frequently controlled by radiotherapy the smaller the volume of a tumor. This explains why 70% of all local failures occurred in the vicinity of the primary tumor in our patients treated with breast-conserving therapy, the figure being comparable to that found in other studies. From these histomorphological investigations, it can be concluded that, for breast-conserving therapy, a boost dose beyond the normal total breast dose of 50–55 Gy is appropriate if there are signs of residual tumor (i.e., in one in five patients).

It must be borne in mind that residual tumors of more than 3 cm from the resection margin were found in 8% of all patients. In these patients, the boost dose is only appropriate if a relatively large volume extending for more than 6 cm is covered.

The importance of residual tumor (one-fifth of all patients) makes it appear appropriate to carry out secondary resection at resection margins not free of tumor. It is to be expected that with surgical reduction of the residual tumor mass, the rate of local failure will also fall. In the literature, the relatively radical surgical technique of VERONESI et al. quadrant resection; VERONESI et al. [27] also led to the lowest rate of local failure (4% within 5–12 years). With a less radical surgical technique, RECHT et al. [24], for example, found local failure in 8.2% of patients within a follow-up period of 4.5 years.

If the thesis of HAYWARD (this volume) that local clearance of the carcinoma affects the rate of survival, especially in small tumors, is correct, it is to be inferred from our investigations that local resection in wide excision should be as extensive as possible in order to keep the rate of residual tumor low. Experience shows that radiotherapy cannot prevent local recurrences arising from these frequently extensive residual tumor in all cases.

References

1. Bonadonna G, Rossi A, Valagussa P (1985a) Adjuvant CMF chemotherapy in operable breast cancer. Ten years later. World J Surg 9:707–713
2. Bonadonna G, Valagussa P, Rossi A, et al. (1985b) Ten year experience with CMF-based adjuvant chemotherapy in resectable breast cancer. Breast Cancer Res Treat 5:95–115
3. Calle R (1978) Conservative management of operable breast cancer. Ten years experience at the Foundation Curie. Cancer 42:2045
4. Calle R, Vilcoq JR, Pilleron JP, et al. (1983) Conservative treatment of operable breast carcinoma by irradiation with or without limited surgery – ten-year results. In: Harris JR, Hellman S, Silen W (eds): Conservative management of breast cancer. Lippincott, Philadelphia, pp 3–9

5. Connolly JL, Schnitt SJ, Harris JR, Hellman S, Cohen RB (1983) Pathologic correlates of local tumor control follow primary radiation therapy in patients with early breast cancer. In: Harris JR, Hellman S, Silen W (eds) Breast cancer. New surgical and radiotherapeutic techniques. Lippincott, Philadelphia, pp 123–130
6. Finzi NS (1927) X-rays and radium in the treatment of carcinoma of the breast. Br Med J 2:728–733
7. Fisher B, Bauer M, Margolese R, et al. (1985a) Five-years results of a randomized clinical trial comparing total mastectomy and segmental mastectomy with or without radiation in the treatment of breast cancer. N Engl J Med 312:665
8. Fisher B, Redmond C, Fisher ER, et al. (1985b) Ten-year results of a randomized clinical trial comparing radical mastectomy and total mastectomy with or without radiation. N Engl J Med 312:674
9. Fletcher G (1972) Local results of irradiation in the primary management of localized breast cancer. Cancer 29:545
10. Fournier vD, zum Winkel K, Kuttig H, Kubli F (1986) Strahlentherapie als adjuvante Maßnahme beim Mammakarzinom. In: Kadach U, Kaufmann M, Kubli F (eds) Hormone Antihormone Zytostatika zur aduvanten Therapie des Mammakarzinoms. Zuckschwerdt, Munich, pp 82–97
11. Gocht H (1897) Therapeutische Verwendung der Röntgenstrahlen. Fortschr Gebiete Röntgenstr 1:14–22
12. Harris JR, Hellman S (1987a) Adjuvant radiotherapy. In: Harris JR, Hellman S, Henderson IC, Kinne DW (eds) Breast diseases. Lippincott, Philadelphia, pp 284–299
13. Harris JR, Hellmann S (1987b) Conservative surgery and radiotherapy. In: Harris JR, Hellman S, Henderson IC, Kinne DW (eds) Breast diseases. Lippincott, Philadelphia, pp 299–324
14. Hayward JL (1983) The Guy's Hospital trials on breast conservation. In: Harris JR, Hellman S, Silen W (eds) Conservative management of breast cancer. Lippincott, Philadelphia, pp 77–90
15. Hayward L (1985) Trials of wide excision and radiation therapy at the breast unit, Guy's Hospital, London. In: Zander J, Balzer J (eds) Early breast cancer. Springer, Berlin Heidelberg New York, pp 253–263
16. Høst H, Brennhovd JO (1977) The effect of post-radiotherapy in breast cancer. Int J Radiat Oncol Biol Phys 3:1061
17. Høst A, Brennhovd IO, Loeb M (1986) Post-operative radiotherapy in breast cancer – long-term results from the Oslo study. Int J Radiat Oncol Biol Phys 12:727
18. Marcial VA, Velez-Garcia E, Moore M, et al. (1985) Radiotherapy related adjuvant chemotherapy initiation delay in breast cancer with positive nodes: Does it affect prognosis? A Southeastern Cancer Study Group report. Int J Radiat Oncol Biol Phys 11 (suppl 1):150
19. Palmer MK, Ribeiro GG (1985) Thirty-four year follow-up of patients with breast cancer in a clinical trial of postoperative radiotherapy. Br Med J 291:1088
20. Pfahler GE, Parry DL (1931) Roentgen therapy in carcinoma of the breast. Ann Surg 93:412
21. Pierquin B (1983) Conservative treatment for carcinoma of the breast. Experience of Creteil – ten-year results. In: Harris JR, Hellman S, Silen W (eds) Conservative management of breast cancer. Lippincott, Philadelphia, pp 11–14
22. Pierquin B, Otmetzquine Y, Lobo PA (1985) Conservative management of breast carcinoma. In: Zander J, Balzer J (eds) Early breast cancer. Springer, Berlin Heidelberg New York, pp 276–284
23. Rao AR, Murthy AK, Hendrickson FR, et al. (1985) Analysis of risk factors for locoregional failure in stage II (T1N1Mo and T2N1Mo) breast carcinoma treated with mastectomy and adjunctive chemotherapy. Int J Radiat Oncol Biol Phys 11 (suppl 1): 151
24. Recht A, Connolly JL, Schnitt SJ, Cady B, Love S, Osteen RT, Patterson WB, Shierley R, Silen W, Come S, Henderson JC, Silver B, Harris JR (1986) Conservative surgery and radiation therapy for early breast cancer: Results, controversies, and unsolved problems Semin Oncol 13:434–449

25. Veronesi U (1985) Randomized trails comparing conservation techniques with conventional surgery: an overview. In Tobias JS, Peckham MJ (eds) Primary management of breast cancer: Alternatives to mastectomy management. Arnold, London, pp 131–152 (Management of malignant disease series)
26. Veronesi U, Zucali R, Luini A, Belle F, Crispino S, Merson M (1985) Conservative treatment of breast cancer with the "Qu.A.RT" technique. In: Zander J, Baltzer J (eds) Early breast cancer. Springer, Berlin Heidelberg New York, pp 264–270
27. Veronesi U, Banfi A, Vecchio M, Saccozzi R, Clemente C, Greco M, Luini A, Marubini E, Muscolino G, Rilke F, Sacchini V, Salvadori B, Zecchini A, Zucali R (1986) Comparison of Halsted mastectomy with quadrantectomy, axillary dissection, and radiotherapy in early breast cancer: long-term results. Eur J Cancer Clin Oncol 22:1085–1089
28. von Hagens G (1979) Impregnation of soft biological specimens with thermosetting resins and elastomers. Anat Rec 194:247–256
29. Wallgren A, Arner O, Bergström J et al. (1986) Radiation therapy in operable breast cancer: – results from the Stockholm trial on adjuvant radiotherapy. Int J Radiat Oncol Biol Phys 12:533–537
30. Wellings SR, Jensen HM, Marcum RG (1975) An atlas of subgross pathology of the human breast with special reference to possible precancerous lesions. J Natl Cancer Inst 55:237–273

Treatment of Breast Cancer with Breast Preservation

S. HELLMAN

The treatment of breast cancer is based on the surgical treatments designed by MEYER [11], and HALSTED [6], and the notion that the disease is orderly in its spread, and that any treatment should maximize local and regional control, since loco-regional persistence of disease acts as a source of distant metastases. This view has been questioned by a number of investigators [3,13], most recently by FISHER [4]. The alternative view of breast-cancer treatment suggests that local and regional control are of little or no importance as they do not effect the ultimate frequency of metastasis, or outcome. In studying which of these two hypotheses best explains breast cancer, different treatment techniques have been applied, some of which preserve the breast.

It is important to separate questions concerning the natural history of breast cancer from questions concerning the efficacy of breast-preservation techniques as they affect local control. Evidence for the importance of local and regional control has come from two studies of breast preservation. The first, by the Guy's Hospital Group, compared mastectomy with tumor excision and irradiation of the breast and axilla [9]. The techniques used were inadequate by today's standards, since they undertreated the axilla. This study showed that axillary recurrence was more frequent in the group receiving irradiation. Importantly, this was associated with reduced survival. More recently, the National Surgical Adjuvant Breast Project (NSABP) compared segmental resection of the tumor with and without breast irradiation [5]. In this randomized trial, breast recurrence was more frequent in the group not receiving radiation. This was associated with a significant increase in the frequency of distant metastasis. Both these studies, therefore, indicate the importance of achieving local and regional control, since this appears to affect the incidence of distant metastasis, leading to differences in survival. The technique to be recommended here for breast preservation accepts the premise that local and regional recurrence is to be avoided; the technique is *radical* in intent.

Shortly after the discovery of X-rays by ROENTGEN, their efficacy in the treatment of breast cancer was appreciated. There are a number of reports from both Europe and North America describing the results of irradiation in the treatment of breast cancer. These studies uniformly indicate that this tumor is quite responsive to radiation and that local control can be achieved under a variety of circumstances. The radiation facilities available were not able to deliver tumoricidal doses of radiation without causing significant undesirable sequelae in the skin and soft tissues. For this reason, radiotherapy was not a satisfactory alternative to mastectomy.

If the goal of treatment was to cure the tumor with the least cosmetic deformity, radiation using these early orthovoltage techniques had little to offer. The use of radium needle implants, however, did provide the opportunity for local tumor control and acceptable cosmesis. This technique was pioneered at the Curie Institute in France and by JEFFREY KEYNES in Great Britain. KEYNES [10] wrote extensively on this subject, describing results equivalent in survival to those of mastectomy, with acceptable cosmetic results. A significant problem with the technique was the extensive and time-consuming manipulation of radium, resulting in significant exposure of the operator. After the Second World War, supervoltage radiation became more readily available in the form of electrical generators producing X-rays of 2 MeV or greater, and cobalt units. These facilities provided the opportunity to reconsider the efficacy of radiation treatment. Since its tumoricidal properties were already known, interest was in providing the optimal cosmetic results. Exposure to ionizing radiation was greatly reduced for interstitial therapy with the development of afterloading techniques using radioactive iridium. Both supervoltage radiation and these afterloading interstitial techniques were applied to breast cancer at a number of centers, perhaps earliest and most importantly in France. Results by CALLE et al. [2], PIERQUIN [14], ALMARIC et al. [1], and their colleagues in France; MONTAGUE et al. [12] and her colleagues at the M.D. Anderson Hospital; and HARRIS and HELLMAN [7] at the Joint Center for Radiation Therapy all demonstrate efficacy in terms of tumor control and satisfactory cosmetic results. Randomized controlled clinical trials by VERONESI et al. [15] and FISHER [5] confirmed the efficacy of such breast-preservation techniques as compared to different forms of mastectomy. The current position, therefore, appears to be that it is possible to preserve a cosmetically acceptable breast and still embark upon radical treatment of breast cancer.

There are a number of questions regarding this technique which must be asked in order to develop a standard treatment of breast cancer. First, with regard to the primary lesion, it has become increasingly clear that the gross tumor should be removed. It is unclear how much more than this should be excised in the initial surgery. Randomized studies by VERONESI et al. [15] used the quadrantectomy technique. This required removal of a very large volume of tissue. The FISHER [5] study required removal of the tumor with a clear and distinct margin. If this margin was not confirmed by the pathologist, the patient was offered only mastectomy. On the other hand, some American and French groups used much smaller excisions, and for large tumors the French used no excision at all. A workshop was held in New York in 1985 [8] to develop a consensus on the appropriate treatments combining radiotherapy and breast preservation. It was agreed that the tumor should be removed in a manner sufficient to allow adequate evaluation of the resected specimen by the pathologist. The extent of surgery, and the dose of radiation required for local tumor control are complementary: the more extensive the surgical procedure, the less radiation required for tumor control. Our current recommendation is excision that is wide enough to produce negative margins of resection. If the margins are positive after such an excision, further resection should be considered before starting radiotherapy, unless such resection would result in a major cosmetic deformity. If that is the case, then one should consider a more extensive, "radiation-boost" technique.

The entire breast should be treated with a total dose of 45–50 Gy at 18–20 Gy per day for 5 days per week utilizing a cobalt unit or a 4–6 MeV linear accelerator. Nothing should be placed on the skin during treatment. The use of a bolus will raise the skin dose, thus compromising the cosmetic effect. The breast is irradiated utilizing opposed tangential fields. The lateral border lies between the mid axillary and posterior axillary lines. The medial border is the midline, unless internal mammary nodes are to be included. We do not recommend that the whole breast receive more than 50 Gy. There is some controversy regarding the need for supplementary radiation of the primary site. If the surgery is quite extensive, this may not be necessary. At present, however, we do recommend a boost using either electrons or a radioactive iridium implant. It is important that the boost technique should not appreciatively diminish the cosmetic result. Where the breast tissue is thin, especially in the inner quadrants, we recommend that the boost be carried out using electron-beam techniques. A total boost dose of 14–16 Gy in 2-Gy fractions is administered with a technique which uses two field sizes so that the edge of the boost is not clearly demarcated. This helps to improve the cosmetic result. In thicker areas of breast tissue or where the margins are quite uncertain, we recommend a radioactive-iridium implant to a total dose of 18–20 Gy, being sure to direct the irradiation well below the skin surface. Care must be taken to limit the volume and yet encompass the tumor bed. The dose rate should be approximately 0.4–0.5 Gy/h.

The use of radiation to treat regional lymph nodes is an area of uncertainty. The appropriate treatment for the axilla is axillary dissection, as this serves several functions. Since patients found to have positive axillary nodes are at greater risk of distant metastasis than patients with negative nodes, this information is important if such patients are to be considered as candidates for adjuvant systemic hormone therapy or chemotherapy. Axillary dissection is indicated in all patients for whom such adjuvant therapy is being considered; dissection provides both diagnosis and treatment. It is important, however, that the dissection be extensive enough to provide local tumor control, thus avoiding the need to apply both radiation and surgery to the axilla. Dissection should avoid producing cosmetic deformity. The radiotherapist must be aware of the extent of the surgical procedure so that overlapping of the radiation and surgical fields can be avoided. Patients with outer-quadrant lesions in whom axillary dissection reveals no evidence of lymph-node metastasis do not need nodal irradiation. Patients with positive axillary lymph nodes should receive irradiation of the internal mammary and supraclavicular nodes. We make every effort to localize the internal mammary lymph nodes using lymphoscintigraphic techniques. Once located, the ipsilateral internal mammary nodes are included in the tangential breast field unless such treatment irradiates an excessive amount of lung. If this is the case, then a portion of the treatment is given utilizing this technique (20–25 Gy) and the remainder is given using a separate internal mammary electron field or mixed electron-photon field. Care should be taken to accurately match the dose distribution of the internal mammary and tangential fields, avoiding both underdosing and overdose areas. This can be done by careful treatment planning and inclining the electron field toward the involved side. We find this "mix-and-match technique" useful, but not as desirable as including all these nodes in the tangential breast fields. When their treatment is indicated, the supraclavicular fossa and apex of the axilla are included in an *en fosse* field. Care is taken to avoid overlap of the axillary dissection. This is facilitated by having the surgeon place a clip at the apex of the dissection. For patients with inner quadrant and central lesions it is our current recommendation to treat the internal mammary nodes, if this can be done without exposure of unnecessary amounts of normal tissue, using the techniques described above. We recognize that the data to support irradiation of the internal mammary nodes are limited. In treating this area, therefore, one must be confident that neither the functional nor the cosmetic result will be compromised.

There is still much to learn about the proper interdigitation of surgery and radiotherapy. They are clearly complementary. In a large majority of patients satisfactory cosmetic results can be obtained with excellent local control. The interdigitation of chemotherapy with breast-preservation procedures still needs a great deal of investigation. We currently initiate chemotherapy following the surgical procedure, administering one cycle of multidrug chemotherapy to patients with less than four positive nodes. Following radiotherapy, the remainder of the chemotherapy course is administered. For patients with four or more positive lymph nodes, the entire course of chemotherapy is given (over approximately 5 months) prior to radiotherapy. So far, this has been delivered without difficulty. It remains to be seen whether such treatment will affect either local control or cosmetic results.

References

1. Almaric R, Santamaria F, Robert F, et al. (1983) Conservation therapy of operable breast cancer – results at five, ten, and fifteen years in 2216 consecutive cases. In: Harris JR, Hellman S, Silen W (eds) Conservative management of breast cancer. Lippincott, Philadelphia, pp 15–22
2. Calle R, Vilcoq JR, Pilleron JP, et al. (1983) Conservative treatment of operable breast carcinoma of irradiation with or without limited surgery – 10 year results. In: Harris JR, Hellman S, Silen W (eds) Conservative management of breast cancer. Lippincott, Philadelphia, pp 3–9
3. Crile G Jr (1967) A biological consideration of the treatment of breast cancer. Thomas, Ft Lauderdale
4. Fisher B (1979) Breast cancer management: Alternatives to radical mastectomy. N Engl J Med 301:326–328
5. Fisher B, Bauer M, Margolese R, et al. (1985) Five year results of a randomized clinical trial comparing total mastectomy and segmental mastectomy with or without radiation in the treatment of breast cancer. N Engl J Med 312:665–673
6. Halsted WS (1894/1895) The results of operations for the cure of cancer of the breast performed at the Johns Hopkins Hospital from June, 1889 to January, 1894. Johns Hopkins Hosp Bull 4:297
7. Harris JR, Hellman S (1983) The results of primary radiation therapy for early breast cancer at the Joint Center for Radiation Therapy. In: Harris JR, Hellman S, Silen W (eds) Conservative management of breast cancer. Lippincott, Philadelphia, pp 47–52
8. Harris JR, Hellman S, Kinne DW (1985) Limited surgery and radiotherapy for early breast cancer. N Engl J Med 313:1365–1368

9. Hayward JL (1983) The Guy's Hospital trials on breast conservation. In: Harris JR, Hellman S, Silen W (eds) Conservative management of breast cancer. Lippincott, Philadelphia, pp 77–90
10. Keynes G (1937) Conservative treatment of cancer of the breast. Br Med J 2:643–647
11. Meyer W (1894) An improved method of the radical operation for carcinoma of the breast. Med Rec 46:746
12. Montague ED, Schell SR, Romsdahl MM, Ames FC (1983) Conservation surgery and irradiation in clinically favorable breast cancer – the M.D. Anderson Experience. In: Harris JR, Hellman S, Silen W (eds) Conservative management of breast cancer. Lippincott, Philadelphia, pp 53–60
13. Park WW, Lees VC (1951) The absolute curability of cancer of the breast. Surg Gynecol Obstet 93:129–157
14. Pierquin B (1983) Conservative treatment for carcinoma of the breast: Experience of Creteil – ten-year results. In: Harris JR, Hellman S, Silen W (eds) Conservative management of breast cancer. Lippincott, Philadelphia, pp 11–14
15. Veronesi U, Saccozzi R, del Vecchio M, et al. (1981) Comparing radical mastectomy with quadrantectomy, axillary dissection and radiotherapy in patients with small cancer of the breast. N Engl J Med 305:6–11

First Experiences in Würzburg of Interstitial Low-Dose Afterloading for Breast-Conserving Therapy with the Microselectron

K. Rotte and E. Löffler

In Germany, manual interstitial brachytherapy was abandoned for many years due to the radiation hazard associated with it. There is now a return of this mode of treatment with the introduction of remote-controlled afterloading machines [4, 7-9, 14, 15]. Compared with teletherapy, two great advantages favor contact therapy. One is that, for the same reference volume, the integral dose within the target is higher. The other advantage is that the treatment volume can be kept smaller. In breast-conserving therapy, this enables us to administer a high dose within the tumor bed and simultaneously spare skin and lung.

The treatment of early breast cancer (stages T1 and T2) at our hospital consists of lumpectomy combined with dissection of the axillary lymph nodes followed by a boost of approximately 20 Gy into the tumor bed, administered by an implant of 192-Ir wires and external-beam therapy of 45 Gy to the whole breast. In patients with positive axillary nodes, six cycles of chemotherapy follow the completion of radiotherapy.

In accordance with the Paris system [2, 11-13] we implant 1.5-mm rigid guide needles in parallel order with the help of perspex templates. The templates are perforated so as to keep the needles in a triangular arrangement to obtain a homogeneous dose distribution and are placed symmetrically on both sides of the implants. According to the target volume, we insert the needles 14-20 mm apart. In most cases the implantation of two layers of needles is sufficient. Before final adjustment of each needle's position to provide a constant distance between the proximal end of the needle and the skin, stainless-steel clips are clamped onto the needles. Subsequently, each needle is fixed in its place with immobilization buttons. Finally, the distal end of the unloaded needles is trimmed so that it is a few centimeters longer than the future radioactive implant (Figs. 1 and 2).

After this procedure, a set of isocentric stereoradiographs of the needles is taken. These radiographs are used to reconstruct the positions of the needles and skin points within the patient [8]. With additional lead markers placed on the skin, the outline of the breast is also reconstructed. Afterwards, the exact length of each iridium wire is computed. A few millimeters of healthy tissue should be left unirradiated at the entry and exit point of each needle to spare the skin at these points.

In the computerized dosimetry [6] based on this stereo reconstruction, the iridium core and platinum capsule are handled together like an unencapsulated linear source. In accordance with the Paris system of dosimetry [2], the reference dose is assessed in a plane perpendicular to the parallel wires from the mean dose

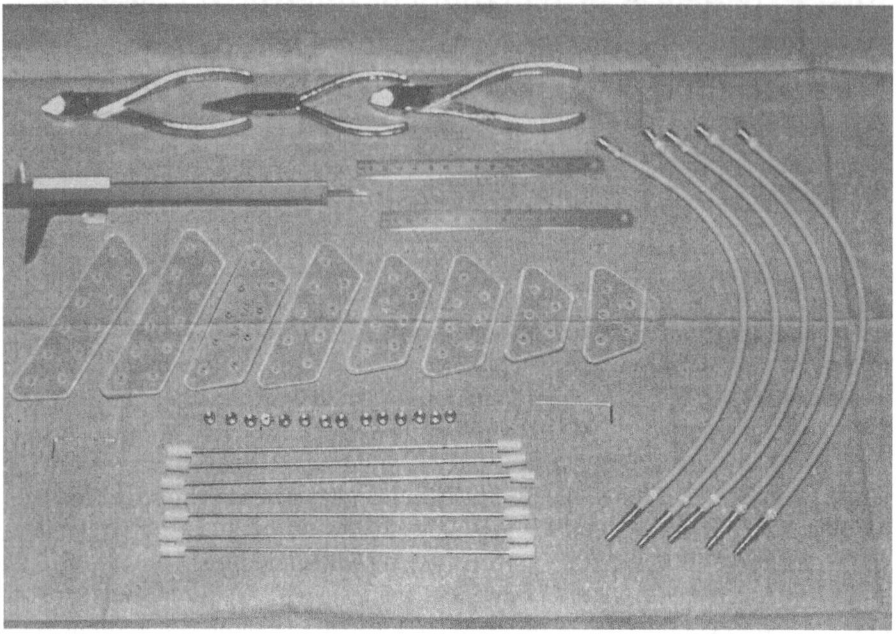

Fig. 1. Instruments

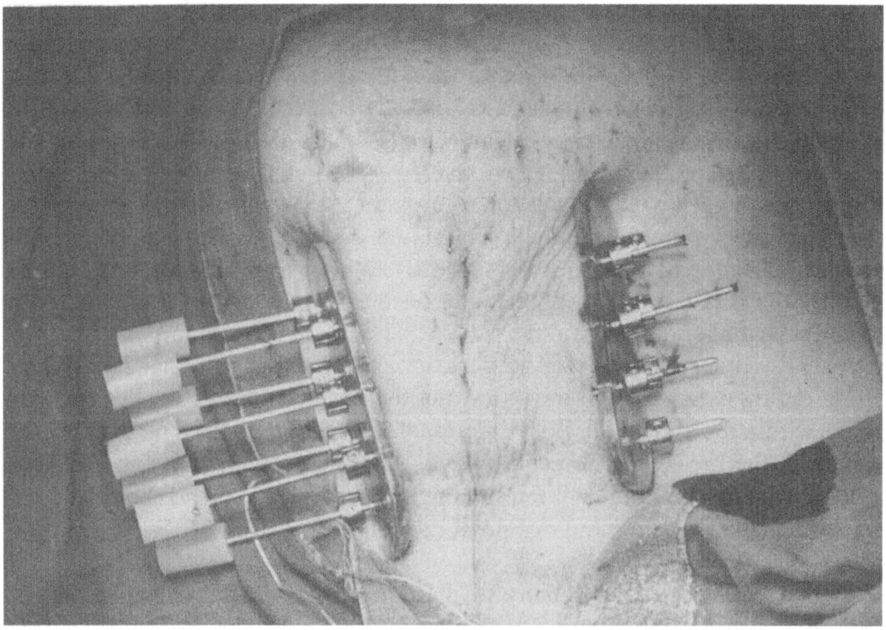

Fig. 2. Implantation technique

rates at the points midway diagonally between the wires (Fig. 4). The reference dose rate is set as 85% of the mean basic dose. The treatment time is based on this dose rate. The dose distribution midway between the planes of the needles (Fig. 5) is used to determine the reference volume, which is 30–120 cm^3 and is assessed clinically.

The position of the active wires relative to the specified skin points on the radiograph allows accurate control of the needle position (Fig. 3). All source assemblies should be prepared with the same inactive length relative to the positioning pellet. This is important if the sources will be reused. The distance from the proximal end of the needle to the skin must be the same for all implants; the needles are therefore marked.

In order to reduce the number of sources to be prepared, we assemble wires with active lengths of 10–100 mm, numbered according to our experience of the frequency with which they are needed. The sources are cut from a 50-cm iridium wire in a special preparation station (Fig. 6) without exposure of the personnel, and sealed in a thin plastic tube which is crimped on an inactive guide.

As determinations of source strength are the basic data for computed dosimetry, all sources are measured in a well-type ionization chamber (Fig. 7). The chamber current is calibrated against a reference 192-iridium wire air kerma rate. In an initial check, the linear activity is also measured, using a ring-shaped ionization chamber (Fig. 8). This allows the distribution of activity of the whole iridium wire to be checked.

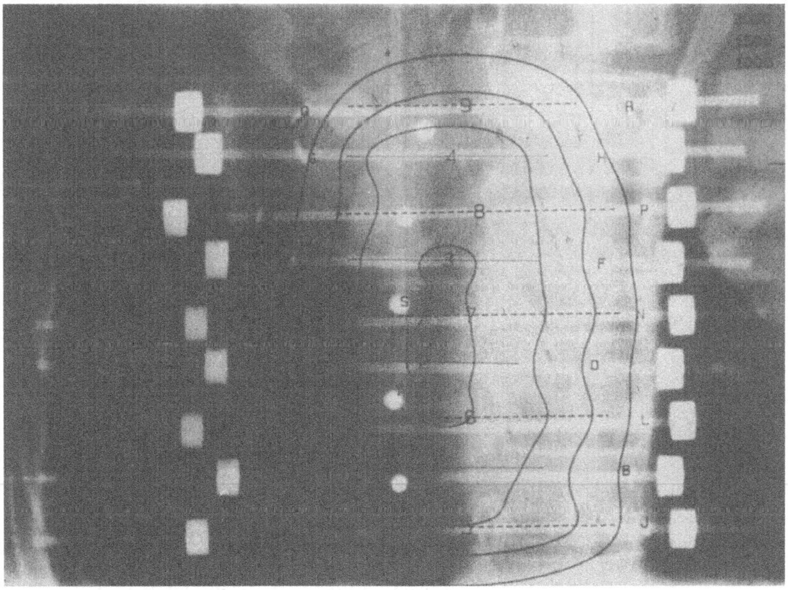

Fig. 3. Anteroposterior radiograph with overlay of dose distribution midway between the needle planes

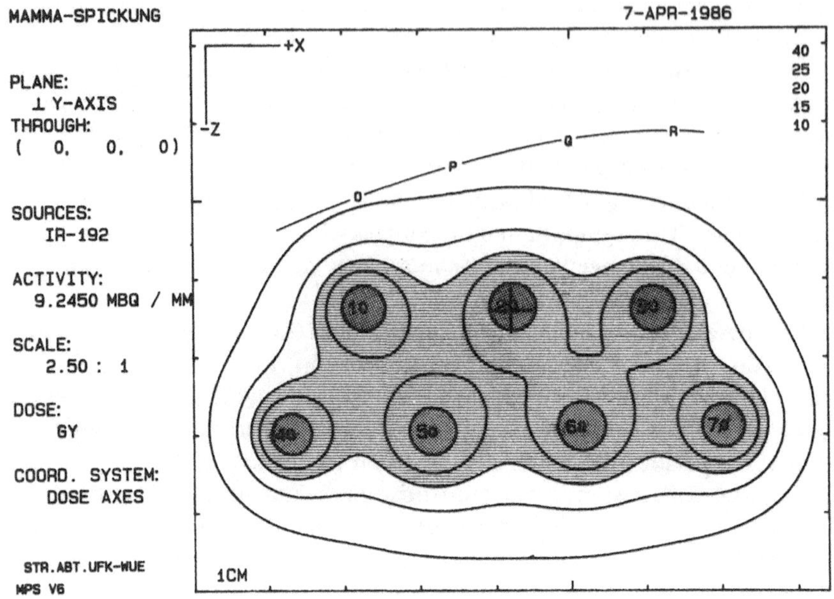

Fig. 4. Dose distribution of a ^{192}Ir implant in the central plane. The reference volume is shaded

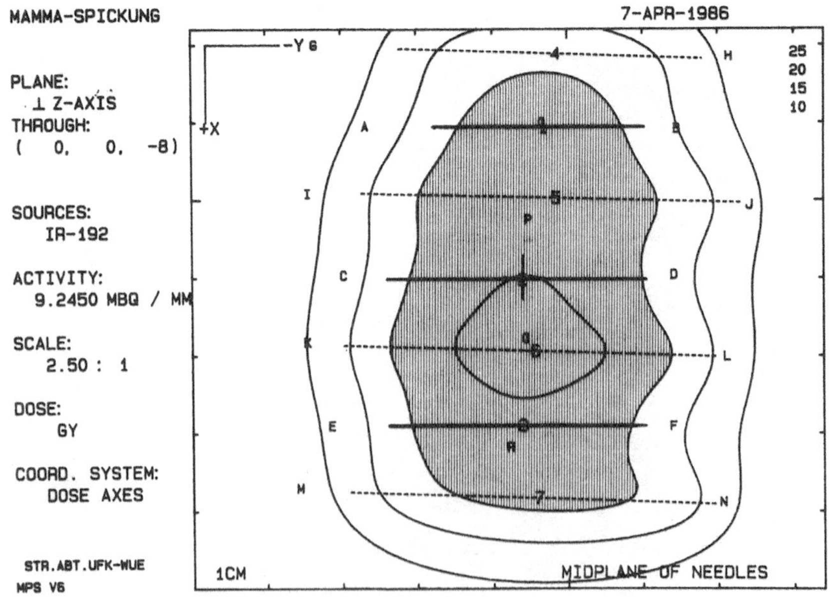

Fig. 5. Dose distribution of a ^{192}Ir implant midway between the needle planes; the reference volume is *shaded*

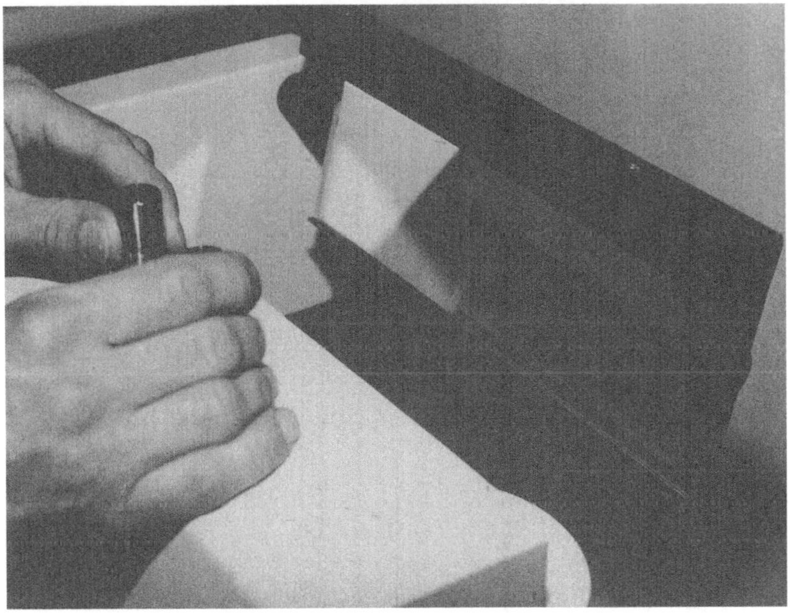

Fig. 6. Exposure-free station for preparation of sources

For the microselectron, a set of up to 45 prepared sources is loaded in a storage container. The microselectron can pick up 15 sources and transfer them into the intermediate safe by remote control for the patient's treatment. Before treatment, a check film is made from the loaded sources to confirm their lengths and positions. The afterloading device is then connected to the patient by a quick-release coupling. A fiber-drive mechanism provides a highly reliable source transfer into the implanted needles.

We reuse the iridium source assemblies for about 100 days. The linear activity of a later application is considerably lower than that of an earlier application. This, together with variation in reference volume, number of needles, source length, and needle separation will result in a reference dose rate of 0.25–1 Gy/h. This marked dosage variation can be compensated for with the help of biologic treatment planning, using the linear quadratic model. On the basis of this simple formula relating the cell survival and induction of cellular effects to the dose, KELLERER and ROSSI [5] introduced a time-effect correction factor. They assumed an exponential repair function of the subeffective lesions with a half-life of about 2 h. Barendsen [1] proposed an α/β ratio of 5 Gy if connective tissue is the critical tissue. Normalizing the extrapolated tolerance dose to 0.50 Gy/h (20 Gy in 40 h) the correction factor for the treatment time or prescribed dose is 1.2–0.8 for 0.25–1 Gy/h.

We have now treated 43 patients by the method described, with an observation period of 4–18 months after cessation of treatment. So far we have seen no locoregional recurrences or distant metastases. Figures 9 and 10 show the cosmetic results of this therapy.

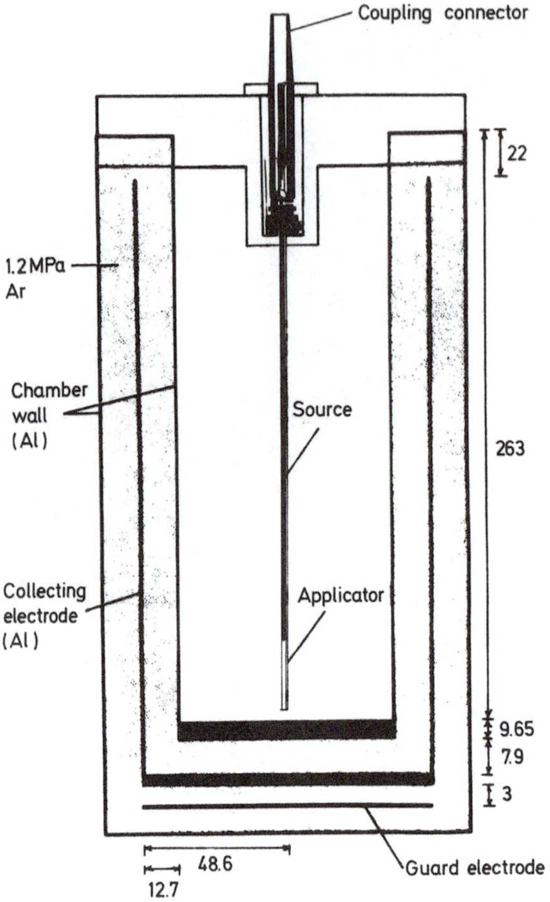

Fig. 7. Well-type ionization chamber for initial dosimetry of ^{192}Ir sources

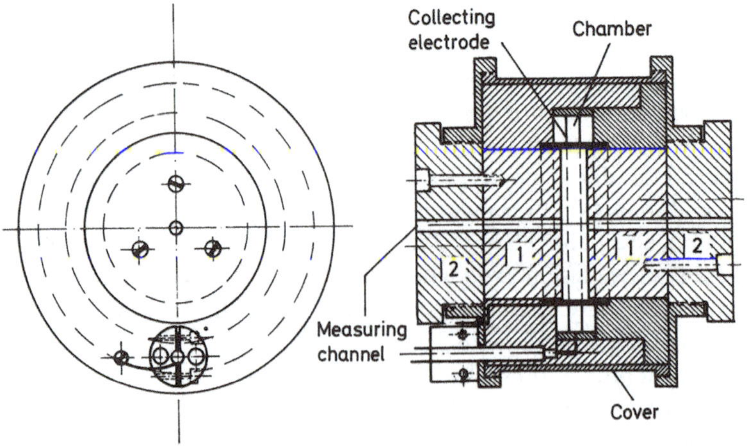

Fig. 8. Ring-shaped ionization chamber for determination of linear activity of ^{192}Ir wires. *1*, Tungsten primary diaphragm; *2*, diaphragm holder

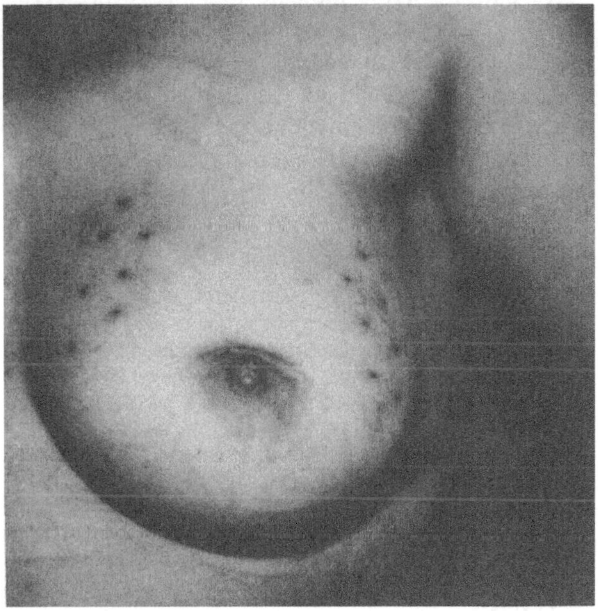

Fig. 9. Diseased breast 8 days after removal of implants

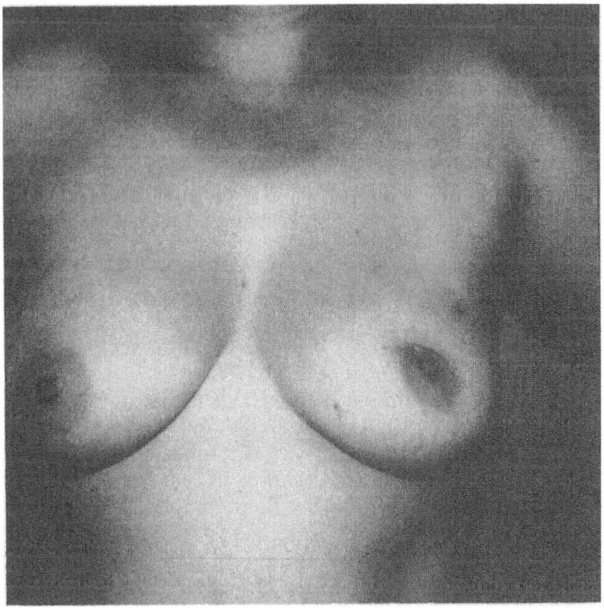

Fig. 10. Diseased breast 12 months after cessation of treatment

All data available indicate that breast-preserving procedures for primarily operable carcinomas of the breast have the same results in tumor control as the classical surgical management of this disease. However, breast-preserving procedures, as outlined, give the patient the chance to be treated without mutilation. Therefore, women with a tumor of the breast not exceeding stage T2N0M0 should be advised of this kind of treatment and be referred to a clinical center with the appropriate facilities.

References

1. Barendsen GW (1982) Dose fractionation, dose rate and iso-effect relationships for normal tissue response. Int J Radiat Oncol Biol Phys 8:1981
2. Dutreix A, Marinello G, Wambersie A (1982) Dosimétrie en curiethérapie. Masson, Paris
3. Hall EJ (1972) Radiation dose-rate: a factor of importance in radiobiology and radiotherapy. Br J Radiol 45:81
4. Jacobs H, Teusch P, Schleppi V, Schmieder A, Moncke G (1984) Interstitielle Brachytherapie – Erste Erfahrungen mit 192-Iridium in der Kurzzeittherapie. Strahlentherapie 160:8
5. Kellerer AM, Rossi HH (1972) The theory of dual radiation action. Curr Top Radiat Res Q 8:85
6. Laarse R (1985) Treatment planning of interstitial radiotherapy (MPS) with the selectron treatment planning system. In: Mould RF (ed) Brachytherapy 1984. Nucletron, Leersum, p 286
7. Löffler E, Rotte K (1987) Die Würzburger Methode der ferngesteuerten interstitiellen low-dose-rate Brachytherapie bei der brusterhaltenden Behandlung des Mammakarzinoms. Arch Gynecol Obstet 242:301–303
8. Löffler E, Sauer O (1987) 3-D Rekonstruktion von Brust-Implantaten zur Applikationskontrolle und Bestrahlungsplanung mittels isozentrischer stereoskopischer Röntgenaufnahmen (ISR) unter Berücksichtigung einer ferngesteuerten interstitiellen Nachlademethode. Strahlentherapie, (in press)
9. Löffler E, Sauer O, Rotte K (1986) Interstitielle Low-Intensity Afterloading-Therapie mit ^{192}Ir-Drähten. In: von Klitzing L (ed) Medizinische Physik 1986. DGMP, Lübeck, p 433
10. Meertens H, Bartelink H (1985) First experience with the microselectron in breast conserving therapy implants. In: Mould RF (ed) Brachytherapy 1984. Nucletron, Leersum, p 271
11. Pierquin B, Baillet F, Wilson JF (1976) Radiation therapy in the management of primary breast cancer. A J R 127:645
12. Pierquin B, Dutreix A, Paine CH, Chassagne D, Marinello G, Ash D (1978) The Paris system in interstitial radiation therapy. Acta Radiol [Oncol] 17:33
13. Pierquin B, Owen R, Maylin C, Otmezguine Y, Raynal M, Mueller W, Haunoun S (1980) Radical radiation therapy of breast cancer. Int J Radiat Oncol Biol Phys 6:17
14. Rotte K, Löffler E (1986) Strahlentherapeutische Möglichkeiten bei der Behandlung des primär operablen Mammakarzinoms. Gynäkol Prax 10:695
15. Schulz U, Busch M, Bormann U (1984) Interstitial high doserate brachytherapie: Principle, practice and first clinical experiences with a new remote-controlled afterloading system using Ir-192. Int J Radiat Oncol Biol Phys 10:915

V. Results

Long-Term Survival Following Breast-Conserving Therapy in Comparison to Radical Surgical Treatment: An Overview

J. M. Spitalier, J.M. Kurtz, R. Amalric, H. Brandone, Y. Ayme, C. Bressac, and D. Hans

Introduction

It is generally accepted that proper comparison between the results obtained with different forms of therapy requires scientific prospective randomized clinical trials. Such trials seldom give rise to new types of treatment, but formally test therapeutic approaches which may in fact be long-established. Breast-conserving therapy was extensively practised long before the era of the clinical trial, beginning in the 1930s and 1940s with the pioneering work of Keynes [13], Baclesse et al. [4], Mustakallio [16], and Peters [17]. These investigators were encouraged by their own retrospective analyses of their results, which seemed to be comparable to those of primary radical surgery. With the introduction of megavoltage radiotherapy, their work stimulated important activity in this field, beginning around 1960 in Europe, especially in France, and in America during the 1970s [2,6,8,11,15,18]. Five-year-survival figures from this new generation of studies began to appear in the early 1970s, and the first 10-year results around 1980 [2,6,8,18]. This experience with thousands of patients over several decades, referred to as "anecdotal" by those dedicated exclusively to prospective randomized trials [10], provided the clinical basis for the inception of the Milan Trial in 1973 [23], the World Health Organization Trial in 1972 [20], and the National Surgical Adjuvant Breast Project (NSABP) trial in 1976 [10]. The pioneering clinical trial at Guy's Hospital also deserves mention in this context [17].

The Cancer Institute in Marseille, with its associated clinics, is one of the world's most experienced centers in performing breast-conserving therapy, with more than 5500 patients treated by radiotherapy (alone or following breast-conserving surgery) since 1960. We are convinced that long-term survival in operable breast cancer is not prejudiced by treatment which preserves the breast. The purpose of this paper is to examine the evidence which supports this conviction, based upon our own experience and that reported in the literature.

Outside the context of a prospective clinical trial, comparison of the results obtained from conservative management with those of radical surgery is associated with certain difficulties, principally related to staging and patient selection. During the 1960s and early 1970s, patients treated conservatively seldom had axillary surgery, which became mandatory only during the mid-1970s with the advent of adjuvant chemotherapy. The long-term results of conservatively-treated series were therefore based on clinical staging, since lymph-node histology was largely undetermined. Moreover, there is relatively limited literature on the long-term results of primary radical surgery in clinically staged patients, making a satisfactory comparison difficult. Problems of selection are even more difficult to account for. In many centers, the indication for tumorectomy has been limited to a maximal clinical tumor size of 3 cm, and most centers are reluctant to treat patients with clinically apparent extensive adenopathy conservatively. A clinical impression of rapid tumor growth has always discouraged us from surgery, and we have tended to treat such patients primarily with radiotherapy [22].

After 10 Years Treatment Results

Clinical Stage I

Problems of staging and selection are minimal in clinical stage I, as defined by the American Joint Committee (T1N0, or T1N1a). This represents a rather homogeneous group of favorable patients, about 25%–30% of whom have histologic evidence of nodal involvement, almost always with less than four positive nodes [23]. Table 1 presents the uncorrected 10-year-survival rates for patients treated with either breast conservation or primary radical therapy. Not only is the absolute equivalence of these results remarkable, but it is also noteworthy how well the results from the retrospective studies correspond to the data, from the randomized Milan trial. This suggests that less-radical forms of tumor excision than quadrantectomy will yield equivalent long-term results.

We are convinced that the equivalence of radical and breast-conserving treatments for clinical-stage-I patients will continue to be substantiated by longer follow-up, since we have found that locoregional recurrence in these patients does not prejudice survival. For 65 clinical-stage-I patients receiving salvage surgery for recurrence at Marseille, the corrected 15-year-survival rate following primary therapy was 81%, which was not significantly different from the 83% corrected 15-year-survival rate for 557 patients who did not require salvage surgery.

Table 1. Results of therapy in clinical stage I (T1N0, T1N1a)

Type of therapy		*n*	Crude 10-year survival
Breast-conserving			
Milan*	[24]	352	79%
Marseille	[22]	201	82%
Curie[a]	[7]	173	81%
Houston	[15]	134	78%
Radical surgery			
Milan*	[24]	349	78%
Chicago	[9]	178	75%
Houston	[15]	224	80%

n, no. of patients
*prospective randomized trial
[a]includes tumors up to 3 cm

Clinical Stage II

In contrast to stage I, an analysis of long-term results in clinical stage II is decidedly more problematic. First, there are no 10-year results available from randomized clinical trials, with the exception of the Guy's Hospital Trial, which included insufficient radiotherapy [3]. The poor results of breast-conserving therapy in this latter trial suggest that treatment inadequate to control local or regional disease will be prejudicial to survival in some patients. In contrast, the 5-year results from the NSABP Trial B-06, testing the equivalence of radical and breast-conserving therapies for tumors 4 cm or smaller, have been most encouraging [10]. This suggests that the good 10-year results achieved in selected conservatively managed stage-II patients will be borne out by this large prospective study, which has been based upon well-defined eligibility criteria.

In contrast to stage I, 10-year results for breast-conserving surgery combined with irradiation in clinical stage II are sparsely documented in the literature, with most series reporting few patients with long follow-up. The strongest argument in favor of extending the indications for conservative surgery to include larger tumors is that the local recurrence rate is not strongly dependent upon tumor size, provided that the primary tumor is resected by wide excision. We ourselves have found a significant tendency to higher breast recurrence rates only for tumors clinically larger than 4 cm. It should also be borne in mind that, in contrast to chest wall recurrences after radical surgery, local recurrences following breast-conserving therapy can be quite successfully managed by further surgery [22]. Nonetheless locoregional recurrence in clinical-stage-II patients is correlated with an unfavorable prognosis. For 77 clinical-stage-II patients treated by salvage surgery at Marseille, the corrected 15-year-survival rate was 50%, which is significantly less than the corrected 15-year-survival rate of 68% for 604 clinical-stage-II patients not requiring salvage surgery.

As mentioned above, selection criteria for stage-II patients vary considerably from center to center. In general, one can assume that conservatively treated stage-II patients represent a relatively favorable subgroup, with less-extensive axillary involvement, and a better prognosis, than an unselected group of stage-II patients from a radical surgical series. In addition, clinical stage II is inherently a very heterogeneous stage grouping (T1N1b, T2N0–T2N1), containing many patients with an excellent prognosis, which is better defined through pathologic staging.

With these reservations in mind, we have represented the uncorrected 10-year-survival rates for clinical stage II in Table 2, for both conservatively and radically treated patients. The results from Marseille include only those cases treated with breast-conserving surgery and radiotherapy, eliminating the less-favorable patients treated by radiotherapy alone, since the latter approach is very seldom employed today. On the other hand, it should be pointed out that the Marseille series contained patients with clinical tumor sizes up to 5 cm, as well as patients with early clinical axillary adenopathy [22]. It is apparent that 10-year survival in these selected conservatively treated patients compares favorably with the results of radical surgical therapy.

Table 2. Results of therapy in clinical stage II (T1N1b, T2N0, T2N1)

Type of therapy		*n*	Crude 10-year survival
Breast-conserving			
Marseille	[22]	296	78%
Creteil	[18]	67	68%
Houston	[15]	157	73%
Radical surgery			
New York	[21]	175	57%
Chicago	[9]	459	55%
Houston	[15]	370	65%

The results of breast-conserving therapy in stages III and IV are best dealt with in the framework of a discussion of the management of locally advanced breast cancer. Although such patients are not uncommonly treated with preservation of the breast, this paper will principally emphasize the management of clinical stages I and II.

Results Beyond 10 Years

The overwhelming majority of surgical reports do not provide survival data after 10 years, beyond which evaluation of results is considerably complicated by an ever-increasing percentage of intercurrent deaths, and increasing numbers of patients lost to follow-up. In order to take these factors into account, long-term results are frequently expressed in terms of corrected overall survival rates or relative survival rates [19]. Either of these statistical techniques can be accepted as a measure of breast-cancer mortality. FERGUSON observed a 20-year relative survival of 72% for stage-I patients and 40% for stage-II patients following radical mastectomy [9], and ADAIR calculated a 20-year relative survival rate of 40% for all operable stages [1]. For RUTQVIST and WALLGREN, the 20-year corrected overall survival rates were 65% in patients with negative nodes, and 27% in patients with positive nodes [19] (Table 3).

We are unaware of any published studies of long-term results (beyond 10 years) for significant numbers of conservatively operated patients treated according to the principles of modern radiotherapy. Since a literature review is of little value in this regard, we will limit this part of the discussion to our own results. Figure 1 shows the corrected actuarial overall survival curves (Kaplan-Meier) for 2806 consecutive patients with clinical-stage-I, -II and -III breast cancer treated with breast conservation at Marseille between September 1960 and September 1980. Patients treated with radiotherapy alone, without operation, were included in order to eliminate selection bias. The 20-year corrected overall survival of 59% for this large series of operable cases compares favorably with the data cited above for radical surgical therapy. As a function of clinical stage, the corrected rates of 20-year survival are 75% for stage I, 57% for stage II, and 45% for stage III (Fig. 2). The

Table 3. Long-term (20-year) results of treatment for operable breast cancer

		20-Year survival
Radical surgery		
Chicago [9]*	(n=1,259)	
Stage I		72%
Stage II		40%
Stage III		24%
New York [1]*	(n=1,458)	
All operable stages		40%
Stockholm [19]**	(n=458)	
Negative nodes		65%
Positive nodes		27%
Conservative management		
Marseille**	(n=2,806)	
Clinical stage I		75%
Clinical stage II		57%
Clinical stage III		45%

*Relative survival rate
**Corrected actuarial survival rate

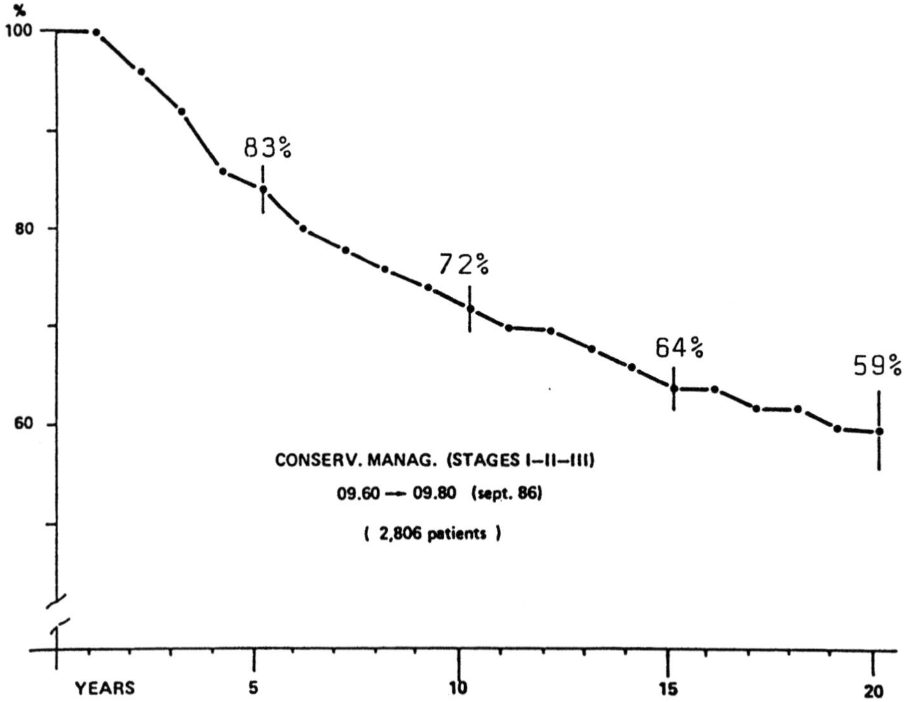

Fig. 1. Corrected actuarial overall survival curves (Kaplan-Meier) for 2806 consecutive patients with tumors of clinical stage I–III treated by curative radiotherapy, with or without breast-conserving surgery between September 1960 and September 1980. Minimum follow-up was 5 years. Results of patients dying from intercurrent disease while free of breast cancer were deleted from the study at time of death

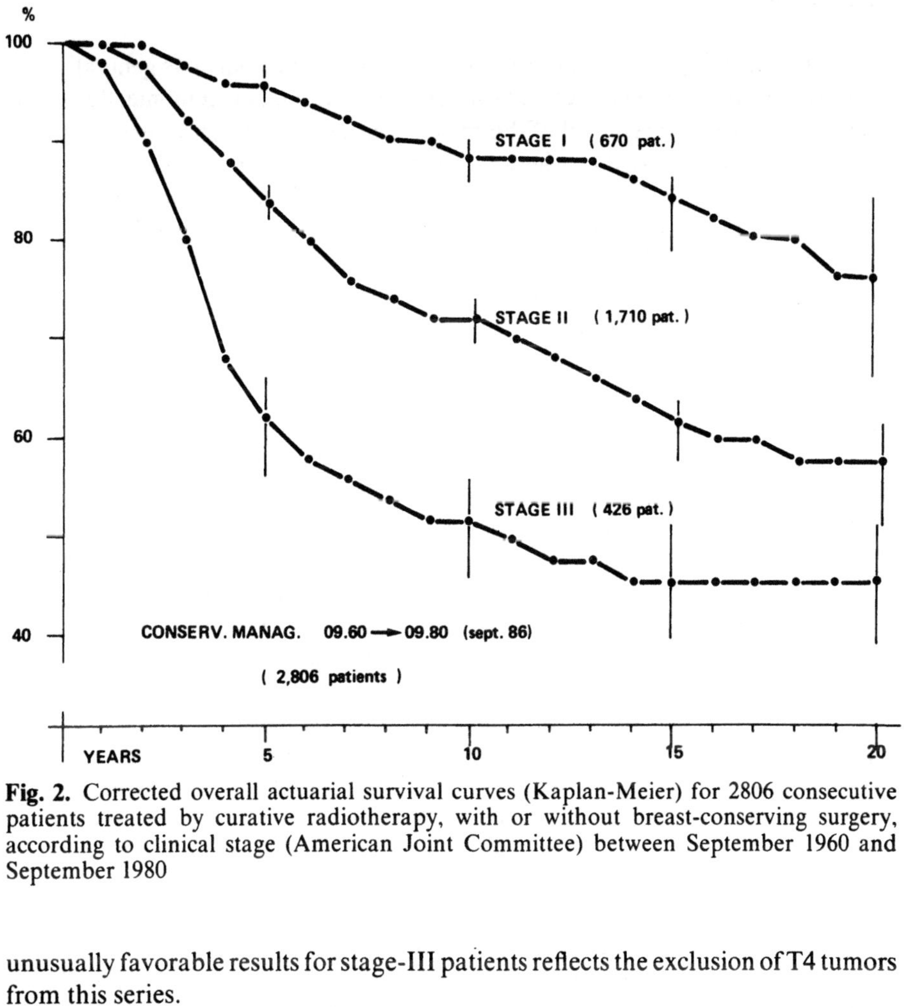

Fig. 2. Corrected overall actuarial survival curves (Kaplan-Meier) for 2806 consecutive patients treated by curative radiotherapy, with or without breast-conserving surgery, according to clinical stage (American Joint Committee) between September 1960 and September 1980

unusually favorable results for stage-III patients reflects the exclusion of T4 tumors from this series.

Another approach to the evaluation of long-term results would be to compare the evolution of disease-related events during the second decade following therapy. Ferguson observed that 10.6% of stage-I patients who were disease-free 10 years after radical mastectomy developed recurrent breast cancer by the 20th year; the corresponding figure for stage-II patients was 20.6% [9]. The excess breast-cancer mortality during the second decade was calculated to be 18%, according to HIBBERD et al. [12]. Similarly, RUTQVIST and WALLGREN determined that radically treated patients who were apparently disease-free at 10 years had a residual breast-cancer mortality of 12% [19]. For comparison, we recently evaluated the long-term results of treatment for a group of 300 stage-I and -II patients who were apparently cured 10 years after breast-conserving therapy [14]. The actuarial probability of remaining free of distant metastases was 91% at 20 years, which compares favorably with the data cited above for radically treated patients. It is therefore quite likely that the favorable 10-year results achieved by breast-conserving treatments will be borne out by longer follow-up.

Discussion

Since the early days of this century, some form of mastectomy has generally been accepted as the treatment of choice for operable mammary carcinoma, despite the lack of evidence that removal of the breast is either a necessary or even desirable step in primary breast-cancer therapy. Evidence has been accumulating for many decades that treatment approaches which preserve the breast can provide adequate local control and equivalent long-term survival to that achieved by primary radical surgery [5,7,8,11,15,17,18,22,24]. Breast-conserving surgery provides the same diagnostic and prognostic information as mastectomy, and the preservation of the breast interferes neither with adequate treatment of the axilla, nor with the delivery of adjuvant systemic therapy [10,23]. The form of therapy, therefore, differs from radical surgical treatment only in conservation of the involved breast, and in the requirement for breast irradiation.

The favorable results of conservative therapy in clinical stage I (Table 1) are so convincing that one might question whether it is ethically acceptable to recommend mastectomy to patients in this favorable subgroup. Using modern surgical and radiotherapeutic techniques, local control and 10-year survival have been reproducibly excellent, substantiated by a large prospective clinical trial [24]. In addition, we have found that locoregional recurrences in stage-I patients can be effectively treated, without any unfavorable influence on long-term survival, at least up to the 15th year.

Although long-term survival results are less extensively documented in the literature, available evidence also supports the application of breast-preserving surgery to selected stage-II tumors, provided that the relationship between tumor extent and breast size allows a satisfactory breast-conserving operation to be performed. The option of radiotherapy alone without surgery will not be discussed here [2]. With the exception of the Guy's Hospital Trials, in which inadequate radiotherapy was employed, 10-year-survival statistics available for clinical stage-II patients have been encouraging (Table 2). We have found that modern radiotherapy ensures adequate local control of tumors up to 4 cm or even 5 cm in clinical size, provided that a satisfactory excision has been performed [22]. In addition, for patients with histologically positive nodes, prospective randomized trials suggest that patients treated with breast conservation may have survival superior to that achieved by primary radical surgery, provided that all such patients receive adjuvant chemotherapy [10,24]. It also appears from the NSABP Trial B-06 that the addition of chemotherapy to breast irradiation results in superior local control in the group of patients with more agressive tumors [10]. Hence, neither a tumor size greater than 2 cm, nor histologically positive axillary nodes, may be considered a contraindication to breast-conserving treatment.

Long-term results beyond 10 years have not been extensively documented in the literature. However, our own data, as well as those from other centers, suggest that breast-conserving therapy is associated with a similar breast-cancer mortality during the second posttreatment decade to that observed in stage-I and -II patients treated primarily with radical surgery [14]. There is good reason to believe, therefore, that the favorable 10-year results cited above will continue to be borne out by longer follow-up.

Opponents of breast conservation are fond of pointing out that the benefits of such treatment, if any, are "merely" cosmetic and psychological, at the expense of possible survival disadvantages. After long experience with both mutilating and conservative surgery, it is clear to us that the quality of life is generally superior following limited surgery and irradiation. However, it should be stressed that ongoing randomized clinical trials suggest a possible survival *advantage* for conservatively treated patients, at least in some subgroups [10,24]. In addition, one must not forget the unquantifiable "failures" of radical mastectomy, namely those patients with advanced breast cancer in whom diagnosis as delayed because the patient was afraid of surgical mutilation. The ever-increasing percentage of women presenting with the earliest stages of breast cancer in our institutions has convinced us that this is a very real phenomenon. Breast-conserving therapy can play a significant role in encouraging early detection and diagnosis, thereby further reducing breast-cancer mortality. For these reasons treatment which preserves the breast does not simply offer "imaginary" advantages, but must be recognized as a significant advance in breast-cancer therapy. It is our conviction that breast amputation will be practised with ever-decreasing frequency in the years to come.

References

1. Adair F, Berg J, Joubert L, Robbins GF (1974) Long-term followup of breast cancer patients: the 30-year report. Cancer 33:1145–1150
2. Amalric R, Santamaria F, Robert F, et al. (1982) Radiation therapy with or without primary limited surgery for operable breast cancer. A 20-year experience at the Marseille Cancer Institute. Cancer 49:30–34
3. Atkins H, Hayward JL, Klugman DJ, et al. (1972) Treatment of early breast cancer: A report after 10 years of a clinical trial. Br Med J 2:423
4. Baclesse F, Ennuyer A, Cheguillaume J (1960) Est-on autorisé à pratiquer une tumorectomie simple suivie de radiothérapie en cas de tumeur mammaire? J Radiol Electrol 41:137–139
5. Bluming AZ, Dosik G, Lowitz B, et al. (1986) Treatment of primary breast cancer without mastectomy. Ann Surg 204:136–147
6. Calle R, Pilleron JP, Schlienger P, et al. (1978) Conservative management of operable breast cancer. Ten years' experience at the Foundation Curie. Cancer 42:2045–2053
7. Calle R (1985) Experience with breast conserving approaches at the Curie Institute. In: Tobias JS, Peckham MJ (eds) Primary management of breast cancer. Arnold, London, pp 59–79
8. Delouche G, Bachelot F (1980) Tumorectomie et radiothérapie pour les petits cancers du sein opérable d'emblée – résultats à 5 et 10 ans. J Eur Radiother 1:133–140
9. Ferguson DJ, Meier P, Karrison T, et al. (1982) Staging of breast cancer and survival rates. An assessment based on 50 years of experience with radical mastectomy. JAMA 248:1337–1341
10. Fisher B, Bauer M, Margolese R, et al. (1985) Five-year results of a randomized clinical trial comparing total mastectomy and segmental mastectomy with or without radiation in the treatment of breast cancer. N Engl J Med 312:674–681
11. Harris JR, Beadle GF, Hellman S (1984) Clinical studies on the use of radiation therapy as primary treatment of early breast cancer. Cancer 53:705–711

12. Hibberd AD, Horwook LJ, Wells JE (1983) Long-term prognosis of women with breast cancer in New Zealand. Study of survival to 30 years. Br Med J 286:1777–1779
13. Keynes G (1937) Conservative treatment of cancer of the breast. Br Med J 2:643–647
14. Kurtz JM, Amalric R, Delouche G, et al. (1987) The second ten years: Long-term risks of breast conservation in early breast cancer. Int J Radiat Oncol Biol Phys, (in press)
15. Montague ED (1984) Conservation surgery and radiation therapy in the treatment of operable breast cancer. Cancer 53:700–704
16. Mustakallio S (1972) Conservative treatment of breast carcinoma. Review of 25-year followup. Clin Radiol 23:110–116
17. Peters MV (1977) Wedge resection with or without radiation in early breast cancer. Int J Radiat Oncol Biol Phys 2:1151–1156
18. Pierquin B (1983) Conservative treatment for carcinoma of the breast: Experience of Créteil – Ten-year results. In: Harris JR, Hellman S, Silen W (eds) Conservative management of breast cancer. Lippincott, Philadelphia, pp 11–14
19. Rutqvist ER, Wallgren A (1985) Long-term survival of 458 young breast cancer patients. Cancer 55:658–665
20. Sarrazin D, Le M, Rouesse J, et al. (1984) Conservative treatment versus mastectomy in breast cancer tumors with macroscopic diameter of 20 millimeters or less. Cancer 53:1209–1213
21. Schottenfeld D, Nash AG, Robbins GF, Beattie EJ (1976) Ten-year results of the treatment of primary operable breast carcinoma. A summary of 304 patients evaluated by the TNM system. Cancer 38:1001–1007
22. Spitalier JM, Gambarelli J, Brandone H, et al. (1987) Breast-conserving surgery with radiation therapy for operable mammary carcinoma: a 25-year experience. World J Surg, (in press)
23. Veronesi U, del Vecchio M, Greco M, et al. (1983) Results of quadrantectomy, axillary dissection, and radiotherapy (QUART) in T1N0 patients. In: Harris JR, Hellman S, Silen W (eds) Conservative management of breast cancer. Lippincott, Philadelphia, pp 91–99
24. Veronesi U, Zucali R, Luini A (1986) Local control and survival in early breast cancer: the Milan trial. Int J Radiat Oncol Biol Phys 12:717–720

Breast-Conserving Treatment: Experience Derived from the National Surgical Adjuvant Breast Project

R. G. MARGOLESE

A 20-year debate about the appropriate surgery for breast cancer has resulted in two successive clinical trials comparing radical, intermediate, and breast-conserving operations (National Surgical Adjuvant Breast Project Protocols B-04 and B-06). Before this process began, surgical tradition and teaching favored radical operations. When it became apparent that cure rates were no longer improving, many surgeons thought that surgery should become more radical. The extended and superradical mastectomies were implemented for this purpose. Several studies were reported in the 1950s comparing variations on the radical theme. Almost all of these showed no significant difference between radical mastectomy and other procedures which were more, and sometimes less, extensive. This should have suggested the now-obvious conclusion that variations of local and regional treatment would not improve survival and that most treatment failures were due to the existence of distant metastases.

This concept, however, was long in coming and was eventually addressed in the first National Surgical Adjuvant Breast Project (NSABP) protocol, B-04. Patients were randomly assigned radical mastectomy, total mastectomy with irradiation, and total mastectomy alone with subsequent axillary dissection only for those patients who developed evidence of carcinoma in the nodes (Fig. 1). Analyses of results at 5 and 10 years indicated no discernible difference between any of the treatment options (Fig. 2). For patients with clinically positive axillary nodes, either radical mastectomy alone or total mastectomy with irradiation were employed; no difference in outcome was seen. The simple conclusion is that removing the lymph nodes or irradiating them does not improve the prognosis. The converse, however, must also be appreciated. Leaving the lymph nodes untreated does not harm the prognosis. This confirms the biologic principle being tested: variations in locoregional treatment will have no impact on patients with established metastases, even if they are not yet visible.

Although the use of radiotherapy decreased the incidence of recurrences in the chest wall and supraclavicular nodes, survival was not altered. Even for patients with involvement of internal mammary nodes, radiation treatment was of no benefit (Fig. 3). This sheds further light on the importance of lymph-node treatment in preventing dissemination of cancer. It is known that patients with primary tumors in the medial or central part of the breast have a higher likelihood of internal mammary node metastases, yet when these patients were compared with other patients who had laterally placed tumors, there was no difference between of the three results, regardless of whether or not the patients received nodal radiotherapy.

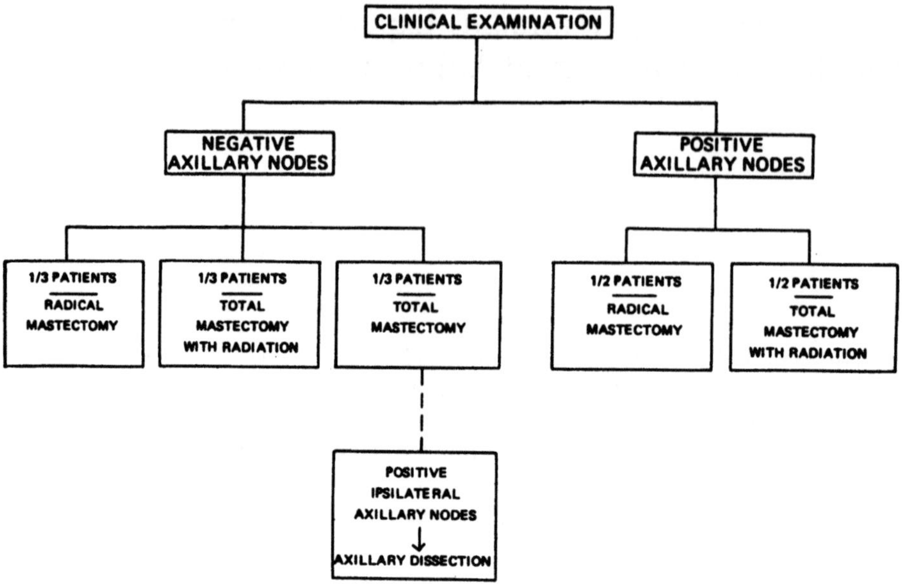

Fig. 1. Schema for protocol B-04

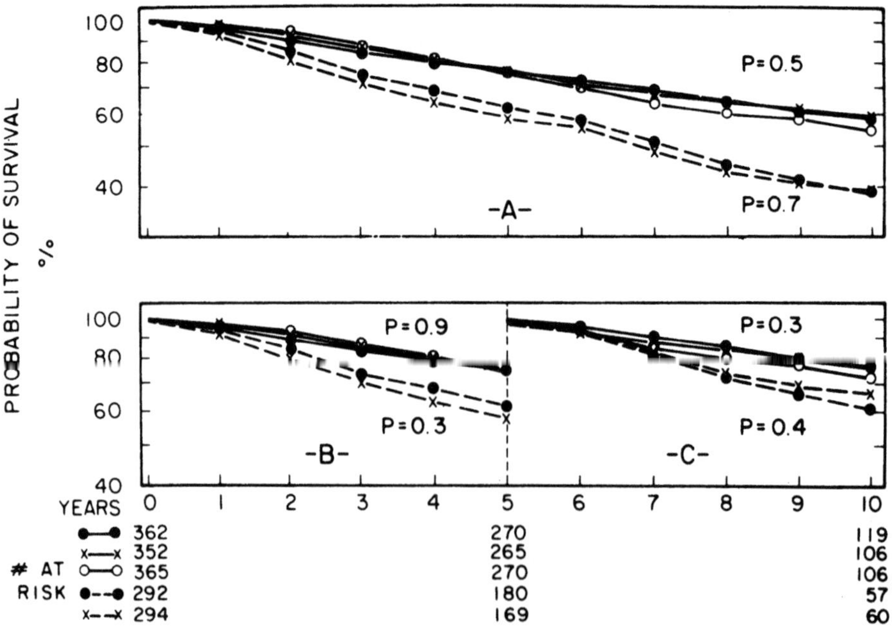

Fig. 2A-C. Survival over 10 years (**A**), during the first 5 years (**B**), and during the second 5 years for patients alive at the end of the fifth year (**C**). Patients were treated by radical mastectomy (●), total mastectomy and radiation (X), or total mastectomy alone (○). There were no significant differences among the patients with clinically negative nodes (*continuous lines*) or between the two groups with positive nodes (*dashed lines*)

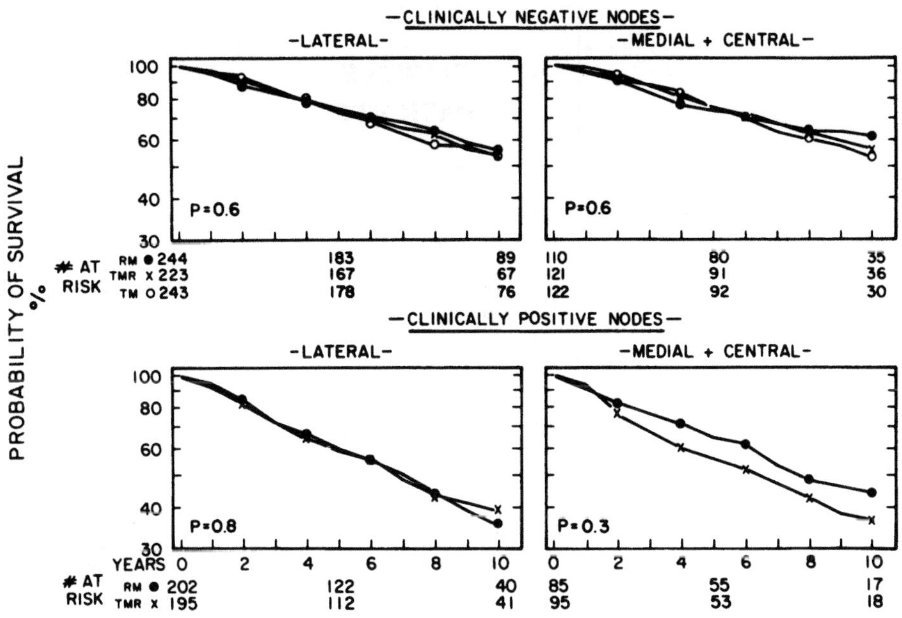

Fig. 3. Relation of treatment and survival according to tumor location. Treatments and symbols are as in Fig. 2. The outcome for patients with clinically negative or positive nodes and lateral tumors or medial and central tumors was not affected by treatment

Again, this shows there is no benefit in treating nodes which may harbor a metastasis. It indicates that the nodes are not the source of distant metastases, but simply one of the places where metastatic disease occurs when dissemination is present. The word "early" refers to a biologic state and not a time frame.

The second protocol (B-06) compared total mastectomy to segmental mastectomy with and without radiation (Fig. 4), a logical extension of the first study. Total mastectomy was the new reference operation, having supplanted radical mastectomy. In the first study, the focus had been treatment of lymph nodes. They were treated surgically, the radiation, or left untreated. In protocol B-06, the focus was the remaining breast parenchyma, which was similarly treated surgically, by irradiation, or left untreated. All patients with positive axillary nodes were subjected to a standard two-drug adjuvant chemotherapy program consisting of 5-fluorouracil (5-FU) and 1-phenylalanine mustard.

The initial 5-year analysis showed no significant difference in rate of metastasis or overall survival. Patients who had not received breast irradiation had a higher incidence of local breast recurrence, which was then treated by salvage mastectomy (Fig. 5). This difference in local recurrence rates, however, had no impact on disease-free survival, distant disease-free survival, or on overall survival. The results were the same for the three treatment groups (Fig. 6). These findings extend and support the original hypothesis that it is disseminated disease, and not the primary tumor, that causes ultimate failure. Systemic therapy must therefore be an integral part of breast-cancer treatment.

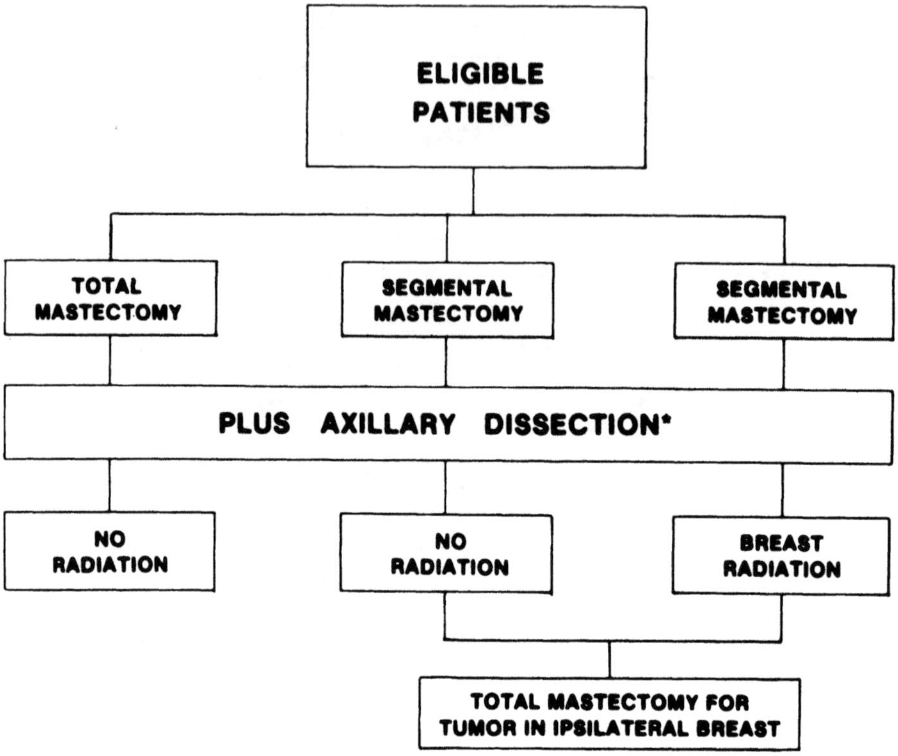

Fig. 4. Schema for protocol B-06 (segmental mastectomy)

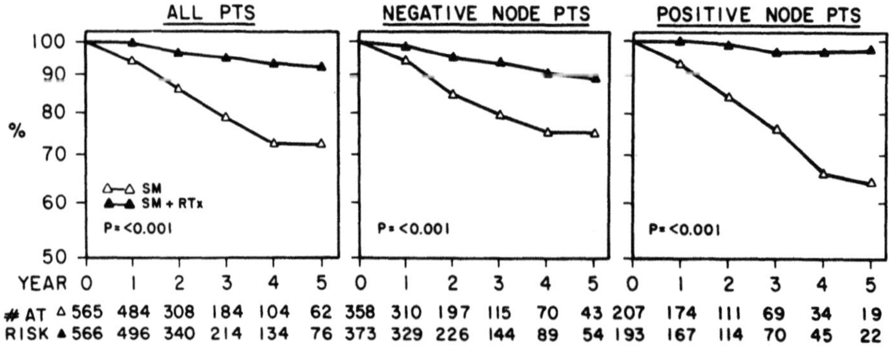

Fig. 5. Life-table analysis showing the percentage of patients remaining free of breast tumor after segmental mastectomy (*SM*, △) or segmental mastectomy with breast irradiation (SM + RTx,▲). The data for all patients (*left*) are adjusted for the number of positive nodes

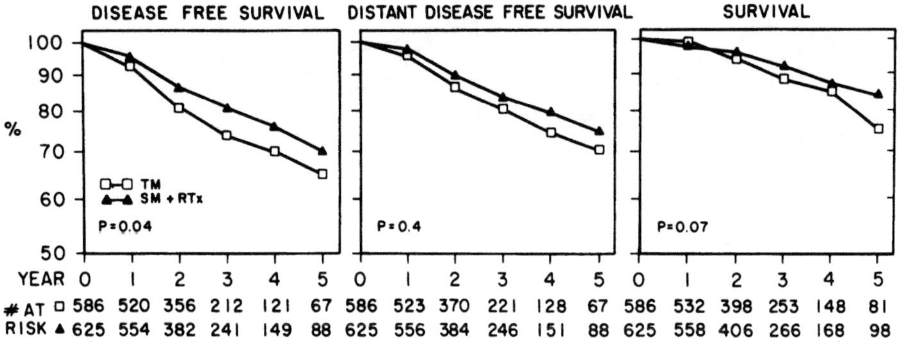

Fig. 6. Life-table analysis showing disease-free survival, distant disease-free survival, and overall survival of patients treated by total mastectomy (*TM*, □) or segmental mastectomy with radiation (*SM* + *RTx*, ▲). The data are adjusted for the number of positive nodes

Local recurrence rates in patients with nodal involvement who received chemotherapy in addition to radiotherapy were much lower than those in patients without nodal involvement who received radiotherapy alone. This suggests a form of synergism between chemotherapy and irradiation, to produce a lower local recurrence rate even in patients with positive nodes.

The two surgical protocols follow a consistent theme and suggest that any improvement in survival following breast cancer will have to come from effective treatment of metastatic disease. Adjuvant chemotherapy is predicated on the idea that some patients harbor micrometastases that can be eliminated by prompt use of chemotherapy. The same chemotherapy would not be curative if it was withheld until clinical evidence of metastases was seen. The NSABP embarked on a sequence of adjuvant-therapy protocols comparing first one drug against placebo, then various combinations of two and three drugs in an attempt to find more successful programs. It soon became evident that pretreatment selection variables could be used to focus the treatment for better response. The age of the patient and the estrogen-receptor (ER) content were the most useful of these variables. With pretreatment ER and progesterone-receptor (PR) determination, it was possible to select suitable patients for chemotherapy regimens, others for antiestrogen therapy, and others for combined chemohormonal therapy.

The most conspicuous benefits occur with chemotherapy in premenopausal women, especially those with few positive nodes. There has been a 64% reduction in mortality (P, 0.009; Fig. 7). In the initial chemotherapy studies there was no apparent benefit for patients over 50 years of age. However, subsequent studies with two- and three-drug combinations have changed this original finding. Disease-free survival and overall survival are prolonged for patients over the age of 50 years treated with two and three drugs, especially those with more than four positive nodes.

With the addition of tamoxifen (T) to SFU and 1-phenylalanine mustard (PF) therapy, there was a significant prolongation of disease-free survival, which seemed

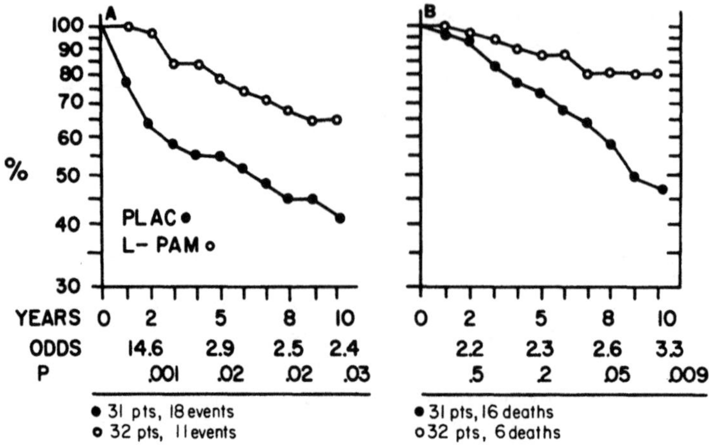

Fig. 7A,B. Results of protocol B-05 in patients less than 49 years of age with one to three positive lymph nodes **A** Events, **B** deaths

restricted to those over 50 years of age. When the advantage from tamoxifen was related to estrogen-receptor levels, patient age, and nodal status, the improvement was seen to be most significant in patients with ER and PR levels above 10 fM (Fig. 8). Following the NSABP plan of designing subsequent studies on the basis of earlier findings, the next NSABP Protocol allocated patients to treatment groups according to preliminary ER and PR status. Protocols B-11 (for ER-negative patients) and B-12 (for ER-positive patients) evaluated the addition of adriamycin to existing regimens. Preliminary results indicated the addition of adriamycin prolonged disease-free survival compared to PF or PFT alone. It is particularly significant that this benefit included patients over 50 years of age, and that overall survival was improved as well as disease-free survival (Fig. 9).

Conclusions

Clinical trials have provided clear evidence that breast-conserving surgery can replace more-radical procedures with no loss in control of disease. The addition of adjuvant chemotherapy has improved statistics of disease-free and overall survival for all groups of patients with positive nodes. While this may be an oversimplification, it does accurately describe the trends in these studies. Systemic adjuvant therapy is beneficial in premenopausal and postmenopausal women with primary breast cancer. All patients do not respond uniformly. There are both specific and nonspecific factors influencing outcome. Specific factors include tumor size, menopausal and nodal status, estrogen- and progesterone-receptor content, and tumor differentiation. Nonspecific host and tumor factors also exist and have yet to be elucidated by subsequent protocols. The NSABP experience has resulted in improved results with successive protocols, because each study is designed to answer a question raised by previous protocols.

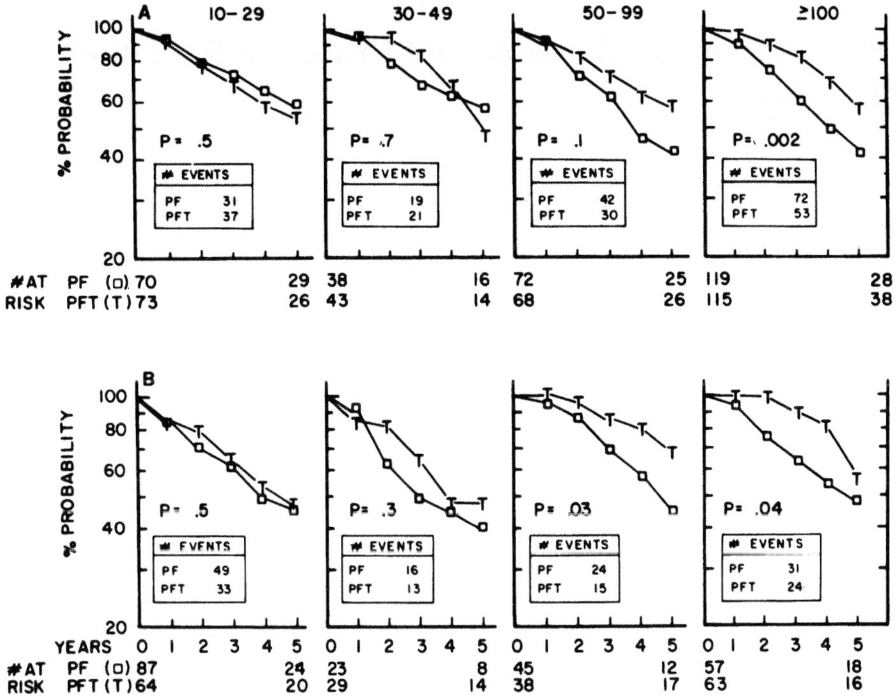

Fig. 8A,B. Results of protocol B-09: 5-fluorouracil (5 FU) and 1-phenylalanine mustard, i.e., *PF*, versus PF plus tamoxifen (*PFT*) according to estrogen-(**A**) and progesterone-receptor (**B**) status

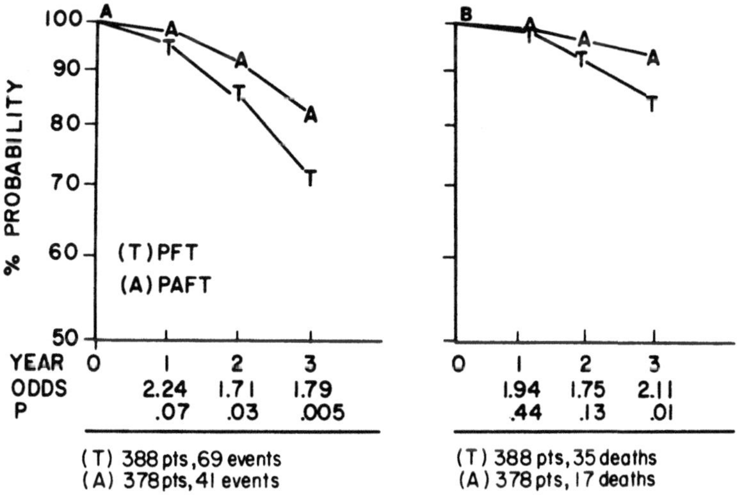

Fig. 9A,B. Results of protocol B-12 (addition of adriamycin, *A*, to PFT therapy). **A** Events, **B** deaths

Local Recurrence After Breast-Conserving Treatment: Results from the Harvard Joint Center for Radiation Therapy

J.R. HARRIS, A. RECHT, S.J. SCHNITT, B. SILVER, and J.L. CONNOLLY

Breast-conserving treatment using radiation therapy has been established as an important alternative treatment to mastectomy for patients with early breast cancer. The increased use of this approach is based on results obtained from both retrospective and prospective studies which indicate that the rates of local tumor control and survival obtained are comparable to those seen with mastectomy, but are achieved with preservation of a satisfactory cosmetic appearance.

During the period from July, 1968 to December, 1980, 524 patients with clinical stages I or II breast carcinoma were treated at the Joint Center for Radiation Therapy (JCRT). We have documented the results of treatment in these patients in an attempt to assess the effectiveness of this approach and to determine avenues for improved results [5–8]. In August, 1986, we reanalyzed the results; the median follow up was then 74 months, with a range of 33–185 months. In this report, we present our results emphasizing local recurrence after breast-conserving treatment, with consideration of frequency and clinical course, classification, prognostic factors, treatment, and prognosis.

All of the patients had invasive carcinoma as diagnosed by the original hospital pathologist and confirmed by the study pathologists (Schnitt and Connolly). In ten patients, (second, contralateral breast cancer was treated, yielding a total of 534 breast cancers treated. The breakdown by TN subclassification was as follows: T1N0, 248; T1N1, 29; T2N0, 202; and T2N1, 55. The median age of the group was 52 years, with a range of 25–93 years.

The details of treatment in our patients have been described previously. Variations in treatment were often substantial and have been analyzed; 508 breasts were treated after excisional biopsy, and 26 after incisional or needle biopsy. Of the patients treated after excisional biopsy, 411 received supplemental radiation (a "boost") of 6000 cGy or greater to the primary site, and 97 patients did not. It is important to emphasize that most patients treated with excisional biopsy in this series simply had the tumor grossly removed without an attempt to obtain microscopically negative margins of resection.

Figure 1 shows the probability of local recurrence. Local recurrence was scored whenever tumor was noted in the breast or the skin overlying the breast after treatment. In 57 patients there was an isolated local recurrence, and 2 patients had simultaneous local and distant recurrence. Eight patients had suspected or proven local recurrence after distant recurrence, but were withdrawn from the study at the time of distant recurrence. By 10 years, the probability of local recurrence was 20%, with 23 patients still at risk after this time. The crude incidence of local recurrence

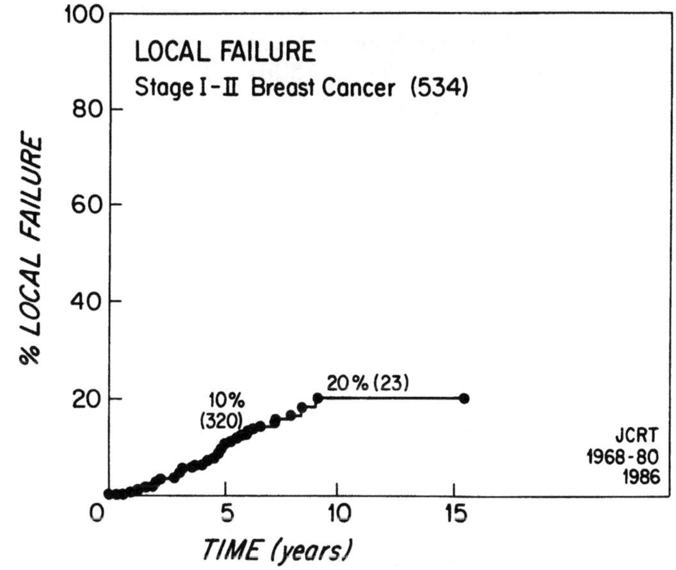

Fig. 1. Actuarial probability of local failure in all treated patients. The numbers in parenthesis in all figures indicate the numbers of patients still at risk at that time

was 11%. When this curve was plotted semilogarithmically as local tumor control against time (not shown), a straight line was obtained. This means that the risk of local recurrence was constant for at least the first 10 years after treatment.

Figure 2 shows the effect of excisional biopsy on the probability of local recurrence. The 10-year probability of local recurrence was 9% for patients treated with excisional biopsy and 43% for patients treated with incisional or needle biopsy ($P < 0.0001$). It is likely that the probability of local recurrence for patients treated without excisional biopsy could have been improved by the use of more-aggressive radiotherapy, but this would have been achieved at the expense of the cosmetic result. Excisional biopsy facilitates the use of radiation therapy, and is now routinely recommended in all our patients. The optimal extent of the resection to be performed prior to radiation therapy is a more complicated matter, as will be discussed.

Local recurrence after breast-conserving treatment was classified on clinical and pathologic grounds as a true recurrence (TR) a marginal miss (MM), occurring elsewhere in the breast (E), or in skin (S). A TR was a recurrence within the borders of the boost or at the site of the primary in the absence of a boost. MM was scored for a recurrence near the primary site, but just outside the borders of the boost. A recurrence elsewhere in the treated breast was scored as recurrence at a site at least several centimeters from the boost volume or at a substantial distance from the primary tumor site. A skin recurrence was scored when the recurrence was confined to the skin of the breast without parenchymal recurrence being found. We viewed either TR or MM as a recurrence of the original cancer.

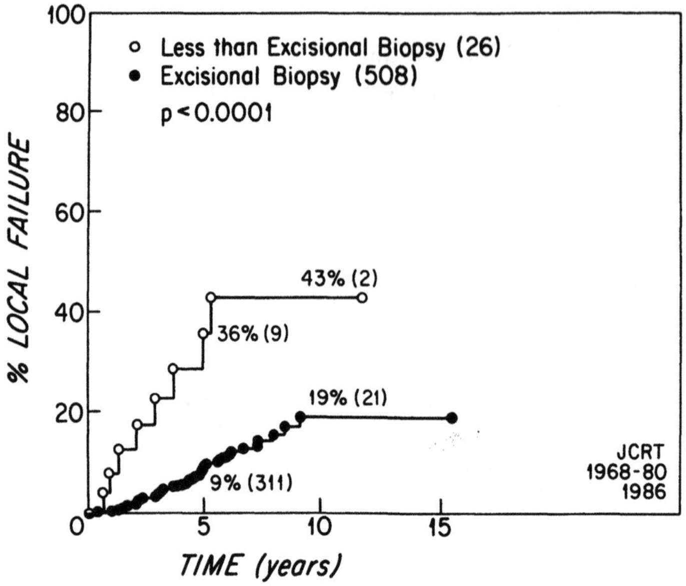

Fig. 2. Actuarial probability of local failure by type of biopsy

Figure 3 shows the probability of TR following breast-conserving treatment in patients treated with irradiation after excisional biopsy of the tumor. The probability of TR was 4% at 5 years and 11% at 10 years. We compared the probability of TR in the 411 patients treated with a boost at the primary site of 6000 cGy or greater to that in the 97 patients treated without a boost. (The validity of this comparison was limited by selection bias, because patients at greater risk of local recurrence more often received a boost). Patients treated with a boost had a lower probability of TR (7% at 10 years) than patients treated without a boost (15% at 10 years, P, 0.19). This result suggests that a boost to the primary site is useful in decreasing the likelihood of TR.

Figure 4 shows that the probability of MM in patients treated with excisional biopsy of the tumor and radiation therapy including a boost to the primary site was 4% at both 5 and 10 years. We compared the probability of MM among the subset of patients with infiltrative ductal carcinoma for whom there was sufficient tissue available to assess the presence of an extensive intraductal component (EIC). EIC is defined as the presence of *both* intraductal carcinoma comprising 25% or more of the tumor (as defined by its infiltrating margin) *and* intraductal carcinoma clearly extending beyond the infiltrating margin or present in sections of grossly normal adjacent breast tissue. There were 107 patients who had EIC and 188 who did not. The 5- and 10-year probability of MM was 13% for patients with EIC and 0% for patients without EIC ($P < 0.0001$). These results suggest that MM is rare except in patients with EIC, and that the presence of EIC indicates a form of the disease which is more locally extensive than can be appreciated by clinical means. The implications of EIC will be discussed in greater detail.

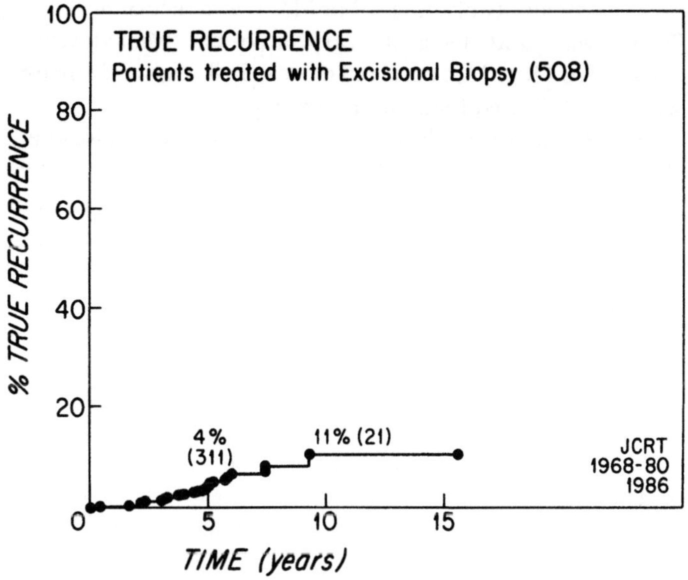

Fig. 3. Actuarial probability of developing a true recurrence for 508 patients treated with excisional biopsy and radiotherapy

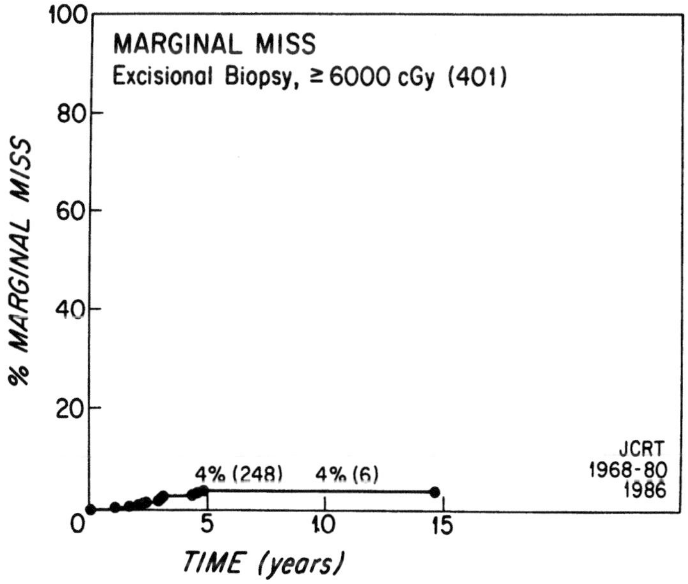

Fig. 4. Actuarial probability of developing a marginal miss for 401 patients treated with excisional biopsy and radiation therapy including a boost dose to the primary tumor site to 6000 cGy or more

The probability of either TR or MM (i.e., a recurrence of the primary tumor) was 7% at 5 years and 10% at 10 years for patients treated with excisional biopsy and a boost. No TR or MM occurred more than 8 years after treatment in the 30 patients who were followed for at least that long.

Figure 5 shows that the probability of a recurrence elsewhere in the treated breast (E) was 1% at 5 years and 7% at 10 years. The time course of this type of recurrence was different from that of TR or MM. TR and MM were more common in the first 5 years and less common after 5 years, whereas E was less common in the first 5 years and more common after 5 years. The number of patients with E was small, and the chance of developing such a recurrence did not appear to be related to any clinical or pathologic feature. The probability of E was greater for patients aged 49 years or younger than for patients aged 50 years or older, but this difference did not reach statistical significance (8% vs. 5% at 10 years, P, 0.08). The probability of E was not related to the presence of EIC. We compared the probability of developing a metachronous breast cancer in the contralateral breast to the probability of E (Fig. 5). The usefulness of this comparison can be questioned, since the remainder of the ipsilateral breast is at risk for the subsequent development of new cancers, the late clinical appearance of multicentric cancers existing at the time radiotherapy was given, and recurrences due to inapparent extensions of the primary tumor, whereas the contralateral breast is at risk only for the subsequent development of a new or multicentric cancer. The probability of metachronous contralateral breast cancer was 4% at 5 years and 10% at 10 years. The use of whole-breast irradiation appeared

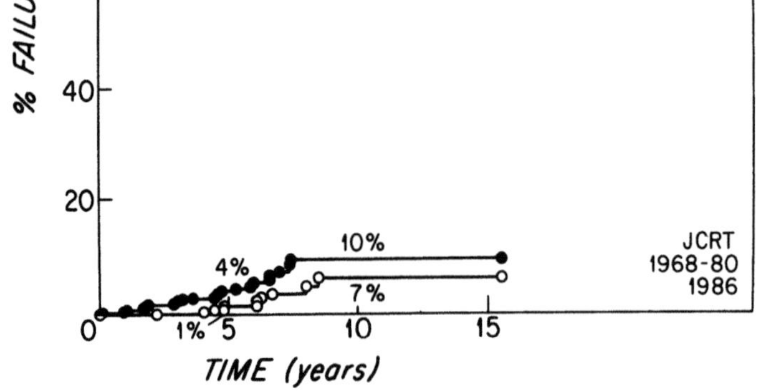

Fig. 5. Actuarial probability of developing a metchronous contralateral breast cancer compared with the probability of developing a failure in the ipsilateral breast away from the primary site

to decrease (or delay) the subsequent appearance of E, but further follow-up is required to assess this effect more accurately.

Skin recurrence was uncommon in our series, occurring in only three patients. The 5- and 10-year probability of skin recurrence was 0.7%. All three skin recurrences were seen in patients who had pathologically positive axillary nodes on initial presentation. The 5-year probability of skin recurrence was 2.5% for node-positive patients, compared to 0% for node-negative patients (P,0.03).

The influence of EIC on the probability of local recurrence in our experience has been previously described. We have updated these results, and they are shown in Fig. 6. Patients whose tumors contain significant intraductal carcinoma only within the primary tumor *or* had intraductal carcinoma only in the adjacent breast tissue (or neither) had a very low risk of local recurrence, whereas patients whose tumors show significant intraductal carcinoma within the primary tumor *and* in the adjacent tissue EIC had a high risk of local recurrence. As noted above, patients with EIC had an appreciable risk of MM (13% at 10 years, compared with 0% for other patients). It is also notable that patients with EIC had a higher probability of TR (23% at 10 years, compared to 2% for patients without EIC, $P < 0.001$). In this latest analysis, neither axillary-node status, tumor size, nuclear grade, nor dose to the primary site significantly influenced these results. However, patients with EIC and poorly differentiated nuclei failed at a faster rate than did patients with EIC and well or moderately differentiated nuclei.

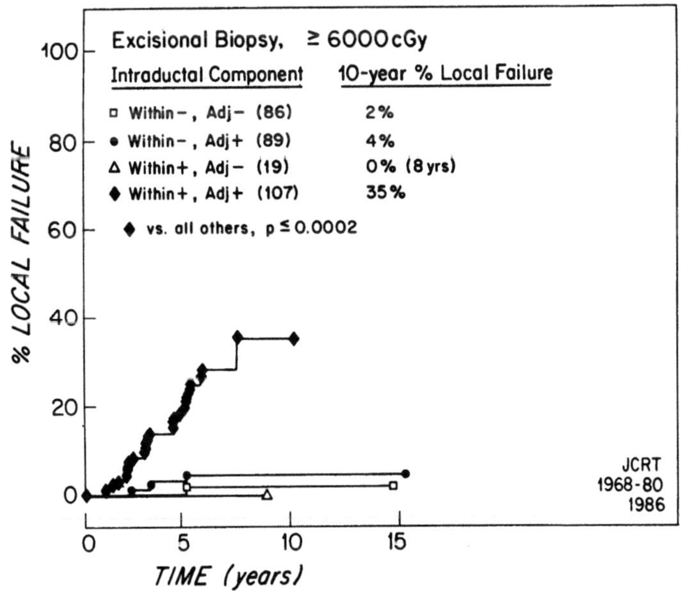

Fig. 6. Actuarial probability of local failure by the extent of intraductal cancer in the primary tumor. *Within–*, no intraductal cancer within the infiltrating borders of the tumor; *Within+*, ≤ 25% of the tumor within the infiltrating borders is intraductal; *ADJ–*, no intraductal cancer beyond the infiltrating borders of the tumor; *ADJ+*, intraductal cancer present beyond the infiltrating borders of the tumor; Within+, ADJ+ = EIC

These observations on the frequency and pattern of local recurrence in patients with EIC suggest that patients with EIC have a more extensive tumor burden after excision than patients without EIC. This view is also supported by our recent results concerning the pathologic findings on reexcision of the primary site in 71 patients previously treated by gross excision of the tumor. Reexcision was performed in 46 patients who, despite initial margins of resection that were felt to be positive or suspicious, did not have EIC, and in 25 patients with EIC demonstrated on the initial excision. Residual carcinoma (infiltrating or intraductal) was seen in 62% of all patients, but was more frequent among the 25 patients with EIC than among the 46 without EIC (88% vs. 48%, P, 0.002). The nature of this residual carcinoma was different for patients with and without EIC in the primary excision specimen. The residual carcinoma in patients without EIC was usually limited in quantity, consisting of scattered microscopic foci of either infiltrating or intraductal carcinoma. In contrast, the residual carcinoma in patients with EIC was often widespread and was composed predominantly of intraductal carcinoma. Of patients with EIC, 44% had extensive residual intraductal carcinoma on reexcision, compared with only 2% of patients without EIC ($P < 0.0001$). These results indicate that patients with EIC treated with a gross excision of the tumor frequently had considerable residual intraductal carcinoma near the primary site. This provides additional support for the view that tumors with EIC have a more extensive residual tumor burden after excision than other tumors do, and are therefore more likely to recur following radiation therapy.

Our current approach for patients with EIC is to widely resect the tumor in order to obtain negative margins of resection prior to recommending radiation therapy. We are currently evaluating our results using this treatment approach in patients with EIC, but our follow-up time is, at present, too short to provide meaningful results. It is encouraging, however, that the results from institutions which routinely practice wide excision with negative margins of resection fail to show a higher local recurrence rate in patients with EIC [2–4].

The standard treatment for an isolated local recurrence after breast-conserving treatment in the United States has been mastectomy. Figure 7 shows the probability of subsequent distant failure in the 41 patients in this series who developed an isolated local recurrence and subsequently underwent mastectomy. The 5-year probability of freedom from distant relapse in these patients was 67%. These results were substantially better than those for patients with local recurrence after mastectomy. In a recent review from our institution of 90 patients with isolated local recurrence after mastectomy treated with high-dose radiation, the probability of freedom from distant failure was 30% at 5 years and only 7% at 10 years [1]. These results indicate that treatment of an isolated local recurrence can be associated with a high probability of long-term disease-free survival, and that close surveillance of patients treated with breast-conserving treatment is necessary in order to detect such recurrence promptly.

Figure 8 shows the probability of survival in our series. The 10-year probability of survival was 84% for patients with clinical stage I disease (T1N0) and 63% for patients with clinical stage II disease (T1N1, T2N0, and T2N1). These results are comparable to those seen with mastectomy.

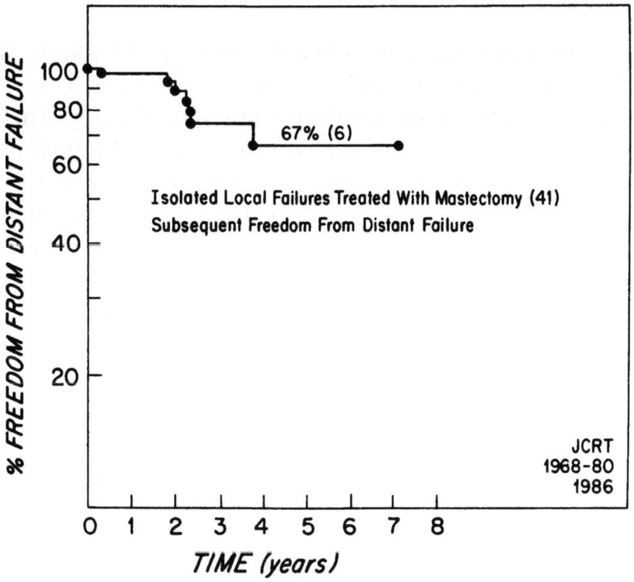

Fig. 7. Actuarial probability of freedom from distant failure in 41 patients treated with mastectomy for local failure following initial conservative surgery and radiotherapy

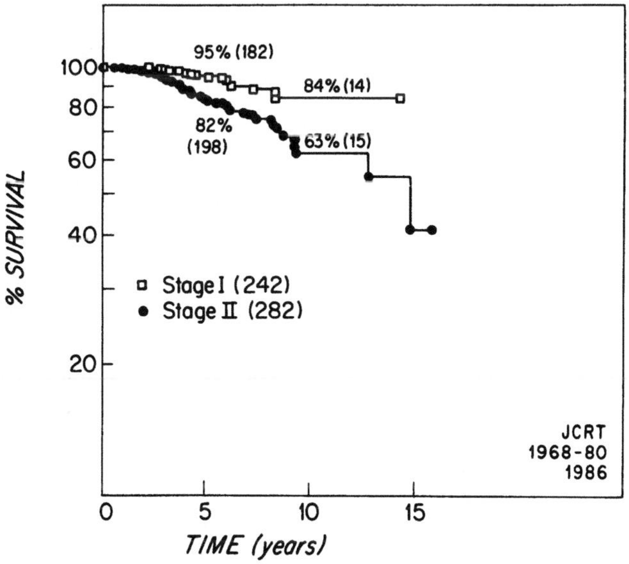

Fig. 8. Actuarial probability of survival by clinical stage for all treated patients

Assessment

The retrospective results obtained from our institution indicate that high levels of local tumor control and long-term survival can be obtained by the use of breast-conserving treatment employing radiation therapy. These results stress, however, that the time course of local recurrence after this treatment is protracted and that long-term results are essential to assess the outcome accurately. The analysis of failure presented here has provided us with a format for the selection and treatment of patients with early breast cancer. Patients who present with suspicious breast masses typically undergo excision of the tumor under local anesthesia as an outpatient. The incision is placed over the tumor and a small rim of adjacent breast tissue is taken to assess the degree of intraductal involvement. If the tumor does not show EIC, then only axillary dissection is indicated prior to radiation. (In practice in this situation, however, a very modest reexcision is frequently performed if it will not diminish the cosmetic appearance significantly). If the tumor does show EIC, then reexcision of the primary site is indicated prior to radiation, along with axillary dissection. If the new margins of resection are clear, then radiation therapy appears to be a reasonable approach. If the new margins of resection are involved, then mastectomy is generally recommended.

Radiotherapy typically consists of 4500 cGy in 25 fractions over 5 weeks to the entire breast followed by a boost of 1600 cGy in eight fractions by electron beam to the primary site. This approach provides a very high rate of local tumor control and generally excellent cosmetic results. Finally, the use of breast-conserving treatment requires that the patient be followed up closely in order to detect a treatable local recurrence promptly.

References

1. Aberizk WJ, Silver B, Henderson IC, et al. (1986) The use of radiotherapy for treatment of isolated local-regional recurrence of breast cancer after mastectomy. Cancer 58:1214–1218
2. Calle R, Vilcoq JR, Zafrani B, et al. (1986) Local control and survival of breast cancer treated by limited surgery followed by irradiation. Int J Radiat Oncol Biol Phys 12:873–885
3. Clarke DH, Le MG, Sarrazin D, et al. (1985) Analysis of local-regional relapses in patients with early breast cancers treated by excision and radiotherapy: Experience of the Institut Gustave-Roussy. Int J Radiat Oncol Biol Phys 11:137–145
4. Fisher ER, Sass R, Fisher B, et al. (1986) Pathologic findings from the national surgical adjuvant breast project (protocol no 6). II. Relation of local breast recurrence to multicentricity. Cancer 57:1717–1724
5. Harris JR, Connolly JL, Schnitt SJ, et al. (1985) The use of pathologic features in selecting the extent of surgical resection necessary for breast cancer patients treated by primary radiation therapy. Ann Surg 201(2):164–169
6. Harris JR, Recht A, Schnitt S, et al. (1985) Current status of conservative surgery and radiotherapy as primary local treatment for early carcinoma of the breast. Breast Cancer Res Treat 5:245–255
7. Recht A, Silver B, Schnitt S, et al. (1985) Breast relapse following primary radiation therapy for early breast cancer. I. Classification, frequency, and salvage. Int J Radiat Oncol Biol Phys 11(7):1271–1276
8. Schnitt SJ, Connolly JL, Recht A, et al. (1985) Breast relapse following primary radiation therapy for early breast cancer. II. Detection, pathologic features and prognostic significance. Int J Radiat Oncol Biol Phys 11(7):1277–1284

Local Recurrence and New Primary Ipsilateral Carcinomas After Conservative Treatment of Breast Carcinoma

U. VERONESI, A. LUINI, and M. DEL VECCHIO

One of the greatest concerns in conservative treatment of breast cancer is the increased risk of local recurrence of the disease. In fact, local recurrence not only represents treatment failure and creates serious psychological distress to the patient [4], but ultimately leads, in most cases, to mastectomy, defeating the object of the original project, i.e., avoidance of mutilation. Moreover, it is not unlikely that an increased rate of local recurrence may negatively influence survival and obscure the prognosis [2]. For all these reasons, it appears that the avoidance of local recurrence must be regarded as a major objective in breast-conservation programs.

At the Milan Cancer Institute, conservative breast treatment is largely applied; the results of a randomized trial, comparing radical mastectomy with quadrantectomy, axillary dissection, and radiotherapy, have been published. The trial showed that in the quadrantectomy patients the incidence of local recurrence was no higher, and the survival no worse, than that observed in the Halsted mastectomy patients (Figs. 1–3). However, it appears important to evaluate results from a larger series of patients, including patients treated outside the clinical trial, as they are more representative of routine practice. For this reason 1041 patients treated with quadrantectomy, axillary dissection, and radiotherapy from 1973 to 1982 were reviewed in order to evaluate the rates of local recurrence and to analyze the parameters connected with this unfavorable event.

Patients and Methods

From June 1973 to December 1982, 1128 patients with breast cancer were treated with a conservative procedure defined as QUART (quadrantectomy, axillary dissection, and radiotherapy). The details of this method have been repeatedly described [3,5], and may be summarized as follows. Quadrantectomy consists of a large resection of the quadrant in which the primary tumor is located, including a large portion of the skin and underlying fascia. The excision is performed in normal breast tissue, 2–3 cm from the edge of the primary carcinoma. Axillary dissection is always completed, with removal of the lymph nodes of the three levels up to the apex of the axilla. Radiotherapy is given only to the breast submitted to the quadrantectomy at a dosage of 50 Gy to the whole breast with high-energy equipment through two opposite tangential fields, with a boost of an additional 10 Gy to the scar delivered by an orthovoltage machine. No irradiation is applied to regional lymph nodes.

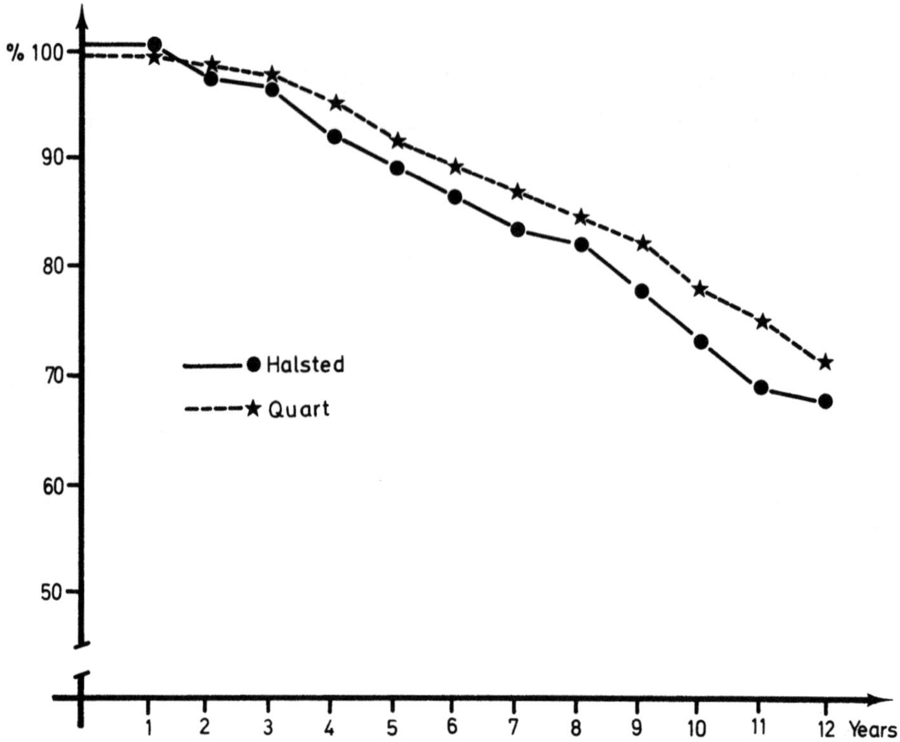

Fig. 1. Milan Trial I: survival according to type of treatment; *QUART*, quadrantectomy, axillary dissection, and radiotherapy; *HALSTED*, Halsted mastectomy; P, 0.13

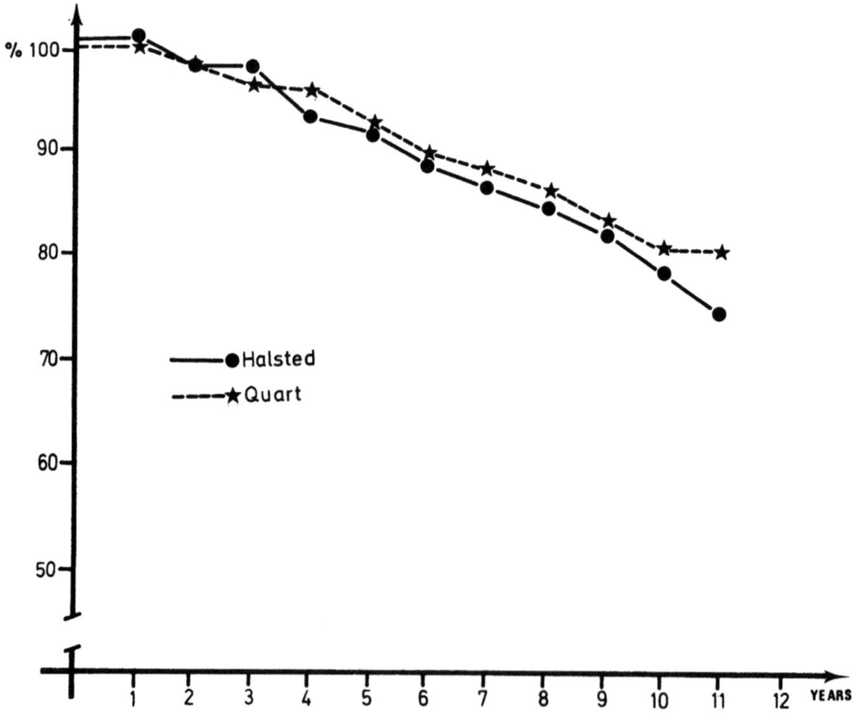

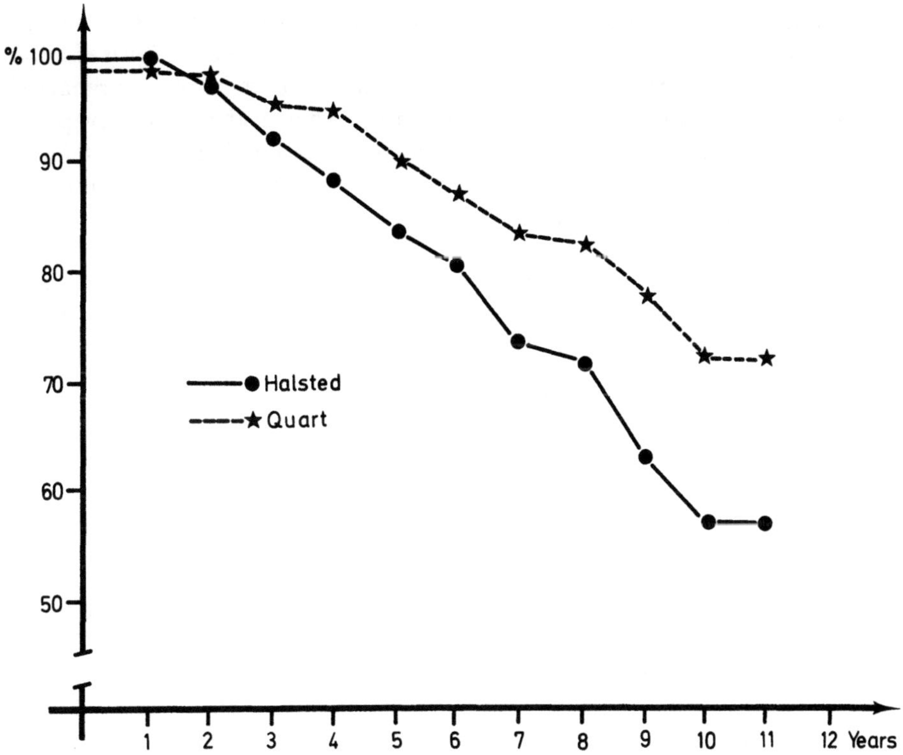

Fig. 3. Milan Trial I: survival of patients with axillary-node metastases, who were treated with Halsted mastectomy (*HALSTED*) or with *QUART*

Out of 1128 patients, 87 were excluded from the analysis either because they had a previous or concomitant contralateral breast cancer, a previous malignant tumor in another organ, or a noninfiltrating carcinoma; or because they were submitted to a type of conservative treatment other than QUART. In 982 patients the tumor was smaller or equal to 2 cm. in its largest pathologic diameter, while in 59 patients the pathologic diameter was larger than 2 cm. The average age of the patients was 49 years; 644 patients (62%) were premenopausal, 311 (30%) had positive axillary nodes. Most of the patients with axillary metastases were submitted to adjuvant chemotherapy, mainly cyclophosphamide, Methotrexate, Fluorouracil (CMF). All the patients were followed up regularly with a clinical examination twice per year and chest radiography, bone scan, and bilateral mammography once per year.

All cases who had local recurrence were carefully analyzed by a joint team (surgeon, radiotherapist, pathologist) with the aim of subdividing them into those

Fig. 2. Milan Trial I: survival of patients without axillary-node metastases, who were treated with Halsted mastectomy (*HALSTED*) or with quadrantectomy, axillary dissection and radiotherapy (*QUART*); P, 0.62

with local recurrences and those with second ipsilateral carcinomas. Although it is not always possible to make such a subdivision, an effort in this direction is essential, as the rate of true local recurrences (i.e., reappearance of the original primary tumor) will measure the adequacy of the treatment, whereas the rate of new primary carcinomas will measure either the ability of radiation therapy to inhibit the proliferation of new carcinomatous foci in the breast tissue or, on the contrary, the possible carcinogenic effect of radiation. The main criterion with which to separate the two entities is the site of tumor reappearance: if it was in the same quadrant, it was likely to be a true recurrence, but if it appeared in distant quadrants it was likely to be a new primary carcinoma. Other criteria were the appearance of a nodule in the subcutaneous tissue (obviously a local recurrence) or a difference in histologic type (obviously a new carcinoma). All data were stored in a computed, automated system, and survival rates were calculated up to December 1986, according to the method of KAPLAN and MEIER.

Results

The initial unfavorable events are listed in Table 1. Among them we observed 33 local recurrences (3.2%) and 18 new primary ispilateral carcinomas (1.7%). The average age of the patients with local recurrence was higher (44 years) than that of those with new ipsilateral carcinoma (39 years). The distribution of local recurrences according to nodal status was similar (3.2% in node-negative and 3.1% in node-positive patients). Patients with tumors located in the outer quadrants were exposed to twice the risk of local recurrence as patients with tumors in other parts of the breast. The risk of local recurrence was correlated to the size of the primary carcinoma: 1.9% for tumors less than 1 cm, 2.7% for tumors 1–2 cm, and 5.0% for tumors more than 2 cm in diameter.

From the clinical point of view the newly appeared nodule was always discovered during careful palpation of the breast. In 3 of 26 cases in which a mammogram was taken, the result was positive in 18 cases and (false-) negative in 8 cases. Local reexcision of the breast was possible in 6 cases of local recurrence and in 2 cases of ipsilateral primary carcinoma, whilst in 27 cases of local recurrence and 16 of a second primary, total mastectomy was performed. The survival after treatment was 80% at 3 years, both for patients who had a true local recurrence and

Table 1. First unfavorable event in 1041 patients treated with quadrantectomy, axillary dissection and radiotherapy (QUART) 1973–1982

Event	*n* (%)
Local recurrence	33 (3.2%)
Second ipsilateral tumor	18 (1.7%)
Contralateral tumor	39 (3.7%)
Distant metastases	133 (12.8%)

Median follow-up, 67 months; *n*, no. of patients

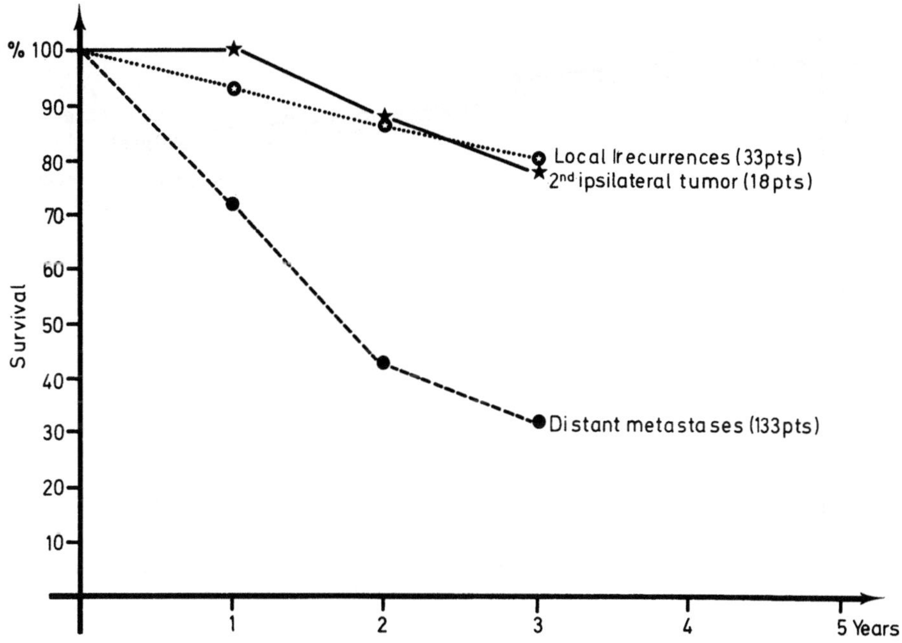

Fig. 4. Survival according to the type of first unfavorable event (from the time of occurrence of the event); *pts,* patients

patients who developed a new primary carcinoma, whilst the 133 patients who showed a distant metastasis, as the first unfavorable event had a 3-year survival of 31% (Fig. 4). The overall 8-year survival of the 51 patients, calculated from the time of the first treatment, was not different from that of the remaining 990 patients of our series (Fig. 5).

As regards regional-node recurrences, there were no axillary recurrences in any of the 1041 cases; 22 patients (3.6%) had supraclavicular metastases, and only 2 had metastases of the internal mammary nodes (0.2%). The latter figure appears particularly low compared to previous series of patients. Finally, it must be recorded that of 1041 cases, 39 (5.5%) developed a new carcinoma in the contralateral breast.

Discussion

The overall incidence of disease recurrence after quadrantectomy, axillary dissection, and radiotherapy appears to be around 5%. However, if one separates the 18 cases identified as new primary carcinomas appearing in the residual mammary tissue, true local relapses of the breast occurred in 33 out of 1041 patients (3.3%). This low rate of local recurrence, roughly of the same order as the rate observed after radical mastectomy or modified radical mastectomy, is likely to be due to the association of extensive local excision (quadrantectomy), with vigorous radiotherapy.

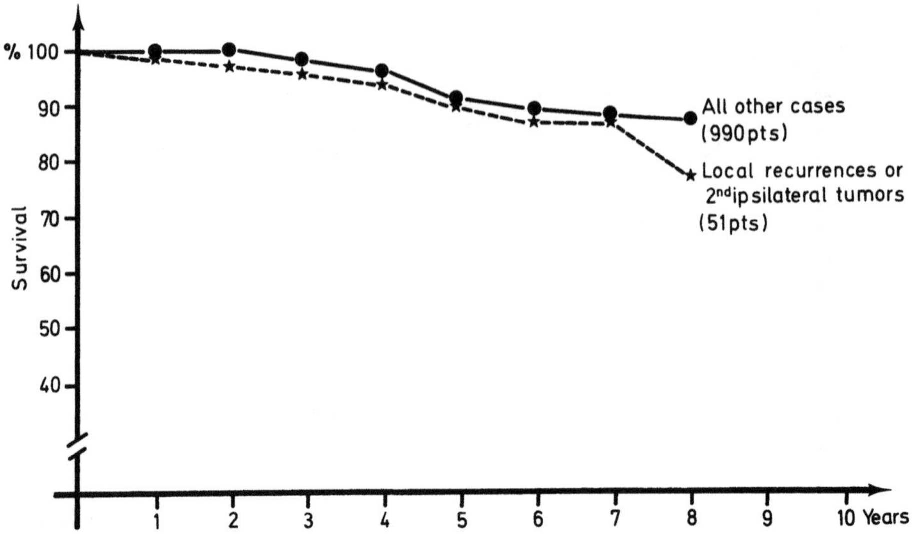

Fig. 5. Survival from the time of primary surgery, in patients who developed local recurrences or second ipsilateral tumors, and in all other patients; *pts*, patients

The survival of patients who had suffered local recurrence and been treated with a second operation (in most cases total mastectomy) does not seem to be worse than that of the remaining patients who did not develop a relapse. If one considers that local recurrence may be an expression of a particularly aggressive type of cancer, this not-unfavorable evolution of our cases may appear surprising. Although careful follow-up of these patients during the years to come appears fundamental, our observation is, however, consistent with the recent results of FISHER et al. [1], which showed that the considerable increase in recurrence rate in one of the arms of Trial 06 did not influence the overall survival. The fact that primary carcinomas localized in the upper-outer quadrants had an higher rate of recurrence cannot be reasonably explained and may in fact be due to chance. It is, however, an important observation that the rate of local recurrence increases according to the size of the primary carcinoma. This observation is a warning against the excessive use of conservative treatment in patients with primary tumors larger than 2 cm. One must be aware that large tumors pose a significant risk of local failure if treated with limited surgery and radiotherapy.

From the clinical point of view, detection of a local recurrence and/or a new primary carcinoma after quadrantectomy and radiotherapy is not easy. The frequent sclerosis of tissue, although generally mild, is fairly often associated with persistent breast edema (due to radiotherapy and axillary dissection), and makes the diagnosis of recurrence difficult, especially as granulomas and fibrotic nodules are not rare after conservative procedures. In addition, mammography loses some of its efficacy, as shown by our experiences. Follow-up of these cases must therefore be very meticulous, with frequent thorough physical examination and cytology with fine-needle biopsy.

References

1. Fisher B, Bauer M, Margolese R, et al. (1985) Five-year results of a randomized clinical trial comparing total mastectomy and segmental mastectomy with or without radiation in the treatment of breast cancer. N Engl J Med 312:665–673
2. Hayward JL (1983) Prospective studies, the Guy's Hospital trials on breast conservative. In: Harris JR, Hellman S, Silen W (eds) Conservative management of breast cancer. Lippincott, Philadelphia, pp 77–90
3. Veronesi U, Banfi A, Saccozzi R, et al. (1977) Conservative treatment of breast cancer. Cancer 39:2822–2826
4. Veronesi U (1984) Current status of primary surgery in the management of breast cancer. In: Bonadonna G (ed) Cancer investigation and management. Wiley, New York, pp 169–209 (Breast cancer: Diagnosis and management, vol 1)
5. Veronesi U, Saccozzi R, del Vecchio M, et al. (1981) Comparing radical mastectomy with quadrantectomy, axillary dissection, and radiotherapy in patients with small cancers of the breast. N Engl J Med 305:6–11

Pathoanatomical Characteristics of Local Treatment Failure Following Breast-Conserving Therapy

A. MÜLLER and D. VON FOURNIER

In recent years carcinoma of the breast has been treated increasingly frequently with forms of therapy allowing conservation of the breast. The key factor that has made it possible largely to abandon more radical surgical procedures is a completely new understanding of the biology of the breast [1]. According to this concept, in the majority of cases disseminated disease is already present when primary treatment is started. The patient's fate is therefore determined not by what happens in the locoregional area, but by early metastasis to distant sites. The results of numerous prospective and retrospective studies are now available to show that removal of the primary tumor, with varying degrees of radicality, followed by radiation to the residual breast tissue can give survival rates comparable to those achieved with modified radical mastectomy [2, 9, 13]. Nevertheless locoregional clearance of the tumor process is important. HAYWARD's studies have shown that inadequate control of the tumor in the breast region has a negative influence on the survival rates, especially in the case of a heavy tumor burden [7]. On the other hand, local recurrences can cause serious problems with treatment, as a result of fulminant tumor spread in the irradiated breast itself [8]. Thus it is important to find tumor characteristics that correlate with a high local relapse rate, in order to allow surgical or radiological treatment to be adapted in future to take account of the risk of relapse in the individual patient.

We studied the patients who had undergone breast-conserving therapy as primary treatment for carcinoma of the breast at the University Hospital for Women in Heidelberg up to 1984 to check whether the risk of local recurrence is linked with any particular morphological characteristics of the primary tumor.

Patients and Course of Therapy

Primary breast-conserving therapy for invasive carcinoma of the breast was started in 254 patients at the University Hospital for Women in Heidelberg during the period from June 1976 to December 1984 (Table 1). In all these cases, lumpectomy or segmentectomy with axillary lymphadenectomy was performed. In 50 cases the carcinoma had been confirmed by biopsy in another hospital, and these patients underwent subsequent resection of the tumor bed amounting to segmental resection in addition to dissection of the regional lymph nodes. After the histological examination a secondary mastectomy was performed in 17 patients, since the

Table 1. Breast-conserving treatments planned and carried out (including postoperative radiotherapy), for invasive carcinoma of the breast at the University Hospital for Women in Heidelberg during the study period (1976-1984). Position of carcinomas relative to the margins of the segmental tissue removed

	n	%	
Therapy planned	254	100	
Therapy carried out	237	93	
Ductal carcinoma in situ to edge of tissue resected	23	9	
Invasive carcinoma to edge of tissue resected	8	3	19
Secondary mastectomy (no healthy tissue margins)	17	7	

invasive carcinoma had not been removed with a margin of healthy tissue. The present study is concerned with the remaining 237 patients in whom the radiotherapy of the breast residue usual in our clinic was carried out in full in addition to the conservative surgical treatment. This patient sample includes 31 patients in whom the tumors were not removed with healthy tissue margins but who refused the recommended mastectomy when the risk was explained to them. Patients with histologically demonstrated axillary lymph node metastases also received adjuvant hormone therapy and/or chemotherapy. The study was completed in February 1987. The average follow-up period was 48 months.

Morphological Examination

The margins of the segments to be removed were marked by the surgeon with thread. After fixation with formalin the specimens were laminated into 2.5-mm-thick slices. These slices were then X-rayed. The lamellae were subjected to full histological examination, except for a few tissue regions that clearly contained fat. The sequential position of the each block of tissue taken from the lamellae was recorded on the X-ray pictures. In light of our experience in the preparation of subcutaneous mastectomy specimens, it was thus possible to reconstruct the spatial relations of pathoanatomical changes at any time [10]. Since about 1 year ago we have been using an inking technique to mark the edges of the tissue segments to be removed, which has made the topographic allocation less laborious.

The system of nomenclature published by the World Health Organization in 1982 was used for histological classification of the carcinomatous tumors. Particular attention was paid to any cases of lymphangiosis carcinomatosa, to the positions of the primary tumors relative to the margins of the tissue to be removed, to intratumoral intraductal portions and to peritumoral intraductal tumor extensions.

Results

In all, 11 relapses occurred in the breast, four of which had a clinically and histologically inflammatory course of growth with pronounced subcutaneous lymphangiosis carcinomatosa (Table 2). In these cases it was impossible to link the site of recurrence topographically with the primary tumor. In seven patients the relapse occurred in the operation scar or in the same quadrant as the primary tumor. According to the pathoanatomical classification of the primary tumors, invasive ductal carcinomas were present in 67% of the evaluable cases. Lobular and tubular invasive carcinomas were each present in 10% and 9% of cases respectively. In 12% of the patients, invasive ductal carcinomas with a predominant intraductal component were diagnosed. This diagnosis was recorded when the intraductal tumor components took up over 50% of the entire invasive tumor region. We found medullary carcinomas in 1% of these patients and mucinous carcinomas in 1%. In the group with relapses, invasive ductal carcinoma was found in 10 cases. One patient had a biopsy specimen removed for examination at another hospital. In this patient there was no residual tumor in the tissue removed from the same segment in our own clinic.

Table 2. Distribution of various morphologic characteristics of the primary tumors in the entire patient population and in the subgroup of patients with local recurrence

	Total patient population		Group with local recurrences	
	n	%	*n*	%
	237	100	11	100
Positive lymph nodes	69	29	5	45
Ductal carcinoma in situ extending to margin of resected tissue	23	10	6	55
Lymphangiosis carcinomatosa	52	22	5	45
Invasive carcinoma to margin of resected tissue	8	3	–	–

In 69 patients, or 29% of the total study population, axillary lymph node metastases were present. This finding was recorded in five (45%) of the patients with local recurrences. Peritumoral lymphangiosis carcinomatosa was observed in 22% of cases in the entire group. In 23 cases of the entire sample (10%), intraductal components were found reaching the margins of the segments. In six of these patients a breast recurrence occurred during the follow-up period. So far no intramammary recurrences have been observed in any of the 8 patients in whom the invasive tumor extended to the margin of the segment.

Discussion

According to the literature, local recurrences that arise after breast-conserving therapy for invasive carcinoma of the breast have a better prognosis than relapses in the chest wall after mastectomy [4, 6]. There are also differences in their timing: while about 80% of the recurrences after a regular mastectomy arise within the first 3 years after the primary operation [12], HARRIS reports a constantly increasing relapse rate, rising by about 2% per year over a follow-up period of 15 years [6]. Radioresistant residual tumor and multifocal carcinomas still occult at the time of the operation are thought to be possible origins of these recurrences in the breast. Finally, they can be due to glandular epithelia that start to undergo malignant degeneration after the operation; such degeneration may be triggered by the radiotherapy. The follow-up periods so far are too short to allow detailed answers. It is certain, however, that these recurrences are difficult to diagnose because of the postoperative and radiogenic changes in the breast tissue [6, 8] and can take a progressive course in the breast subjected to radiotherapy, thus becoming practically incurable [8]. The literature contains few data as yet on tumor characteristics that would allow the definition of patient groups with an elevated risk of local relapse. SCHNITT and CONOLLY report an elevated risk when extensive intraductal tumor components are present [11]. They also feel there is an additional risk with a poor differentiation of the primary tumor. In the study conducted by FISCHER et al. [3] only peritumoral lymphangiosis carcinomatosa was found to correlate with an elevated risk of local recurrence. In view of the short observation period our figures can be referred only to relapses occurring in the breast relatively soon after the primary treatment. In our group of patients with recurrence, positive axillary lymph node status and peritumoral lymphangiosis carcinomatosa was encountered approximately twice as frequently as in the entire group of breast carcinoma patients who had undergone conservative treatment. Particular emphasis must be placed on the fact that the 23 patients in the entire patient population in whom histology documented intraductal tumor extension reaching to the segmental margin included six who were found to have recurrences in the breast within the observation period. In all six cases these tumor extensions reached over 1 cm beyond the periphery of the invasive part of the carcinoma. In contrast, the intraductal parts within the primary carcinoma seemed to have no influence on the risk of local recurrence in our patient population.

According to our studies, then, a small subgroup of patients can be defined in whom the risk of developing early local recurrence is almost 30%. Further studies will be needed to clarify whether this elevated risk correlates with the extent of intraductal tumor extensions or exclusively with their extension to or beyond the segmental margins. Among those of our patients who suffered local recurrence, both these findings were recorded simultaneously. Such tumor extensions need to be recognized in order to allow modification of the surgical or radiological treatment in keeping with the level of risk obtaining in each case. Since ductal extensions cannot generally be macroscopically observed, histopathological preparation of the surgical specimens must be carried out with the utmost care to allow accurate microscopic assessment of the tumor margins. If the topography of the margin affected by tumor is precisely known and if the breast remnant is large enough, a secondary resection can be undertaken in a controlled manner without detriment to the cosmetic result. If the above conditions are not present, we are of the opinion that a secondary mastectomy should be performed, possibly with primary breast reconstruction.

References

1. Fisher B, Redmond C, Fisher ER (1980) The contribution of recent NSABP clinical trials of primary breast cancer therapy to an understanding of tumor biology – an overview of findings. Cancer 46:1009–1025
2. Fisher B, Bauer M, Margolese R (1985) Five year results of a randomized clinical trial comparing total mastectomy and segmental mastectomy with or without radiation in the treatment of breast cancer. N Engl J Med 312:665–673
3. Fisher ER, Sass R, Fisher B, Gregorio R, Brown R, Wickerham L (1986) Pathologic findings from the national surgical adjuvant breast project (protocol 6) II. Relation of local breast recurrence to multicentricity. Cancer 57:1717–1724
4. Genz T (1985) Kritische Analyse der Brustkrebsbehandlung (1963–1982) unter Bestimmung identischer morphologischer Prognosefaktoren und besonderer Wertung der brusterhaltenden Operation. Habilitationsschrift, Universität Berlin
5. Harris JR, Connolly JL, Schnitt SJ, Cohen RB, Hellman S (1983) Clinical-pathologic study of early breast cancer treated by primary radiation therapy. J Clin Oncol 1:184–189
6. Harris JR, Recht A, Amalric R, Calle R, Clark RM, Reid JG, Spitalier JM, Vilcoq JR, Hellman S (1984) Time course and prognosis of local recurrence following primary radiation therapy for early breast cancer. J Clin Oncol 2:37–41
7. Hayward JC (1983) Guy's hospital trials on breast conservation. In: Harris JR, Hellman S, Silen W (eds) Conservative Management of Breast Cancer. Lippincott, Philadelphia
8. Kubli F, v. Fournier D (1986) Brusterhaltende Therapie des Mammakarzinoms. In: Melchert F, Beck L, Hepp H, Knapstein PG, Kreienberg R (Hrsg). Aktuelle Geburtshilfe und Gynäkologie. Springer, Berlin Heidelberg New York Tokyo
9. Montague ED, Fletcher GH (1985) Local regional effectiveness of surgery and radiation therapy in the treatment of breast cancer. Cancer 55:2266–2272
10. Müller A, Tschahargane C, Kubli F (1984) Subkutane Mastektomie: Bedeutung der histopathologischen Aufarbeitungstechnik. Dtsch Med Wschr 109:50–54
11. Schnitt SJ, Connolly JL, Harris JR, Hellman S, Cohen RB (1984) Pathologic predictors of early local recurrence in stage I and II breast cancer treated by primary radiation therapy. Cancer 53:1049–1057
12. Valagussa P, Bonadonna G, Veronesi U (1978) Patterns of relaps and survival following radical mastectomy. Cancer 41 1170–1178
13. Veronesi U, Zucali R, Luini A, Belli F, Crispino S, Merson M (1985) Conservative treatment of breast cancer with the "Qu.A.R.T." technique. In: Zander J, Balzer J (eds) Early Breast Cancer, Springer Verlag Berlin, Heidelberg

Selective Issues in the Evaluation of the Efficacy of Breast-Conserving Therapy

J.A. VAN DONGEN, N.K. AARONSON, and H. BARTELINK

Introduction

The HALSTED-MEIER approach has been the standard treatment of early breast cancer for over 100 years. The efficacy of any new therapy must be weighed carefully against this classical approach before it can be considered a viable treatment alternative. This typically means the carrying out of prospective, randomized clinical trials. Yet, even with the aid of a randomized trial, evaluation of the relative efficacy of new approaches to the treatment of early breast cancer may be difficult. While we are quick to note the methodological limitations inherent in research employing nonexperimental designs, it is less often recognized that the use of a randomized design does not solve all of our interpretive problems. Rather, the randomized clinical trial provides us only with a sound starting point for comparative clinical evaluations. To ensure the robustness of our results, we must consider carefully the numerous pitfalls to which even this most elegant of research models may be prone.

Pitfalls of Noncontrolled Studies

Before turning to the randomized trial model, it should be emphasized that non-randomized studies can yield important preliminary data regarding the efficacy of alternative treatment modalities. For example, since 1979 some 900 patients of the Netherlands Cancer Institute with stage I and stage II breast cancer have been treated with breast-conserving therapy. Only a subset of these patients have been included in a randomized study protocol. To date, in the total group of 900 patients, only 18 locoregional recurrences have occurred. Furthermore, the survival curves for these patient groups do not deviate from those derived from mastectomized patient groups [2]. Nevertheless, such comparisons with historical controls must be viewed cautiously, even when cohort composition (age, disease stage, etc.) and the length of follow-up are taken into consideration.

Unfortunately, many reports of nonrandomized studies do not attend to even the most basic of methodological considerations. Information on disease stage is often missing, with some reports mixing operable and inoperable cases. Other problems include the use of different staging systems, short follow-up, and failure to report locoregional recurrence in addition to overall survival data.

In general, the abundant data available from nonrandomized studies are encouraging with regard to the efficacy and safety of breast-conserving therapy [4,6,8]. No data have emerged from such studies to suggest that the more conservative procedures result in increased risk to the patient. Nevertheless, final judgment regarding the effect of conservative treatments for early breast cancer await the results of ongoing randomized clinical trials.

Pitfalls of Randomized Clinical Trials

The prospective, randomized clinical study represents the methodologically soundest approach to evaluating new treatment schedules in early breast cancer. It should be emphasized, however, that the results of such studies are valid only for the specific patient groups and clinical procedures under investigation. For this reason it is essential that a complete description of both patient eligibility and treatment procedures be provided in the study protocol itself, as well as in any reports of study results.

Even given positive results from several randomized trials, it would be inappropriate to state that "breast-conserving therapy" is safe for "breast cancer patients". Due to the many variations in patient characteristics and breast-conserving techniques, a large number of randomized studies would be required before we could make such a generalized statement with any degree of confidence. The reality is that only a very few randomized studies are investigating the efficacy of breast-conserving therapy [3,5,7,9,11], and each of these has some limitations with regard to external validity.

As stated earlier, even when considering the randomized clinical trial, we should attend carefully to the varied methodological shortcomings – some of which may be unavoidable – when interpreting results and drawing conclusions. In many trials quite large study samples are needed in order to achieve statistical robustness. This is particularly the case when one is attempting to confirm a null research hypothesis; for example, that a particular method of breast-conserving therapy is as clinically effective as mastectomy.

In order to accrue sufficient numbers of patients within a reasonably short time-frame, researchers are increasingly turning to multicenter, cooperative trials. For example, in 1980 the European Organization for Research and Treatment of Cancer (EORTC) activated a prospective, randomized, multicenter trial to compare breast-conserving therapy (i.e., lumpectomy, axillary dissection, and radiotherapy of the breast, including boost techniques with iridium implantation) with (conservative) radical mastectomy [9,10] (see Fig. 1). This trial, which was closed to entry in May 1986, has accrued a total of 900 patients, 755 of whom have stage II disease. This latter group is most interesting in that no previous trial has investigated such a large number of stage II patients. A preliminary report of the results of this trial shows equal survival curves and equal local recurrence rates for both groups [10].

The fact that this trial is being conducted in six clinical centers has resulted in some unavoidable variations in both patient selection and treatment procedures.

Breast cancer stage I and II Randomization < (modified) radical mastectomy / breast-conserving therapy (BCT)

BCT:
- lumpectomy
- axillary dissection
- RT breast (60 Gy over 5 weeks)
- RT booster – iridium implant (25 Gy)

Indication for adjuvant chemotherapy and adjuvant parasternal RT same in both arms

Evaluation endpoints:
- survival
- locoregional control
- time to distant recurrence
- cosmesis and quality of life

Activated May 1980
Intake closed May 1986
Accrual: 903 patients

Stage of disease	No. of patients	
T1 N0-1a	153	stage I (153 patients)
T1 N1b	34	stage II (755 patients)
T2 N0–1a	569	
T2 N1b	152	

Fig. 1. Design of EORTC phase III trial 10801: breast-conserving therapy in operable breast cancer. (This information, as well as information in the text regarding this trial, is provided on behalf of the EORTC Breast Cancer Cooperative Group)

Necessarily, such variations in trial procedures can present problems in aggregating the study data. To minimize such problems, the centralized randomization procedure was so organized that there were equal numbers of patients in both study groups in each participating center. Nevertheless, it remains an empirical question as to whether it is appropriate to aggregate the data across treatment settings for purposes of statistical analysis. If this proves not to be the case, then it may be necessary to carry out the analyses based on particular substrata of the total sample. While this would yield a number of interesting "substudies" within the larger trial, it could also dilute the statistical power of the study (i.e., result in insufficient sample sizes).

This problem of interinstitutional variation in protocol procedures has led some to argue in favor of greater reliance on unicenter studies. Indeed, one would expect fewer protocol violations in a unicenter trial than is often the case in multicenter studies. Yet, in situations where very large sample sizes are required, or where the trial concerns a relatively rare tumor, a single center may not be capable of generating a sufficient number of patients within a realistic time. It is our general impression that a clinician's motivation to enter patients into a trial is inversely related to the length of time a trial has been running. Thus, one should not underestimate the impact of slow patient accrual on overall trial efficiency and quality.

A further potential disadvantage of unicenter studies concerns the issue of generalizability of findings. It is true that we can expect greater uniformity in the performance of clinical procedures within a single institution than across institutions. Such uniformity will increase the internal validity of a trial. Yet, in reality, interinstitutional variations do exist in the manner in which clinical procedures are carried out. For this reason, results derived from a multicenter trial may have greater external validity or generalizability than is the case with single-center studies.

An additional consideration that has become increasingly relevant when evaluating the validity of phase III clinical trials concerns the impact of informed consent procedures on the representativeness of study samples. While informed consent requirements currently vary from center to center, and from country to country, the trend is in the direction of the American model, which requires full informed consent, including information regarding the randomization procedures employed. While there is a good deal of controversy surrounding the ethics of informed consent, few would argue with the projection that more stringent informed consent requirements will result in an increase in the number of patients refusing to participate in trials. This can certainly be anticipated in trials such as those undertaken in early breast cancer, where there is a major difference in the degree of mutilation produced by the competing clinical procedures. If, as a result of informed consent, there is differential refusal to participate in trials on the basis of certain patient characteristics (e.g., age), then study conclusions may be valid for only a subset of the patient population of interest.

Survival and Local Recurrence as Evaluation Endpoints

Survival data (distant disease-free survival, recurrence-free survival) represent the primary evaluation endpoints in phase III trials. The most up-to-date actuarial curves provide us with the best information on survival and local recurrence, and inform us of the risk of treatment failures in relation to the period of follow-up.

To date, the few randomized studies where breast-conserving therapy is compared with radical mastectomy show superimposable curves, although the follow-up periods for these studies are still short [3,5,7,9,11]. The trial with the longest follow-up – 11 years – is the Milan study in which patients with T1 N0 disease receive either modified radical mastectomy or QUART (wide quadrantectomy, axillary dissection, and radiotherapy) [11].

An important feature of the Milan study is that a distinction is being made between true recurrences and new tumor formation (reoccurrence). This is particularly important in breast-conserving therapy, where reoccurrence is an unavoidable consequence of not removing all "at-risk" tissue. While it is sometimes difficult to distinguish between these two cases, a long disease-free interval, different histology, and localization in another quadrant strongly hint at the formation of a new tumor.

True local recurrences should appear later in the breast-conserving therapy group than in the mastectomy group due to the introduction of radiotherapy. Even if the overall number of true local recurrences is higher in the breast-conserving therapy group, they will appear at a later point in time than in the mastectomy group. This difference in time to recurrence is noted in many studies, and can explain the slightly better early survival rate for breast-conserving therapy noted in some trials. When breast-conserving surgery is performed without additional radiotherapy (e.g., as is the case in one of the subgroups of the NSABP trial) [3], locoregional recurrences occur more quickly. In the NSABP trial the number of such cases is relatively large, and in all probability will show an effect on survival. If so, this will confirm the findings of the first trial at Guy's Hospital, where inadequate local treatment resulted in a poorer prognosis [5].

As noted by VERONESI, following breast-conserving therapy in which radiotherapy is included, new tumors (reoccurrences) emerge later than the second primaries in the opposite breast [11]. When such new tumors are included in the analysis, the breast re(oc)currences will, in the long run, outnumber the local recurrences after mastectomy. However, because additional surgery can be performed following breast-conserving therapy, the effect of these re(oc)currences on survival will hopefully be small. To estimate more precisely the extent of the risk, large patient groups are needed with longer follow-up periods than have yet been achieved in the currently running randomized trials.

There is controversy regarding the expected cure rate following treatment of re(oc)curring breast cancer among patients treated with breast-conserving therapy. It has been postulated that the effectiveness of the additional treatment may be impaired by the previous disturbance of the lymph draining fields [8]. In any case, even if the prognosis of patients treated for re(oc)currences is as good as that found for any other new breast cancer, there is less than a 100% chance of cure. Hence, with breast-conserving therapy there is a fundamental elevation in risk as compared with those cases where no breast tissue has been left. It is clear that the risks associated with the formation of a new tumor are highest for young patients with small tumors (i.e., patients with less risk of death due to distant metastases). These patients have a greater number of years at risk for new tumor formation.

Quality of Life and Cosmesis as Evaluation Endpoints

Many investigators expect that survival and final local failure rate (accepting a number of secondary surgery patients) will be the same for patients treated with breast-conserving therapy and those receiving a mastectomy. In a certain sense it is not unreasonable to view such trials as "quality of life" investigations. Therefore, it is quite important that maximum effort be made to evaluate in a systematic manner the psychosocial impact of these two treatment approaches. Toward this end, the EORTC breast conservation trial includes an evaluation of a number of psychosocial endpoints of treatment – body image, fear of disease recurrence, overall satisfaction with treatment and, for the breast-conserving therapy group, satisfaction with the cosmetic results. These data are being collected via a short questionnaire administered 2 and 4 years following treatment.

While the quality of life data for the full trial have not yet been analyzed, a smaller, more intensive study of trial patients treated at the Netherlands Cancer Institute provides some illuminating findings [1]. Seventy-five women (31 radical mastectomy, RM; 44 breast-conserving therapy, BCT) were interviewed 2–4 years following treatment in the EORTC trial. The two groups were comparable with regard to age, marital status, social class, and time elapsed between treatment and interview. The results indicated that, compared to the RM group, the BCT group reported a significantly better body image and greater acceptance of bodily change, significantly fewer sexual problems, and less employment disability. There were no significant differences between the groups with regard to psychological status, pain, or quality of marital relationship. Contrary to expectations, heightened fear of disease recurrence was noted more frequently among the RM patients than among those receiving BCT (30% vs 18%), with differences in the reporting of such fears increasing as a function of patient age and time elapsed since treatment.

Approximately 90% of the BCT group reported one or more advantages associated with their treatment, as compared with only 50% of the RM patients. Avoidance of mutilation was the treatment advantage most frequently cited by the BCT patients, while greater confidence that the cancer had been adequately treated was the benefit most frequently mentioned by the RM patients.

Although 50% of the BCT patients reported substantial differences in feeling and appearance between the treated and the untreated breast, 88% reported moderate to high satisfaction with the cosmetic results of their treatment. With regard to overall satisfaction with treatment, 84% of the BCT group reported preference for the same treatment (i.e., BCT) should the need arise, while only one-third of the RM group would opt for RM again. These differences in satisfaction were even more pronounced when the question was framed in terms of what the patients would recommend to a friend or a daughter.

While these data indicate a significant psychosocial advantage of breast-conserving therapy over radical mastectomy, we await the results of the questionnaire used in the larger trial, as well as those from in-depth interviews conducted at other participating centers, before drawing final conclusions.

In addition to the patient-based data on quality of life, the EORTC trial will allow for independent ratings of cosmetic results. For all patients in the breast-conserving therapy arm of the trial, three photographs of the treated breast are taken at 2 and 4 years post treatment. These photos will be rated by a panel composed of surgeons, radiotherapists, and plastic surgeons. Standard evaluation forms will be used to assess the breast size and shape, skin color, nipple location, scar appearance, and overall cosmetic results (see Fig. 2). Eventually, we hope to have ratings performed by a lay panel as well.

It should be noted that a 4-year follow-up period for rating of cosmetic results was chosen primarily for reasons of practicality. However, this follow-up period may be inadequate for assessing the long-term cosmetic results of the treatment. If side effects such as fibrosis, tissue wasting, and teleangiectasias are noted at the

Instructions: For each of the breast characteristics presented below, please rate the treated breast *as compared to the untreated breast.*

a. Breast Size

0	1	2	3	4
no difference	a small difference	a moderate difference	a large difference	not evaluable

b. Breast Shape

0	1	2	3	4
no difference	a small difference	a moderate difference	a large difference	not evaluable

c. Skin Color

0	1	2	3	4
no difference	a small difference	a moderate difference	a large difference	not evaluable

d. Location of Areola and Nipple

0	1	2	3	4
no difference	a small difference	a moderate difference	a large difference	not evaluable

e. Shape of Areola and Nipple

0	1	2	3	4
no difference	a small difference	a moderate difference	a large difference	not evaluable

f. How would you rate the appearance of the surgical scars?

0 = Very unobtrusive
1 = Visible but not affecting cosmetic results
2 = Visible and detracting somewhat from cosmetic results
3 = Visible and detracting a great deal from cosmetic results
4 = Not evaluable

g. Overall, how would you rate the cosmetic results of this patient's breast treatment?

0 = Excellent
1 = Good
2 = Fair
3 = Poor
4 = Not evaluable

Fig. 2. EORTC Breast Cancer Cooperative Group protocol 10801: rating of cosmetic results of breast-conserving treatment

4-year mark, it may be desirable to extend the follow-up in order to evaluate long-term radiation effects.

An important set of data that will not be available from the EORTC trial concerns the cosmetic benefits of breast-conserving therapy versus breast reconstruction following mastectomy. In the EORTC trial breast reconstruction was not a standard procedure in the mastectomy arm. In fact, as far as we know, no trials are currently being conducted where such reconstruction is a standard part of the treatment. With the recently developed techniques of breast reconstruction with muscle-skin flaps, such a comparative study would be quite valuable. Figure 3

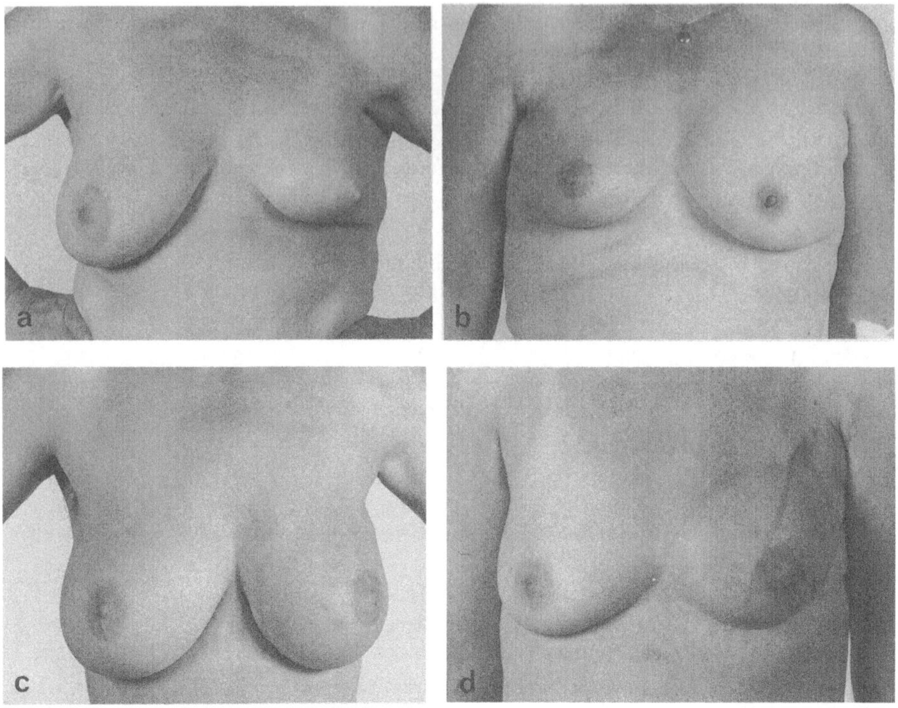

Fig. 3a-d. Cosmetic results of breast-conserving therapy and breast reconstruction. Variation in the quality of the cosmetic results presented in these photographs is based primarily on differences in breast shape and size: **a** poor cosmetic results; **b** fair/good cosmetic results; **c** excellent cosmetic results; **d** successful breast reconstruction

illustrates the range of cosmetic outcomes associated with breast-conserving treatment (poor, fair/good, and excellent), as well as an example of successful breast reconstruction.

Finally, it should be noted that the evaluation of cosmetic results should take patient subgroups into consideration. It is expected that the cosmetic quality of the surgery will vary as a function of certain patient characteristics. For example, we will be stratifying the sample according to tumor size. By means of such subgroup analyses we may be able to identify subsets of patients for whom breast-conserving therapy should not necessarily be advocated, at least from the perspective of improved cosmetic outcome.

Pooling Data of Subgroups

As has been hinted at several times in this paper, the pooling of data from patient subgroups can contribute importantly to establishing treatment policy for early breast cancer. Identification of the characteristics of patients with local re(oc)currences (which are postulated to result in a poorer long-term prognosis) may only be possible if data regarding this hopefully rare group of patients are pooled across trials. The reference population is easily available. We need only to collect data regarding the patient and tumor characteristics of all trial patients. Efforts in this direction have already been initiated by the EORTC Breast Cancer Cooperative Group. Similarly, if comparable data on trial patients who have undergone breast reconstruction were collected across studies, the type of cosmetic comparisons mentioned previously would be possible. This implies, of course, a standardization of data collection procedures across clinical trial groups. While this is no simple task, there is clearly much to be gained by working toward such a goal.

Conclusion

The evaluation of breast-conserving therapy is a complex undertaking. Of particular importance is long-term follow-up of trial patients. While we hope that the risk of re(oc)currence associated with such therapy is small, we know that such events often occur after a long period of time. It is essential that we obtain such data, as they can have important implications for the choice of treatment, particularly for younger patients with small tumors.

A second priority in evaluating the efficacy of breast-conserving therapy is to integrate assessment of quality of life into the standard battery of endpoints used in the evaluation of clinical outcome. This requires careful attention to the development of valid, reliable and standardized measures, as well as willingness to undertake the additional work associated with such assessment.

Finally, the desirability of undertaking more sophisticated subgroup analyses suggests the need for pooling of data from a number of trials. This is particularly important if we hope to undertake meaningful analyses of some of the rare events associated with early breast cancer and its treatment.

References

1. Aaronson NK, van Dongen JA, Bergman R, et al. (1987) The cosmetic results of breast conserving therapy. 4th EORTC Breast Cancer working conference, London
2. Bartelink H, van Dongen JA, Went G, et al. (1987) Does local control differ between stage I and II disease after breast conserving therapy? 4th EORTC Breast Cancer Working Conference, London
3. Fisher B, Bauer M, Margolese R, et al. (1985) Five-year results of a randomized clinical trial comparing total mastectomy and segmental mastectomy with or without radiation in the treatment of breast cancer. N Engl J Med 312(11):665–673
4. Harris JR, Recht A, Schnitt S, et al. (1985) Current status of conservative surgery and radiotherapy as primary local treatment for early carcinoma of the breast. Breast Cancer Res Treat 5(3):245–255
5. Hayward J (1978) Limited treatment in the management of early breast cancer. Cancer Treat Rep 62(7):983–987
6. Pierquin B, Mazeron JJ, Glaubiger D (1986) Conservative treatment of breast cancer in Europe, a review. Radiother Oncol 6(3):187–198
7. Sarrazin D, Dewar JA, Arriagada R, et al. (1986) Conservative management of breast cancer. Br J Surg 73(8):604–606

8. van Dongen JA (1983) Breast conserving therapy in operable breast cancer, a review. Eur J Cancer Clin Oncol 19(12):1741–1749
9. van Dongen JA, Bartelink H, van Dam FSAM, et al. (1985) EORTC 10801: the value of breast conserving therapy in operable breast cancer. 3rd EORTC Breast Cancer Working Conference, Amsterdam
10. van Dongen JA, Bartelink H, Aaronson N, et al. (1987) Randomized clinical trial to assess the value of breast conserving therapy in Stage I and Stage II breast cancer (EORTC trial 10801). 4th EORTC Breast Cancer Working Conference, London
11. Veronesi U, Banfi A, del Vecchio M, et al. (1986) Comparison of Halsted mastectomy with quadrantectomy, axillary dissection and radiotherapy in early breast cancer: long term results. Int J Cancer Clin Oncol 22(9):1085–1089

VI. Complications

Long-Term Complications of Surgery and Associated Irradiation as Breast-Conserving Therapy

G. KINDERMANN and T. GENZ

Introduction

A form of breast-conserving therapy for breast carcinoma initiated by H. LAX in 1963 has proved as good as radical surgery with respect to the patients' chances of survival in our long-term study comparing identical patient populations by means of the retrospective analysis technique of matched samples (matched for tumor size, nodal status, age, degree of histological differentiation, histological type, tumor localization etc.). The patients who underwent the breast-conserving therapy had no worse a result in 5- to 15-year survival than did patients subjected to ablative procedures [2,3]. The problem of local recurrence, however, was greater in the women treated with the breast-conserving therapy. Women who had undergone lumpectomy with subsequent radiotherapy had local recurrence twice as frequently [3] as women in whom ablation was performed, although local recurrence did not worsen the chances of survival [3]. These long-term results of the Berlin retrospective study are confirmed by prospective studies over a period of about 10 years so far: they also show a considerably higher rate of local recurrence but no lower chances of survival with breast-conserving therapy [1,4].

Patients

The breast-conserving operation performed as part of the treatment strategy between 1963 and 1985 was lumpectomy or quadrantectomy. From 1979 onward quadrantectomy was preferred whenever there were grounds for suspecting that ductal or lobular carcinoma was present. Concomitant lymphadenectomy was superficial up to 1979 (only sampling). From 1979 onward the type of lymphadenectomy performed was systematic dissection of the axillary and lower infraclavicular lymph nodes (levels I–II).

Radiotherapy, with a low focal dose compared with those given in the literature (telecobalt; 40–45 Gy) was delivered over two tangential fields to ensure homogeneous irradiation throughout the entire breast. Systemic treatment on the basis of lymph node status was not incorporated into the treatment design until 1979. These patients are not evaluated in the study.

Between January 1963 and December 1985, 354 patients underwent breast-conserving therapy (Table 1). The further course required a secondary mastectomy in 5% (17 patients) and later resection with retention of the breast remnant in 2%

Table 1. Course following lumpectomy, January 1963 to December 1985

	n	%
Patients subjected to surgery	354	
secondary mastectomy	17	5
secondary resection	8	2
Patients monitored	337	
Lost to follow-up	8	2
died	68	
still alive in June 1986	261	

(eight patients). All 354 patients were considered evaluable for postoperative sequelae. With reference to the long-term sequelae of the therapy as a whole and in particular of the radiotherapy, it is important to note that eight women (2%) were lost to follow-up in the observation period of up to 22 years.

In June 1986, 261 patients were still living and under observation; 66 had meanwhile died of the original illness.

Postoperative Sequelae

The term postoperative sequelae was considered to apply to all complications that occurred up to the start of radiotherapy – as a rule 4–6 weeks after the operation. Table 2 gives a review of the changes, some of which were treated by surgery and others by conservative procedures. Breast edema was diagnosed as a postoperative complication because of the mandatory mammogram performed before radiotherapy was started. Hematomas or seromas and postoperative hemorrhage were considered to include all alterations treated by conservative means (compression) or by an operative procedure (hemorrhage immediately after the operation, puncture of a hematoma/seroma).

Table 2. Breast-conserving therapy ($n=354$); postoperative sequelae

	n	%
Postoperative hemorrhage:		
corrective surgery	2	0.6
Hematoma	16	4.5
Seroma	2	0.6
Infection	8	2.3
Mammary edema	7	2.0
Impaired wound healing: slight	8	2.3

Sequelae of Irradiation

The sequelae of cobalt irradiation of the breast remnant are listed in Table 3. They were diagnosed by clinical or mammographic examination. While erythema, dermatitis and altered pigmentations were severe and caused the patients affected a great deal of distress, this was not true to the same degree for induration/sclerosis of the breast or for breast edema. The 45 patients with breast edema include seven in whom this had already been noted as a postoperative complication, since it was markedly exacerbated by the radiotherapy. The seven patients concerned therefore figure in both the postoperative and the postirradiation analyses. The breast edema improved or disappeared in 44 cases after some weeks or months of treatment. The same was true of the symptoms (heaviness of the breast, feeling of heat, increased size). Only one patient, who had very pronounced and also very painful breast edema, insisted on secondary mastectomy after conservative therapy had failed to provide any relief.

Despite the timing of its occurrence relative to the therapy, the pathogenesis of this postirradiation breast edema cannot be considered without reference to the lymphadenectomy performed before the radiotherapy. Edema was not verifiable by clinical or mammographic examination in the patients concerned in the early weeks after the operation; nonetheless a correlation with the extent of the lymphadenectomy can be documented (Table 4). While definite breast edema was seen in only 11 (6.8%) of the 162 patients who underwent the superficial lymphadenectomy practiced in the early years (sampling), it developed in 34 (17.7%) of the 192 patients subjected to the more radical lymphadenectomy performed since 1979.

Table 3. Breast-conserving therapy ($n = 354$): sequelae of radiation in breast remnant

	n	%
Edema	45	12.7
Erythema (pronounced)	6	1.7
Radiodermatitis	4	1.1
Altered pigmentation	5	1.4
Induration, sclerosis (apparent on mammography)	33	9.3
Teleangiectasia	7	1.9
Necrosis of skin	1	0.3

Table 4. Incidence of breast edema after radiotherapy, referred to extent of earlier lymphadenectomy performed as part of breast conserving therapy ($n = 354$)

Lymphadenectomy	Edema of breast	Therapy	
Superficial $n = 162$	11 (6.8%)	Conservative	44
Extensive $n = 192$	34 (17.7%)	Mastectomy	1

The second most frequent sequela of radiotherapy was the mammary induration and sclerosis revealed by the radiological examination. In this connection it was rare for the results of clinical examination or an impairment in the patient's well-being to correspond to the mammographic picture. So far as subjective well-being is concerned this sequela of irradiation, while recognizable within the breast, is not important for the vast majority of patients, though it does pose problems with diagnosis in the after-care period.

Extramammary Complications Following Breast-Conserving Surgery and Subsequent Radiotherapy

Table 5 shows that 10.5% of the patients had complications affecting vessels, nerves, joints and lungs, some of which were unequivocally interpreted as postoperative sequelae (sensitive nerves on the inner side of the upper arm) and others as complications of the radiotherapy (pulmonary fibrosis). The low proportion of patients with edema of the arm is probably attributable not least to the very superficial type of lymphadenectomy performed up to 1979. With increasingly radical lymphadenectomy an increase in the proportion of patients with subsequent edema of the arm must also be expected. It was also striking that in some cases edema started a long time after surgery and radiotherapy (Table 6), so that it was difficult to interpret it as a direct sequela of surgery.

Table 5. Breast-conserving therapy ($n=354$): extramammary complications after primary therapy

	n	%
Muscles	0	
Vessels: edema of arm	13	3.7
Nerves: sensitivity	4	1.1
Bones	0	
Joints: periarthritis	1	0.3
Lungs: fibrosis	19	5.4
Heart	0	

Table 6. Breast-conserving therapy ($n=354$): complications

	n	Months after operation Range	Median	Duration (months) Range	Median
Breast edema	45	0– 20	2.8	4–106	22.8
Induration, sclerosis	33	1– 57	6.0	10–204	90.5
Pulmonary fibrosis	19	2– 41	7.4		
Edema of arm	13	2– 12	4.7	7–36	17.0
Local relapse	21	6–120	37.0		

Onset and Duration of Complications

If local recurrence is included as the most important complication of breast-conserving therapy, the interval during which sequelae and complications can arise after the therapy is a particularly long one. The time to diagnosis of intramammary local recurrence varied between 6 and 120 months, with an average of 37 months. In the case of pulmonary fibrosis diagnosed by radiological examination after radiotherapy, the diagnosis was made between the 2nd and the 41st month after the primary therapy. There were also wide differences in the time of diagnosis of edema of the breast or induration/sclerosis by mammography, ranging from the immediate postoperative period to years after completion of the entire combination therapy. This phenomenon was paralleled by a very variable duration of the changes, which ranged from 4 to 104 months, with an average of 22.8 months, in the case of breast edema, and from 10 to 204 months, with an average of 90.5 months, in the case of induration and sclerosis of the breast.

Summary

Among 354 women who underwent breast-conserving therapy between 1. 1. 1963 and 31.12. 1985 (lumpectomy, lymphadenectomy, postoperative irradiation to the breast remnant with telecobalt) intramammary local recurrence was observed as the most significant complication in 6%. Postoperative complications were observed in 12.1% of patients, among whom surgical correction was necessary in 0.6% because of postoperative hemorrhage and in 5.1% because of puncture of a hematoma or seroma. In 10.5% of patients there were complications resulting partly from surgery and partly from radiotherapy, including pulmonary fibrosis in 5.4% of cases and edema of the arm in 3.7%. Among the complications that did not appear until after radiotherapy or became much worse following radiotherapy the most common was breast edema, occurring in 12.7% of patients; this improved or disappeared altogether in all patients but one. It was possible to document a connection between postirradiation breast edema and the degree of radicality of the preceding lymphadenectomy. The long-term study showed that some of the complications did not appear until many months or years after completion of the treatment. The exceptionally wide range in the time interval between the completion of therapy and the onset of complications suggests that predisposing factors may also play a part in their occurrence. It was not, however, possible to clarify this point in the course of the study.

References

1. Fischer B, Bauer M, Margolese R, Poisson R, Pilch Y, Redmond C, Fisher E, et al. (1985) Five-year results of a randomized clinical trial comparing total mastectomy and segmental mastectomy with or without radiation in the treatment of breast cancer. N Engl J Med 312:665
2. Genz T, Schmidt-Gollwitzer M, Pachaly J, Meyer RD, Lax H, Kindermann G (1986) Die brusterhaltende Karzinomtherapie. Geburtshilfe Frauenheilk 46:567–572
3. Kindermann G, Genz T (1985) A comparison between the results of simple mastectomy and tumorectomy for breast cancer: the problem of local recurrence. Arch Gynecol 237:67–73
4. Veronesi U, Costa A (1982) The role of surgery. In: Baum M (ed) Clinics in oncology. Saunders, Philadelphia

Long-Term Complications of Breast-Conserving Treatment: Experience with the Basel Lumpectomy Protocol

R. Hünig, E. Walther, F. Harder, A.C. Almendral, J. Torhorst, and J. Roth

The effectiveness of a cancer therapy can be measured by the following criteria:

1. The oncological result as expressed by locoregional control, disease-free survival and overall survival
2. Treatment-related side effects

Among similarly effective treatment methods, the best is the one with the lowest incidence of morbidity and least discomfort for the patient. The oncological result of breast-conserving treatment in suitable patients corresponds today to that of radical mastectomy with axillary dissection [1, 4–6, 8, 10, 11, 13, 14]. Our aim should therefore be not only to improve disease-free survival, but also to reduce the incidence of treatment-related side effects to a minimum.

The duration of the radiation treatment seldom poses problems for the patient, although a few prefer a mastectomy for this reason. Nonetheless, it is principally the non-oncological treatment effects which determine the practicability of breast-conserving therapy as well as the quality of the result.

Potential radiation-induced side effects are categorized into acute (occurring during irradiation), intermediate (occurring days or weeks after completion of radiotherapy) and late (occurring months to years after completion of radiotherapy). An acute reaction is characterized by hyperthermia, erythema of the skin, lymphedema of the breast and hyperpigmentation. The intermediate reaction also presents with hyperthermia, hyperpigmentation and lymphedema of the breast, as well as induration at the site of the primary and radiation pneumonitis. Late side effects are hyperpigmentation, lymphedema of the ipsilateral arm, teleangiectasias in the boost region, fibrosis of the tumor bed, the whole breast or the overlapping area of two irradiation fields ("matchline effect"), osteoradionecrosis of ribs, lung fibrosis, a second primary or a tumor in the contralateral breast.

There is a probability that all the mentioned non-oncological local radiation-induced side effects can be enhanced by the administration of a simultaneous or sequential adjuvant chemotherapy [2, 3, 7, 9, 12]. By the same token, the extent of the surgical procedure determines the likelihood of lymphedema – not only of the arm but also of the breast, as well as the degree of fibrosis in the region of the primary.

The oncological result of a breast-preserving therapy is influenced by a multitude of factors, including unknown specific characteristics of the patient herself, location, extent and specific qualities of the tumor and treatment technique. Treatment-related side effects are also strongly influenced by unknown individual qualities of the patient, a fact which becomes very obvious in a strictly defined treatment. Furthermore, the treatment concept and the anatomy of the treated breast also influence side effects and risks of treatment.

The Basel Protocol

In 1976, at the University Hospital in Basel, a team consisting of a surgeon, a gynecologist, a pathologist and two radiation oncologists defined a protocol for breast-preserving therapy, after visiting medical centers with experience in the field. The following two goals were defined:

1. Locoregional recurrences, cosmetically unsatisfying results and treatment-related non-oncological side effects should be reduced to a minimum.
2. Strict adherence to protocol guidelines should provide the possibility of recognizing risk factors and lead to an improvement of protocol design.

The previous valid eligibility criteria are as follows:

- Unilateral carcinoma
- Maximum age 70 years
- Pathological tumor stage T_{1-2} (maximum diameter 3 cm), N_{0-1}
- Breast size and composition suitable for radiotherapy
- No pregnancy
- No lactation within previous 6 months
- No multicentric, retroareolar or inflammatory cancers
- No Paget's disease
- No distant metastases
- Patient agreeable to submit to specified follow-up examinations
- Informed consent signed

The maximal tumor diameter should not exceed 3 cm in the pathological specimen, breast size and consistence should allow a homogeneous distribution of the irradiation dose and the follow-up should be performed by one of the two radiation oncologists involved.

In defining the radiotherapeutic part of the protocol we had two aims in mind: (1) To achieve optimal dose homogeneity in the target volume. (2) To apply intensive radiation treatment with maximal sparing of healthy tissue.

The radiotherapy concept of the protocol which was activated in 1977 is shown in Table 1. This concept was applied to all patients treated with breast-preserving surgery, independent of tumor site and stage. According to protocol guidelines the breast and chest wall were irradiated with 4 MV Linac photons using opposing tangential fields corrected with wedge filters if necessary, up to a dose of 50 Gy with a daily dose of 2 Gy applied five times per week. The dose was calculated to the isodose encompassing the target volume. This corresponded in most cases to the

Table 1. Basel protocol: original radiotherapy concept

Target volume	Dose	Dose calculation	Treatment duration (days)	Radiation type
Breast	50	Isodose	33	Linac photons
Boost	21	Isodose	9–11	Betatron electrons
Internal mammary	48	Isodose	32	Linac photons Betatron electrons
Axilla	52	Midplane	50[a]	Linac photons
Supraclavicular	52	Midplane	50[a]	Linac photons

[a] Including 2-week break

90% isodose, assuming that 100% represented the maximum dose within the treated volume.

An optimal homogeneous dose distribution for the breast and chest wall is shown in Fig. 1. The boost was applied with Betatron electrons to a minimal field size of 6 × 6 cm. The energy chosen lay between 5 and 15 MeV and was adapted to breast size, enabling the 80% isodose to reach the chest wall. The dose calculated at the 80% isodose was 3 Gy for seven sessions (Fig. 2).

All regional lymph nodes were also irradiated. The ipsilateral axillary and supraclavicular regions received 52 Gy Linac photons in 50 days (with a break of

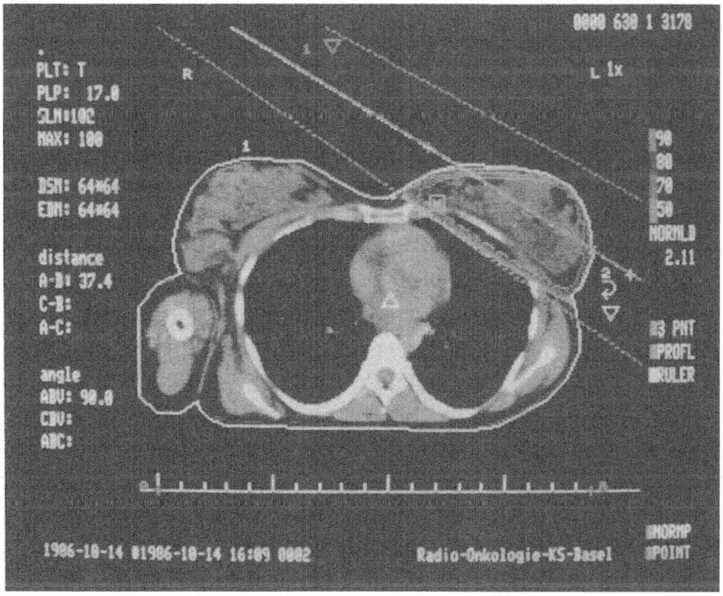

Fig. 1. Dose distribution in the breast and chest wall for 4 MV linac photons with opposing wedged fields (dose maximum = 100%). The target volume is encompassed by the 90% isodose

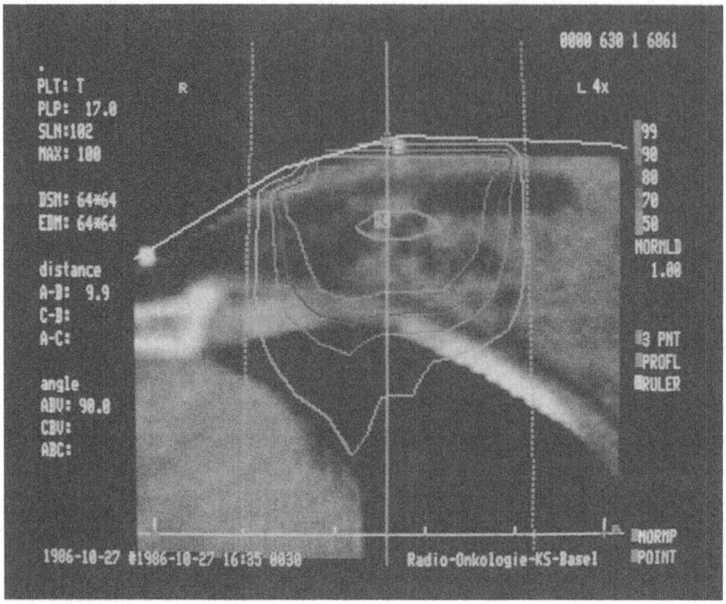

Fig. 2. Boost irradiation of the primary tumor site according to the original 1977 concept: with 20 MeV electrons the 80% isodose reaches the chest wall. The maximum dose is in the center of the target volume

14 days), calculated midplane in the central axis using parallel opposed fields. The internal mammary lymph nodes were treated with 48 Gy in 32 days. Half of the dose was applied with Linac photons, the other half with Betatron electrons, the dose was calculated for the encompassing isodose; for the electrons this was at least the 80% isodose. We chose to mix electrons and photons in order to minimize treatment-induced morbidity to the sternum and mediastinal structures. Figure 3 shows the dose distribution of 4 MV photons, illustrating the deep-lying 50% isodose. Figure 4 demonstrates the advantages of the combined photon and electron isodose in a 1:1 relation. The target volume is encompassed by the 90% isodose.

We decided to treat the axillary and supraclavicular lymph nodes using parallel opposed fields in order to reduce dose inhomogeneities in the target volume and avoid the ugly matchline effect toward the border of the breast field. As illustrated in Fig. 4 a direct ventral field allows only 82% of the 4 MV photon dose to reach a depth of 7 cm, which on the average corresponds to the midplane of the axilla. With the application of 200 cGy to the target volume the ventral dose maximum reaches 244 cGy. The somewhat painstaking technique of parallel opposed fields (Fig. 4b) allows the axillary lymph nodes to be encompassed by the 90% isodose, 100% corresponding to the maximum dose.

In all techniques using parallel opposed fields, both ventral and dorsal fields were treated daily.

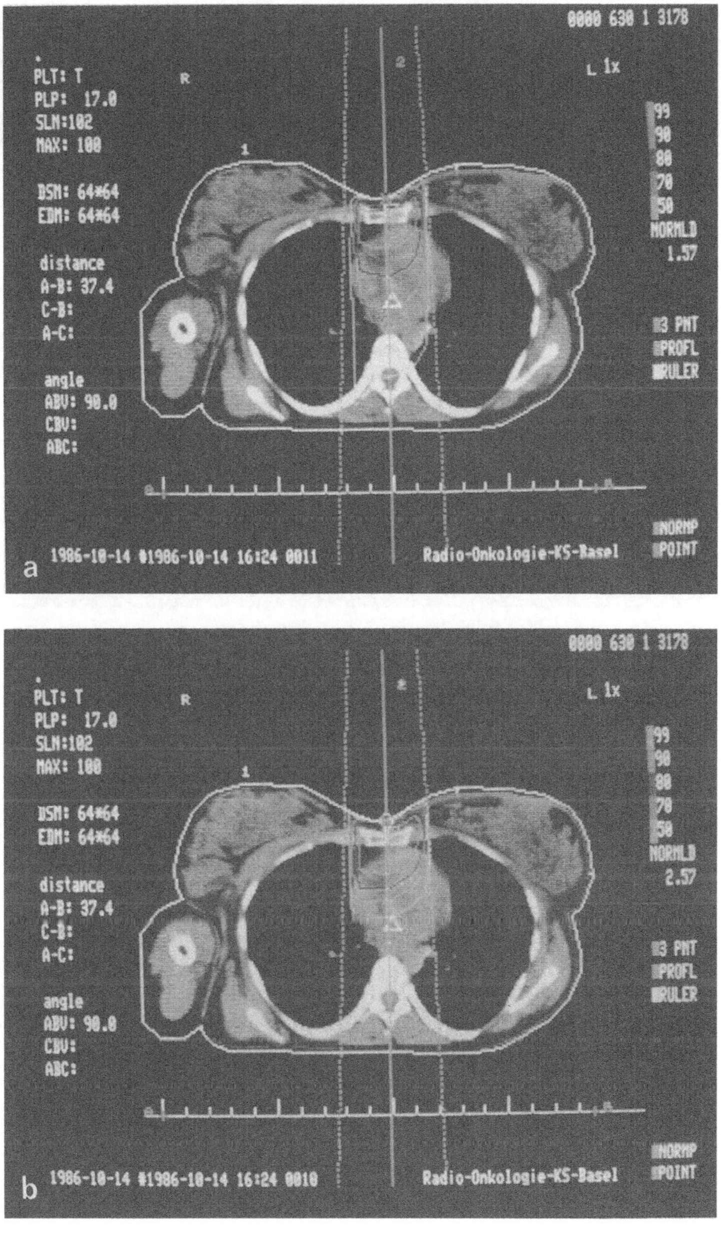

Fig. 3a,b. Dose distribution in the internal mammary lymph nodes. **a** For 4 MV photons: The 50% isodose reaches the spinal cord, the mediastinum receives a high radiation dose. **b** For 50% 4 MV Linac photons and 50% 15 MeV Betatron electrons: The 90% isodose encompasses the target volume, the 50% hardly reaches the middle of the thorax

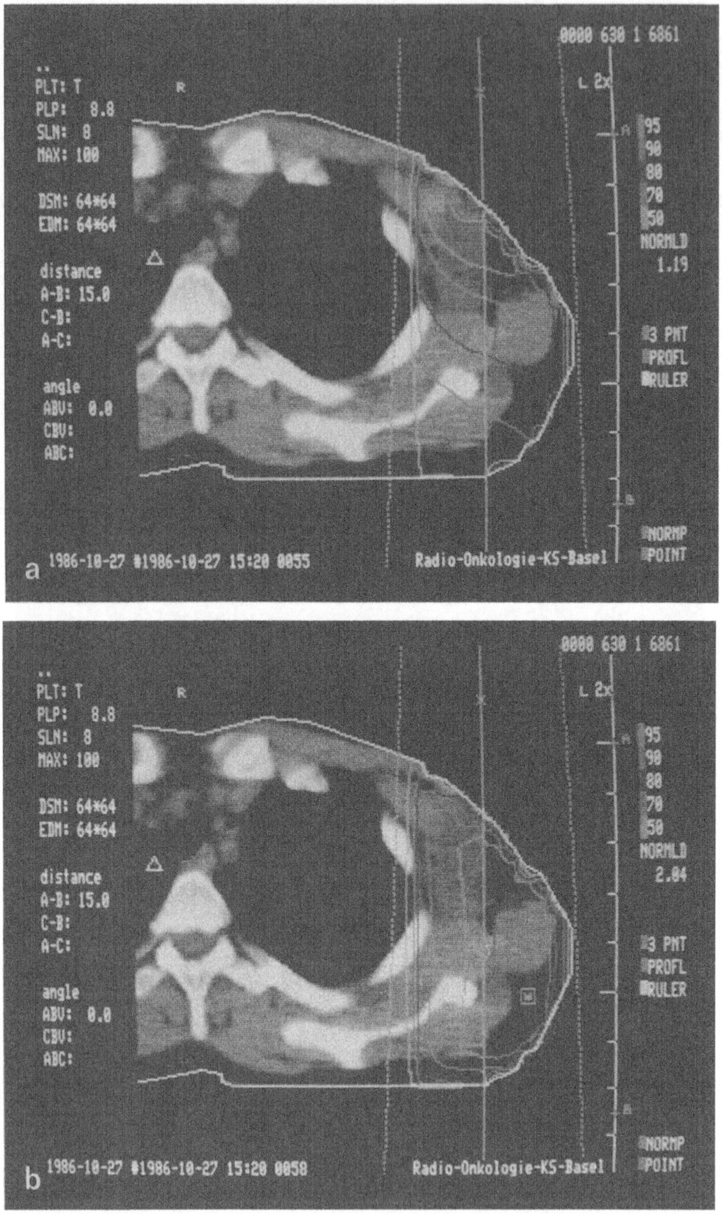

Fig. 4a,b. Dose distribution in the axillary lymph nodes for 4 MV Linac photons. **a** Irradiation with a direct ventral field: the difference between maximum dose and target dose (middle of the axilla) is 18%. **b** Irradiation with opposing ventral and dorsal fields: the difference between maximum dose and target dose (90% isodose) is only 10%

Clinical Data

Of the 369 patients treated according to the Basel protocol between 1.1.77 and 31.12.86, 201 patients treated up to 31.12.84, with 31.12.85 serving as cut-off date, have been evaluated. Of these 201 patients, 198 (99%) had a complete follow-up. Three patients had an incomplete follow-up; two of them were living abroad and one could not be motivated to appear for regular check-ups. The median follow-up for this group was 46 months.

Table 2 shows the age distribution. The largest subgroup (39%) was in the 40- to 49-year range. The stage distribution as depicted in Table 3, with 24% T_2 and 32% N_1 cases, is comparable to other studies including T_2 tumors. It is interesting to note that a meticulous examination of the pathologic specimen showed that the tumor reached the resection margin in 18.5% of cases. In 4.5% of patients the resection margin could not be evaluated reliably.

Only seven patients had less than five axillary lymph nodes excised, as required in the protocol. On average, 13 lymph nodes were excised.

Table 2. Age distribution of the first 201 patients treated

Age (years)	*n*	%
20–29	8	4
30–39	40	20
40–49	78	39
50–59	50	25
60–69	23	11
70–79	2	1
Total	201	100

Table 3. Stage distribution of the first 201 patients treated

	N_0	N_1	Total
T_{is}	11		11 (5%)
T_1	92	30	122 (61%)
T_2	34	34	68 (34%)
Total	137 (68%)	64 (32%)	201 (100%)

Treatment Results

Table 4 illustrates the pattern of first relapse in relation to pathologic tumor stage and shows that seven patients developed a malignancy in the contralateral breast. With a median follow-up period of 46 months the local recurrence rate was 6.5%, of which 4% were in the region of the primary tumors, 1.5% manifested themselves in a different quadrant of the breast and 1% were inflammatory. This result corresponds well to the recurrence rate expected under strict adherence to protocol guidelines. This also holds true for disease-free survival (Fig. 5a) and locoregional recurrence-free survival rates (Fig. 5b) as shown with the life-table analysis in the KAPLAN-MEIER curves as well as for the result of a multivariant analysis of various risk factors, which cannot be discussed further here. It should be mentioned, however, that with a maximum follow-up of 9 years no secondary radiation-induced malignancy was observed.

The frequency and severity of late treatment side effects can be appreciated only in the context of the technical and clinical data presented above. Table 5 describes the post-therapeutic complications encountered. A grading system was established to measure the extent of telangiectasis and induration in the primary tumor area: grade I, none; grade II, mild; grade III, moderate; grade IV, severe. A complication was defined as a distinct, esthetically relevant reaction (grade II–III) present during the last 4 months preceding cut-off date.

The normal outcome of a treatment according to our protocol is illustrated in Fig. 6a, a discrete reaction (grade II) in the boost region in Fig. 6b. Figure 6c shows a patient with a grade III reaction. Telangiectasis is distinctly recognizable; the outline of the breast and subcutis in the boost region, however, are unaltered. A severe reaction, grade IV, is shown in Fig. 6d, where extensive telangiectasis is combined with a subcutaneous induration and deformation of the breast.

Arm edema is defined as a complication when the increase in circumference compared to the contralateral arm exceeds 3 cm. Postoperative measurements often

Table 4. Pattern of first relapse and contralateral cancers among the first 201 patients treated (median follow-up 46 months)

Pathologic stage	n	Ipsilateral Near primary	Distant primary	Unknown[a]	Contra lateral breast	Axilla	Distant metastasis
T_{is}	11	1			1		
$T_1 N_0$	92	3			2	1	6
$T_1 N_1$	30	1	1	1[a]	3[b]		5
$T_2 N_0$	34		1			1	1
$T_2 N_1$	34	3	1	1	1	2	9
Total	201	8	3	2	7	4	21
%	100	4	1.5	1	3.5	2	10

[a] Inflammatory recurrence
[b] Simultaneous breast recurrence and contralateral cancer

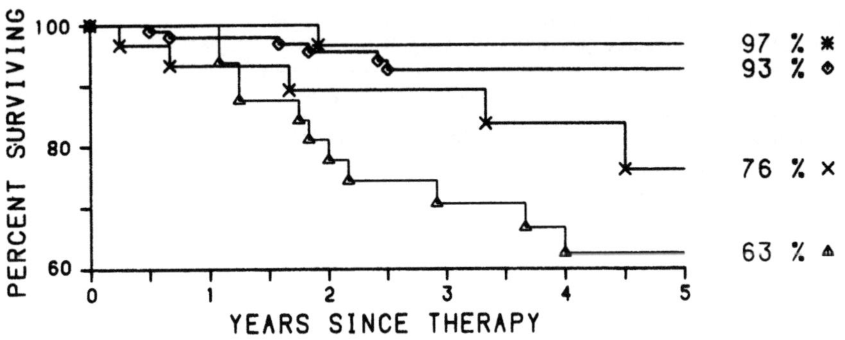

—◆—	103	103	100	85	73	62	54	51	43	38	34	TO-1 NO
—✱—	34	34	34	31	28	24	23	18	1.5	1.2	9	T2 NO
—×—	30	29	28	24	22	20	16	14	12	11	8	T1 N1
—▲—	34	34	34	27	24	21	19	18	16	14	1.2	T2 N1

CALCULATION ACCORDING TO KAPLAN AND MEIER (1958).

a THE SMALL NUMBERS BELOW THE TIME-AXIS INDICATE THE PATIENTS AT RISK.

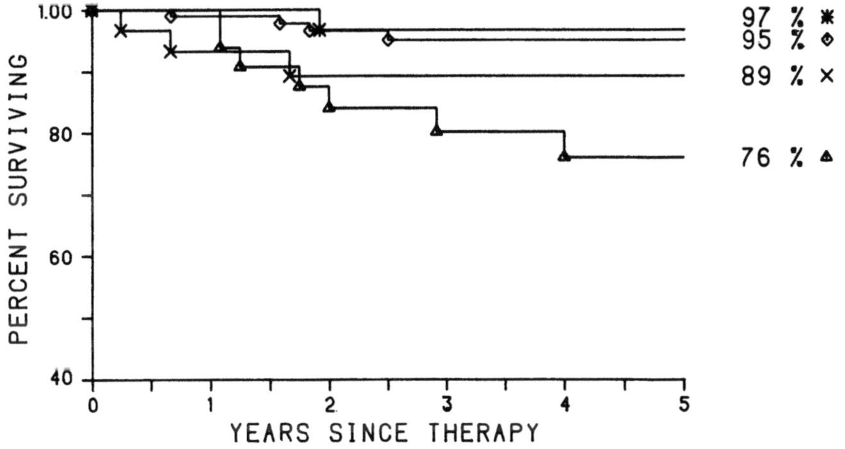

—◆—	103	103	101	86	74	64	56	53	44	38	34	TO-1 NO
—✱—	34	34	34	31	28	24	23	18	15	12	9	T2 NO
—×—	30	29	28	24	22	20	16	15	13	12	10	T1 N1
—▲—	34	34	34	28	25	23	21	20	19	17	14	T2 N1

CALCULATION ACCORDING TO KAPLAN AND MEIER (1.958).

b THE SMALL NUMBERS BELOW THE TIME-AXIS INDICATE THE PATIENTS AT RISK.

Fig. 5a,b. Kaplan-Meier curves for **a** disease-free and **b** locoregional recurrence-free survival, calculated for the first 201 patients treated according to the Basel protocol (original 1977 concept). Cut-off date 31.12.1985, median follow-up 46 months, no adjuvant chemotherapy

Table 5. Incidence and type of the late complications among the first 201 patients treated (median follow-up 46 months)

Type	*n*	%
No complications	147	73
Teleangiectasias and/or induration in the primary tumor area	43	21
Rib fractures	6	3
Arm edema	9	4.5
Breast fibrosis	4	2
Mastectomy for breast fibrosis	1	0.5
Erysipelas	7	3.5

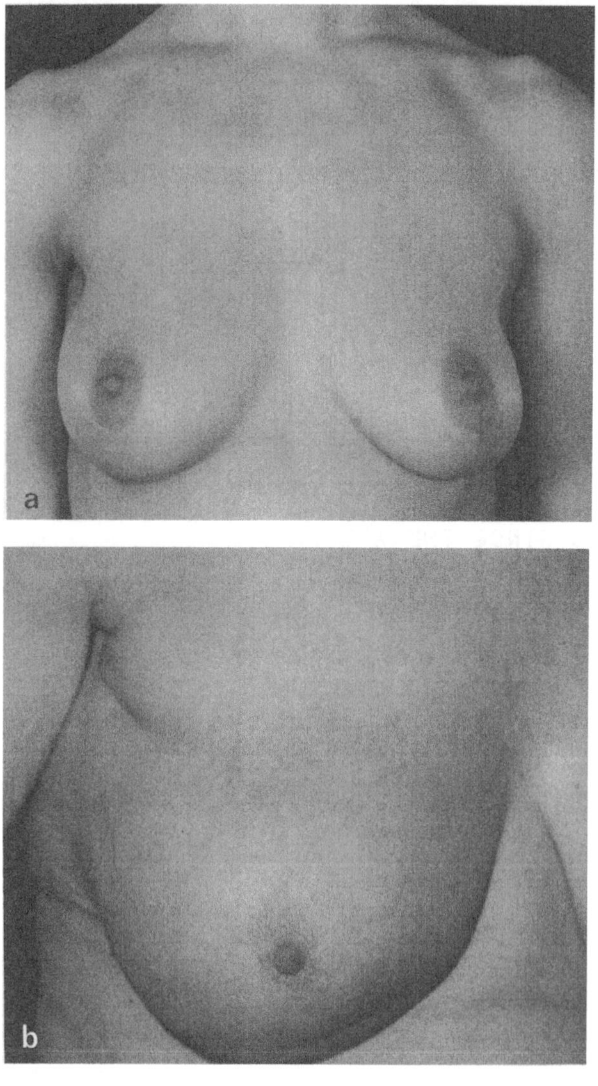

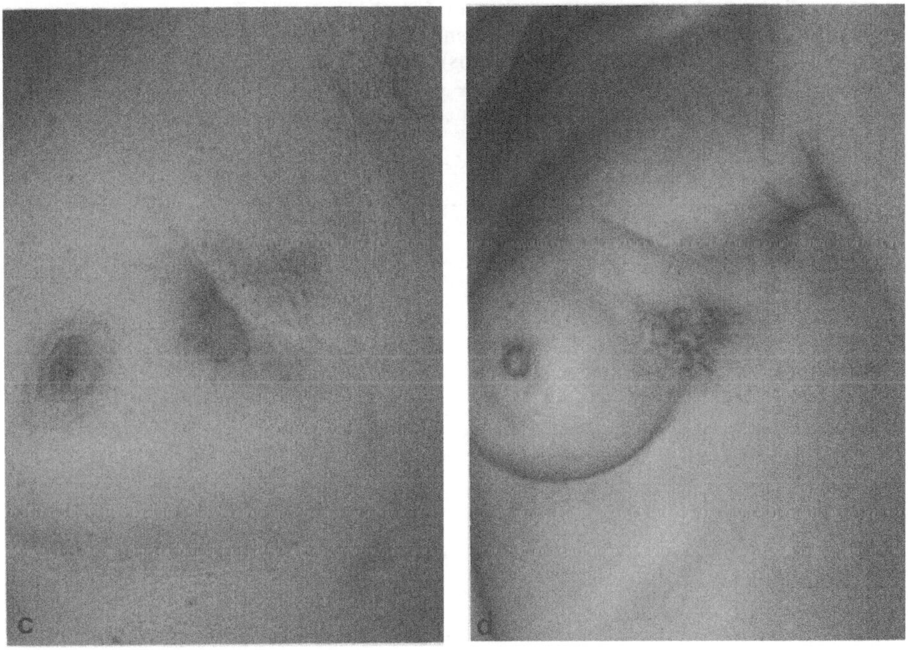

Fig. 6a-d. Late sequelae in the boost region. **a** Grade I: no treatment sequelae; **b** grade II: discrete telangiectasis and/or fibrosis; **c** grade III: moderate telangiectasis and/or fibrosis; **d** grade IV: severe telangiectasis and/or fibrosis

reveal preexisting small differences in circumference, sometimes even to the disadvantage of the contralateral arm.

Relatively severe fibrosis and shrinkage of the treated breast was observed in three heavy smokers and in one non-smoker with a normal-sized breast and good surgical result. One of the heavy smokers developed persistent pains in the fibrotic breast, which had to be amputated. There was no tumor in the pathological specimen.

As shown in Table 5, 73% of all patients had no complications, 21% developed severe telangiectasis and /or induration at the site of the primary which received the booster dose, 3% had asymptomatic osteoradionecrosis of the ribs and 4.5% had arm edema. It is interesting that 3.5% of the patients, who did not necessarily have lymphedema of arm or breast, developed erysipelas.

It is obvious that the risk of arm edema increases with the number of excised lymph nodes. Of the patients who had more than 20 lymph nodes excised, 13% developed a lymphedema in the ipsilateral arm (Table 6).

We had no cases of symptomatic radiation pneumonitis or lung fibrosis. Chest X-rays of numerous patients, however, showed opacification in the ipsilateral lung apex, resembling that of tuberculosis, due to irradiation of supraclavicular nodes.

The cosmetic results after a median follow-up of 46 months can be considered as good to excellent in 60% of patients and satisfactory in 24% (Table 7). The reason for this not entirely satisfying outcome might lie in the fact that one-third of our patients were operated on by surgeons and gynecologists outside of our hospital

Table 6. Relationship between number of lymph nodes dissected and incidence of lymphedema in the ipsilateral arm (median follow-up 46 months)

Lymph nodes	No. of patients	Arm edema	
		n	%
1-4	22	0	0
5-10	70	2	3
11-20	86	4	5
Over 20	23	3	13
Total	201	9	4,5

Table 7. Medical judgment of the cosmetic result in the first 201 patients treated (median follow-up 46 months)

	n	%
Good to excellent	117	58.5
Moderate	49	24.5
Poor	23	11.5
Secondary breast amputation	11	5.5

who were not acquainted with surgical protocol guidelines and did not have the necessary experience. A comparative study was initiated to quantify this impression.

Conclusions

What were the consequences for the development of new protocol guidelines, considering the complications described earlier and benefiting from the experience accumulated in other medical centers throughout the years? This question is answered by the description of our 1985 modified protocol, in which premenopausal patients with a stage pN_1 tumor also receive adjuvant chemotherapy (Table 8). The breast and chest wall receive 50 Gy in 5 weeks as before. A boost is not applied when adjuvant chemotherapy for stage pN_1 is given and the primary had been excised with histologically negative margins. The boost-dose is: 20 Gy in 10 fractions in 2 weeks for a pN_0 stage and histologically positive or questionable excision margins; 10 Gy in five fractions in 1 week for a pN_0 stage and negative excision margins and for a pN_1 stage with histologically suspect or positive excision margins.

The impact of the modified fractionation and differentiation of the boost dose on the cosmetic outcome is not yet clear. The accumulated data allow the application of 10 Gy or total omission of the boost in certain cases. Thus far there is no convincing argument for giving up our technique of boost application with electrons in favor of interstitial iridium implantation.

Table 8. Basel protocol: modified radiotherapy concept

Target volume	Radiotherapy indicated	Dose (Gy)
Breast	Always	50
Boost	N_0; N_1, if resection margins positive or uncertain[a]	10 or 20[b]
Internal mammary	Central or medial tumor	48
Axilla and supraclavicular	Tumor infiltration of axillary fat	48

[a]In conjunction with adjuvant chemotherapy
[b]For "low-risk" and "high-risk" cases respecticely

The internal mammary lymph nodes are irradiated only if the primary was situated centrally or in a medial quadrant of the breast and no adjuvant chemotherapy is employed. Continuation of this procedure is, however, uncertain. The irradiation of the axillary and supraclavicular lymph nodes is omitted unless the tumor invades the axillary fat or less than eight lymph nodes have been resected. The applied dose is 48 Gy.

In conclusion, the relation between the frequency and severity of complications and the oncological result in patients treated since 1976 according to the Basel protocol is encouraging. The protocol modifications realized in 1985 will hopefully influence this relation favorably. The impact of the combined radio- and chemotherapy of pN_1 patients on the manifestation of late reactions and complications remains unclear. In order to collect sufficient data to answer these questions as soon as possible, cooperation between groups active in this field is very desirable.

References

1. Amalric R, Santamaria F, Robert F, Seigle J, Altschuler C, Kurtz JM, Spitalier JM, et al. (1982) Radiation therapy with or without primary limited surgery for operable breast cancer: a 20-year experience of the Marseilles Cancer Institute. Cancer 49:30–34
2. Beadle GF, Come S, Henderson C, Silver B, Hellman S, Harris JR (1984) The effect of adjuvant chemotherapy on the cosmetic results after primary radiation treatment for early stage breast cancer. Int J Radiat Oncol Biol Phys 10:2131–2137
3. Botnick LE, Come S, Rose CM, Goldstein M, Lange R, Tishler S, Schnipper L (1983) Primary breast irradiation and concomitant adjuvant chemotherapy. In: Harris J, Hellman S, Silen W (eds) Conservative management of breast cancer. Lippincott, Philadelphia, pp 321–328
4. Calle R, Vilcoq JR, Pilleron JP, Schlienger P, Durand JC (1983) Conservative treatment of operable breast carcinoma by irradiation with or without limited surgery – ten-year results. In: Harris JR, Hellman S, Silen W (eds) Conservative management of breast cancer. Lippincott, Philadelphia, pp 3–9
5. Danoff BF, Haller DG, Glick JH, Goodman RL (1985) Conservative surgery and irradiation in the treatment of early breast cancer. Ann Intern Med 102:634–642
6. Fisher B, Bauer M, Margolese R, Poisson R, Pilch Y, Redmond C, Fisher E, et al. (1985) Five-year results of a randomized clinical trial comparing total mastectomy and

segmental mastectomy with or without radiation in the treatment of breast cancer. N Engl J Med 312:665–673

7. Glick JH, Danoff B, Haller D, Weiler C, Hurwitz S, Richter M, Goodman R (1984) Integration of adjuvant chemotherapy with definitive radiotherapy for primary breast cancer. In: Jones SE, Salmon SE (eds) Adjuvant therapy of cancer IV. Grune and Stratton, New York, pp 291–300
8. Harris JR, Beadle GF, Hellman S (1984) Clinical studies on the use of radiation therapy as primary treatment of early breast cancer. Cancer 53:705–711
9. Lichter AS, Lippman ME, Gorrell CR, d'Angelo TM, Edwards BK, DeMoss EV (1983) Adjuvant chemotherapy in patients treated primarily with irradiation for localized breast cancer. In: Harris J, Hellman S, Silen W (eds) Conservative management of breast cancer. Lippincott, Philadelphia, pp 299–310
10. Montague ED, Gutierrez AE, Barker JL, Tapley ND, Fletcher GH (1979) Conservation surgery and irradiation for the treatment of favorable breast cancer. Cancer 43:1058–1061
11. Pierquin B, Owen R, Maylin C, Otmezguine Y, Raynal M, Mueller W, Hannoun S (1980) Radical radiation therapy of breast cancer. Int J Radiat Oncol Biol Phys 6:17–24
12. Ray GR, Fish VJ, Marmor JB, Rogoway W, Kunshlan P, Arnold C, Lee RH, Marzoni F (1984) Impact of adjuvant chemotherapy on cosmesis and complications in stage I and II carcinoma of the breast treated by biopsy and radiation therapy. Int J Radiat Oncol Biol Phys 10:837–841
13. Sarrazin D, Le M, Rouesse J, Contesso G, Petit J-Y, Lacour J, Viguier J, Hill C (1984) Conservative treatment versus mastectomy in breast cancer tumors with macroscopic diameter of 20 millimeter or less. The experience of the Institut Gustave-Roussy. Cancer 53:1209–1213
14. Veronesi U, Saccozzi R, Del-Vecchio M, Banfi A, Clemente C, De-Lena M, Gallus G, et al. (1981) Comparing radical mastectomy with quadrantectomy, axillary dissection, and radiotherapy in patients with small cancers of the breast. N Engl J Med 301 (1):6–11

The German Breast Cancer Study I: Preliminary Results of Breast-Conserving Treatment Dependent on Radiation Technique*

R. SAUER, J. DUNST, H. RAUSCHECKER, A. SCHAUER, and
M. SCHUMACHER

Recruitment of patients for the national multicenter treatment project began on 1 November 1983, following a pilot period of over 3 years. The protocol is designed to allow comparison of simple mastectomy against excision of the primary tumor with subsequent radiation of the breast with reference to the local recurrence rate and disease-free survival in patients with breast cancer classified pathohistologically as pT1 pN0 M0. [13]. The results of several controlled studies comparing simple mastectomy with the ROTTER-HALSTED procedure [2,7,9] justified the early view of simple mastectomy as standard therapy in this early tumor stage. Retrospective studies, especially in France, Scandinavia, and the USA, subsequently gave rise to the suspicion that breast-conserving treatment might be just as satisfactory as radical surgery [1,3–5,10–12,14,15,17]. But even now the NSABP-06 protocol (National Surgical and Breast Project) has been published [8], the equal value of the two procedures still cannot be regarded as confirmed.

Study Design

Following the usual clinical diagnostic examinations to exclude the presence of distant metastases, patients with clinically proven early breast cancer T1 N0 M0 initially undergo tumorectomy with resection of all palpable tumor and a small amount of surrounding tissue. A lower axillary dissection (level I and II) with removal of at least six lymph nodes is also performed.

Only patients presenting pathohistologically confirmed pT1 pN0 M0 breast cancer may enter the protocol. Multifocal and multicentric tumors are excluded.

Following the pathohistological staging, the patients are informed that they will be participating in a clinical trial and also told about the treatment modalities and their advantages and possible disadvantages. After informed consent, patients are randomized to one of two treatment arms: mastectomy or breast irradiation. Women who refuse randomization (more than 90% of these eligible) but are willing to be treated according to the protocol can choose one of the two treatment modalities and are then considered as the cohort group. A prerandomization as performed in other protocols [8,17] is considered inappropriate in clinical trials because of the legal situation in our country.

*Sponsored by the Bundesministerium für Forschung und Technologie (BMFT)

Irradiation Technique and Dosage

The radiation volume includes the whole breast. If the tumor is sited medially or centrally, the parasternal and the supra- and infraclavicular lymph drainage regions are also irradiated, regardless of the treatment modality to which the patient has been allocated. We do not include the surgically treated axilla in the radiation volume because of the low risk of axillary recurrences in node-negative patients.

The radiation therapy is performed using 4- to 6-MV linear accelerators or cobalt-60 machines, employing tangential opposing portals with wedge filters for treating the breast. The total dose to the whole breast should not exceed 50 Gy in 25 fractions during a period of 5 weeks. A boost of 12 Gy in four fractions is given to the tumor bed.

To standardize the dosage in the participating institutions, the single dose and the total dose are calculated for a reference point in the middle of the breast at least 2 cm below the skin. The dose inhomogeneity within the target volume should be less than 10% when using a linear accelerator and less than 20% with a cobalt machine (Fig. 1).

The supraclavicular and parasternal lymphatics are treated using an AP portal, with a total dose of up to 50 Gy at a depth of 3 cm. In the parasternal field, half of the dose is given by 12- to 15-MeV electrons.

Patient Recruitment

At the time of writing, 59 institutions are taking part in the study (Table 1). From November 1983 until January 1988, 762 patients were recruited, of whom 537 (69%) received breasts conserving therapy and 225 (31%) were treated by mastectomy.

As shown in Table 2, the entry of patients into the study has been increasing. Unfortunately, the randomization rate has decreased, and at the moment only about 10% of the women have been randomized.

It is very disappointing, though not unexpected, that so few patients consented to randomization. We see four reasons for this:

1. Prejudice in the doctor first consulted, with a critical attitude to randomization for so-called ethical reasons.
2. Inadequate or unsuitable patient information, or inadequate knowledge in staff conducting discussions designed to give information.
3. The patients' uneasiness at the idea of submitting to a random decision made by a computer, when what they would really like is individual personal advice from the doctor drawing on the wealth of his or her experience. The patients are thinking people who can make their own decisions.
4. The strict legal restrictions applying to the conduct of randomized clinical trials: potential equivalence of the investigation modalities, requirement to inform of random nature of decision, fact that decisions will be made by a centrally located computer.

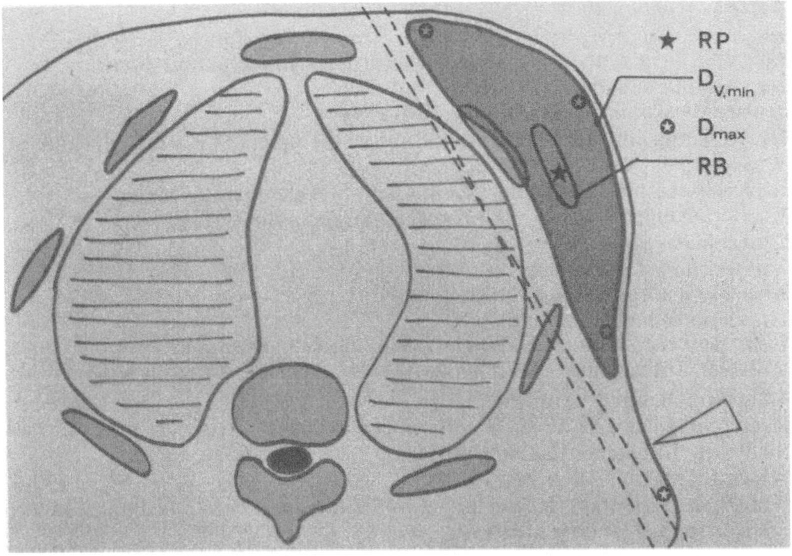

Fig. 1. Dose calculation for irradiation of the breast. The daily single dose is calculated with reference to a point within a reference area in the center of the breast at least 2 cm below the surface of the skin. The minimum dose to the target volume (D_{Vmin}) is then 5%–10% lower than the dose at this reference point, according to the quality of irradiation. The maximum dose can be only roughly estimated and is approximately at the point marked with *open circles*

Table 1. Institutions participating in the study

Krankenhaus Hetzelstift, Neustadt a.d. Weinstr.; Strahlentherapie Mannheim
Mutterhaus, Trier
Frauenklinik Hartmannstift, Bremen; Radiologische Klinik "Links der Weser"
Knappschaftskrankenhaus, Dortmund
Städtische Kliniken, Duisburg
Marienhospital, Essen-Altenessen; Universitäts-Strahlenklinik Essen
Universitätskliniken, Frankfurt
Kreiskrankenhaus, Albstadt; Universitäts-Strahlenklinik Freiburg
Universitätskliniken, Freiburg
Städtisches Krankenhaus, Ludwigshafen; Radiologische Klinik Konstanz
Universitätskliniken, Gießen
Evang. Krankenhaus, Göttingen-Weende; Universitäts-Strahlenklinik Göttigen
Neu Mariahilf, Göttingen; Universitäts-Strahlenklinik Göttingen
Universitätskliniken, Göttingen
Allgem. Krankenhaus; Harburg; Strahlentherapie, Allgem. Krankenhaus St. Georg Hamburg
Universitätskliniken, Innsbruck
Diakonissen-Krankenhaus, Karlsruhe; Strahlentherapie, St. Vincentius Krankenhaus Karlsruhe
Frauenklinik im Klinikum, Karlsruhe; Strahlentherapie, Städtische Kliniken Karlsruhe
Universitätskliniken, Kiel
Städtische Krankenanstalten, Konstanz
Universitätskliniken, Köln
Kreiskrankenhaus, Lahr; Universitäts-Strahlenklinik Freiburg
St. Vincents-Krankenhaus, Limburg

Table 1. *(continued)*

Diakonie-Krankenhaus, Marburg; Universitäts-Strahlenklinik Marburg
Klinikum Großhadern, München
Universitätskliniken rechts der Isar, München
Evang. Krankenhaus, Oberhausen; Strahlentherapie, Mühlheim a.d. Ruhr
Kreiskrankenhaus, Rottalmünster
St. Josefs-Hospital Sterkrade, Oberhausen; Strahlentherapie, Mühlheim a.d. Ruhr
Kreiskrankenhaus, Rinteln; Universitäts-Strahlenklinik Hannover
Universitätskliniken, Ulm
Knappschaftskrankenhaus, Würselen
Medizinische Hochschule, Lübeck
Universitätskliniken, Mannheim
Franz-Hospital, Dülmen; Strahlentherapie, Recklinghausen
Krankenhaus, Siegburg; Strahlentherapie, Robert-Janker-Klinik Bonn
Kliniken Innenstadt, München
Kreiskrankenhaus, Wittlich; Strahlentherapie, Trier
Städtische Krankenanstalten, Konstanz
Kreiskrankenhaus, München-Pasing
Krankenhaus Benrath, Düsseldorf; Strahlentherapie: Dr. Kühnemann, Hilden
Städtisches Krankenhaus, Passau
Krankenhaus Feuerbach, Stuttgart; Strahlentherapie, Katharinenhospital Stuttgart
Klinik "Links der Weser", Bremen
St. Katharinen-Hospital, Frechen; Universitäts-Strahlenklinik Köln
Kreiskrankenhaus, Eckernförde; Strahlentherapie, Rendsburg
St. Vincentius-Krankenhaus, Karlsruhe
Stadtkrankenhaus, Wolfsburg
Kreiskrankenhaus, Helmstedt; Strahlentherapie, Wolfsburg
Universitätskliniken, Homburg
Kreiskrankenhaus, Ebersburg; Strahlentherapie, München-Schwabing
Kliniken Herzogin-Elisabeth-Heim, Braunschweig
Kreiskrankenhaus, Kronach; Universitäts-Strahlenklinik Erlangen
Kreiskrankenhaus, Landshut-Achdorf
Städtisches Krankenhaus, München Neu-Perlach; Strahlentherapie, München-Schwabing
Städtisches Klinikum, Bamberg; Universitäts-Strahlenklinik Erlangen

Where no radiotherapy institution is named, radiotherapy was carried out in the hospital where surgery took place.

These reasons weigh particularly heavily in the balance when one therapy makes it possible for the woman to keep the breast, the main symbol of womanhood, while the other means she will lose it.

Up to the time of writing (January 31, 1988), the return of follow-up data to the data center in Freiburg is insufficient for conclusions to be drawn. Table 2 demonstrates that a remarkable amount of patients entered the protocol in 1987; in some of them, the therapy has not yet been completed. The rate of incomplete follow-up data is 29% in both treatment arms. These facts explain the relatively short median follow-up time of 15 months.

Table 2. Patient recruitment November 1983–January 1988 with complete and incomplete follow-up and according to the treatment performed

	Mastectomy		Breast-conserving treatment	
Year of entry	Follow-up Complete	Follow-up Incomplete	Follow-up Complete	Follow-up Incomplete
1983	6	3	10	11
1984	27	14	70	34
1985	31	13	93	27
1986	48	20	95	52
1987	48	14	110	32
1988	1	–	3	–
Total	161	64	381	156

Preliminary Results

The study has now been running for 4½ years. It is not yet possible to make any definite statements about the treatment of breast carcinoma, but a few impressions are already emerging: Cooperation among the various specialties, i.e., surgeons, radiotherapists, pathologists, and statisticians, is excellent.

The group is working well. Patient recruitment is increasing constantly. The quality of treatment and/or examination has improved considerably in all disciplines concerned while the protocol has been in force. Thus, a significant educative effect has been achieved.

Quality of Radiation Therapy

In the Radiotherapeutic Reference Center, we check the dosimetric data, the treatment protocols, the localization films, and the verification portals for each patient. Radiotherapy is considered correct if performed exactly according to the protocol with dose deviations of less than 5%. Minor protocol deviations concerning time-dose relationship or variation in treatment technique are considered acceptable if an impact on local control or cosmesis is not to be expected (Table 3).

So far, 95% of the reviewed documents of patients who have undergone radiation therapy of the breast have demonstrated that treatment was correct and acceptable treatment. In only 5% of the patients was radiation therapy not acceptable, i.e., there were major deviations from the protocol, including delayed start of treatment, marked dose deviations, or refusal of radiation therapy. During the last 2 years no further major protocol deviations have been observed (Table 4).

Table 3. Quality criteria in radiation therapy

(time after operation)	Correct	Acceptable	Major Deviations from protocol
Start of RT	< 6 weeks	6–8 weeks, due to postoperative complications	> 8 weeks
Irradiation technique	Standard	Other techniques with adequate dose distribution	Inadequate dose distribution
Dose deviation	< 5%	5–10%	> 10%
Total treatment time	< 6–7 weeks	7–8 weeks	> 8 weeks
Regional irradiation	Correct	Overtreatment	–

Table 4. Quality control of radiation therapy in breast-conserving treatment (date of analysis 31.1.88)

Total number of patients	537	
Data available	455	(85%)
Radiotherapy correct	309	(68%)
Radiotherapy acceptable	119	(27%)
Protocol deviations (including refusal of treatment)	27	(5%)
Documents not reviewed (RT not completed, lost cases)	82	(15%)

Recurrences

At present, the recurrence rate is very low; this might be explained by the short follow-up period. Table 5 summarizes the cases of first recurrences after breast-conserving therapy and after mastectomy recurrence only. As of January 1988 there was an even distribution of local and distant relapses, as well as intercurrent disease, in: nine vs six local recurrences, two vs one axillary recurrences, eight vs two distant metastases, etc.

Table 5. First recurrences (date of analysis: 31.1.88)

	Breast-conserving therapy	Mastectomy
Local recurrence	9	6
Axillary recurrence	2	1
Supraclavicular recurrence	1	–
Distant metastases	8	2
Contralateral breast cancer	2	2
Other malignancy	3	–
Non-cancer death	1	3
Overall	26	14

Protocol violation is implicated in four recurrences following breast-conserving therapy. In one case multifocal carcinoma was present. In another case the radiotherapy was discontinued after 14 Gy and residual tumor was found on subsequent mastectomy. In a third case treatment was extended to twice the usual duration, i.e., to 10 weeks, and the individual radiation doses were correspondingly lower. Finally, in one case the interval between surgery and the commencement of radiotherapy was, at 3 months, unjustifiably long. In the mastectomy group there were six recurrences in the nonirradiated chest wall and also one case of lymph node recurrence in the nonirradiated axilla.

Cosmetic Results

So far we have reviewed 100 patients with a follow-up of more than 2 years. Questions related to eight parameters: pigmentation, telangiectasia, subcutaneous fibrosis, disfigurement of the bosom owing to the surgical intervention, unsightly scars, rib fractures, arm plexus damage and lymphedema.

Table 6 shows that results so far are very good. The only severe sequelae are five cases of circumscribed fibrosis and two of rather pronounced fibrosis of the breast. So far, there have been no cases of plexus damage, rib fracture, significant lymphedema, or fibrotic change of the chest muscles. The evaluation was conducted by gynecologists and surgeons, with the result that the sequelae of surgery (asymmetry of bosom, scar formation, etc.) were presumably more leniently assessed than those of irradiation.

In the case of conservative therapy, the cosmetic result depends mainly on six influential parameters:

- Tumor size: better, tumor size in relation to volume of the breast.
- Surgical technique. Unfortunately, segmental resection and quadrantectomy were performed instead of the prescribed procedure of lumpectomy in some of the patients in our group too. Both these procedures disfigure the breast, and neither leads to a higher rate of local tumor control.

Table 6. Cosmetic results in 100 patients at least 2 years after lumpectomy and radiotherapy

Late sequelae	Slight	Moderate	Severe
Hyperpigmentation	10%	2%	–
Teleangiectasia	13%	2%	–
Subcutaneous fibrosis	14%	7%	–
Breast disfigurement	33%	9%	–
Scars	3%	6%	–
Rib fractures	1%	–	–
Plexus damage	2% (?)	1% (?)	–
Arm edema	4%	–	–

Combination of various sequelae: 23%
No late sequelae: 41%

Results assessed by gynecologists and surgeons

- Postoperative wound healing.
- Technique used in radiotherapy.
- Simultaneous, previous or subsequent chemotherapy.
- Exogenous noxae such as nicotine and alcohol.

It is not our intention to go into detail on the operative premises for adequate conservative therapy; these are more properly discussed by surgeons. In addition to the importance of the radiation technique, however, we do wish to draw attention to the fact that more pronounced cutaneous reactions and fibrotic changes of the breast must be expected in smokers and alcoholics.

Radiation Technique and Cosmetic Results

In many cases cosmetically disturbing disfigurements of the breast and local recurrences are attributable to the radiation technique used. The five most important contributing factors are discussed below.

Dose Administered

The total dose administered and the time over which it is spread must be considered, but so must the level of individual doses and the volume of breast tissue irradiated. Unfortunately, there is far too little awareness of the fact that calculation of the dose in the breast is hard in the case of tangential incidence if the difficulties with our computer systems are not taken into account. The distribution of the dose in the breast can theoretically be estimated using very complicated measuring procedures, but it cannot be calculated by the computers used in planning of radiotherapy. As information on scatter dose from the air with different radiation beam qualities is lacking, these computer systems cannot even calculate the maximum reliably. The isodose including the tumor is nonetheless referred to the maximum dose, and this is what makes for the uncertainties in dosimetry. As part of the BMFT protocol, we have therefore introduced a third reference quantity, viz. a reference point at a precisely definable location, 2 cm below the surface of the skin in the center of the breast (Fig. 1). The dose aimed at this point corresponds to the central radiation calculation used earlier, whose cosmetic and tumor control effects are known. The minimum isodose including the target volume is 5%–10% lower than the dose at the reference point, depending on the energy of the radiation beam. The maximum dose can be estimated only roughly, as already mentioned.

Tables 7 and 8 explain how we calculate the dosage. We always give single doses of 2 Gy at the reference point. When telecobalt is used we have a difference of 10% in either direction in the dose to the target volume, while the use of linear accelerator photons leads to a difference of 5% either way. There are corresponding differences in the total dose administered. In this way, we can be sure that a dose of 2 Gy per fraction is not substantially exceeded. When radiogenic complications arise, it is precisely to high single doses of over 2–2.5 Gy that they are attributed.

Table 7. Single radiotherapy doses used (Gy)

	Linac 4–6 MV	Cobalt 60
Reference	2.0	2.0
Minimum	1.9	1.8
Maximum	2.1	2.2

Table 8. Total radiotherapy doses delivered (Gy)

	Linac 4–6 MV	Cobalt 60
Reference	50 (56)	50 (56)
Minimum	47.5 (53)	45 (50)
Maximum	52.2 (59)	55 (62)

Figures in parentheses: without booster dose

Irradiation of All Fields Daily

SARRAZIN et al. recently drew attention to the importance of treating all radiation fields daily. For many years they treated the breast with single doses of 2.5 Gy, calculated at the center of the breast, but only one field was irradiated daily. This led to a daily maximum dose of over 3 to over 4 Gy on the side where the radiation entered. As a result, over the years the satisfactory cosmetic results declined constantly, while the unsatisfactory ones (hyperpigmentation, telangiectasia, fibrosis of the breast) increased [6]. If all irradiation portals are used at every treatment session – and the isodose plan is based ultimately on the correct estimation of the importance of these entry portals – overdosage at the maximum point can be avoided and a satisfactory cosmetic result obtained.

Quality of Radiation Beam

The type of irradiation used is the next important factor affecting dose distribution in the target volume. Typical examples illustrating this are shown in Figs. 2–5.

Figure 2 shows the dose distribution when cesium irradiation is used. The inhomogenity in the irradiated organ is clearly seen. This can lead to underdosage, with the risk of tumor recurrence and of dosage peaks with subsequent radiation sequelae. Nor do we have a computer program that we could use for cesium irradiation. The difficulties described above concerning dose calculation in the breast in the case of tangential irradiation are particularly serious in this case. We have therefore rejected cesium irradiation for homogeneous irradiation to the breast.

SPITALIER (1985) reported the cosmetic results obtained in Marseilles after 5, 10, and 15 years. Unfortunately fibroses, hyperpigmentation and telangiectasia were

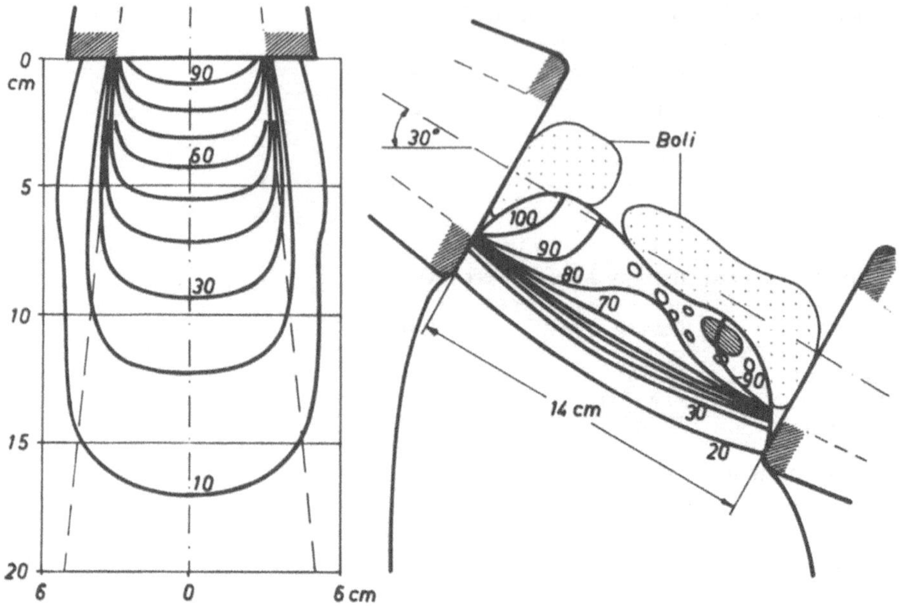

Fig. 2. Dose distribution with cesium-137 irradiation. *Left*, isodose distribution in water phantom; *right*, isodose distribution in breast with use of bolus material. There is very unfavorable dose distribution in the breast

found with increasing frequency as follow-up continued. It is our opinion that the cesium irradiation was responsible for this phenomenon.

Figure 3 illustrates the dose distribution in a medium-sized breast with telecobalt. Satisfactory distribution can be obtained, particularly if wedge filters are used in addition. However, the figure shows that the maximum dose is already reached close to the entry portals. This is more pronounced with large breasts, which is why we advise against telecobalt irradiation in such cases.

Figure 4 shows the isodose distribution when linearly accelerated photons at 10 MV are used. This type of radiation is also unsuitable for homogeneous irradiation of the breast, because the quality of the rays is too hard. This leads to an area where the dosage is too low in the tissue a few centimeters below each entry portal.

Figure 5 shows a CT plan for irradiation with linearly accelerated photons at 6 MV. We think that photons at 4–6 MV give irradiation of a quality that is particularly suitable for irradiation of the breast. The effective dose begins immediately beneath the skin, and there are no harmful excess doses.

Booster Technique

The following basic points can be made concerning the delivery of a booster dose in and around the tumor bed:

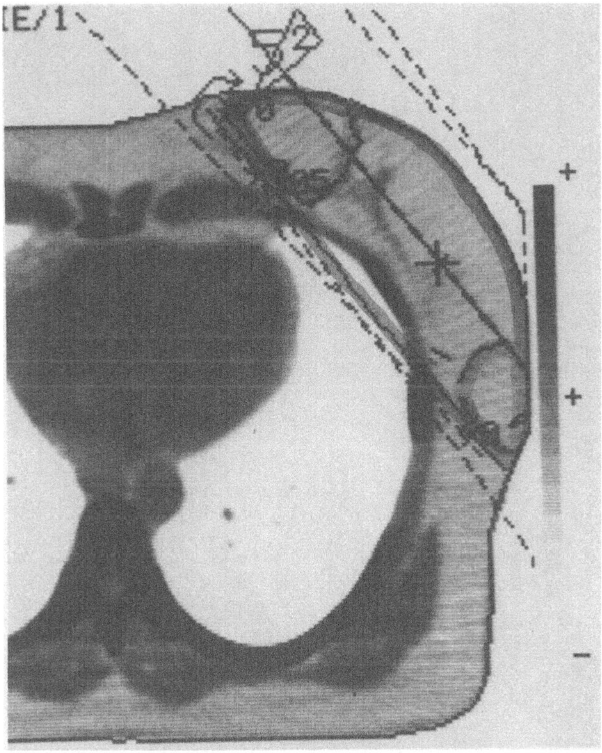

Fig. 3. Dose distribution in a medium-sized breast on irradiation from a telecobalt source. Immediately below the point of entry there is a circumscribed area where the dose is excessively high (CT section)

- The value of boosting is controversial. The need for it is not demonstrated beyond doubt in the literature. Nonetheless, the fact that 70%–85% of local recurrences in the breast are in the immediate vicinity of the site of the original primary tumor does suggest that a procedure of this kind is basically necessary if the tumor-bearing quadrant has not been totally removed.
- It has not yet been decided what boosting technique should best be used. We prefer a direct electron field. The depth of penetration of the irradiation can be determined very precisely by selection of the most suitable electron energy. The effective dose reaches the ribs without any irradiation burden to the parenchyma of the lung below them. This dose distribution cannot be achieved with photon rays. We are also not ready to recommend interstitial iridium boosting at present. The technique is very complicated and the dosimetry difficult. Neither the sophistication of the technique nor the effort involved in dosimetry is in any relation to the result of treatment.
- If a booster dose is, however, given, care must be taken to see that it genuinely reaches the tumor bed. This may be impossible if the surgeon has not marked the tumor bed with clips that will show up as shadows; the position of the scar(s), the findings on palpation and the patient's memory do not allow accurate

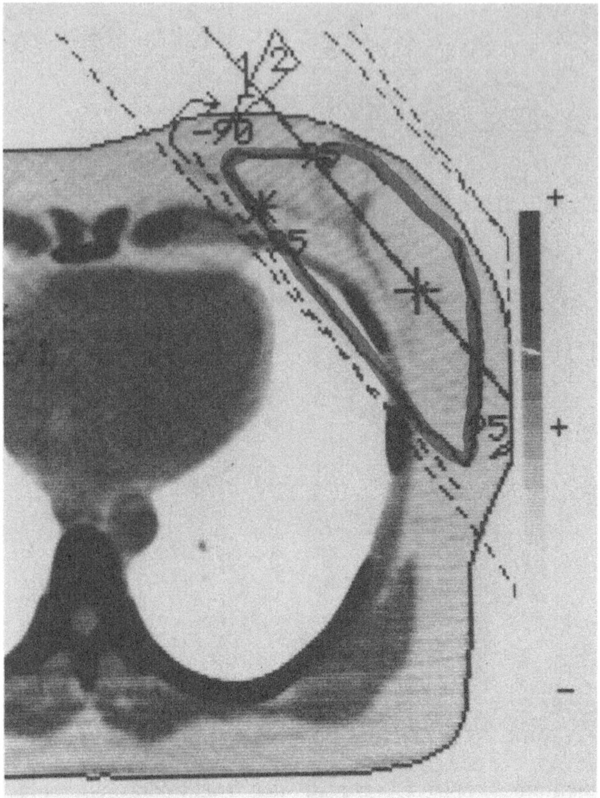

Fig. 4. When linear accelerator photons at 10 MV are used the cumulative effect is so great that underdosage becomes visible in the superficial layers of tissue (CT section)

localization. As absorbable clips that show up as shadows are now commercially available, the use of clips no longer leads to scatter in the computer tomogram. Thus, the only argument against marking the original tumor site with clips during surgery no longer applies.

Field Junction

In efficient radiotherapy institutions a great deal of effort is devoted to avoiding overlapping of the adjacent radiation fields. For this purpose various satellite and/or block techniques are used which prevent divergence at the point of entry. With the patient in a semi-inclined position the breast lies optimally at the lateral chest wall, but this position can only be recommended if the breast alone is to be irradiated. If the lymph drainage regions or regions affected are also going to be irradiated, the semi-inclined position is not suitable, as it would mean repositioning the patient during the radiotherapy session. This would lead either to gaps between fields, with consequent underdosage at the field borders, or to hot spots, which

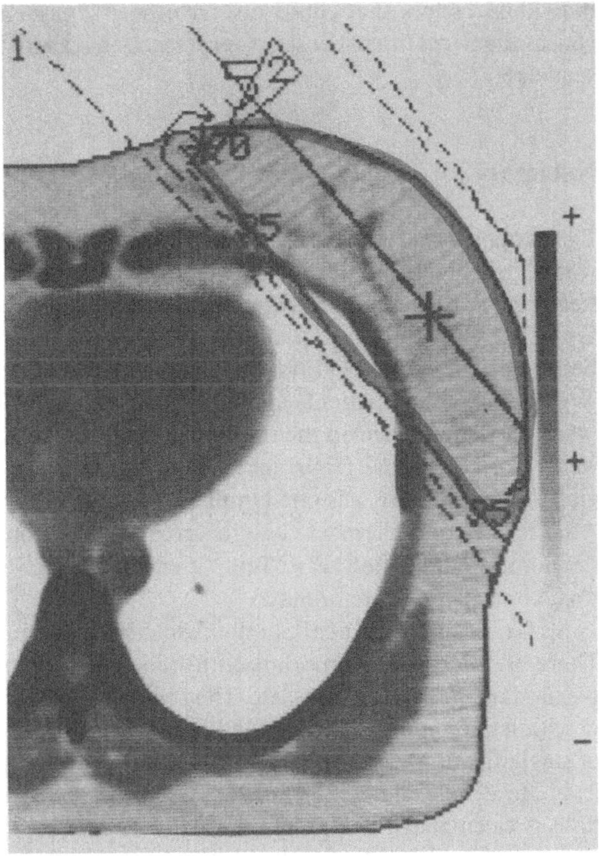

Fig. 5. Ideal dose distribution with use of linear accelerator photons at 4–6 MV (CT section)

would result in circumscribed fibrotic changes, hyperpigmentation, and telangiectasia.

Conclusions

The so-called radiation damage is not attributable to the conservative procedure as such. Owing to the complicated structure of the target volume, radiotherapy of breast carcinoma is one of the most difficult tasks within the whole field of radiation therapy. Not everyone can master conservative therapy: this is true both of surgeons and of radiotherapists. The Deutsche Röntgengesellschaft offers postgraduate training courses in which one of the techniques that can be learned is that of radiotherapy of breast carcinoma. One purpose of the BMFT protocol discussed in this paper is assurance of uniform quality for radiotherapy throughout the Federal Republic of Germany.

Unpleasant sequelae of radiotherapy can also be due to exogenous noxae and to individual factors that could not have been foreseen. In general, with suitable concomitant treatment the short-term reaction is slight and there are no serious late sequelae.

Summary

The national breast cancer protocol is designed to investigate whether lumpectomy with subsequent irradiation of the breast is as good as simple mastectomy for the treatment of breast cancer staged by pathohistological examination as T1 N0 M0. Up to 31.1.88 a total of 762 patients had been enrolled in the trial. The trial has now been in progress for 4½ years, and the median follow-up period is 15 months.

Only 10% of the patients agreed to random allocation to one treatment or the other: the others selected the therapy themselves. In the lumpectomy group there were 12 locoregional recurrences. Four of these were attributable to protocol violations, and there was one lymph node recurrence in the nonirradiated axilla. After mastectomy there was one recurrence in the nonirradiated axilla, and six at the nonirradiated chest wall. Ten patients developed pulmonary metastases and four, contralateral carcinomas.

So far, we are hopeful about the cosmetic aspects of the result of radiotherapy. There are no cases of pronounced fibrotic changes, marked skin reactions, arm plexus damage, rib fractures, etc. The following five factors must be taken account of within the context of the irradiation techniques: size of dose (total dose and size of single fraction); type of irradiation; booster technique; field junctions; care to irradiate all fields daily. To avoid dose inhomogeneity as far as possible, the tumor dose is calculated for a precisely definable reference area that was specifically introduced for the BMFT protocol. The isodose including the target volume and the estimated maximum dose vary by 10% either way when telecobalt irradiation is used, and by 5% either way when linear accelerator photons at 4–6 MV are used.

References

1. Amalric R, Santamaria F, Robert F, Seigle J, Altschuler C, Kurtz JM, Spitalier JM, Brandore H, Ayme Y, Pollet JF, Burmeister R, Abed R (1982) Radiation therapy with or without primary limited surgery for operable breast cancer. A 20 year experience at the Marseilles Cancer Institute. Cancer 49:30–34
2. Atkins SH, Hayward JL, Klugman DJ, Wayte AB (1972) Treatment of early breast cancer: A report after ten years of clinical trial. Brit Med J 2:423–429
3. Brady LW, Damsker JI, Schatanoff D, Micaily B (1981) Primary radiation therapy for carcinoma of the breast. Phila Med 77:53–55
4. Calle R, Vilcoq R, Pilleron JP, et al. (1985) Conservative treatment of operable breast carcinoma by irradiation with or without limited surgery – Ten years results. In: Harris J, Hellman S, Silen W (eds) Conservative management of Breast Cancer. Lippincott, Philadelphia, pp 3–10
5. Clark RM, Wilkinson RH, Mahoney LJ, Reid JG, MacDonald WD (1982) Breast cancer: A 21 year experience with conservative surgery and radiation. Int J Radiat Oncol Biol Phys 8:967–975

6. Dewar JA, Sarrazin D, Arriagada R, Benhamour S, Benhamour E, Petit JY, Fontaine F (1986) Cosmetic results following lumpectomy and radiotherapy for small breast cancer. Proceedings of the 5th Annual Meeting ESTRO, p 235, 8–10 Sept
7. Fisher B, Montague E, Redmond C, Deutsch M, Brown GR, Zauber A, Hanson WF, Wong A (1980) Findings from NSABP Protocol No. B-04 – Comparison of radical mastectomy with alternative treatments for primary breast cancer. Cancer 46:1–13
8. Fisher B, Bauer M, Margolese R, et al. (1985) Five-year results of a randomized clinical trial comparing total mastectomy and segmental mastectomy with or without radiation in the treatment of breast cancer. N Engl J Med 312:665–673
9. Forrest APM, Gleave EN, Roberts MM, Henk JM, Glavelle IH (1970) A controlled clinical trial of conservative treatment for early breast cancer. Proc R Soc Med 63:107
10. Harris JR, Connolly JL, Schnitt SJ, Cohen RB, Hellman S (1983) Clinical-pathologic study of early breast cancer treated by primary radiation therapy. J Clin Oncol 1:184–189
11. Hünig R, Walther E, Harder F, Almendral AC, Torhorst J, Roth J (1983) The Basel lumpectomy protocol: 5 year experience with a prospective study for conservative treatment of breast cancer. In: Harris JR, Hellman S, Silen W (eds) Alternative to mastectomy. Lippincott, Philadelphia, pp 23–35
12. Mustakallio S (1972) Conservative treatment of breast cancer – review of 25 years follow-up. Clin Radiol 23:110–116
13. Rauschecker H, Sauer R, Schauer A, Scheurlen H, Peiper HJ (1985) Our experiences in setting up BMFT-Multicenter trial: therapy of small breast cancer. In Zander J, Baltzer J (Hrsg) Early Breast Cancer. Springer-Verlag, Berlin-Heidelberg-New York Tokyo, pp 310–316
14. Rissanen PM (1969) A comparison of conservative and radical surgery combined with radiotherapy in the treatment of stage I carcinoma of the breast. Br J Radiol 42:423–426
15. Sarrazin D, Le M, Mouriesse H, Contesso G, Fontaine F, Arriagada R, Tubiana M (1982) Radiotherapeutic studies on breast cancer at Villejuif. Cancer Bulletin 34:242–249
16. Spitalier JM, Gambarelli J, Brandone H (1986) Breast-conserving surgery with radiation therapy for operable mammary carcinoma: a 25-year experience. World J Surg 10:1014–1020
17. Veronesi U, Delvecchio M, Greco M (1983) Results of quadrantectomy, axillary dissection and radiotherapy (QUART) in T1 N0 patients. In: Harris J, Hellman S, Silen W (eds) Conservative management of breast cancer. Lippincott, Philadelphia, pp 91–99

Long-Term Results and Late Complications After Breast-Preserving Therapy of Breast Cancer in Vienna

A. Staffen

In the last 10 years breast-preserving therapy in breast cancer has become a standardized procedure in regard to surgical technique, axillary dissection, and necessary radiotherapy. All centers which followed this procedure from the beginning now have more than 10 years' experience in this field. Discussion of the experience gained should enable the optimization of surgical and irradiation technique both to improve cancer treatment and to avoid late complications.

At the Second Department of Surgery in Vienna we started with breast-preserving surgery in 1974, and together with the Department of Radiotherapy and Radiobiology we treated 230 patients, of whom 214 received irradiation. The 26 nonirradiated patients were N0 cases of the upper external quadrant, who we initially thought would not need radiation therapy.

We divide our long-term results and late complications as follows:

1. Dependent on the disease itself: results, local recurrence, survival time in relation to irradiation or nonirradiation and to the status of lymph nodes
2. Experience with surgical therapy
3. Experience with postoperative irradiation therapy

Disease-Dependent Factors

From 1974 to May 1986, 141 patients from our clinic were treated with the above-described therapeutic concept. Table 1 depicts the division of cases by histology, localization, status of lymph nodes and number of patients who received postoperative radiation. Table 2 shows the results of the last follow-up examination after 12 years. During this time we observed 18 local recurrences, and 18 patients died from carcinoma. It is significant that no more cases of local recurrence were found at follow-up examination in 1984 than in 1986 (Table 3). This means that the rather high rate of local recurrences is caused by the incidence among the 26 patients without postoperative radiation therapy. Table 4 shows significantly that the greatest number of local recurrences was observed in these nonirradiated N0 cases. The initially performed frozen section examination of the dissected axilla was abandoned because of its inexactness. Furthermore, dissection of the axilla is just a staging procedure; the finding of positive axillary glands does not demand radical surgery of the breast, but rather adequate adjuvant postoperative treatment.

Table 1. Quadrant resection with axillary dissection at the Second Surgical University Clinic, Vienna, January 1974 – May 1986 ($n = 141$)

						Postoperative radiotherapy
Duct cancer	123	External quadrants	106	N0	68	57
				$N \leq 3$	28	27
				$N > 3$	10	7
		Internal quadrants	17	N0	12	5
				$N \leq 3$	4	2
				$N > 3$	1	1
Lobular cancer	18	External quadrants	15	N0	6	6
				$N \leq 3$	7	6
				$N > 3$	2	2
		Internal quadrants	3	N0	2	2
				$N \leq 3$	1	0
				$N > 3$	0	0

Postoperative radiotherapy: 115
No postoperative radiotherapy: 26

Table 2. Follow-up examination after quadrant resection with axillary dissection at the Second Surgical University Clinic, Vienna ($n = 127$)

Local, regional, and mammographic NAD	80	(postoperative radiotherapy 75)
After second operation (local recurrence, second carcinoma) NAD	16	(radiotherapy after first operation 10; after second operation 16)
Alive with carcinoma or metastases	6	(postoperative radiotherapy 5)
Local recurrence	18	Mastectomy 8
		Re-resection 10
Metastases		
Bones	2	
Liver	3	
Lung	3	
Other	6	
Multiple location	4	
Died	25	Because of carcinoma 18
		Other/unknown reasons 7

Surgical Therapy

Circular or radial incisions displayed no differences in late results. The decision on which incision to employ should depend on the circumstances. We remove the axilla whenever possible using a separate incision, except in lateral tumors of the upper external quadrant. The cosmetic result is far better. We also discontinued

Table 3. Follow-up examinations in 1984 and 1986

1984 ($n = 102$; evaluated 92)			
Local recurrence	18	17.6%	(of 102)
		19.5%	(of 92)
Died of carcinoma	12	11.7%	(of 102)
1986 ($n = 141$; evaluated 127)			
Local recurrence	18	12.7%	(of 141)
		14.1%	(of 127)
Died of carcinoma	18	12.7%	(of 141)

Table 4. Local recurrence and second carcinomas after quadrant resection with axillary dissection at the Second Surgical University Clinic, Vienna

Local recurrence: findings at first operation					Postoperative radiotherapy
18	Ductal	17	N0	13	4
			$N \leq 3$	3	2
			$N > 3$	2	0
	Lobular	1	N0	0	0
			$N \leq 3$	1	0
			$N > 3$	0	0
Second carcinoma: findings at second operation					**Radiotherapy after first operation**
10 (8 contralat., 2 ipsilat.)	Ductal	7	N0	3	3
			$N \leq 3$	1	1
			$N > 3$	3	2
	Lobular	3	N0	2	2
			$N \leq 3$	1	1
			$N > 3$	0	0

reconstruction of the gland body, as it results in considerable scar distortion which is made even worse by radiation. Without reconstruction of the breast better results could be achieved. For venous preparation of the axilla the same rules apply as for radical procedures. The lower venous edge should be the limit of all surgical intervention. Furthermore, no disproportion should exist between breast size and tumor size. Tumor diameter of 2 cm is the utmost limit to us, as we try to resect 1 cm of healthy breast tissue all around. Submamillary tumor localization, as well as clinically proven massive axillary involvement with adherent glands, represents a contraindication for this therapeutic protocol.

Postoperative Irradiation Therapy

Late changes partly involve slowly proliferating tissue, with fibroses, indurations, and teleangiectasias caused by the boost of electrons; skin atrophies may also occur in the boost area. The intensity of acute effects does not allow any conclusions concerning the intensity of late changes, which depend on the size of the individual radiation dose. Therefore the individual dose should be reduced to 1.7–1.8 Gy and both breast areas irradiated each day, which means half dose per area. Field overlapping may cause tumorlike fibrosis which often mimics local recurrence. Even mammography complicates differential diagnosis. Excision of such areas reveals fatty tissue necrosis with strong tissue induration on histological examination. Healing of these wounds is rather prolonged and accompanied by secondary infections. Since 1981 some of our patients received interstitial brachytherapy with iridium-191 wires in an afterloading procedure, which makes it possible to focus a greater radiation dose directly into the tumor bed (Table 5).

At the follow-up examinations we evaluated our patients not only in regard to local recurrence and survival rate, but also for the cosmetic results of symmetry, consistency and skin change. Ninety per cent of 214 patients, of whom a great many had received boost of electrons, showed very good or good results which were absolutely satisfactory for the patients. Only 19 patients (8.9%) showed unsatisfactory results, the reasons for which are depicted in Tables 6–8.

Table 5. Late changes after breast-preserving surgery and percutaneous radiation (Second Surgical Clinic and Clinic for Radiotherapy and Radiobiology, University of Vienna)

Pigmentation: radiotherapy
Teleangiectasis: radiotherapy: boost area
Dermatrophy: radiotherapy

- Indurations
  - Fibrosis
    - Whole breast (radiotherapy)
    - Parts (radiotherapy boost)
    - Localized (radiotherapy: field overlapping)
  - Edema
    - Remaining breast (operation + radiotherapy)
    - Branchial edema (operation or recidiv) differential-diagnosis: ultra soundexamination

Scarf distortion: operation

Table 6. Changes leading to classification of results as unsatisfactory

Category	Changes
Symmetry	Scarf distortion
Consistency	Whole breast
	Parts of breast
Skin changes	Pigmentation
	Teleangiectasis
	Dermatrophy

Table 7. Results after percutaneous radiation (Clinic for Radiotherapy and Radiobiology, University of Vienna) ($n=214$)

Result	*n*	%	
Very good	141	65.8	91
Satisfactory	54	25.2	
Unsatisfactory	19	8.9	

Table 8. Breakdown of 19 poor results (Clinic for Radiotherapy and Radiobiology, University of Vienna)

Result	*n*
Induration of the whole remaining breast	5
Teleangiectasias	2
Distortion of the whole remaining breast	2
Edema of the remaining breast	3
Tumorlike induration with reoperation	3

Table 9. Summary of Results in 141 breast cancer patients (Second Surgical Clinic, University of Vienna)

Result	*n*	%	
Very good	117	82.9	93.5
Good	15	10.6	
Unsatisfactory	9	6.4	
Induration of whole remaining breast	5		
Tumorlike fibrosis with reoperation	2		
Scarf distortion	2		

The results in patients exclusively operated on at our clinic seem to be even better, but it cannot be ignored that they include some nonirradiated patients (Table 9). It was significant that the patients were content with results which were unsatisfactory to us. We were never forced to remove the breast for cosmetic reasons.

Assuming correct indication, adequate excision and postoperative irradiation in this increasingly common carcinoma, – which can, however, be diagnosed rather earlier, and therefore smaller, by modern measures – breast-preserving therapy is superior to mutilating interventions in regard to local recurrence, survival time, cosmetic result and late complications. Furthermore, the compliance of the patients was excellent under adequate guidance.

Possible Risk of Second Primary Cancers Associated with Irradiation in Breast-Conserving Therapy

J.D. Boice

The incidence of breast cancer exceeds that of practically all other cancers among women, and in the United States approximately one in 11 women will develop this disease in their lifetime. The relatively good survival following an initial diagnosis of breast cancer, i.e., over 70% at 5 years, provides ample opportunity for women to develop second primary cancers over time, particularly at sites which may be associated with initial treatment or with common risk factors. The combination of surgical therapy of breast cancer with locoregional radiation has become an increasingly important treatment approach today [10,12]. While it is too early to evaluate directly the potential adverse health effects associated with breast-conserving therapy, inferences can be made from previous studies of women treated with radiation for breast cancer [4–6,9,11] and from studies of women exposed to ionizing radiation for reasons unrelated to cancer therapy [3,13,15].

Etiologic Factors Involved in Multiple Primary Cancers

The study of multiple primary cancers has led to the identification of tumor constellations which have been subject to a variety of possible etiologic interpretations. When evaluating the possible effects of radiotherapy for breast cancer, it is thus important to appreciate that there are other factors increasing a woman's risk of developing a new primary cancer. For example, the constellation of multiple cancers of the breast, uterine corpus, ovary, and colon has long intrigued investigators. Because reproductive factors (such as nulliparity) and dietary habits (such as high fat intake) appear involved in these cancers, it is thought that nutritional and hormonal interactions may contribute to the development of multiple primaries of these sites. Previous studies have also demonstrated that women with breast cancer are at a more than threefold excess risk of developing a new primary cancer in the opposite breast. Studies of multiple primary cancers have also reported an excess of thyroid, colon, ovarian, uterine, and connective tissue neoplasms, as well as melanoma following breast cancer. Factors suggested to explain these associations include genetic influences, common environmental exposures, endogenous hormones, increased medical surveillance among cancer patients, and treatments for the initial primary cancer [2,11].

Treatment for breast cancer was associated with the development of second primary cancers as early as 1948, when Stewart and Treves [14] linked lymphangiosarcoma with the partial lymphedema of the upper extremities that may accompany radical mastectomy. Cancer of the uterine corpus has been associated with both nonsteroidal estrogen treatment for breast cancer and ovarian radiotherapy [4]. An excess of leukemia following chemotherapy and/or radiotherapy for breast cancer has been reported [6]. Radiotherapy has been suggested as a possible factor in the etiology of bilateral breast cancer [9].

Population Studies of Multiple Primary Cancers Following Breast Cancer

A comprehensive monograph on the risk of developing multiple primary cancers was recently prepared by the USA National Cancer Institute in conjunction with the Connecticut Tumor Registry and the Danish Cancer Registry [5,11,13]. Among 41 109 women diagnosed as having breast cancer in Connecticut between 1935 and 1982, almost 4000 developed a second cancer, whereas only 2426 were expected based on population rates (relative risk (RR) = 1.64). Table 1 presents the observed and expected numbers of second primary cancers by years after diagnosis of an initial cancer of the breast among females given radiotherapy, and Table 2 presents similar data for women not given radiotherapy. The increased risk of developing a second cancer persisted for 30 years and was highest in women under 55 years of age at the time of breast cancer diagnosis. Second primary breast cancers (RR = 3.0) accounted for almost 50% of all new primary cancers. Interestingly, if subsequent breast cancers were excluded, the risk for all other second cancers was only 1.15, i.e., a 15% excess over expectation, and no excess risk was seen among women over age 55 at initial breast cancer. Women who received initial radiotherapy compared with those who did not were at slightly higher risk of developing a second cancer, most notably acute nonlymphocytic leukemia, non-Hodgkin's lymphoma, and cancers of the esophagus, kidney, and connective tissue. The nature of these associations, however, was not always clear. Women treated with radiation were at higher risk of developing a second breast cancer (RR = 3.9) than nonirradiated women (RR = 2.8). Figure 1 indicates the elevated risk of a second cancer of the female breast over time following an initial primary breast cancer for the entire population. These high risks could be associated with hormonal, dietary, and/or genetic influences, as well as heightened medical surveillance and possibly the effects of treatment.

In Denmark, approximately 55 000 women diagnosed with breast cancer between 1943 and 1980 were evaluated for the risk of second cancers [5]. Unfortunately, contralateral breast cancers were not recorded by the Danish Cancer Registry and thus this major site has been excluded from the analyses (Table 3). Overall, 2480 second cancers, not counting the second breast cancers, were reported compared with 2398 expected based on rates from the general population. While a breakdown by treatment, i.e., whether radiotherapy was given or not, was not possible, over 75% of treatments do include radiation (in contrast to Connecticut where the percentage is only about 25%), and thus the data in Table 3 can be interpreted as derived from a largely irradiated population. Significant excess cancers of the lung, bone, and connective tissue were observed. The risk of cancers

Table 1. Observed (O) and expected (E) numbers of second primary cancers by years after diagnosis of an initial cancer of the breast (ICD-O code 174) among females given radiotherapy in Connecticut, 1935–1982 [11]

	Years after first primary cancer diagnosis														
	< 1			1–4			5–9			10+			Total		
No. starting interval	11 691			9 750			4 366			2 002			11 691		
Person-years in interval	8 865			25 846			15 102			13 283			63 096		
Second primary cancer site	O	E	O E	O	E	O E	O	E	O E	O	E	O E	O	E	O E
All second cancers	**129**	**61.98**	**2.1**[a]	**407**	**193.78**	**2.1**[a]	**245**	**126.57**	**1.9**[a]	**259**	**132.41**	**2.0**[a]	**1040**	**514.41**	**2.0**[a]
All excluding site of initial cancer	**48**	**44.56**	**1.1**	**154**	**139.55**	**1.1**	**131**	**91.91**	**1.4**[a]	**163**	**98.21**	**1.7**[a]	**496**	**374.00**	**1.3**[a]
Buccal cavity, pharynx	**2**	**1.12**	**1.8**	**4**	**3.58**	**1.1**	**2**	**2.39**	**0.8**	**4**	**2.45**	**1.6**	**12**	**9.53**	**1.3**
Lip	0	0.06	0.0	0	0.18	0.0	0	0.12	0.0	1	0.13	7.6	1	0.50	2.0
Tongue	0	0.23	0.0	0	0.74	0.0	1	0.48	2.1	2	0.51	4.0	3	1.95	1.5
Salivary gland	0	0.14	0.0	1	0.44	2.3	0	0.28	0.0	0	0.28	0.0	1	1.14	0.9
Gum, other mouth	2	0.38	5.3	2	1.23	1.6	1	0.84	1.2	0	0.86	0.0	5	3.30	1.5
Pharynx	0	0.26	0.0	1	0.84	1.2	0	0.56	0.0	0	0.57	0.0	1	2.23	0.4
Digestive system	**14**	**17.07**	**0.8**	**56**	**53.35**	**1.0**	**54**	**35.41**	**1.5**[a]	**54**	**39.81**	**1.4**[a]	**178**	**145.55**	**1.2**[a]
Esophagus	1	0.41	2.5	0	1.30	0.0	3	0.88	3.4	2	0.93	2.2	6	3.51	1.7
Stomach	4	2.24	1.8	10	6.66	1.5	8	4.20	1.9	4	4.56	0.9	26	17.65	1.5
Colon	3	7.87	0.4	22	24.92	0.9	27	16.77	1.6[a]	28	19.17	1.5	80	68.68	1.2
Rectum	6	3.37	1.8	15	10.55	1.4	11	6.98	1.6	7	7.72	0.9	39	28.61	1.4
Liver, biliary	0	1.12	0.0	4	3.42	1.2	2	2.23	0.9	2	2.55	0.8	8	9.32	0.9
Pancreas	0	1.69	0.0	5	5.41	0.9	1	3.64	0.3	8	4.14	1.9	14	14.87	0.9
Respiratory system	**2**	**3.86**	**0.5**	**9**	**12.94**	**0.7**	**10**	**9.14**	**1.1**	**26**	**9.44**	**2.8**[a]	**47**	**35.36**	**1.3**
Nasal cavities, sinuses	0	0.11	0.0	0	0.33	0.0	0	0.21	0.0	1	0.22	4.6	1	0.87	1.1
Larynx	0	0.24	0.0	1	0.79	1.3	1	0.55	1.8	1	0.55	1.8	3	2.13	1.4
Trachea, bronchus, lung	2	3.46	0.6	8	11.66	0.7	9	8.28	1.1	24	8.57	2.8[a]	43	31.94	1.3
Female breast	81	17.42	4.7[a]	253	54.23	4.7[a]	114	34.66	3.3[a]	96	34.20	2.8[a]	544	140.41	3.9[a]

cont'd.

Table 1. *(continued)*

	Years after first primary cancer diagnosis														
	< 1			1–4			5–9			10+			Total		
No. starting interval	11 691			9 750			4 366			2 002			11 691		
Person-years in interval	8 865			25 846			15 102			13 283			63 096		
Second primary cancer site	O	E	O E	O	E	O E	O	E	O E	O	E	O E	O	E	O E
Female genital tract	**18**	**11.29**	**1.6**	**49**	**34.10**	**1.4**[a]	**33**	**21.36**	**1.5**[a]	**37**	**20.92**	**1.8**[a]	**137**	**87.61**	**1.6**[a]
Cervix uteri	0	2.49	0.0	6	6.98	10.9	3	3.98	0.8	5	3.49	1.4	14	16.93	0.8
Corpus uteri	6	4.43	1.4	25	14.09	1.8[a]	15	9.29	1.6	13	9.42	1.4	59	37.21	1.6[a]
Uterus, NOS	1	0.78	1.3	1	2.08	0.5	1	1.17	0.9	2	1.05	1.9	5	5.07	1.0
Ovary, fallopian tubes	11	3.05	3.6[a]	12	9.29	1.3	13	5.85	2.2[a]	14	5.77	2.4[a]	50	23.94	2.1[a]
Kidney, renal pelvis, ureter	3	0.93	3.2	7	2.95	2.4	3	1.97	1.5	2	2.14	0.9	15	7.98	1.9[a]
Bladder, other urinary	1	1.52	0.7	4	4.93	0.8	3	3.37	0.9	3	3.81	0.8	11	13.63	0.8
Melanoma of the skin	1	0.80	1.2	6	2.56	2.3	0	1.66	0.0	3	1.54	1.9	10	6.57	1.5
Eye	0	0.11	0.0	2	0.32	6.2	0	0.20	0.0	1	0.21	4.7	3	0.85	3.5
Brain, central nervous system	2	0.69	2.9	1	2.14	0.5	0	1.38	0.0	1	1.40	0.7	4	5.61	0.7
Thyroid gland	1	0.51	2.0	0	1.53	0.0	2	0.93	2.2	3	0.86	3.5	6	3.83	1.6
Bone	0	0.10	0.0	1	0.28	3.5	0	0.17	0.0	1	0.16	6.1	2	0.71	2.8
Connective tissue	0	0.27	0.0	2	0.82	2.4	3	0.51	5.8[a]	4	0.53	7.6[a]	9	2.12	4.2[a]
Lymphatic, hematopoietic system	**3**	**3.70**	**0.8**	**9**	**11.83**	**0.8**	**13**	**7.95**	**1.6**	**18**	**8.80**	**2.0**[a]	**43**	**32.26**	**1.3**
Non-Hodgkins lymphoma	2	1.42	1.4	4	4.59	0.9	7	3.15	2.2	8	3.42	2.3[a]	21	12.58	1.7[a]
Hodgkin's disease	0	0.32	0.0	0	0.92	0.0	0	0.55	0.0	1	0.56	1.8	1	2.35	0.4
Multiple myeloma	0	0.62	0.0	0	2.05	0.0	0	1.41	0.0	2	1.62	1.2	2	5.70	0.4
Leukemias	1	1.34	0.7	5	4.25	1.2	6	2.82	2.1	7	3.18	2.2	19	11.59	1.6
Chronic lymphocytic	0	0.36	0.0	0	1.17	0.0	2	0.80	2.5	2	0.95	2.1	4	3.27	1.2
Acute nonlymphocytic	1	0.45	2.2	3	1.47	2.0	3	0.99	3.0	3	1.11	2.7	10	4.02	2.5[a]

[a] $p < 0.05$

Table 2. Observed (O) and expected (E) numbers of second primary cancers by years after diagnosis of an initial cancer of the breast (ICD-O code 174) among females not given radiotherapy in Connecticut, 1935–1982 [11]

	Years after first primary cancer diagnosis														
	< 1			1–4			5–9			10+			Total		
No. starting interval	29 418			26 318			14 243			7 304			29 418		
Person-years in interval	23 177			77 428			51 060			56 763			208 428		
Second primary cancer site	O	E	OE	O	E	OE	O	E	OE	O	E	OE	O	E	OE
All second cancers	**284**	**185.93**	**1.5**[a]	**1005**	**648.43**	**1.5**[a]	**719**	**462.41**	**1.6**[a]	**936**	**615.59**	**1.5**[a]	**2944**	**1,911.27**	**1.5**[a]
All excluding site of initial cancer	**124**	**136.53**	**0.9**	**504**	**476.79**	**1.1**	**366**	**341.41**	**1.1**	**567**	**461.28**	**1.2**[a]	**1561**	**1,415.22**	**1.1**[a]
Buccal cavity, pharynx	3	**3.23**	**0.9**	**19**	**11.39**	**1.7**[a]	**7**	**8.23**	**0.9**	**15**	**10.94**	1.4	**44**	**33.77**	**1.3**
Lip	1	0.20	5.0	1	0.69	1.5	1	0.49	2.0	1	0.65	1.5	4	2.03	2.0
Tongue	1	0.65	1.5	8	2.31	3.5[a]	1	1.69	0.6	1	2.25	0.4	11	6.90	1.6
Salivary gland	0	0.42	0.0	3	1.45	2.1	1	1.03	1.0	5	1.31	3.8[a]	9	4.21	2.1
Gum, other mouth	0	1.12	0.0	6	3.967	1.5	3	2.87	1.0	4	3.93	1.0	13	11.87	1.1
Pharynx	1	0.71	1.4	1	2.51	0.4	1	1.82	0.5	4	2.38	1.7	7	7.42	0.9
Digestive system	**60**	**56.22**	**1.1**	**207**	**196.63**	**1.1**	**140**	**141.86**	**1.0**	**243**	**195.99**	**1.2**[a]	**650**	**590.37**	**1.1**[a]
Esophagus	0	1.28	0.0	4	4.48	0.9	2	3.20	0.6	4	4.40	0.9	10	13.35	0.7
Stomach	8	7.74	1.0	29	26.33	1.1	21	18.32	1.1	18	22.87	0.8	76	75.21	1.0
Colon	24	26.02	0.9	92	91.76	1.0	77	66.99	1.1	138	94.96	1.5[a]	331	279.58	1.2[a]
Rectum	17	10.66	1.6	38	37.33	1.0	19	26.90	0.7	46	36.97	1.2	120	111.80	1.1
Liver, biliary	4	3.83	1.0	13	13.22	1.0	8	9.44	0.8	12	12.71	0.9	37	39.17	0.9
Pancreas	6	5.53	1.1	26	19.50	1.3	8	14.20	0.6	23	20.50	1.1	63	59.69	1.1
Respiratory system	**5**	**11.04**	**0.5**	**45**	**39.28**	**1.1**	**32**	**28.48**	**1.1**	**64**	**41.00**	**1.6**[a]	**146**	**119.74**	**1.2**[a]
Nasal cavities, sinuses	0	0.32	0.0	1	1.09	0.9	2	0.77	2.6	1	0.99	1.0	4	3.16	1.3
Larynx	1	0.66	1.5	2	2.34	0.9	1	1.70	0.6	2	2.27	0.9	6	6.95	0.9
Tranchea, bronchus, lung	3	9.93	0.3[a]	42	35.38	1.2	28	25.67	1.1	61	37.29	1.6[a]	134	108.21	1.2[a]
Female breast	160	49.40	3.2[a]	501	171:64	2.9[a]	353	121.00	2.9[a]	369	154.31	2.4[a]	1,383	496.05	2.8[a]

cont'd.

Table 2. *(continued)*

	Years after first primary cancer diagnosis														
	< 1			1–4			5–9			10+			Total		
No. starting interval	29 418			26 318			14 243			7 304					29 418
Person-years in interval	23 177			77 428			51 060			56 763					208 428
Second primary cancer site	O	E	O E	O	E	O E	O	E	O E	O	E	O E	O	E	O E
Female genital tract	**34**	**31.17**	**1.1**	**127**	**107.06**	**1.2**	**113**	**74.59**	**1.5**[a]	**124**	**91.09**	**1.4**[a]	**398**	**303.73**	**1.3**[a]
Cervix uteri	9	6.62	1.4	26	21.78	1.2	16	14.20	1.1	11	14.78	0.7	62	57.35	1.1
Corpus uteri	13	11.94	1.1	51	42.17	1.2	50	30.59	1.6[a]	54	40.51	1.3[a]	168	125.13	1.3[a]
Uterus, NOS	0	2.46	0.0	6	7.93	0.8	3	5.04	0.6	8	4.71	1.7	17	20.12	0.8
Ovary, fallopian tubes	10	8.41	1.2	40	29.13	1.4	37	20.46	1.8[a]	46	25.25	1.8[a]	133	83.19	1.6[a]
Kidney, renal pelvis, ureter	2	2.81	0.7	9	9.92	0.9	6	7.14	0.8	4	9.90	0.4	21	29.77	0.7
Bladder, other urinary	4	5.06	0.8	25	17.91	1.4	12	13.09	0.9	21	18.84	1.1	62	54.87	1.1
Melanoma of the skin	4	2.22	1.8	12	7.72	1.6	8	5.37	1.5	9	6.69	1.3	33	21.99	1.5[a]
Eye	0	0.32	0.0	4	1.09	3.7	0	0.77	0.0	3	1.00	3.0	7	3.17	2.2
Brain, central nervous system	0	1.83	0.0	6	6.42	0.9	3	4.57	0.7	8	5.93	1.3	17	18.73	0.9
Thyroid gland	5	1.40	3.6[a]	7	4.78	1.5	6	3.26	1.8	4	3.89	1.0	22	13.32	1.7[a]
Bone	[illegible]	0.29	3.4	0	0.97	0.0	0	0.64	0.0	1	0.74	2.4	2	2.64	0.8
Connective tissue	0	0.80	0.0	7	2.76	2.5[a]	4	1.93	2.1	3	2.46	1.2	14	7.94	1.8
Lymphatic, hematopoietic system	**5**	**11.52**	**0.4**	**25**	**40.62**	**0.6**[a]	**26**	**29.56**	**0.9**	**38**	**42.43**	**0.9**	**94**	**124.06**	**0.8**[a]
Non-Hodgkin's lymphoma	3	4.35	0.7	11	15.40	0.7	10	11.18	0.9	9	15.92	0.6	33	46.82	0.7[a]
Hodgkin's disease	0	0.85	0.0	3	2.89	1.0	2	2.02	1.0	2	2.53	0.8	7	8.82	0.8
Multiple myeloma	2	1.92	1.0	3	6.86	0.4	3	5.13	0.6	4	7.93	0.5	12	21.83	0.5[a]
Leukemias	0	4.37	0.0[a]	8	15.38	0.5	11	11.20	1.0	23	16.02	1.4	42	46.94	0.9
Chronic lymphocytic	0	1.19	0.0	1	4.25	0.2	0	3.16	0.0	4	4.85	0.8	5	13.44	0.4[a]
Acute nonlyphocytic	0	1.44	0.0	4	5.10	0.8	7	3.74	1.9	8	5.55	1.4	19	15.81	1.2

[a] $p < 0.05$

Table 3. Observed (O) and expected (E) numbers of second primary cancers by years after diagnosis of an initial cancer of the breast (ICD-7 code 170) among females in Denmark, 1943–1980 [5]

	Years after first primary cancer diagnosis														
	< 1			1–4			5–9			10+			Total		
No. starting interval	54 964			46 362			22 421			11 273			54 964		
Person-years in interval	50 710			128 756			79 452			86 180			345 098		
Second primary cancer site	O	E	OE	O	E	OE	O	E	OE	O	E	OE	O	E	OE
All second cancers	**251**	**309.16**	**0.8**[a]	**811**	**818.58**	**1.0**[c]	**601**	**547.16**	**1.1**[c]	**817**	**722.86**	**1.1**[a]	**2480**	**2397.75**	**1.0**
All excluding site of initial cancer	**251**	**309.16**	**0.8**[a]	**811**	**818.58**	1.0	**601**	**547.16**	**1.1**[a]	**817**	**722.86**	**1.1**[a]	**2480**	**2397.75**	**1.0**
Buccal cavity, pharynx	**2**	**5.23**	**0.4**	**10**	**13.80**	0.7	**13**	**9.21**	**1.4**	**16**	**12.23**	1.3	**41**	**40.46**	**1.0**
Lip	2	0.77	2.6	1	2.04	0.5	2	1.37	1.5	2	1.88	1.1	7	6.06	1.2
Tongue	0	0.92	0.0	2	2.39	0.8	2	1.58	1.3	1	2.10	0.5	5	6.99	0.7
Salivary gland	0	1.16	0.0	2	3.02	0.7	1	1.97	0.5	7	2.21	3.2[a]	10	8.37	1.2
Gum, other mouth	0	1.41	0.0	3	3.82	0.8	4	2.61	1.5	6	3.95	1.5	13	11.79	1.1
Pharynx	0	0.97	0.0	2	2.53	0.8	4	1.67	2.4	0	2.09	0.0	6	7.26	0.8
Digestive system	**105**	**130.87**	**0.8**[a]	**315**	**344.64**	**0.9**	**242**	**230.88**	**1.0**	**347**	**315.58**	**1.1**	**1009**	**1021.97**	**1.0**
Esophagus	1	3.71	0.3	6	9.56	0.6	7	6.34	1.1	15	8.65	1.7	29	28.25	1.0
Stomach	31	34.41	0.9	87	86.69	1.0	62	55.35	1.1	64	67.25	1.0	244	243.70	1.0
Colon	29	40.20	0.7	105	108.19	1.0	87	74.08	1.2	130	106.65	1.2[a]	351	329.11	1.1
Rectum	21	23.23	0.9	61	61.33	1.0	41	41.14	1.0	64	55.22	1.2	187	180.93	1.0
Liver, biliary	8	10.80	0.7	16	29.50	0.5[a]	17	20.58	0.8	21	30.71	0.7	62	91.59	0.7[a]
Pancreas	13	12.77	1.0	25	34.93	0.7	20	24.30	0.8	46	36.33	1.3	104	108.32	1.0
Respiratory system	**16**	**19.68**	**0.8**	**63**	**54.01**	**1.2**	**60**	**37.39**	**1.6**[a]	**82**	**53.41**	**1.5**[a]	**221**	**164.49**	**1.3**[a]
Nasal cavities, sinuses	1	0.60	1.7	1	1.56	0.6	0	1.03	0.0	0	1.36	0.0	2	4.56	0.4
Larynx	2	0.86	2.3	1	2.33	0.4	3	1.60	1.9	1	2.09	0.5	7	6.89	1.0
Tranchea, bronchus, lung	13	16.56	0.8	57	45.78	1.2	53	31.84	1.7	76	46.12	1.6[a]	199	140.30	1.4[a]
Female breast[a]	–	–	–	–	–	–	–	–	–	–	–	–	–	–	–

cont'd.

Table 3. (*continued*)

	Years after first primary cancer diagnosis														
	< 1			1–4			5–9			10+			Total		
No. starting interval	54 964			46 362			22 421			11 273			54 964		
Person-years in interval	50 710			128 756			79 452			86 180			345 098		
Second primary cancer site	**O**	**E**	**OE**	**O**	**E**	**OE**	**O**	**E**	**OE**	**O**	**E**	**OE**	**O**	**E**	**OE**
Female genital tract	**70**	**79.51**	**0.9**	**218**	**208.63**	**1.0**	**145**	**136.08**	**1.1**	**190**	**159.99**	**1.2**[a]	**623**	**584.20**	**1.1**
Cervix uteri	21	28.44	0.7	64	72.20	0.9	36	44.20	0.8	43	44.27	1.0	164	189.11	0.9
Corpus uteri	22	21.67	1.0	61	58.37	1.0	44	39.85	1.1	51	50.14	1.0	178	170.03	1.0
Uterus, NOS	5	1.75	2.9	9	4.30	2.1	5	2.68	1.9	1	3.13	0.3	20	11.85	1.7[a]
Ovary, fallopian tubes	21	22.92	0.9	75	61.19	1.2	50	40.91	1.2	76	51.07	1.5[a]	222	176.09	1.3[a]
Kidney, renal pelvis, ureter	10	9.90	1.0	34	26.82	1.3	24	18.46	1.3	29	25.72	1.1	97	80.91	1.2
Bladder, other urinary	10	10.35	1.0	30	28.27	1.1	19	19.65	1.0	23	28.52	0.8	82	86.79	0.9
Melanoma of the skin	6	5.56	1.1	24	14.98	1.6[a]	13	9.93	1.3	16	12.68	1.3	59	43.15	1.4[a]
Eye	2	1.10	1.8	3	2.90	1.0	1	1.94	0.5	3	2.38	1.3	9	8.31	1.1
Brain, central nervous system	4	7.83	0.5	20	20.87	1.0	14	13.96	1.0	13	17.49	0.7	51	60.16	0.8
Thyroid gland	3	2.63	1.1	9	7.02	1.3	7	4.72	1.5	4	6.39	0.6	23	20.76	1.1
Bone	0	0.68	0.0	2	1.72	1.2	5	1.10	4.6[a]	4	1.33	3.0	11	4.83	2.3[a]
Connective tissue	1	1.35	0.7	5	3.46	1.4	3	2.16	1.4	11	2.59	4.3[a]	20	9.56	2.1[a]
Lymphatic, hematopoietic system	**17**	**19.89**	**0.9**	**62**	**53.69**	**1.2**	**47**	**36.77**	**1.3**	**60**	**51.90**	**1.2**	**186**	**162.25**	**1.1**
Non-Hodgkin's lymphoma	6	5.90	1.0	16	16.02	1.0	7	11.04	0.6	21	15.89	1.3	50	48.85	1.0
Hodgkin's disease	1	1.52	0.7	1	3.97	0.3	2	2.60	0.8	2	3.24	0.6	6	11.32	0.5
Multiple myeloma	1	3.89	0.3	6	10.61	0.6	7	7.39	0.9	10	10.75	0.9	24	32.65	0.7
Leukemias	9	8.40	1.1	39	22.58	1.7[a]	29	15.40	1.9[a]	26	21.59	1.2	103	67.97	1.5[a]
Chronic lymphocytic	4	3.61	1.1	9	9.72	0.9	10	6.68	1.5	6	9.63	0.6	29	29.64	1.0
Acute nonlymphocytic	4	2.41	1.7	18	6.67	2.7	13	4.65	2.8	16	6.96	2.3[a]	51	20.69	2.5[a]

[a] ICD-7 code = 170
[b] $p < 0.05$
[c] Second breast cancers were not available on the Danish Cancer Registry computer files

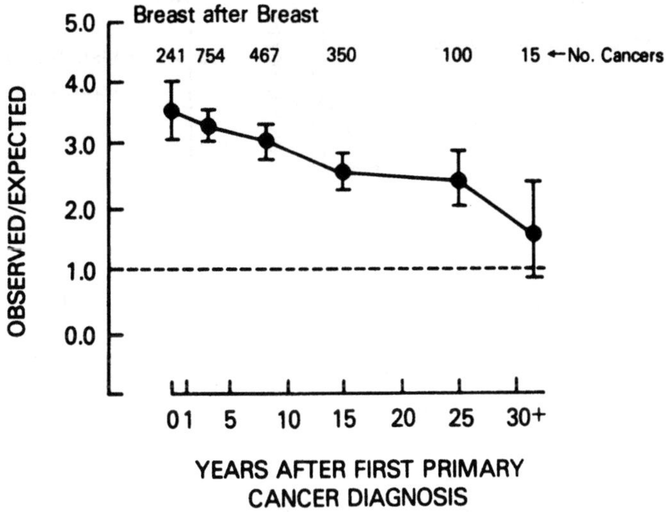

Fig. 1. Observed and expected rates for second breast cancer by time since diagnosis of an initial primary breast cancer in Connecticut, 1935–1982. *Bars*, 95% confidence intervals [2]

of the salivary gland and esophagus also increased with time and suggest that radiation may have been involved. Radiation or chemotherapy, or both, may also have influenced the risk of acute nonlymphocytic leukemia (51 cases observed vs 20.7 expected). A significant excess of malignant melanoma might indicate a common hormonal etiology with breast cancer.

Studies of Radiation-Induced Breast Cancer

Excess breast cancers have been reported in surveys of tuberculosis patients who had multiple fluoroscopic examinations of the chest, mastitis patients given radiotherapy, and atomic bomb survivors [3,13,15]. These studies indicate that the risk is greatest for persons exposed in childhood or early adolescence, that the risk decreases with increasing age at exposure, that the dose-response relationship is consistent with linearity for doses under about 6 Gy (Fig. 2), that the risk remains high even 45 years after the exposure, and that fractionation does not appear to diminish risk.

Practically all studies indicate that the risk of radiogenic breast cancer among women over the age of 40 years when first exposed is small, and no elevation in risk has been reported among atomic bomb survivors or women with tuberculosis of this age. Data from women irradiated for benign breast disorders in Sweden suggest a risk among those over age 40 [1], but there was no comparison group and many of the women were treated for fibroadenomatosis or chronic mastitis, which may predispose toward breast cancer. Interestingly, among women treated for mastitis who received over 8 Gy (Fig. 3), there was a significant decrease in risk, suggesting that the induction of malignancy at high doses may be modified by the increased frequency of cell death.

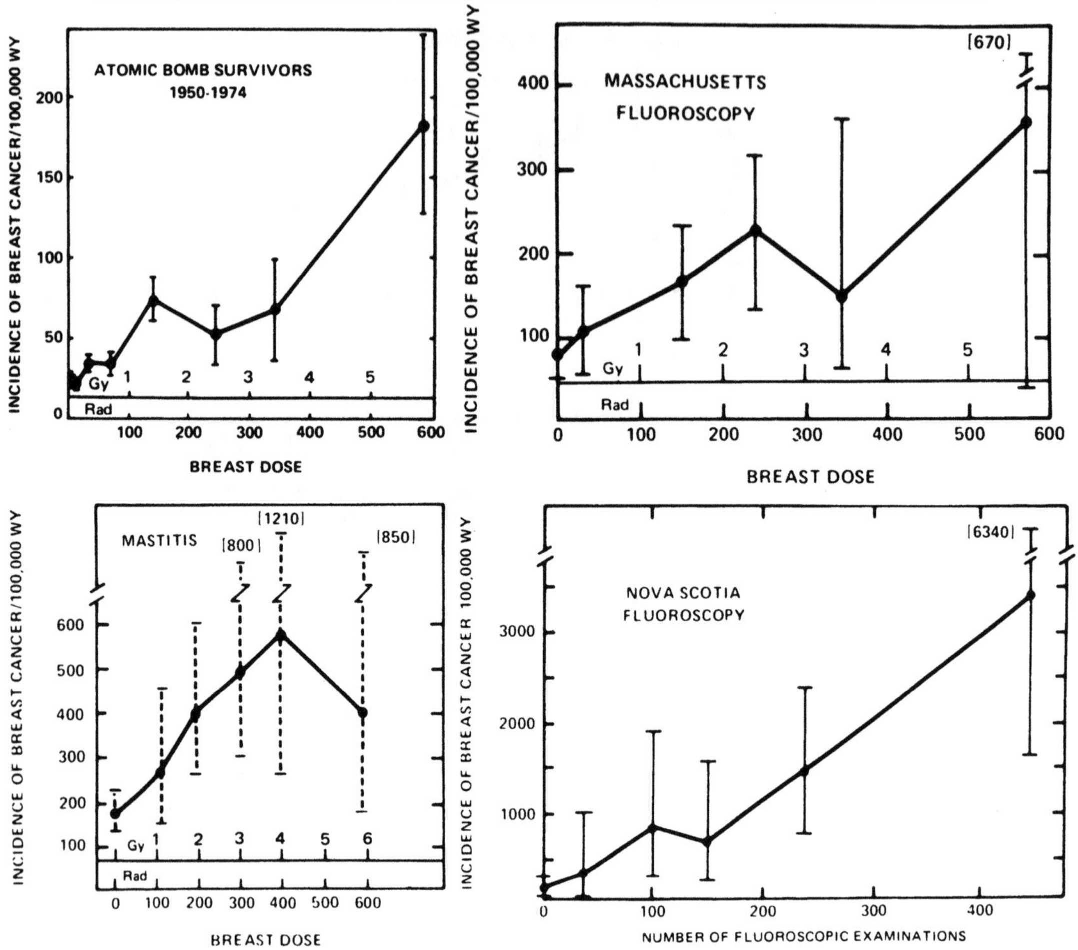

Fig. 2. Dose-response curves of breast cancer incidence by radiation dose or number of fluoroscopic examinations for atomic bomb survivors [11], Massachusetts tuberculosis patients receiving multiple chest fluoroscopies, Rochester mastitis radiotherapy patients, and Nova Scotia tuberculosis patients [3]. *WY*, woman years

Discussion

There is no doubt that radiation in sufficient amounts can increase the risk of cancer in irradiated populations. However, it is unclear whether the radiation treatments accompanying breast-conserving therapy would be associated with a detectable increase in risk of developing a second cancer. With or without radiotherapy, a women with breast cancer is three times more likely to develop a second breast cancer than women in the general population. Would radiation increase the risk of developing a second breast cancer? Perhaps. If the initial cancerous breast is partially conserved, the radiation dose would be over 10 Gy (1000 rad) which might be so large as to kill or render inactive any malignant or premalignant lesions. The

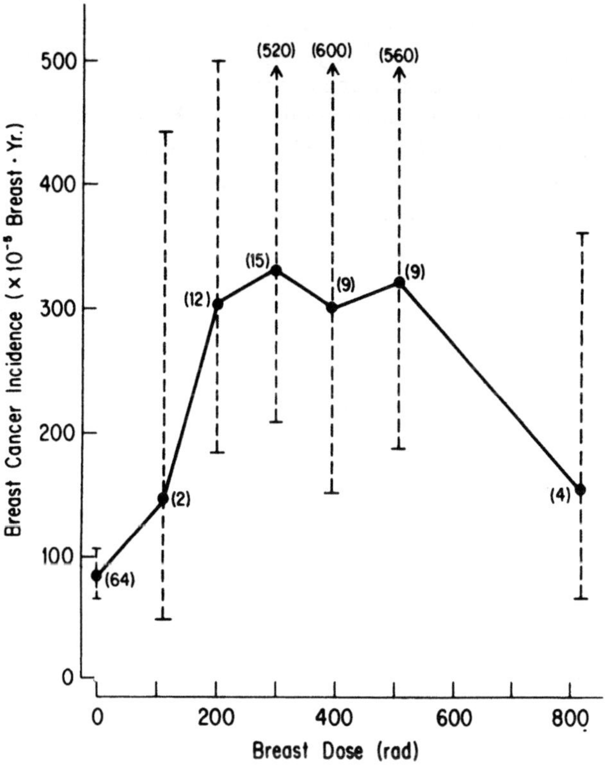

Fig. 3. Radiation dose-response curve for women treated with X-rays for acute postpartum mastitis. Dose to single breast is present along with 90% confidence intervals (*dotted lines*) and the number of breast cancers for each dose group [13]

scatter dose to the contralateral breast ranges from 50 cGy to several hundred cGy [7], and is in the range of doses where excess breast cancers have been reported. However, there is increasing evidence that women over the age of 40 years, i.e., over the age when most women develop breast cancer, are at particularly low risk for the induction of radiogenic breast cancer. It should be kept in mind that these women are at high risk for second breast cancer independent of therapy, and that it is theoretically possible, though not demonstrated, that this underlying increased susceptibility might predispose to radiogenic breast cancer.

Other sites that might receive meaningful doses of radiation during treatment for breast cancer include the bone marrow (chest wall), lung, esophagus, and thyroid. Low doses of radiation can increase the risk of thyroid cancer. Very high doses of radiation can, in rare instances, produce bone cancers and soft tissue sarcomas. High doses of radiation also have been associated with increased rates of cancers of the lung and esophagus. It is unclear, however, to what extent breast-conserving therapy might contribute to increased cancers of these sites. Risk depends on the dose to the organ and the age of the patient, and the period of observation after irradiation is also relevant. In general, the minimum latent period for a radiogenic tumor is approximately 10 years, so that women first treated at an elderly age might

not be expected to live long enough to develop a new cancer. The concern, then, would be with regard to younger women who, perhaps, might be more likely to request breast-conserving treatment.
Surprisingly, excess leukemias have been reported following radiotherapy for breast cancer [6]. The numbers of leukemias were small, but the fact that they occurred in women treated in randomized clinical trials is noteworthy. Excesses have also been seen in Connecticut [11] and Denmark [5] following breast irradiation, but it is unlikely that the magnitude of the risk is comparable to that seen among patients treated with alkylating agents. In fact, for some cancers the risk of leukemia associated with alkylating agent therapy reaches over 100-fold [8]!

In conclusion, the potential adverse effects associated with the use of radiation must always be balanced by the benefits accrued from this treatment modality. It is possible that radiogenic breast cancers could be induced following irradiation during breast-conserving therapy; however, the age of the patients is probably associated with a low overall risk, especially in light of the threefold risk associated with other factors. Leukemia has been reported elevated after breast radiotherapy, despite the fact that only a small portion of the body's bone marrow is exposed. High doses of radiation are known to increase the risk of cancers of the bone, connective tissue, esophagus, lung, and skin. Low doses increase the risk of cancers of the thyroid and salivary gland. Population studies from Connecticut and Denmark, however, indicate that there are likely many factors other than radiation that put a woman with breast cancer at risk of developing a new primary cancer.

References

1. Baral E, Larsson LE, Mattsson B (1977) Breast cancer following irradiation of the breast. Cancer 40:2905–2910
2. Boice JD Jr, Curtis RE, Kleinerman RA, Flannery JT, Fraumeni JF Jr (1986) Multiple primary cancers in Connecticut, 1935–82. Yale J Biol Med 59:533–545
3. Boice JD Jr, Land CE, Shore RE, Norman JE, Tokunaga M (1979) Risk of breast cancer following low-dose radiation exposure. Radiology 131:589–597
4. Ewertz M, Machado SG, Boice JD Jr, Jensen OM (1984) Endometrial cancer following treatment for breast cancer: a case-control study in Denmark. Br J Cancer 50:687–692
5. Ewertz M, Mouridsen HT (1985) Second cancer following cancer of the female breast in Denmark, 1943–80. NCI Monogr 1985; 68:325–329
6. Fisher B, Rockette H, Fisher ER, et al. (1985) Leukemia in breast cancer patients following adjuvant chemotherapy or postoperative radiotherapy: the NSABP experience. J Clin Oncol 3:1640–1658
7. Fraass BA, Roberson PL, Lichter AS (1985) Dose to the contralateral breast due to primary breast irradiation. Int J Radiat Oncol Biol Phys 11:485–497
8. Greene MH, Harris EL, Gershenson DM, Malkasian GD Jr, Melton LJ, Dembo AJ, Bennett JM, Moloney WC, Boice JD Jr (1986) Melphalan may be a more potent leukemogen than cyclophosphamide. Ann Intern Med 105:360–367
9. Hankey BF, Curtis RE, Naughton MD, Boice JD Jr, Flannery JT (1983) A retrospective cohort analysis of second breast cancer risk for primary breast cancer patients with an assessment of the effect of radiation therapy. JNCI 70:797–804
10. Harris JR, Hellman S, Kinne DW (1985) Limited surgery and radiotherapy for early breast cancer. N Engl J Med 305:6–11

11. Harvey EB, Brinton LA (1985) Second cancer following cancer of the breast in Connecticut, 1935-82. NCI Monogr 68:99-112
12. Hellman S, Harris JR (1987) The appropriate breast cancer paradigm. Cancer Res 47:339-342
13. Shore RE, Hildreth N, Woodard E, Dvorestsky P, Hempelmann L, Pasternack B (1986) Breast cancer among women given x-ray therapy for acute postpartum mastitis. JNCI 77:689-696
14. Stewart FW, Treves N (1948) Lymphangiosarcoma in postmastectomy lymphedema: a report of six cases in elephantiasis chirurgica. Cancer 1:64-81
15. Tokunaga M, Land CE, Yamamoto T, Asano M, Tokuoka S, Nishimori EI, Fujikura T (1984) Breast cancer among atomic bomb survivors. In: Boice JD Jr, Fraumeni JF Jr (eds) Radiation carcinogenesis:epidemiology and biological significance. Raven, New York, pp 45-56

Psychological Problems of Women with Carcinoma of the Breast and Possible Means of Treatment

H. BECKER

This chapter is based on an empirical study with a psychoanalytic slant, which was designed to examine to what extent concomitant psychosocial factors in the lives of women with carcinoma of the breast influence the development and, in particular, the course of the illness. At the same time, it was possible to draw on over 10 years' experience in a consultancy for tumor patients, which was concerned particularly with female patients with carcinoma of the breast [2,6].

Apart from the fact of having cancer at all, what does it mean to a woman to have cancer of the breast? First of all we have to ask, for example, to what extent the breast is linked with the woman's sense of identity and how important she considers this organ. The feeling of existential fear arising from the diagnosis of cancer as a physical illness not uncommonly conceals a graduated value structure accepted by both patient and doctor for the various organs. If we name, or consider quite soberly, the different organs in our own body in which a primary tumor could be sited, and the potential feelings we might have about each if it were the one affected, it very quickly becomes clear that it makes a considerable difference whether the lung, the bowel, the breast, the uterus, of the testis is affected. The doctor in charge of treatment, even if guided by the general laws of conventional medicine, is also not completely free of personal feelings about particular parts of the body when assessing the condition and giving advice. This is particularly obvious in borderline situations: when, for example, it can be a matter of discretion whether the uterus is removed as a prophylactic measure or whether a primary therapy allowing conservation of the breast is preferable to amputation in a patient with an early stage of carcinoma of the breast. The sex-specific nature of the feelings of both doctor and patient about the fact of being a physical body will also play a not inconsiderable role in all this: the consultation will take a different course according to whether a male or a female patient is being advised by a male or a female doctor. In addition to the meaning invested in the body and the primary symbolic content of individual organs and body regions and the reactive experience of change, illness, or disablement, we have to ask, first, whether there is such a thing as a specific choice of organ with symbolic expression and then whether such a thing as a *secondary symbolism* and interpretation can begin with the illness [6]. It has been possible to allocate tumors in different sites to more or less specific personality types in psycho-oncologic studies [10]. While this suggests a possible link between personality factors and the organ affected, it might also be regarded as a reaction to affliction of a particular organ or be connected with exogenous factors involved in carcinogenesis, which can include social behavior. Oncologic conditions have to be regarded as generalized rather than organ-specific illnesses, and the patient's initial fear is also a primal and existential one, with fear for the specific organ taking a back seat at first. Let us now consider the meaning invested in the breast and its symbolic and relational significance for the patient and for the doctor-patient relationship.

The female breast is highly invested by the woman herself, in terms of her sexual and physical identity as a woman, partner, and mother; by the man as an object of sexual desire; and by the child as a source of nourishment. The idea of the breast in connection with physical identity and personality, with its actual and symbolic significance, is thus highly invested by the woman herself, by the man, and by the child. For the pubescent girl the development of her breasts is the first sign of a physical change that she will notice herself, and the most obvious sign to the people around her. The most usual response to the change is a mixture of pride and embarrassed modesty, the balance of the two depending on the individual history. This also seems to be the deciding factor in the extent to which this woman in the making will be able to integrate the changes taking place in her body and ultimately adopt a positive attitude to her own body. Hand in hand with the outward physical process of maturation, the breast, as one of the secondary sex characteristics, acquires a new function as an erogenous zone, which the woman experiences with increasing intensity if she feels comfortable with her body. This extensive investment of the breast is determined partly by the way the woman herself experiences this organ but also by her possibly equivocal attitude, which can be subject to more restrictive or more permissive principles. This conflict can express itself in concealment of the breasts by selected clothing or by the posture adopted, feelings of aversion when the breast is touched, and so on. An impaired bodily and sexual identity in a woman is frequently attributable to the deep-rooted feeling that sexuality is taboo or to the woman's failure to identify with her mother or other female reference person. In its glandular function, then, the breast is not only an organ of nutrition but in addition is of decisive importance to a woman's self-esteem in the area of sexual and physical identity. It is very often – mistakenly – assumed that it is mainly younger women who will experience extreme distress if amputation of the breast is necessary. In fact, the great subjective importance of the breast persists into advanced old age. This means that the indications for breast amputation as against conservative treatment, for example, should be strictly defined and adhered to in the treatment of older women, too. If amputation is indicated, for example, psychosocial factors must be considered in addition to the precise scientific data. If we accept that the breast is important to the woman not only in its glandular function but also for her physical identity and self-esteem, the overriding principle in treatment for both elderly and young women should be conservation of the organ, subject to careful balancing of continuation of life against quality of life. In practice, this means that conservative therapy must be preferred over a radical surgical procedure whenever it will not have a negative influence on survival and thus on the patient's prognosis. Even the present-day prospects of reconstruction surgery cannot compensate for loss of the organ. If amputation is indicated, recognition of the individual significance of the organ's loss for the patient concerned is essential if any mutual understanding is to be reached in the context of the doctor-patient relationship, both in the preoperative phase and even more so during aftercare. Not only younger women experience the loss of a breast as an invasion of their self-esteem associated with enormous fear of destruction of the relationship between themselves and their partners; older women are affected in precisely the same way. The breast symbolizes sexual identity and maternity, and these do not seem to be any less important components of self-esteem than in earlier life. The increasingly frequent offer of cosmetic surgery to reverse the loss to some degree is received very differently by different patients. There are women who cannot come to terms with the necessity for amputation at all unless cosmetic reconstruction is offered. This option is thus a great help in individual cases. On the other hand, many women reject the idea of cosmetic reconstructive surgery even when the doctor in charge of the treatment suggests it in very positive terms, and it has to be assumed that this is intimately linked with the individual woman's way of processing her illness; for example, it is bound up with the question of whether a woman can come to terms with her illness and the loss of her breast and can later build up a new physical identity, or whether she completely rejects this process by way of a reversal of what has taken place. The following two brief case histories illustrate what is meant.

Case 1. After a careful and detailed diagnosis, breast amputation was considered to be indicated as the treatment of choice for carcinoma of the breast in a 37-year-old patient. She had said that she would only be prepared to have the breast amputated if cosmetic reconstructive surgery was possible. She connected the loss of her breast with a crisis in the relationship with her partner and also, as was seen later during the psychosocial counseling after the operation, with further confirmation of her feelings of rejection and worthlessness towards her own body. She spontaneously requested psychotherapy as part of the aftercare, and it was also medically indicated. During the course of this therapy a deep-rooted premorbid disturbance of her sense of female identity was revealed, which was treated with a satisfactory result. The patient said no more about reconstructive surgery. For the first time, she was able to build up a new relationship with a partner in which she experienced sexual satisfaction and could expose her body during bathing and in the sauna with relatively little embarrassment.

Case 2. A 62-year-old patient had to undergo amputation of the left breast because of mammary carcinoma. As she was afraid she would have problems with a prosthesis she asked the surgeon to amputate the other breast too, which was done only 11 days after the first operation. According to what was said, the doctor and the patient had agreed on the necessity of prophylactic surgery to avoid carcinoma of the contralateral breast. While relating her life history the patient reported that she had formerly had an exceptionally pretty bosom, which had made her very attractive to men. She herself, however, had wished from the age of 20 onwards that she could have her breasts made smaller. During one of the postoperative counseling sessions it became clear that she was going through an extremely distressing crisis in the relationship to her partner and was acutely suicidal. She said that while she had set a high value on her attractiveness to men, she had always experienced herself as defensive in relationships and had never known any sexual feelings. She declared that she was now having suicidal ideas again, but on the other hand there was a clear tendency for her to deny the situation that was currently causing her such distress. Two months after the bilateral breast amputation she confirmed that she did not regret also having had the healthy breast removed and would make the same decision again now. The criticism and doubts she really felt became obvious, however, because of an observation that was only tentatively implied: that more trouble should have been taken to make the scar resulting from amputation of the right breast less ugly and that a bit had been left sticking out. The patient's history and character structure allowed a clear diagnosis of pronounced masochism, which was also expressed in her tendency towards actual self-mutilation.

These case histories are meant to illustrate how extremely difficult it is to evaluate a patient's request for surgical correction with reference to the psychological diagnosis, even when the patient makes an unequivocal statement. In particular, immediately after any serious operation a patient needs an adequate amount of time to come to terms with the illness, especially in the case of an outwardly mutilating operation, and to build up a new physical identity. The doctor has to adopt an attitude suited to the individual patient when offering advice and should avoid falling prey to the seductive idea of the most extensive operative technique —in the cosmetic sector as in any other [3]. The extremely prevalent trend to recommend breast reconstruction after radical surgery may well spring from a defense mechanism in a male doctor, taking the form of an attempt at reversal on the basis of his own unconscious fears and guilt feelings, in his attitude to the breast as a symbol of female potency and motherhood. Certainly, it would also be possible to object at this juncture that we are not concerned with the numerous women who have a satisfactory self-image following cosmetic reconstructive surgery or correction without malignant disease. In one study, WENDERLEIN and HOFFMANN (1983) questioned women about their well-being 1 year after breast augmentation surgery. Only about 50% of the women felt more self-confident and more able to make new contacts, and only one-third were more satisfied with their sex lives than before. A good half of the women complained, above all, that they experienced hardly any sexual arousal when the area of the nipple was touched. Since a cosmetic operation is also a kind of irreversible mutilation, the indications must be carefully decided on, and particularly strictly a detailed psychological examination is essential; there is absolutely no justification for going ahead with the operation without this. If organ-centered medicine is not to miss the point in the treatment of patients, it will need to draw much more on knowledge derived from psychosomatic medicine both in clinical practice and in the training of medical students.

This empirical study was performed in a total of 143 women, 71 patients with carcinoma of the breast and a control group of 72 with fractures or benign gynecological conditions [2].

Table 1. A Psychosomatic Empirical Study on Carcinoma of the Breast

Test group $n=71$		Control group $n=72$	
20 breast carcinoma patients aged under 50 years, in various clinical stages	51 breast carcinoma patients with comparable clinical stages.	36 women atients with fractures	36 patients from the gynecological outpatient department.

With the intention of detecting cofactors that might be involved in the etiology and the course of the illness, the following methods of examination were also used (in order of administration):

1. Projective test (Holtzman Inkblot Technique; HIT)
2. Personality test (Giessen test; self and ideal)
3. Intelligence test (Multiple Word Test; MWT-B)
4. Questionnaire (social data in objective sector)
5. Psychoanalytic interview with documentation and evaluation by means of
   a) Formal written record of interview
   b) Questionnaire relating to subjective and objective patient data (filled out by interview)
   c) Verbatim record for psycholinguistic analysis after GOTTSCHALK and GLESER and for evaluation of defense mechanisms
   d) Qualitative and quantitative assessment of psychosocial trauma in earlier life (life events)

The most important part of the study was the prospective part relating to the course of the illness, i.e., the question as to how far the psychosocial data differed between the subgroup with a favorable and that with an unfavorable course of disease, since the patients had all been comparable for stage of disease at the time of the initial examination. It was intended that the conclusions reached should be used as a basis on which to plan aftercare.

With respect to the course of the illness, the following points emerged as significant for aftercare strategy: breast cancer patients in whom the illness took an unfavorable course were found in a prospective study to have pronounced inhibitions in the expression of aggressive feelings. In comparison with patients in whom the disease took a favorable course they were characterized significantly more by feelings of hopelessness and had significantly fewer plans for the future. The history of patients with an unfavorable prognosis is more frequently characterized by the loss of primary reference people in childhood, which will also influence their way of dealing with the illness.

Overall, the study showed that older women who had passed the menopause more frequently corresponded to the psychopathological norm than younger, premenopausal, breast carcinoma patients.

If the result of studies performed within the context of prospective psycho-oncological research are considered from the aspects of etiology and prognosis, striking agreements become apparent (these results, however, do not refer exclusively to carcinoma of the breast):

a) Prospective psycho-oncological studies
   Psychosocial risk factors
   "Substable personality" [9]
   Lack of emotional closeness to parents [18]
   Premorbid depression [16]
b) Studies of course (prospective)
   Psychosocial features of prognosis
   Personal adjustment to the illness [15]
   Denial of aggressive feelings [2,7,14,17]
   Stoic acceptance and hopelessness [8]
   Depressive symptoms [1,7]

What are the implications of this for useful psychosocial aftercare? One purpose of psychosocial *aftercare* is to create conditions in which the patient can enjoy an active, sanguine way of life so far as possible. Something that seems particularly important to me is that active or even aggressive behavior on the part of the patient should not be met with rejection but tolerated within the doctor-patient relationship as far as possible. There is of course a problem, insofar as a hopeful attitude and aggressive behavior cannot be simply prescribed; rather, the reasons for despair and for defenses against aggressive feelings need to be systematically worked out.

I have seen in the care of cancer patients that one of the main reasons for despair, resignation, and inhibition of aggression lies in the patients' own ideas about their illness, that is to say in their *subjective naive theory of illness* or in the lay person's ideas about the different forms of cancer, for example. More than a few patients connect their ideas about how and why they have come to be ill with guilt and punishment, even though the connection is hardly a conscious one for most of them.

Thus, during the aftercare period, it is essential for a good doctor-patient relationship that the doctor be aware of the patient's own spontaneous theory of illness. In one study the patients were asked questions about how and why they thought their illness had arisen [4] (Table 2).

Table 2. Subjective theories of cause of illness

	Patients with carcinoma of the breast ($n=71$)	
External traumas (injury, illness, environment, etc.)	39	(55%)
Iatrogenic causes	13	(18%)
Heredity	13	(18%)
Psychosocial theories	49	(59%)
Tending more to assumption of endogenous causes	28	(39%)
Tending more to assumption of causation by external psychosocial stress	14	(19%)
Fate	23	(32%)
Guilt/punishment	21	(30%)

It was striking that almost three-fifths of the patients had some psychosocial theory to account for their illness, one-third thought their illness was their fate, and one-third connected their illness with wrongdoing and punishment. During the interviews it was noticeable that the patients were inclined to put forward rational, socially accepted theories of illness initially, and then later rather irrational, inexplicable, and psychodynamic ideas; this shift might be attributable to increasing intimacy as the interview progressed.

Subjective theories of illness involving guilt and punishment in particular often disturb the doctor-patient relationship in the context of aftercare; that is to say, they are often responsible for noncompliance.

Theories of illness involving guilt and punishment:
As a child I once stole something and I've never been able to forget it. I'm all knotted up – literally – in my breast.

The main thing was when I had the baby. I wanted to keep it inside me and felt we'd been separated too brutally. I'm afraid I'm a bad mother.

I often think it's a punishment – though really I've already been punished enough. I feel such blows of fate enrich me.

I was too late taking my husband into hospital when he had a perforated appendix, and I shouted at my mother too often.

I didn't breast-feed. My husband's mother thinks that's why I've got it.

I've not done anything wicked. It just suddenly happened.

Well, I looked after everybody else and then something like this had to happen. But I'll put up with it.

Why me? I've always lived in a normal decent manner.

We've all got to go sometime; I should have taken more care of myself. You can beat it with willpower.

I've never done anything wrong. Why me? It depends how you've lived.

I don't think it's fair when we've never done anything wrong.

I've taken too many painkillers.

A brief excerpt from the case history of one patient with breast carcinoma illustrates this concept more clearly. A 51-year-old patient had refused postoperative radiotherapy following amputation of the left breast. She spontaneously requested referral to a psychotherapist. The doctor in charge of her treatment told her she was not that crazy yet. She herself had realized that she had wanted to be ill in one sense and saw it as a form of relief, but that on the other hand she wanted to go on living. She reported without being asked that her mother had died of bowel cancer 5 years earlier; shortly before her mother's death, her father had asked her to sit up with her at night, since he felt her mother was being spiteful with him. During the night my patient pretended to be asleep when her mother called her, and her mother died the next morning before they had been able to talk things over together. The patient said she had a terribly guilty conscience about her mother, although she had looked after her for years in a most self-sacrificing manner. Ever since her mother's death she had slept badly all the time and had tried to make up for her sins with good works. She saw her present illness as a result and a welcome relief from her burden of guilt. The opportunity to talk about the whole matter was enough to bring the patient to the point where she was ready to continue with the treatment indicated on the grounds of her physical condition. A consultation of this kind does not need to be conducted by a specialized psychotherapist; the doctor in overall charge of the treatment can also conduct it if the patient is prepared to talk.

This case history clearly shows how the process of coming to terms with the illness is connected with past events in the individual patient's life and how important it can be for the doctor to learn something about this particular lay person's ideas about illness. In years of experience in consultation I have seen that doctors' ignorance of their patients' theories of illness is the main reason for what is called noncompliance and that conversely, precisely if a patient's theory of illness is known when a doctor-patient relationship is initiated, this can be the basis for meaningful communication.

General Criteria for Psychosocial Care of Cancer Patients

The concepts of screening, patient information, therapy, and aftercare imply a tendency to frequent changes of doctor even in the way the words indicate temporal differentiation, thus contradicting the actually progressive nature of the sequence of these steps. On the one hand, this is certainly linked with the increasing level of specialization within scientific medicine; on the other, the family doctor has the very important function of integrating the different aspects of care.

Screening

Participation in screening programs is determined largely by psychological factors. Information designed to frighten patients is not an adequate aid to information, leading rather to a resigned attitude to dealing with such fear, with more pronounced denial [20]. The patient's own family doctor should describe in some detail what to expect during the screening test, give information of the risks and the chances of cure, and appeal to the patient's sense of responsibility. It is clear from the different target groups that a mass information campaign cannot replace an individual talk between doctor and patient. Scaremongering, in particular, makes sensible health behavior less likely, if anything [11]. The patient's own sense of responsibility, his or her attitude to health and illness and therefore to his or her body has a major role precisely in the context of breast cancer screening. A woman knows best herself what her breasts are like and how they change normally in the course of her menstrual cycle. Thus, for example, performance of a mammography without previous palpation, and especially without any findings made by the woman herself during regular self-examination, must be regarded as an incomplete diagnostic procedure (Table 3).

Table 3. Diagnosis of cancer of the breast in the course of screening ($n = 69$; no data on two patients)

60%	(42)	Regular participation in screening programs
39%	(27)	Screening not taken up or only at long intervals
45%	(31)	Discovery of first symptoms by self-examination despite screening
16%	(11)	Diagnosis in course of screening program

Thus, in the present study, over 80% of patients said they had discovered the lump in their breasts themselves, although 60% claimed they had taken part in screening programs regularly. This means that the tumor was diagnosed during a cancer screening program in only 16% of the patient population.

This result re-emphasizes that even with the most excellent equipment, technical medicine cannot replace the individual doctor-patient dialogue and how necessary it is in research to give priority to examining the reasons for the poor motivation of patients in the area of participation in preventive campaigns.

Information

The list below shows individual breast cancer patients' reactions on learning the diagnosis, i.e., in this case, the result of the histological test:

Reaction of individual women with carcinoma of the breast on hearing the diagnosis

It was a terrible shock.

I thought I'd go mad; I felt completely empty.
I thought, "There's a gun to my head now."
I felt as if I were already wrapped in my shroud.
I didn't want to go on living.
The world stopped turning.
Dust to dust.
It was as if I'd been hit over the head; some people would have killed themselves if anything of the sort had happened to them.
It was like being sentenced to death: I just felt like jumping into an open grave.
I felt as though I were being tortured, terrorized.
Everything all rushed in on me.
I wished I could go and bury myself in the ground.
I felt as if nobody could help me.
I suddenly felt I was quite alone.
I just lay about in bed and couldn't move an inch.
I was absolutely devastated; I just hadn't anything left to cling onto.
I felt terribly abandoned; I could have jumped out of the window.

The individual statements, as might be expected, express massive fear of death and, above all, of isolation. Precisely this feeling of isolation is one of the most important points to be borne in mind in the strategy for aftercare; that is, an object constancy within the doctor-patient relationship has a prominent role in the care of cancer patients. This refers to informing the patient of the diagnosis, but it should not be taken to mean that giving the patient information is a single action that has any claim to be considered absolute. The patients' responses in the list are acute reactions to the information given them about the diagnosis by the doctor in charge of treatment once the doctor was certain that cancer was the correct diagnosis, mainly because the histological examination had indicated this. Information, and with this the confrontation with the diagnosis, is not a single act but a long and arduous process starting with observation of the initial symptoms by the patient and continuing in the process of diagnostic testing. There is no question about whether the patient should be told the nature of the illness. Present-day methods of diagnosis and therapy in the oncologic sector are a form of information in themselves for most patients. In the dialogue between doctor and patient, then, the real question involves rather the best way of putting the necessary information across to the particular patient concerned. Neither a routine-type, purely factual, legally correct explanation of the position nor complete suppression of the facts does the patient justice, if the doctor does not take account of the patient's individual pattern of reaction and reaction to the illness. The manner and extent of the explanation given depend on the type of illness and its implication for treatment and the amount of stress the patient and the doctor can tolerate. The doctor must be guided by the necessity for "veracity" at the bedside: this concept is used less in a moral sense than to indicate that the doctor should not tell the patient anything unless personally convinced of it. This does not necessarily imply a brutal presentation of the facts, which may be inappropriate for some patients. The patient can be traumatized by the information given when the doctor devotes time to this on one occasion only and is then no longer approachable on the subject; as we have seen, in addition to real existential fear, cancer patients feel isolated by their illness and abandoned. Complete suppression of the diagnosis or attempts to comfort the patient with unrealistic hopes after the patient has been informed of it impairs the doctor-patient relationship in the long term, making the patient suspicious and leading to even more pronounced feelings of isolation.

Form and Content of Care

Descriptions of psychosocial aftercare with reference to models seldom take enough account of the actual amount of psychological stress a team working exclusively with tumor patients can take. It seems to me that it is not lack of time – as so often claimed – that prevents realization of the demand oncologists are faced with to enter into the fate of each cancer patient in a very personal way: rather the psychological burden is simply too great. This demand should be fulfilled by the

Table 4. Psychological care of cancer patients [5]

Limits	Possibilities
Workload feasible in tumor team	Longer survival – prognosis? Improved *quality of life*
Patient motivation Denial or irrational hopes "Responsibility" and "guilt" following rationalization	*Physical aftercare* Days in hospital, aftercare appointment and diagnostic tests in keeping with strict indications Curative-palliative benefits – quality of life
"Off-loading" onto psychotherapist	Continuity in relationship – changes of doctor Individualized information process *Psychosocial aftercare* Social work, pastoral care, often psychotherapy in primary care phase Subjective theory of illness – dealing with illness Isolation – work, family, etc. Active, aggressive attitude – resignation, adaptation Planning for present and future

family doctor for the most part, since for one thing doctors in general practice do not deal only with cancer patients, and for another they can guarantee continuity in the doctor-patient relationship. Despite this stress limit, in the real world the oncologist is confronted with the patients' fears and hopes and also with their expectations (Table 4). None of this should be delegated to the so-called nerve specialist. The cancer patient's motivation for getting to the bottom of psychosocial problems is quite often extremely ambivalent. For a start, the patient feels increasingly exposed to isolation because of the physical illness, an effect that is experienced more intensely following the offer of psychosocial care if such care is not presented as part of the overall medical care offered. Rationalization that is not understood in the way it is meant can increase the patient's feelings of responsibility and of some fault as the reason for the illness, a phenomenon that looms very large in any case in cancer patients, in the sense of a very strict superego. The doctor in charge of the treatment has to learn how to realize the point at which the rejection allegedly stemming from the patient has actually become his or hers, for example, from fear of being cast in the role of "helpless helper."

There are certainly also limits to the dominant idea that every cancer patient needs psychotherapy. For quite material reasons this is not possible, and it is certainly not desirable either. It would mean a further splitting of the areas of responsibility, and psychosocial care of cancer patients does not generally involve processing the life history or revealing conflicts that have hitherto remained latent. It is rather the exception, to be offered only if strictly indicated, e.g., if old neurotic conflicts are intensified by the current situation with reference to the illness. The main aim of care is not to increase the duration of survival, but to improve the quality of life (Table 5).

The following criteria are based on a follow-up study of one patient population after an average of 2.5–3 years' physical aftercare. As a rule, the stay in hospital should be kept as short as possible, and the number of appointments for aftercare and the extent of examinations directed at a new diagnosis should be considered for each patient in accordance with strict indications. After the relief brought by the initial follow-up examination, aftercare appointments and frequently repeated diagnostic tests lead to an excessive degree of confrontation with the illness, with the

Table 5. Basic schedule proposed for psycho-oncologic care [6]

Patient-oriented aftercare from psychosomatic specialists	Team-oriented tasks for psychosomatic specialists
Offer of therapy in case of *acute reactive crisis* *Individual therapy* if current pathologic process reactivates *neurotic conflicts* from before the illness	*Training for team members in perception and counseling* Help to differentiate individual and collective fears of *illness and* death in the team and in the patient
Family therapy in case of latent or manifest isolation of the patient or *decompensation* in other members of the family	Communicate functions of (e.g.) *defense mechanisms, depression, mourning* Communication *Balint groups*

result that the patient is subject to enormous psychic stress; the quality of life should be given preference over the perfect diagnosis whenever the diagnosis has no implications for the treatment. In addition, as far as organizationally possible, changes of doctor should be kept to a minimum during the aftercare period when patients attend as outpatients. Continuity in the doctor-patient relationship is of the utmost importance for the patients, and to provide this whenever possible the aftercare should revolve around the family doctor. The course of the illness is determined to a large extent by the medical team's constant readiness to accept the patient's fears, despair, and hopes. This does not mean offering unrealistic comfort, which the patient experiences as rejection, so much as standing by and not leaving the patient alone. KÜBLER-ROSS (1973) has described various stages in the emotional reaction of the cancer patients in her studies to their illness. Phases of denial, withdrawal, rage, facing up to the situation, depression, and also acceptance arise in succession. This is true not only of the chronically ill, but also of terminal patients; that is to say, even a dying patient still has the capacity for development and is not bound to go on in total withdrawal or in despair, if only communication with the people round about is not broken off. If a patient initially rejects the diagnosis, it is certainly not the primary duty of the doctor or nurse to confront the patient continually with the serious nature of the illness. The doctor should rather be ready to perceive when the patient starts to signal a desire to know and the ability to accept the diagnosis. Psychosocial aftercare, which includes social work, pastoral care, and psychotherapy, should be offered as early as possible in the primary care phase, since this is one of the essential factors that determine the extent to which the patient will later come to terms with the illness.

It is realistic and necessary for a specialist in psychosomatic medicine to be integrated into an oncology team, though his or her task should not consist so much in psychotherapy offered to individual patients as in team-centered work, i.e., *indirect* care of the patient by counseling work with the team carrying out the direct treatment. Experience so far, however, prompts the critical remark that even in the privileged centers where a psychosomatic specialist is an integral part of the team, it is mainly only the nonmedical team that is ready to adopt this cooperative way of working. The university-trained staff, i.e., the other doctors, frequently expect their colleagues specializing in psychological matters to salvage any patient in whom decompensation in the form of ambivalence arises and deal with the patient's psychic problems in close direct contact with him or her, which quite often gives the patient the feeling of being discriminated against, intensifying the mistrust. Contact between the doctor treating the physical condition and the patient should be maintained precisely at times of crisis. There is no doubt but that in the long term, the care of cancer patients without the achievement of a doctor-patient relationship based on trust requires a much greater time investment.

It is therefore recommended that doctors working in the field of oncology should undertake the psycho-oncological aspect of care themselves even in times of crisis. The nature of the training received in medical schools means that the doctors have missed out on psychosocial training, and they should compensate for this deficiency – which is felt particularly in the dialogue with the patient – as far as possible in an indirect way by being cared for themselves by specialists in psychosomatic medicine attached to their teams. Only in exceptional cases, e.g., when severe pre-existing psychic conditions are reactivated by the concurrent physical illness, does it seem necessary for the psychosomatic specialist to take on the direct psycho-oncologic care of the patient concerned, in close cooperation with the oncologic team concerned with the physical illness.

References

1. Achte KA, Vauhkonen ML (1970) On the significance of psychic factors in the prognosis of cancerous illness. Scandinavian Journal of Clinical and Laboratory Investigation 25:13–14
2. Becker H (1982) Das Mammakarzinom aus psychosomatischer Sicht. Eine empirische Studie zur Ätiologie, Prognose und Nachsorge. Habilitations-schrift, Universität Heidelberg
3. Becker H (1984a) Der Busen: Neid und Sehnsucht des Mannes? – Vom nährenden zum erotischen Beziehungsobjekt. Sexualmedizin 13:519–526
4. Becker H (1984b) Die Bedeutung der subjektiven Krankheitstheorie des Patienten für die Arzt-Patient-Beziehung. Psychother Med Psychol 34:313–321
5. Becker H (1986a) Die psychosoziale Betreuung des Krebskranken. Möglichkeiten und Grenzen. In: Drings P (ed) Bronchialkarzinom: UICC-Fortbildungskurs. Aktuelle Onkologie 26 Zuckschwerdt, München
6. Becker H (1986b) Psychoonkologie. Krebserkrankungen aus psychosomatisch-psychoanalytischer Sicht unter besonderer Berücksichtigung des Mammakarzinoms. Springer, Berlin Heidelberg New York
7. Derogatis LR, Abeloff MD, Melisaratos N (1979) Psychological Coping Mechanisms and Survival Time in Metastatic Breast Cancer. Jama 242
8. Greer S, Morris T (1975) Psychological attributes of women who develop breast cancer. Journal of Psychosomatic Research 19
9. Hagnell D (1966) The premorbid personality of persons who develop cancer in a total population investigated in 1947 and 1957. Ann. NY Acad. Sci 125
10. Hürny C, Adler R (1981) Psycho-onkologische Forschung. In: Meerwein F (Hrsg.): Einführung in die Psycho-Onkologie, 2. Aufl. Huber, Bern, 13–63
11. Janis IL (1953) Effects of fear – a rousing communication. J Abnorm Soc Psychol 48
12. Janis IL, Feshbach S (1953) Effects of fear-arousing communication. J Abnor Soc Psychol 48:78 ff
13. Kübler-Ross E (1973) Interview mit Sterbenden. Kreuz, Stuttgart
14. Nemeth G, Mezei A (1964) Personality traits of cancer patients compared with benign tumor patients on the basis of the Rorschach test. In: Kissen DM, LeShan LL (Hrsg.) Psychosomatic aspects of neoplastic disease. Pitman, New York
15. Rogentine GN, Kammen DP van, Fox BH, Docerty JP, Rosenblatt YE, Boyd SG, Bunney WE Jr (1979) Prospective factor in the prognosis of malignant melanoma: A prospective study. Psychosom. Med. 41/8:647–655
16. Shekelle RB, Raynor WJ, Ostfeld AM et al. (1981) Psychological depression and 17-year risk of death from cancer. Psychosom Med 43/2:117–125
17. Stavraky KM, Buck CN, Lott JS, Wanklin JM Psychological factors in the outcome of human cancer. Journal of Psychosomatic Research 12:251–259
18. Thomas CB, Duszynski KR, Shafer JW (1979) Family attitudes reported in youth as potential predictors of cancer. Psychosomatic Medicine 41:287–302
19. Verres R (1978) Wie beeinflußt Angst vor Krebs die Motivation zur Krebsvorsorge? Medizin-Mensch-Gesellschaft 3:153–160
20. Verres R (1986) Krebs und Angst. Subjektive Theorien von Laien über Entstehung, Vorsorge, Früherkennung, Behandlung und die psychosozialen Folgen von Krebserkrankungen. Springer, Berlin Heidelberg New York
21. Wenderlein JM, Hoffmann E (1983) Augmentation der Brust Münch Med Wochenschr. 125

Side Effects and Major Complications of Breast-Conserving Therapy

K. ENGEL, D. VON FOURNIER, M. KAUFMANN, and F. KUBLI

The increasing degree of adaptation of the treatment administered in general for carcinoma to suit the individual needs of the patients means that in addition to primarily oncological aspects, the patients' quality of life has become a major consideration. As long as the indications for breast-conserving therapy are strictly applied and its limitations are borne in mind, it is an alternative to mutilating amputation of the breast [23,44]. Breast-conserving therapy, however, has not yet been established as a routine procedure, and when it is performed it is important for doctor and patient alike to be aware of the possible complications and side effects.

Heidelberg Patient Population

In the period from 1974 to June 1987, a total of 665 women with carcinoma of the breast underwent breast-conserving therapy at the University Hospital for Women in Heidelberg. A subgroup of 203 nonselected patients was examined for complications and side effects. In addition, the patients' complaints were noted in a standardized questionnaire and considered in conjunction with the assessment of the results of objective examinations performed by the investigators.

The average age of the patients was 48.8 years (median 47 years, min. 25 years, max. 69 years): 56% were premenopausal and 44% postmenopausal. The population examined was also representative of the entire series of 665 patients with reference to tumor stage (T1, 69.3%; T2, 27.2%, T3/4, 2.5%), and nodal status (NO, 7.3%; N+, 26.2%). Patients in whom tumor progression was noted were excluded from the study.

The surgical procedure followed was not uniform. In the early years of the study period the operation most frequently performed was quadrantectomy (55.9%). Later the trend was rather toward wide resection (29.3%) with smaller tumor margins. In 8.7% of all cases lumpectomy was performed, and in 6.1%, tumor-adapted partial mastectomy with adaptation of the contralateral breast. Radical axillary lymphadenectomy including level I, II, and III was performed in 75.3% of all the patients, and a restricted radical lymphadenectomy (level I and II or level I only), in 16.9% and 6.2% of patients, respectively. In 1.6% of cases no axillary surgery was carried out.

The postoperative radiotherapy took the form of homogeneous gamma ray irradiation (mean 50.8 Gy, range 45–70 Gy) delivered to the breast from a cobalt-60 source. Irradiation of the axilla was not routinely carried out; in the case of total or nearly total involvement of the axilla, only a supra-/infraclavicular field was irradiated in 7.7% of patients.

A total of 21% of the patients, who were found to have positive nodes, received adjuvant chemotherapy (LF/CMF/AC/FEC/NOSTE) according to the "sandwich" technique (three cycles of chemotherapy/radiotherapy/three cycles of chemotherapy). The mean follow-up period was 28.9 months (median 21 months, range 3–110 months).

Complications and Side Effects

The subjective complaints and functional changes following breast-conserving therapy depend on the surgical operation performed, the extent of the postoperative radiotherapy, and in the case of node-positive patients, the adjuvant chemotherapy. In addition, factors peculiar to each patient play a role. There is a positive correlation between the complication rate and how radical the surgical procedure has been [22,46]. The primarily radiogenic side effects also increase in severity and frequency with increasing radiation dose. Such subjective complaints as pain, careful posture, or rapid fatigability of the arm are obviously difficult to quantify objectively.

Edema and Fibrotic Tissue Formation in the Breast

According to studies published by BEADLE et al. [2], by 6 months after the irradiation, one-third of all patients had slight edema of the breast, which was still detectable after 60 months in 23% of the patients. The frequency and severity of edema depend on how radical a lymphadenectomy has been performed, but there is a clear trend for it to regress as time goes on [8]. In our own study, 15.3% of all patients had cutaneous edema that was clearly recognizable on clinical examination after a mean follow-up period of 28.9 months, which confirms the results published by BEADLE et al. [2].

The severity of the radiogenic fibrosis of the mammary gland correlates closely with the dose of radiation delivered. According to HARRIS et al. [16]. there are hardly any changes with a total focal dose of 50 Gy. Various investigators [21,30] have shown in this connection that fibrosis occurs significantly more rarely, even with the same total focal dose, if the dose is more highly fractionated. With the fractionation regimen usually used in Heidelberg (200 cGy/day for 5 days per week), 34% of the patients reported slight hardening of the breast and 6.1% pronounced hardening. This individual assessment made by the patients themselves correlated closely with the results of a simple manual pressure test to compare the compressibility of the two breasts between two marked points (Table 1). According to this there was a difference of 3 cm or more between the breasts, reflecting pronounced fibrosis in 9.7% of all cases (Table 1).

Table 1. Primarily radiological side effects and complications of breast-conserving therapy

	Subjective: (patient) (%)	Objective: (doctor) (%)	
Cutaneous edema		15.3	
Fibrosis of the breast			Pressure test (cm)
None	57.9	56.4	≤ 1
Slight	34.4	33.8	2
Pronounced	6.1	9.7	≥ 3
Injury to the brachial plexus		0	
Rib fractures		0	
Pulmonary fibrosis			
Slight		5	
Moderate		3	
Severe		0	

Damage to the Brachial Plexus

Radiologically induced damage to the brachial plexus is observed with increased frequency following irradiation to the supraclavicular region and to the axilla with total focal doses of more than 50 Gy (STOLL 1966; MATCH 1975). According to data published by PIERQUIN [33] and HARRIS and HELLMAN [17], the incidence is around 1% and, depending on the tumor stage, it can be as high as 3% [26]. SALNER et al. [37] observed reversible damage to the brachial plexus quite frequently following radiotherapy associated with adjuvant chemotherapy (4.8%). According to our own experience in Heidelberg, no neurologically demonstrable pathologic conditions of the brachial plexus arose among the patients examined in the course of our study, reported here. Recently, however, a case of reversible paralysis of the plexus was diagnosed directly after surgery, which may have been due to damage sustained as a result of positioning during the operation.

Bone Changes

Radiotherapy can be followed by demineralization of the bone with an increased risk of fractures. This is true especially of the bones of the thorax and the humerus. The frequency of rib fractures after radiotherapy varies between 1% [9] and 5% [17] with a positive correlation between the frequency and dose of radiation. LICHTER et al. [27] observed an elevated incidence of rib fracture in patients who had also received adjuvant chemotherapy (4%). We observed no rib fractures at all in our own patient population. It is extremely rare for radiotherapy to lead to fracture of the humerus; LANGLANDS et al. [25] recorded this in only one of 17 cases of severe osteitis.

Pulmonary Fibrosis

Symptomatic radiation pneumonitis is a rare complication of post-operative radiation delivered in the course of breast-conserving therapy for carcinoma of the breast, occurring in up to 0.8% cases [17] and it depends directly on the volume of lung tissue irradiated and the total focal dose [36]. The risk of radiogenic pulmonary fibrosis is enhanced by irradiation of the lymph drainage regions of the internal mammary artery and the supra- and infraclavicular region by way of perpendicular fields.

In our own patient population, slight or moderate pulmonary fibrosis arose in a total of 8% of our patients. This was only apparent upon radiological examination and did not cause any clinical symptoms.

Impaired Arm Function/Restricted Shoulder Mobility

In breast carcinoma patients, shoulder mobility is more severely restricted after postoperative radiotherapy than after a mastectomy with no irradiation [35,41]. As well as the formation of fibrotic tissue, radiogenic osteitis is also involved in this [25]. HEALEY [18] found restricted shoulder mobility in 34% of his patients, and in 8% of all his cases he actually noted severely inhibited abduction.

In the Heidelberg study, 18.5% of patients complained of shoulder stiffness (Table 2), which it was possible to confirm objectively in a total of 13.4% of all patients. These patients included 3.6% with severely inhibited abduction (up to 90°).

This complication can be decisively reduced by early postoperative mobilization of the arm and carefully planned physiotherapy [34]. Our own experience suggests that the patients' motivation is of decisive significance, as well as regular follow-up examinations. Our results show that almost two-thirds of all patients who had undergone breast-conserving therapy complained of greater or lesser degrees of functional restriction in the arm on the treated side (Table 2).

Table 2. Restriction of arm function

	Subjective: patient (%)	Objective: doctor (%)
Stiffness of shoulder	18.5	13.4
Abduction		
Up to 90°		3.6
Up to 135°		6.2
Almost complete		3.6
Impairment of fine motor function	4.5	
Protection of arm	15.4	
Reduction in absolute force	22.1	
Rapid fatigability	37.4	
	65.6	

Lymphedema of the Arm

The most serious complication following breast-conserving therapy is secondary lymphedema of the arm on the treated side. The incidence rates given in the literature for lymphedema range from 3% to 62.5% (and even higher) (BRITTON et al. 1961; SAY and DONEGAN 1974; JOLLY et al. 1981). The incidence has remained practically unchanged from that of earlier decades [3]. According to recent studies by INGIANNI and HOLZMANN [19], about 30% of all breast carcinoma patients in the Federal Republic of Germany have secondary lymphedema of the arm.

It is difficult to make a direct comparison of the incidence rates of lymphedema, because surgery is not always radical to the same degree, the radiotherapy protocols are not uniform, and there is no uniform standard for evaluation of the results. In addition, low lymphedema rates are found in studies that do not include follow-up examinations with determination of differences in arm circumference [32]. Measurements of the upper arm, forearm, and wrist are usual, but volumetric and plethysmographic measurements [22,24,42] have not been generally accepted. Early diagnosis and the institution of carefully planned physical therapy, even in the case of mild lymphedema, can relieve the patient's symptoms and facilitate her rehabilitation. The prognosis in this condition can be decisively improved and the risk of fixed lymphedema [14], elephantiasis, and hemangiosarcoma (Stewart-Treves syndrome; [1]) clearly reduced.

The incidence of lymphedema following breast-conserving therapy has been variously reported as between 3.1% [45] and 20% [31]. Direct comparison is not possible, because there are different definitions of lymphedema.

According to the experience recorded in Heidelberg, the incidence of lymphedema after breast-conserving therapy is 10.1% [32] when a maximum difference of 2.5 cm is accepted as the cut-off point. The measurement points are 20 cm proximal and 10 cm distal to the olecranon [13], and above the styloid process. The mean maximum difference in circumference was 2.3 cm (range 0.5–5.5 cm; Fig. 1).

After a mean follow-up period of 28.9 months, however, a total of 25.1% of all patients had the subjective feeling that one arm was swollen to a greater or a lesser degree; 17.4% classed the lymphedema as slight and only 2.6% as severe. In all, 23.1% of the patients with subjective symptoms also had an objective difference in the circumference of the arm (Table 3).

The discrepancy between individual symptoms reported and an actual diagnosis of lymphedema (based on a cut-off point arbitrarily fixed at 2.5cm), which was rarer, led us to introduce a lymphedema score taking account of the symptoms reported by the patients, with reference to the degree of severity and the necessity for physical therapy (lymph drainage, compression sleeve, etc.), in addition to the degree of maximum difference in circumference (Table 4). This makes it possible to pick up lymphedema when the difference in circumference is not so pronounced because the nondominant arm, in which the muscles are less well developed, is affected or because lymph drainage has already been carried out.

Comparison of the lymphedema group by differences in circumference and by distribution of points according to the scoring system (Fig. 2) shows that when the

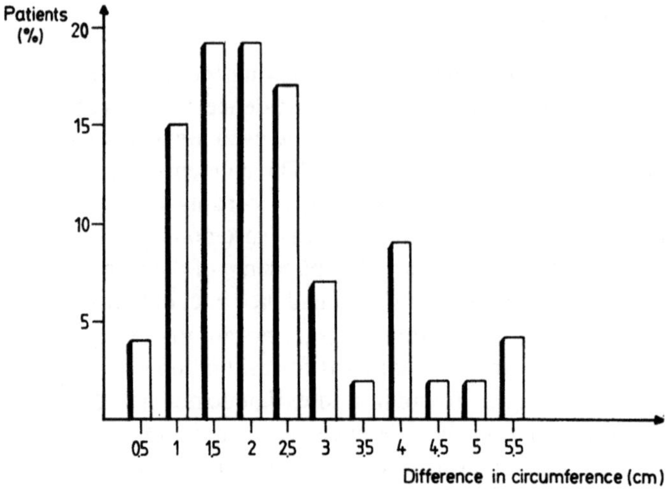

Fig. 1. Percentage distribution of difference in maximum circumference (upper arm, forearm, wrist) among patients with lymphedema ($n = 47$)

Table 3. Lymphedema of the arm

	Subjective: patient (%)	Objective: doctor (%)	Difference in max. circumference of upper arm (cm)
Slight	17.4	8.9	≤ 1.5
Obvious	5.1	7.8	2 – 2.5
Severe	2.6	6.4	≥ 3
Total	25.1	23.1	No cutoff
With chemotherapy		40.1	No cutoff ($p < 0.05$)

individual symptoms and the therapy are both taken into account, the problems associated with lymphedema are seen on average in a more serious light. More cases of edema are then classed as moderate to severe, because patients with only slight differences in upper arm circumference are also included (Fig. 3).

In the patients examined with reference to the lymphedema score, a clear correlation was found between the extent of the difference in upper arm circumference and severity of the symptoms or the degree of handicap noted (Fig. 4). No substantial difference was found among the subgroups in the necessity for or frequency of specific physical therapy (particularly lymph drainage). Introduction of the lymphedema score made it clear that the incidence rates given for any patient population are bound to be too low if they are referred to a threshold value of 2.5, 3, or even 4 cm.

Various studies have shown unequivocally that the incidence of lymphedema rises with increasingly radical surgery. Following a restricted radical operation

Table 4. Lymphedema score (K. Engel, University Hospital for Women, Heidelberg, 1987)

	Difference in maximum circumference (cm)	Symptoms/handicap	Physical therapy	
1	≤ 1.5	None	None (earlier if appropriate)	1
2	–	Slight, no restrictions	–	2
3	2–2.5	Slight, occasional handicap	Occasionally	3
4	–	Obvious, with handicap	–	4
5	≥ 3	Severe, pronounced handicap	Regularly	5
		+	+	= Score

The score is calculated from the total of the individual criteria classed according to their severity:
- Difference in max. circumference (cm) upper arm, lower arm, wrist
- Individual symptoms/degree of handicap
- Necessity for physical therapy (especially lymph drainage)

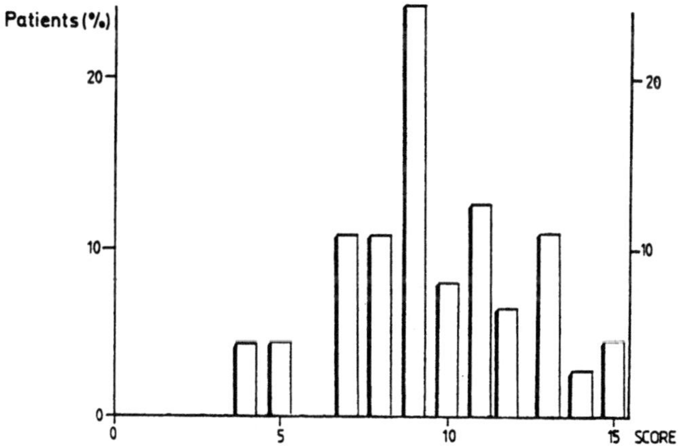

Fig. 2. Percentage distribution of numbers of points per patient according to the lymphedema score among patients with lymphedema ($n=47$)

(simple ablation as against radical mastectomy), the incidence is 9.1% as opposed to 30.9% [39]; other authors have reported a drop in the incidence of lymphedema from 22%–14% to about 6% with modified radical mastectomy [4,6,12].

The frequency and severity of lymphedema of the arm correlate closely with the radicality of the axillary lymph node dissection [22]. SAPALA et al. [38] found in their patient population that there was a direct correlation between the severity of secondary lymphedema and the number of lymph nodes removed. An average of

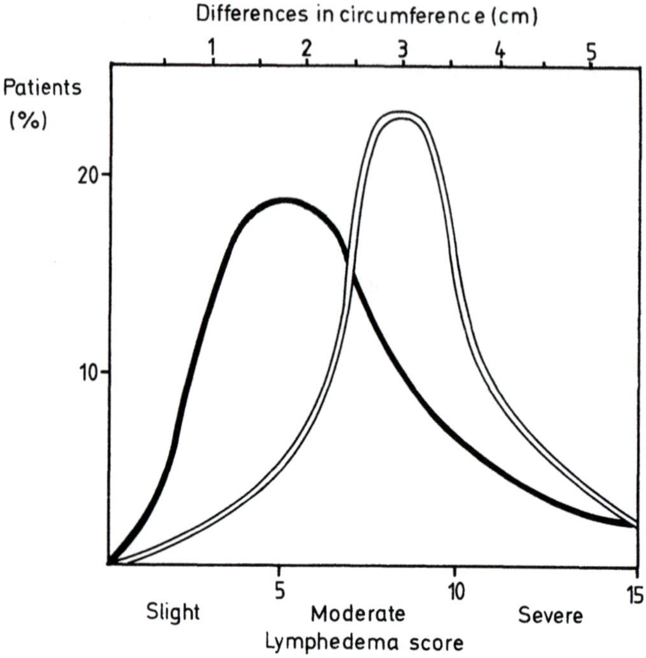

Fig. 3. Comparison of the population with lymphedema by percentage distribution of difference in upper arm circumference and by number of points per patient according to the lymphedema score ($n=47$)

17 lymph nodes per patient had been removed, but in the patients with severe lymphedema, twice as many had been removed. Patients in whom fewer than nine lymph nodes had been removed (axillary sampling) did not develop lymphedema.

In the Heidelberg patient population, the average number of lymph nodes removed was practically the same in patients with lymphedema (19.2, range 7–42) as in those without (18.4, range 5–42). There tended to be a lower rate of incidence of lymphedema following removal of fewer than ten distant lymph nodes and an elevated rate following removal of 30 or more (Fig. 5). If the patients with lymphedema are grouped according to the radicality of the axillary lymphadenectomy (levels I–III), there is no statistically significant difference from patients without lymphedema (Fig. 6). In 75.3% of all our patients the axillary lymph nodes removed included the group III nodes.

According to studies performed by LARSON et al. [26], 37% of all patients in whom radical axillary lymphadenectomy with stripping of the axillary vein was performed developed lymphedema after 6 years, as opposed to 7% of those in whom less radical surgery had been performed.

The results published by PEZNER et al. [32] show a lymphedema incidence of 55% in older patients (over 60 years of age) in whom the lesser pectoral muscle had been separated from its insertion during lymphadenectomy. Only 10% of those in whom the muscle was left intact developed lymphedema. The operation performed in Heidelberg does not include disinsertion of the lesser pectoral muscle; rather,

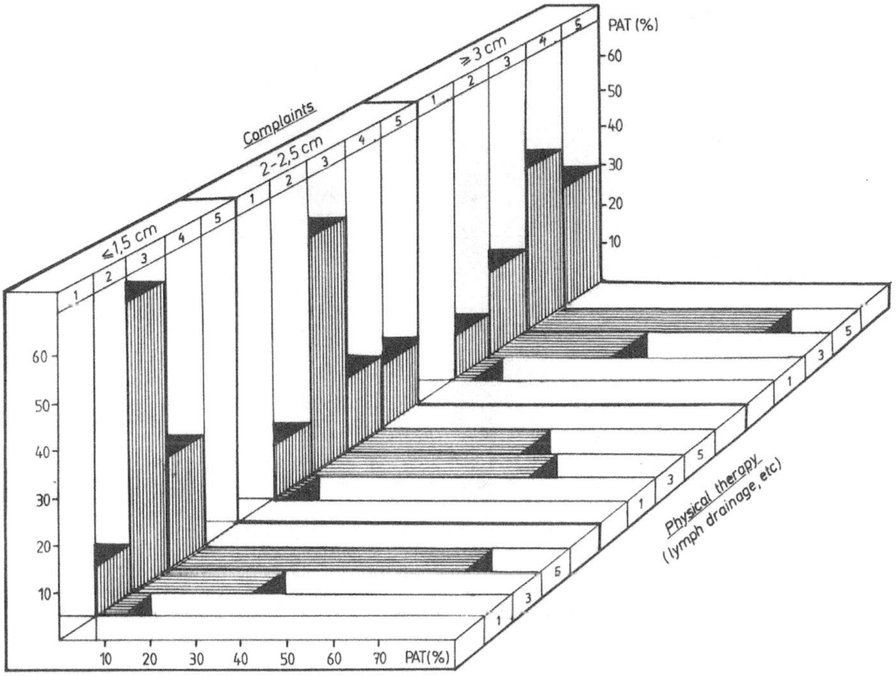

Fig. 4. Three-dimensional representation of individual symptoms and the necessity for physical therapy with reference to the lymphedema score with various differences in arm circumference (≤ 1.5, 2–2.5, ≥ 3 cm) in patients with lymphedema ($n = 47$)

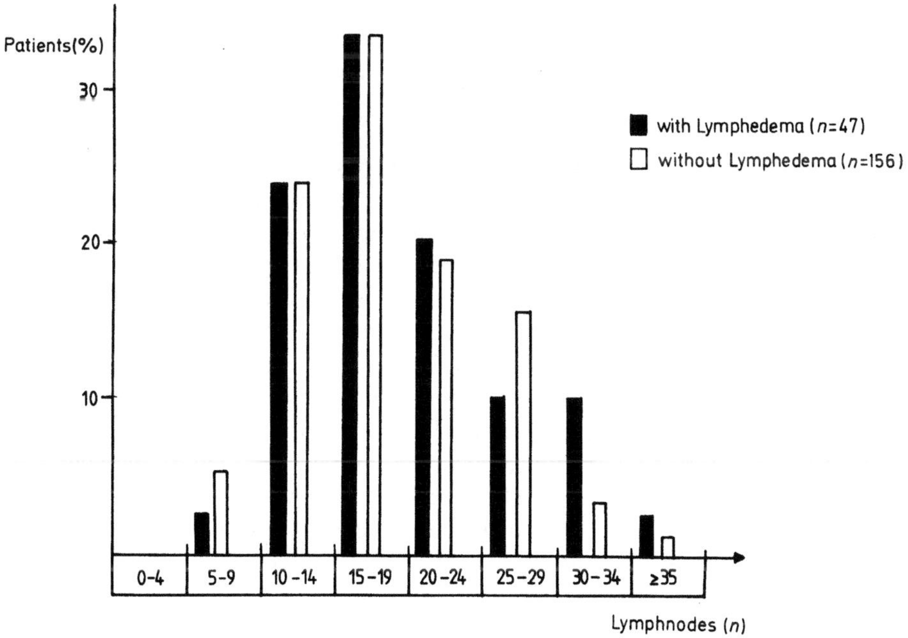

Fig. 5. Number of lymph nodes removed per patient

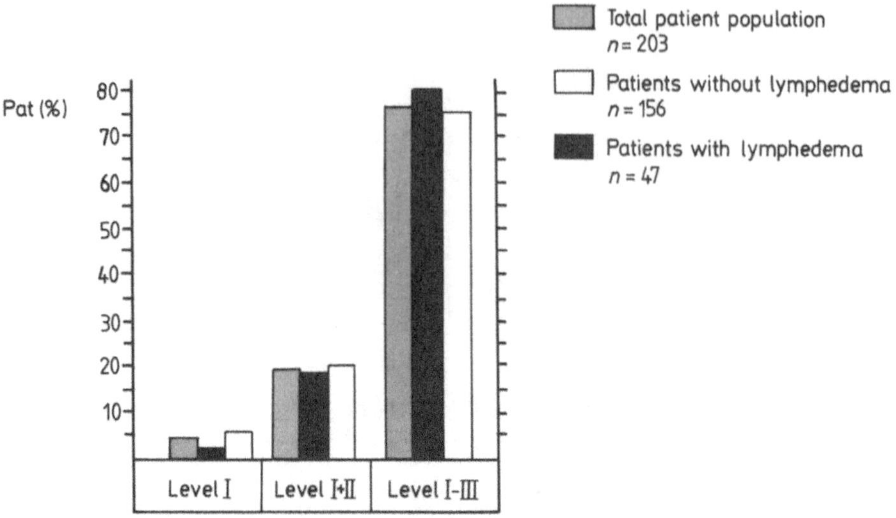

Fig. 6. Radicality of axillary lymph node dissection (level I/I+II/I–III): comparison of patients with lymphedema and without

access to the higher levels of lymph nodes is facilitated by adduction and elevation of the arm following positioning of it in such a way as to allow mobility.

While the risk of lymphedema is minimal after primary irradiation of the axilla [7,26], the incidence of edema rises significantly following postoperative radiotherapy (LOBB 1949; SWEDBORG 1977; DALAND 1986; KISSIN 1986).

The development of secondary lymphedema is dependent not only on surgical and radiological factors, but also on individual factors. Postoperative difficulties with wound healing (local infections, cutaneous necrosis, formation of seromas) are indicative of a predisposition to the development of edema [5,15,20,39]. Increasing age can also have a detrimental influence as far as the development of edema is concerned [11,32], since there is a progressive loss of lymphovenous anastomosis in older patients [43]. An elevated incidence of lymphedema has also been found in obese patients [32,39]. Our results in Heidelberg did not suggest that advanced age and above-average weight were factors predisposing to lymphedema.

A connection between chemotherapy and an elevated incidence of lymphedema has also been suggested [2,32]. Our experience also suggests that the incidence is significantly higher in node-positive patients who receive chemotherapy (40.1%). At the same time, however, more radical surgery (with vein stripping if appropriate) was performed when clinical examination revealed axillary involvement, which is also underlined by the higher number of lymph nodes (23.1 per patient) removed. In these circumstances, however, significance is also attached to problems in the interaction between the type of chemotherapy and the number of cycles administered, and the temporal sequence, fractionation schedule, and total dose of radiation.

Conclusions

In the development of organ-conserving therapy for carcinoma of the breast, efforts must continue to be devoted to further adaptation of the surgical, radiological, and chemotherapeutic procedures to take account of each patient's individual condition. This is essential to reduce the incidence of complications and side effects, especially in low-risk and node-negative patients. In this sector, it is possible that newer methods of tumor-biological staging on the basis of the primary tumor will open up the possibility of modified treatment designs, in particular allowing restriction of the surgical operation in the axilla to determination of the prognosis. The significance of the complications and side effects of breast-conserving therapy for the patient can be seen in perspective once it is realized that, in our experience, patient acceptance of this treatment is significantly better than of amputation plus reconstruction of the breast.

References

1. Amberger H (1983) Die Behandlung des Stewart-Treves-Syndroms. (Treatment of Stewart-Treves syndrome). Chirurg 54, 487
2. Beadle GF, Come S, Henderson IC, Silver B, Hellman S, Harris JR (1984) The effect of adjuvant chemotherapy on the cosmetic results after primary radiation treatment for early stage breast cancer. Int J Radiat Oncol Biol Phys 10, 2131
3. Bell HG (1949) Cancer of the breast. Ann Surg 130, 310
4. Brismar B, Ljundgdahl I (1983) Postoperative lymphedema after treatment of breast cancer. Acta Chir. Scand. 149, 687
5. Britton RC, Nelson PA (1962) Causes and treatment of postmastectomy lymphedema of the arm. JAMA 180, 95
6. Budd DC, Cochran RC, Sturtz DL, et al. (1978) Surgical morbidity after mastectomy operations. Am J Surg 135, 218
7. Calitchi E, Chaula JM, Otmezguine Y, Roucayrol AM, Mazeron JJ, Le Bourgeois JP, Pierquin B (1984) Analyse retrospective a 10 ans des sequelles du traitement locoregional des cancers du seins. (10-year retrospective analysis of the sequelae of locoregional treatment of breast cancer). Bull Cancer (Paris), 71(2), 100
8. Clarke D, Martinez A, Cox RS (1982) Breast edema following staging axillary node dissection in patients with breast carcinoma treated by radical radiotherapy: Cancer 49, 2295
9. Chu AM, Cope O, Russo R, Wang CC, Schultz MD, Wang C, Rodkey G (1980) Treatment of early stage breast cancer by limited surgery and radical irradiation. Int J Radiat Oncol Biol Phys 6, 25–30
10. Daland EM (1950) The incidence of swollen arms after radical mastectomy and suggestions for prevention. N Engl J Med 242, 497
11. Danoff BF, Goodman RL, Glick JH, Haller DG, Pajak Th T (1983) The effects of adjuvant chemotherapy on cosmesis and complications in patients with breast cancer treated by definitive irradiation. Int J Radiation Oncology Biol Phys 9, 1625
12. Feigenberg Z, Zer M, Dintsman M (1977) Comparison of postoperative complications following radical and modified radical mastectomy. World J Surg 1, 207
13. Flew TJ (1979) Wound drainage following radical mastectomy: the effect of restriction of shoulder movement. Br J Surg 66, 302
14. Földi E, Földi M (1986) Die Therapie chronischer Gliedmaßenödeme. Z Allg Med 62, 955

15. Halsted WS (1921) Swelling of the arm after operations for cancer of the breast – elephantiasis chirurgica – its cause and prevention. Bull Johns Hopkins Hosp. 32, 309
16. Harris JR, Levene MB, Svenson G (1979) Analysis of cosmetic results following primary radiation therapy for stages I and II carcinoma of the breast. Int J Radiat Oncol Biol:Phys 5:257
17. Harris JR, Hellman S (1982) Primary radiation therapy for early breast cancer: the experience at the Joint center for Radiation Therapy in Alternatives to Mastectomy, Harris JR, Hellman S, Silen W (Eds), Philadelphia, JB Lippincott Co
18. Healey JE jun (1971) Role of rehabilitation medicine in the care of the patient with breast cancer. Cancer 6, 1666
19. Ingianni G, Holzmann T (1985) Klinische Erfahrungen in der Anwendung von lympho-venösen Anastomosen beim sekundären Lymphödem Handchir Mikrochir Plast Chir 17, 43
20. Jolly P, Viar W (1981) Reduction of morbidity after radical mastectomy. Am Surg 47, 377
21. Kim JHI, Chu FCH, Hilaris B (1975) The influence of dose fractionation on acute and late reactions in patients with postoperative radiotherapy for carcinoma of the breast, Cancer, 35, 1583
22. Kissin MW, della Rovere GQ, Easton D, Westbury G (1986) Risk of lympedema following the treatment of breast disease. Br J Surg 73, 580
23. Kubli F, von Fournier D (1986) Brusterhaltende Therapie des Mammacarcinoms in Aktuelle Geburtshilfe und Gynäkologie, Melchert F, et al. (Eds) Springer Verlag Berlin, 280
24. Kuhnke E (1979) Methodik zur Volumenbestimmung menschlicher Extremitäten aus Umfangsmessungen. Physiotherapie 70, 251
25. Langlands AO, Souter WA, Samuel E (1977) Radiation osteitis following irradiation for breast cancer. Clin Radiol 28, 93
26. Larson D, Weinstein M, Goldberg I, et al. (1986) Edema of the arm as a function of the extent of axillary surgery in patients with Stage I–II carcinoma of the breast treated with primary radiotherapy. Int J Radiat Oncol Biol Phys 12(9), 1575
27. Lichter AS (1982) the National Cancer Institute experience – primary radiotherapy and adjuvant chemotherapy. In Alternatives to Mastectomy, Harris JR, Hellman S, Silen W (Eds), Philadelphia, JB Lippincott Co
28. Lobb AW, Harkins HN (1949) Postmastectomy swelling of the arm with a note on the effect of segmental resection of the axillary vein at the time of radical mastectomy. West J Surg 57, 550
29. Match RM (1975) Radiation-induced brachial plexus paralysis. Arch Surg 110, 384
30. Montague ED (1968) Experience with altered fractionation in radiation therapy of breast cancer, Radiology, 90, 962
31. DeMoss EV, Lichter AS, Lippman ME, Gerber LG, Reichert CM, Edwards BK, Schain WS, Gorrell CR, d'Angelo TM, Rosenberg SA (1983) Complete axillary lymph node dissection before radiotherapy for primary breast cancer. In Conservative Management of Breast Cancer: New Surgical and Radiotherapeutic Techniques, Eds. Harris JR, Hellman S, Silen W (eds) London JB, Lippincott Co, pp 163–182
32. Pezner RD, Patterson MP, Hill LR, Lipsett JA, Desai KR, Vora N, Wong JY, Luk KH (1986) Arm lymphedema in patients treated conservatively for breast cancer: relationship to patient age and axillary node dissection technique. Int J Radiat Oncol Biol Phys 12(12), 2079
33. Pierquin B (1982) Conservative treatment for carcinoma of the breast – Experience of Creteil, 10 years' results. In Alternatives to Mastectomy, Harris JR, Hellman S, Silen W (Eds) Philadelphia JB, Lippincott Co
34. Pollard R, Callum KG, Altman DG (1976) Shoulder movement following mastectomy. Ann Surg 133, 565
35. Ryttov N, Blichert-Toft M, Madjen EL (1983) Influence of adjuvant irradiation on shoulder joint function after mastectomy for breast cancer. Acta Radiol Oncol 22, 29
36. Roberson PL, Lichter AS, Iler V (1983) Dose to lung in primary breast irradiation. Int J Radiat Oncol Biol Phys 9, 97

37. Salner AL, Botnick LE, Herzog AG et al. (1981) Reversible brachial plexopathie following primary radiation therapy for breast cancer. Cancer Treat Rep 65:797
38. Sapala JA, Sapala A, Soto AR, Sharpe D (1980) Lymphedema following modified radical mastectomy. Breast, 6(4), 28
39. Say CC, Donegan W (1974) A biostatistical evaluation of complications from mastectomy. Surg Gynecol Obstet 138, 370
40. Stoll BA, Andrews JT (1966) Radiation-induced peripheral neuropathy. Br Med J 1, 834
41. Swedborg I (1977) Voluminometric estimation of the degree of lymphedema. Scand J Rehabil Med 9, 131
42. Swedborg I, Wallgren A (1981) The effect of pre- and post-mastectomy radiotherapy on the degree of edema, shoulder joint mobility and gripping force. Cancer 47, 877
43. Threefoot SA, Kossover MF (1966) Lymphaticovenous communications in man. Arch Int Med 117, 213
44. Veronesi U, Saccozzi R, Del Vecchio M, Banti A, Clemente C, De Lena M, Gallus G, Greco M, Luini A, Marubini E, Muscolino G, Rilke F, Salvadori B, Zecchini A, Zucali R (1981) Comparing radical mastectomy with quadrantectomy, axillary dissection, and radiotherapy in patients with small cancers of the breast. N Eng J Med 305, 6
45. Veronesi U (1985) Randomized trials comparing conservation techniques with conventional surgery: An overview. In: Tobias JS, Peckham MJ (eds): Primary Management of Breast Cancer: Alternatives to Mastectomy Management of Malignant Disease Series, pp 131–152, London, E Arnold
46. Yeah EK, Denham JW, Davies SA, Spittle MF (1986) Primary breast cancer, complications of axillary management. Acta Radiol (Oncol) 25, 105

Cosmetic Aspects of Breast-Conserving Therapy for Carcinoma of the Breast

K. ENGEL, A. MÜLLER, D. VON FOURNIER, and F. KUBLI

Apart from the primarily oncological aspects, breast-conserving therapy, with the psychological advantages this entails for the patient, is only worthwhile when the result can be expected to be good from the cosmetic and functional aspects. As well as the site of the tumor, the ratio of its size – or rather the extent of the conservative surgical operation – to the volume of the breast is a decisive factor determining the cosmetic outcome. The cosmetic results tend to be rather unsatisfactory when the carcinoma is centrally situated or when the breast is very small [7]. The alternative in such cases is amputation with subsequent reconstruction.

Patient Population in Heidelberg

From 1974 to June 1987, a total of 665 patients with invasive carcinoma of the breast underwent breast-conserving therapy at the University Hospital for Women in Heidelberg. For 203 nonselected patients the cosmetic results were evaluated by two investigators and each patient's own assessment was recorded with the aid of a standardized questionnaire.

The mean follow-up period after the completion of therapy was 28.8 months. The most frequent tumor site in this population was the superior lateral quadrant (56.5%), followed by the superior medial quadrant (19.0%), and then by the inferior lateral (12.8%) and inferior medial (5.1%) quadrants. The central part of the gland was affected in 5.6% of the patients.

In the early years of the study more extensive local surgery was performed (quadrantectomy in 55.9% of cases). In recent years, for cosmetic reasons, we have aimed at local tumor control by means of operations with smaller tumor margins (wide resection in 19.2%, lumpectomy in 8.7%). In 6.1% of all patients macromastia caused us to perform a partial mastectomy specifically adapted to the particular tumor (typical reduction mammaplasty). In 7.7% of cases the contralateral breast was also treated to attain approximate symmetry (reduction mammaplasty). The breast-conserving surgery was performed as a "one-step-procedure" in 62% of the patients (positive puncture cytology in 3.6%, positive "true cut" biopsy in 1%, positive intraoperative fresh frozen section in 57.4%). A "two-step" procedure was required in 38% of cases (biopsy performed elsewhere in 14.9%; biopsy performed in our hospital in 23.1%). For tumors sited laterally in the superior lateral quadrant, a radial incision running into the axilla was made in 37% of cases. In the case of all other incisions (radial 26%, semicircular 21.5%, periareolar 8.7%), radical axillary lymph node dissection was carried out from a separate wide-angled incision in the axilla (56.9%). In 6.1% of cases a typical reduction figure was present.

All patients received postoperative homogenous gamma ray irradiation (mean 50,8 Gy, range 45–70Gy) applied to the whole breast from a cobalt-60 source. In 77,9% of cases an external tumor boost (mean 8,1 Gy, range 5–25 Gy) was also given.

A total of 21% of the patients, who were found to have positive lymph nodes, received adjuvant chemotherapy (LF, CMF, AC, FEC, NOSTE) according to the sequential "sandwich" technique.

Criteria for Assessment of the Cosmetic Results

The cosmetic results of breast-conserving therapy (local tumor control with postoperative radiotherapy) are good to excellent in the majority of cases [10,14]; according to recent reports, good or excellent results are achieved in between 80% and 92% of cases [1,4,9].

In our study in Heidelberg, a total of 87% of all patients described the cosmetic result as good or excellent, while the investigators were generally more critical in their assessment (patients/investigators – excellent: 37,3%/34.9%, good: 47.4%/34.9%, fair: 12.1%/21.5%, poor: 3.2%/8.7%). The generally positive assessment of the cosmetic result is underlined by the fact that subsequent corrective surgery to the treated breast was requested by very few patients (3.1%). On comparison of both breasts most patients (45.6%) found the untreated one preferable in appearance. Among the remaining patients, however, either both breasts were considered to have an equally attractive appearance (19.5%) or the treated breast was described as even having a better appearance (17.4%). Some patients (15.9%) could not decide which looked better.

The investigators based their assessment of the cosmetic result on comparison with the untreated breast, taking note of differences in the size and shape of the breast and in the position and shape of areola and nipple, scar formation, and other cutaneous changes (Table 1).

Size of the Breast. Agreement between investigator and patient was closest when there was only a very slight size difference or none at all. More marked discrepancies were assessed more severely by the investigators, who were also more likely to class them as obtrusive or unacceptable. It must be borne in mind that the patients often refuse surgery to the healthy breast when it is offered as a means of achieving symmetry, accepting even quite pronounced differences in volume (Fig. 1).

Shape of the Breast. The investigators also classed differences in shape as obtrusive or unacceptable more frequently than the patients. In some patients no difference in shape was noted, while in the others the treated breast either looked as though it had been lifted (29.2%), because of fibrosis of the gland, or had a flattened (14.8%) or asymmetrical (11.3%) appearance if there was a sufficiently large tissue deficit or tension on the scar.

Table 1. Assessment of the various cosmetic factors by investigators (Inv.) and patients (Pt.) ($n=203$); comparison of the treated and the contralateral breast

	No/minimal		Visible/not disturbing		Visible/disturbing		Obvious/unacceptable	
	Inv (%)	Pt (%)	Inv (%)	Pt (%)	Inv (%)	Pt (%)	Inv (%)	Pt (%)
Size of breasts not the same	56.4	61.5	17.4	29.7	23.2	8.2	3.1	0.5
Shape of breasts not the same	54.4	63.6	24.1	26.2	16.9	9.7	4.6	0.5
Position/shape of areola and nipple not the same	66.2	72.3	18.5	21.0	12.2	6.7	3.1	0
Obvious scar formation	68.3	63.6	12.8	22.1	17.9	12.8	1.0	1.5
Other cutaneous changes		74.9		21.0		4.1		0

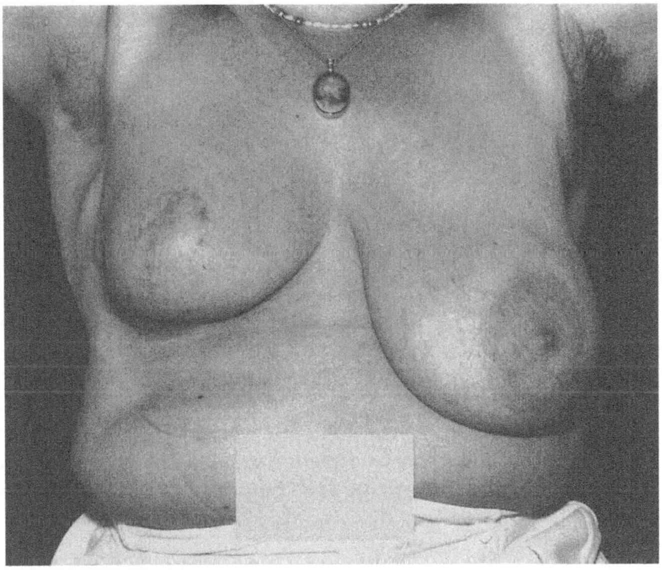

Fig. 1. Result observed 1 year after tumor-adapted partial mastectomy (modified McKissock technique) and irradiation (50 Gy) for a T2 (3 cm) carcinoma of the inferior lateral quadrant of the right breast. The patient refused correction of the left breast and is highly satisfied with the cosmetic result (very good) which was given an overall rating of "fair" by the investigators

Shape and Position of Areola and Nipple. Marked differences from the contralateral breast are more readily accepted by the patients than by the investigators. Upward and/or lateral displacement was the most frequent difference.

Scar Formation, Cutaneous Changes. The scars formed were also more frequently assessed as obtrusive or unacceptable by the investigators. Apart from the cutaneous changes that were objectively verifiable, such as redness (14.3%), edema (11.2%), hyperpigmentation (18.5%), telangiectasia (6.2%), and pronounced loss of pigmentation in the areola (6.7%), three-quarters of all the patients did not notice any difference. Only 4.1% described the cutaneous changes as obvious and obtrusive. Severe skin damage was not recorded in a single case.

Cosmetic Results Referred to Various Influential Factors

"One Step" vs "Two Step" approach in Surgical Procedure. While some specialists recommend surgical treatment in a single session with confirmation of the diagnosis by means of puncture cytology, true cut biopsy, or fresh frozen section examination [6], a two-stage approach with wide excision [8] is preferred by others. After the histological investigation axillary lymph node dissection is then carried out from a new axillary incision in a second operating session, with or without local reexcision

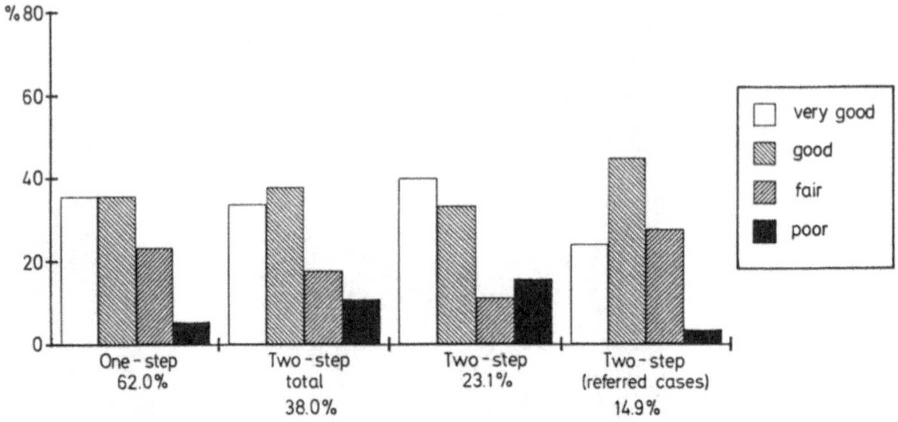

Fig. 2. Distribution (%) of cosmetic results (excellent; good; fair; poor) for different subgroups according to type of procedure. (Referred cases: biopsy was done outside our institution in these cases.)

or amputation. A two-stage approach can lead to a higher local infection rate up to 12.4%; [3], which generally has a negative influence on the cosmetic result.

In our experience, it is possible to restrict the infection rate to 2% even with a two-stage approach if prophylactic antibiotic treatment is administered in the perioperative period. The cosmetic results have not been negatively affected in any significant way by previous biopsy (Fig. 2), although poor or only fair results have tended to be more frequent following a two-stage procedure. Excellent results have been decisively less frequent in those of our patients who had undergone biopsy at other institutions before referral.

Size of the Breasts. The size of the breast is important insofar as a good cosmetic result cannot be expected if the ratio of the size of the breast to the volume of the tumor or the extent of the projected surgery (lumpectomy, wide resection, quadrantectomy) is unfavorable. While this reservation must be borne in mind, it is certainly possible, nonetheless, to achieve good results even in small breasts (Fig. 3); with larger breasts the proportion of poor and only satisfactory results is greater. Other factors certainly play a part in this, such as the larger volume of breast tissue irradiated, with formation of radiogenic fibrosis.

Site of Tumor. In our experience, the results were best when the tumor was sited in the superior lateral quadrant; with other tumor sites there were fewer excellent results and decidedly more poor results (Fig. 4). Even when the bulk of the tumor was centrally situated, making extensive reconstruction of the gland necessary after the breast-conserving therapy in some cases, we were still able to achieve thoroughly acceptable results in contrast to other author's experience [7].

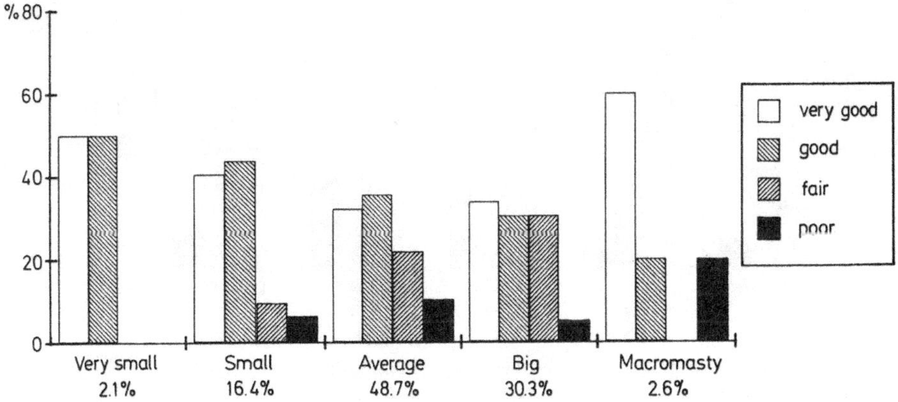

Fig. 3. Distribution (%) of cosmetic results (excellent; good; fair; poor) for different subgroups according to size of breast

Incision. The incision made has to be modified to suit the individual circumstances in each case and should pass directly over the tumor [8]. The procedure followed in Heidelberg also involves removal of a spindle-shaped piece of skin. In general, semicircular incisions are the best. A radial incision extended into the axilla is recommended particularly in the case of larger tumors or a lateral site of the tumor in the area of the superior lateral quadrant. The cosmetic results did not vary significantly with the incision (Fig. 5). They were comparable even after periareolar incisions; such incisions are not, however, suitable for the removal of peripherally situated carcinomas for reasons concerned with different aspects of tumor surgery. Following tumor-adapted partial mastectomy (typical reduction mammaplasty with lifting) the cosmetic appearance was generally given a less positive rating by the investigators.

Scar Formation. Good healing of the wound with a cosmetically unremarkable scar is important for the assessment of the cosmetic result. In our experience the results were considerably more often assessed as good or excellent when the scar was unremarkable than when the scar was wide, retracted, or fixed; the investigators assessed the cosmetic result as poor or fair in the vast majority of cases when such scars were present (Fig. 6).

Radiation. One of the factors with a substantial influence on the cosmetic result of breast-conserving therapy is the mandatory postoperative radiotherapy. Results that are primarily poor from the cosmetic aspect following surgery are not improved by irradiation; a primarily good cosmetic result after surgery, however, can be prejudiced. Besides the irradiation technique, the most vital elements are the total focal dose and the volume of tissue irradiated. No significant changes need be expected with doses up to 50 Gy [7]. With doses of 60 Gy and over HARRIS found severe fibrosis and retraction in every case, which had a detrimental effect on the cosmetic result.

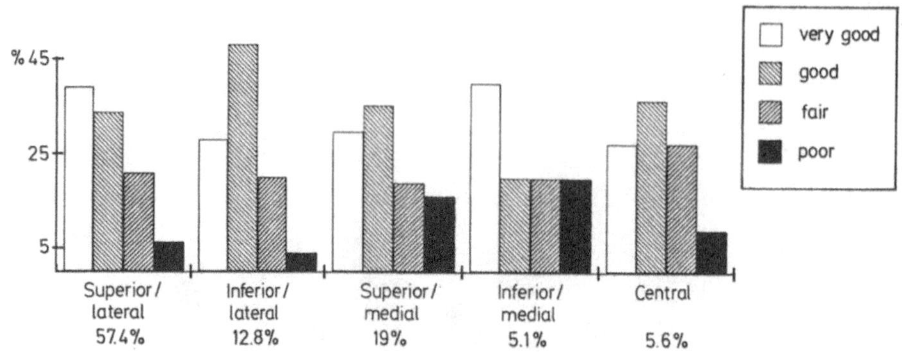

Fig. 4. Distribution (%) of cosmetic results (excellent; good; fair; poor) for different subgroups in relation to localization of primary tumor

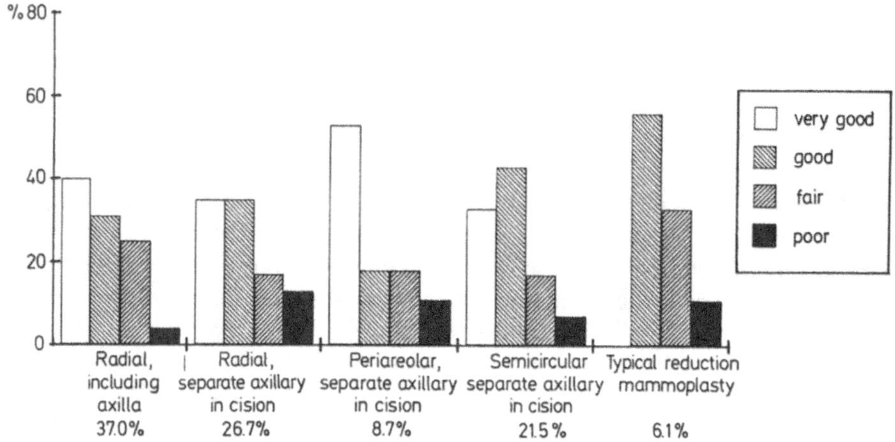

Fig. 5. Distribution (%) of cosmetic results (excellent; good; fair; poor) for different subgroups according to type of incision

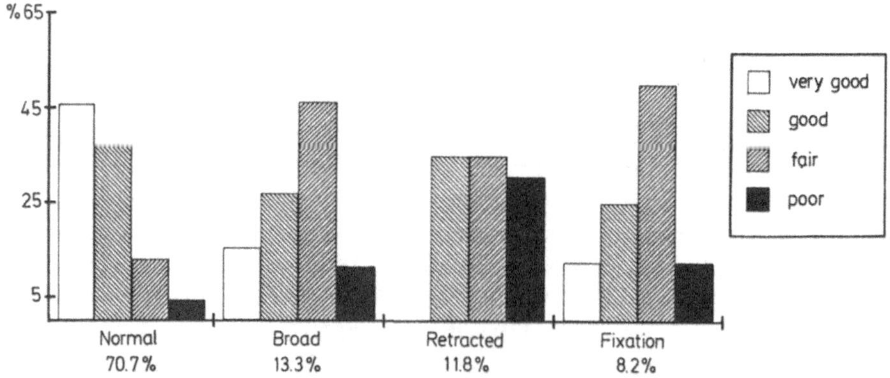

Fig. 6. Distribution (%) of cosmetic results (excellent; good; fair; poor) for different subgroups according to appearance of scar

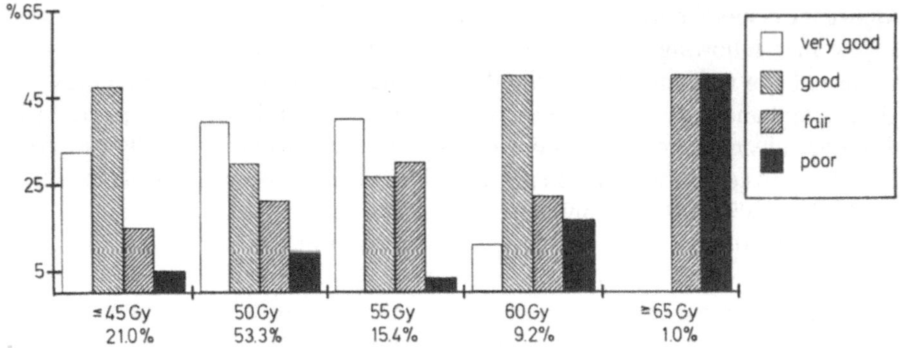

Fig. 7. Distribution (%) of cosmetic results (excellent; good; fair; poor) for the different subgroups according to various ranges of breast irradiation dose (not including tumor boost)

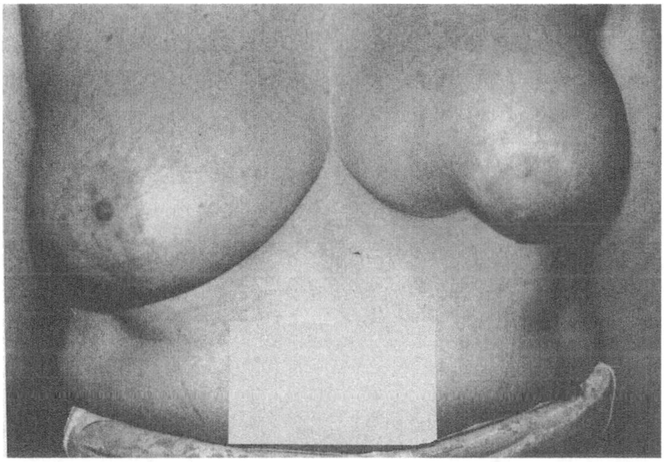

Fig. 8. Result observed 5 years after breast-conserving treatment for a T1 carcinoma of the left breast. The cosmetic result was poor as a consequence of an unfavorable tumor site (inferior medial quadrant) and a high dose of irradiation (60 Gy plus 15 Gy tumor boost)

Our own experience confirms this connection between poor cosmetic results and increasing total focal dose (Fig. 7). When postoperative homogeneous irradiation is delivered to the breast with cobalt-60 gamma rays, the proportion of excellent results remains practically constant, while the fair and poor results tend to increase in frequency, with a corresponding decline in the proportion of good results. We have not known radiation with over 65 Gy to lead to a cosmetic result that could be assessed as anything more than fair or poor (Fig. 8).

The dosing of the external tumor boost (10 Gy on average) with cobalt-60 gamma rays did not have a negative effect on the overall cosmetic result. After an interstitial irradiation boost, the proportion of unsatisfactory cosmetic results increases with increasing size of the implants and rising dose level of the implants [1].

Adjuvant Chemotherapy. The influence of adjuvant chemotherapy on the cosmetic appearance following breast-conserving therapy is a subject of controversy. It seems to be of vital importance whether the chemotherapy and radiotherapy are given simultaneously or sequentially ("sandwich" technique). When cytostatic drugs are given at the same time, worse cosmetic results are generally observed [2,4,12]. LICHTER et al. [9] also noted a reduction in the number of good and excellent results from 80% to 70% in these circumstances.

The cosmetic results can be improved by combining the CMF regimen with prednisone [5]. Overall, however, very good and good results were not significantly more frequent in patients who received radiotherapy only (89%) than in those who received adjuvant chemotherapy at the same time (81%).

The experience recorded in Heidelberg with the "sandwich" technique (3×CHT/radiotherapy/3×CHT) has not shown any significant differences in cosmetic results, as assessed by patients or investigators, from those achieved in the group that did not receive any chemotherapy (Fig. 9). After adjuvant chemotherapy half of all the patients assessed their own result as excellent and a third, as good. The fact that the assessment was even better in this group than in patients who did not receive chemotherapy leads us to suspect that other factors than the purely cosmetic appearance of the breast play a part in the assessment in the case of high risk or lymph-node-positive patients.

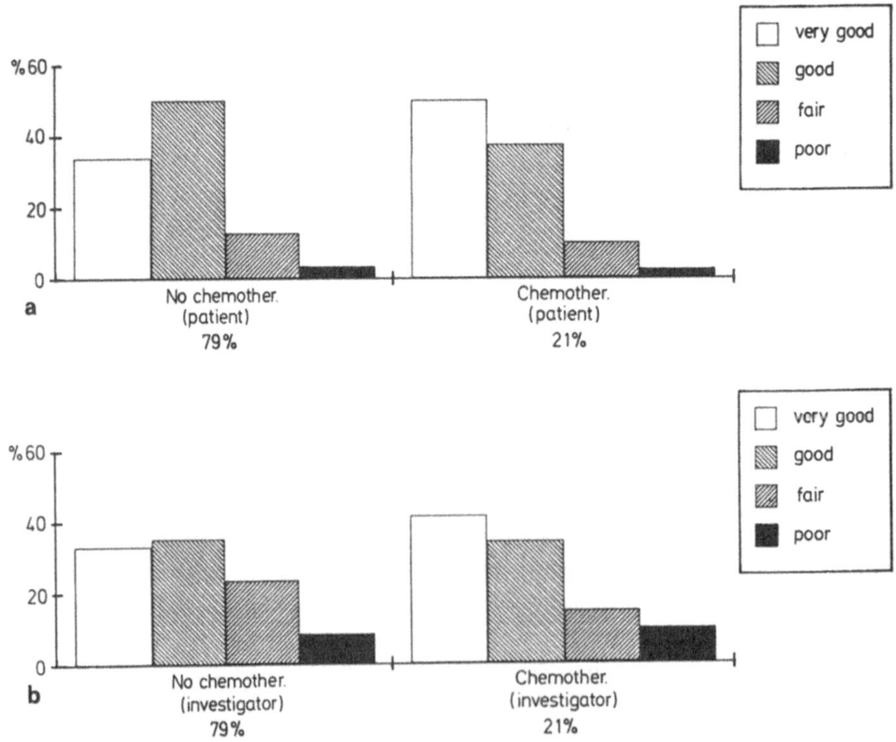

Fig. 9a,b. Distribution (%) of cosmetic results (excellent; good; fair; poor) in patients treated with or without adjuvant chemotherapy, as rated by the patients (**a**) and investigators (**b**)

Time Factor. The comparability of different follow-up studies devoted to the cosmetic aspects of treatment results following breast-conserving therapy is prejudiced insofar as the follow-up periods often vary substantially and are referred to different times after completion of the primary therapy. Longitudinal studies conducted by SPITALIER et al. [13] have shown that there was a progressive worsening of the cosmetic results in his patients. While the results were good to excellent in two-thirds of the patients after 5 years, this proportion had fallen to one-third of all patients by the end of 10 years. In view of this time factor, opinions vary about the best time for a definitive assessment of the cosmetic results. Other investigators [7], in contrast, observed no substantial changes over a follow-up period of 1–4 years. According to the results published by PIERQUIN et al. [11] and DANOFF et al. [5], a final assessment of the cosmetic results after 2–3 years is reasonable.

In the Heidelberg patient population the late cosmetic results were also worse on average (Fig. 10a). The best results were seen after 6 months, when the primary side effects of the radiotherapy and the operation had abated. After 2 years there is a clear trend for the results to be more rarely classed as excellent, and especially after 3 years or more, they are more often classed as fair or poor. This critical evaluation recorded by the investigators is not shared by the patients themselves, whose assessments of the cosmetic results after 3 years and more did not reflect any increase in the proportion of unfavorable cosmetic results (Fig. 10b). However, these observations must still be subjected to further longitudinal studies. Since more extensive local surgery and higher irradiation doses in the past can be expected to affect the cosmetic outcome in a negative way.

Conclusions

The objectives of breast-conserving therapy are maximum local tumor control, with the fewest and mildest side effects possible and the best possible cosmetic result. In any particular case, the cosmetic result is influenced by various individual and therapy-related factors. Advances in irradiation techniques and the trend to restriction of the radiation dose have certainly contributed to the improvements in cosmetic results. Surgical treatment is not yet standardized. Locally restricted surgery, i.e., wide resection, allows better cosmetic results than quadrantectomy, which is a more extensive operation. Questions relating to the optimum surgical technique have still not been definitively answered. While the procedure followed in Heidelberg involves reconstruction of the breast by way of mobilization and readaptation of the gland with suction-free drainage of the wound cavity, other authors recommend primary closure of the wound without reconstruction of the gland and without drainage [8]. In view of the increasingly frequent performance of breast-conserving therapy, further comparative studies could be helpful in the standardization of surgical procedure with reference to the achievement of optimum cosmetic results.

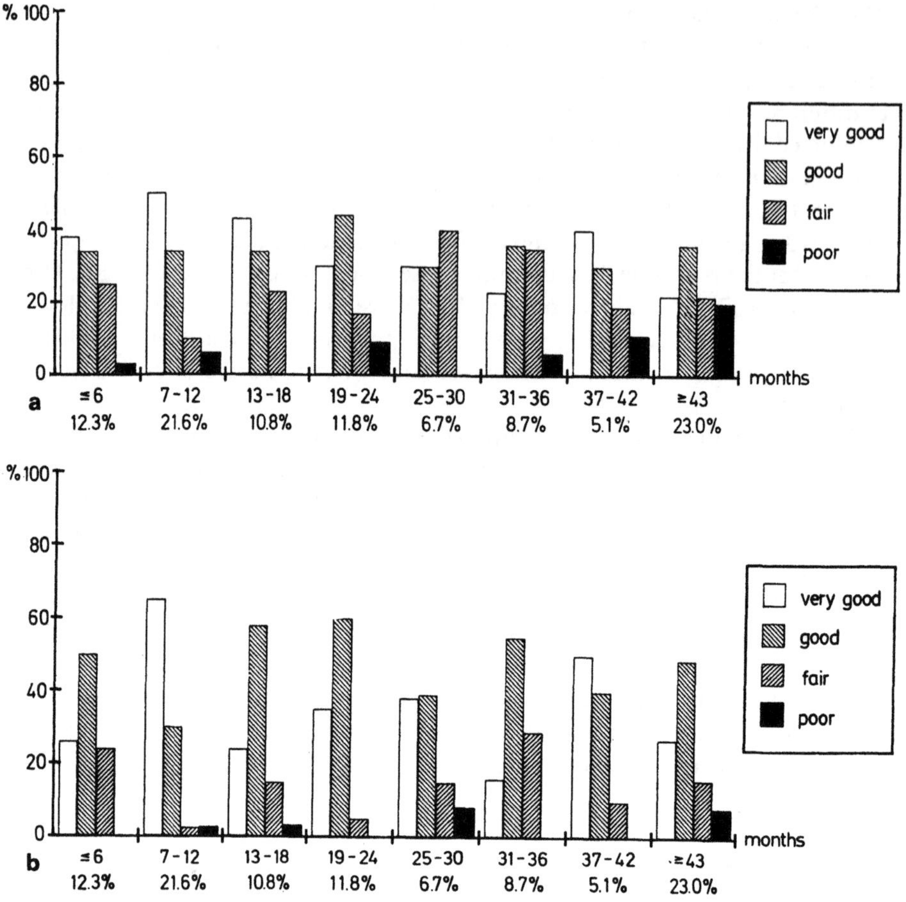

Fig. 10.a,b Distribution (%) of cosmetic results (excellent; good; fair; poor) in relation to mean observation time (months) after termination of treatment as rated by investigators **(a)** and patients **(b)**

References

1. Beadle G, Silver B, Botnick LE et al. (1984a) Cosmetic results following primary radiation therapy for early breast carcinoma. Cancer 54:2911
2. Beadle G, Come S, Henderson IC et al. (1984b) The effect of adjuvant chemotherapy on the cosmetic results after primary radiation treatment for early breast cancer: a preliminary analysis. Int J Radiat Oncol Biol Phys 10:2131
3. Beatty JD, Robinson GV, Zaia JA et al. (1983) A prospective analysis of nosocomial wound infection after mastectomy. Arch Surg 118:1421
4. Botnick LE, Come S, Rose C, Goldstein M, Lange R, Tischler S, Schnipper L (1982) Primary breast irradiation and concomittant adjuvant chemotherapy (CMF). In: Harris JR, Hellman S, Silen W (eds) Alternatives to Mastectomy. Lippincott, Philadelphia

5. Danoff BF, Goodman L, Glick JH, Haller DG, Pajak TF (1983) The effect of adjuvant chemotherapy on cosmesis and complications in patients with breast cancer treated by definite irradiation. Int J Radiat Oncol Biol Phys 9:1625-1630
6. Fisher B (1984) Reappraisal of breast biopsy prompted by the use of lumpectomy, surgical strategy. JAMA 253:3585
7. Harris JR, Levene MB, Svensson G et al. (1979) Analysis of cosmetic results following primary radiation therapy for stages I and II carcinoma of the breast. Int J Radiat Oncol Biol Phys 5:257
8. Kinne DW (1987) Primary treatment of breast cancer, surgery. In: Harris JR, Hellman S, Henderson IC, Kinne DW (eds) Breast disease. Lippincott, Philadelphia
9. Lichter AS (1982) The National Cancer Institute Experience – primary radiotherapy and adjuvant chemotherapy. In: Harris JR, Hellman S, Silen W (eds) Alternatives to Mastectomy. Lippincott, Philadelphia
10. Peters MV (1975) Cutting the "Gordian knot" in early breast cancer. Ann R Coll Phys Surg Can 8:186
11. Pierquin B, Owen R, Maylin C, Otmezguine Y, Raynal M, Mueller W, Hannoun S (1976) Radical radiation therapy of breast cancer. Int J Radiat Oncol Biol Phys 6:17–24
12. Ray GR, Fish VJ, Marmor, JB et al. (1984) Impact of adjuvant chemotherapy on cosmesis and complications in stages I and II carcinoma of the breast treated by biopsy and radiation therapy. Int J Radiat Oncol Biol Phys 10:837
13. Spitalier JM (1982) A 20 year experience at the Marseilles Cancer Institute on conservative management for operable breast cancer. In: Harris JR, Hellman S, Silen W (eds) Alternatives to Mastectomy. Lippincott, Philadelphia
14. Williams IG, Murley RS, Curwen MD (1953) Carcinoma of the female breast: conservative surgery and radical surgery. Br Med J Oct. 10th 787

VII. Adjuvant Chemotherapy and Hormonal Therapy – Results and Complications

The Integration of Radiotherapy and Chemotherapy in the Treatment of Early Breast Cancer

I.C Henderson, D. Hayes, M.A. Rose, S. Come, and J. Harris

Introduction

Conservative surgery (segmental mastectomy or quadrantectomy) followed by radiotherapy to the breast and axillary lymph nodes is now accepted as a standard treatment for early breast cancer and a reasonable alternative to mastectomy for most patients [21]. Even with 10–30 years of observation, the survival of patients treated with conservative surgery equals that of patients with similar clinical characteristics treated with mastectomy and radiotherapy [40]. Thirty-year follow-up on patients treated with primary radiotherapy has revealed no unusual late toxicities. More recently, segmental mastectomy and radiotherapy have been compared in randomized trials with mastectomy, and no significant differences in either local control of the disease or survival have been observed [14,43,47].

Similarly, adjuvant systemic therapy (chemotherapy or endocrine therapy) is now routinely employed following mastectomy for patients with operable breast cancers and histologically involved lymph nodes [25]. In an early adjuvant therapy trial performed in Norway, patients were randomized after mastectomy to either no further therapy or a 6-day course of intravenous cyclophosphamide [37]. With more than 15 years of follow-up, a statistically significant survival advantage remains for all treated patients compared to those treated with mastectomy only. More recent randomized trials have used more intensive chemotherapy programs, including 2 years of L-phenylalanine mustard (L-PAM) in the National Surgical Adjuvant Breast Project (NSABP) trial and a combination of cyclophosphamide, methotrexate, and 5-fluorouracil (CMF) for 1 year in a Milan trial [5,13]. With more than 10 years of follow-up each of these study groups has reported a statistically significant survival advantage for premenopausal women given adjuvant chemotherapy. The benefits of adjuvant therapy in postmenopausal women are less evident in these individual trials, but a recent overview analysis performed by Peto et al. [35] at Oxford demonstrates that adjuvant tamoxifen may prolong the survival of postmenopausal patients.

Almost all of the studies evaluating adjuvant chemotherapy have primarily involved mastectomy patients. The widespread acceptance of segmental mastectomy with primary radiotherapy and the development of adjuvant systemic therapy have proceeded independently during the past two decades. Few data are available concerning the proper integration of these two therapeutic modalities, and in the absence of data, many unfounded assumptions have arisen. Radiotherapists are understandably concerned that delaying radiotherapy may compromise local control of the disease. In addition, they fear that prior or concomitant chemotherapy may compromise cosmesis. On the other hand, medical oncologists are concerned that the initial use of primary radiotherapy will delay chemotherapy, compromising patient survival, and that the maximum tolerated drug dose may be reduced following radiotherapy. Both radiotherapists and medical oncologists are concerned that new or infrequent toxicities associated with either modality may grow in importance when both are used together. In this review we will examine the evidence which has contributed to these concerns of medical oncologists and radiotherapists, and we will assess the current state of the art regarding the optimal integration of these two modalities in patients with early breast cancer.

Delaying Radiotherapy: Effect on Local Control

Historically, physicians have felt a sense of urgency in treating newly diagnosed breast cancer. At one time, most breast cancers were diagnosed by frozen section followed by immediate mastectomy while the patient was still under anesthesia. With the introduction of the "two-step" procedure for the diagnosis and treatment of breast cancer, these initial events became less of a medical emergency. The separation of the initial biopsy and either mastectomy or primary radiotherapy by 1–2 weeks gave the patient time to consider alternatives. A controlled trial has never been performed to determine if this delay in therapy compromises either local control or survival. Patient demand, the lack of evidence to support the traditional one-step procedure, and decreasing emphasis on the importance of local therapy have all led to a general acceptance of this delay in treatment in spite of remaining doubts in the minds of some physicians. While delays of 1–2 weeks have now become standard practice, delays of 1–3 months in the initiation of local therapy are of concern to most physicians. Anecdotal instances of tumor recurrence within the breast during long delays augment physician concern. For example, in a recently reported pilot study, women were initially treated with two courses of CMF followed by primary radiotherapy with both external beam and iridium implant. Sixteen patients were treated, and three (19%) had a locoregional recurrence during the initial 2 months while CMF was being given and before radiotherapy was begun [24].

Two studies from our institution provide data on the effect of delaying the initiation of radiotherapy. The first of these is an assessment of the effect of delaying primary radiotherapy after lumpectomy. At the Joint Center for Radiotherapy (JCRT) we had previously observed that patients with an extensive intraductal component both within the tumor and in grossly normal adjacent tissue have a higher incidence of local recurrence following lumpectomy (without regard to microscopic margins) and radiotherapy than patients who do not have these "high-risk" histologic characteristics [22]. However, we do not find that a delay in the time to initiation of radiotherapy causes a further increase in the local failure rate within these two risk groups. In a retrospective analysis we identified 99 patients *without* high-risk features, i.e., with a limited intraductal component. In 65 of these patients radiotherapy was initiated within 4 weeks of the segmental mastectomy; in

34, radiotherapy was delayed 5 weeks or more while one or more courses of chemotherapy were given. The percentage of patients in these two groups free of local recurrence is almost identical (Fig. 1). An additional 53 patients with an extensive intraductal component were also evaluated, and there was a slight trend for better local control among the 42 patients treated immediately following segmental mastectomy than among the 11 with a delay of 5 weeks or more. However this trend was not statistically significant ($p = 0.26$).

In the other study bearing on this issue, radiotherapy was administered after mastectomy rather than lumpectomy. The Dana-Farber Cancer Institute (DFCI) and the JCRT began a collaborative adjuvant therapy study in 1974. During the first year of this study patients were treated with adjuvant chemotherapy following either mastectomy or a combination of mastectomy and adjuvant radiotherapy. Beginning in 1975, however, patients entered into the study who had not had prior adjuvant radiotherapy were randomized after the completion of all chemotherapy to receive either adjuvant radiotherapy or no further therapy of any type. Patients with four or more histologically involved lymph nodes were considered to be at particularly high risk of recurrence and death from breast cancer, and these patients were treated more intensely than patients thought to be at moderate risk of recurrence. High-risk patients were randomized to receive either 15 or 30 weeks of a combination of cyclophosphamide and doxorubicin (CA). During the first year of this study 25 patients were treated with mastectomy and adjuvant radiotherapy before chemotherapy. One of these 25 patients (4%) had a local recurrence. In subsequent years of the trial, 45 patients received adjuvant radiotherapy after the completion of adjuvant chemotherapy. Four (9%) of these patients relapsed. This

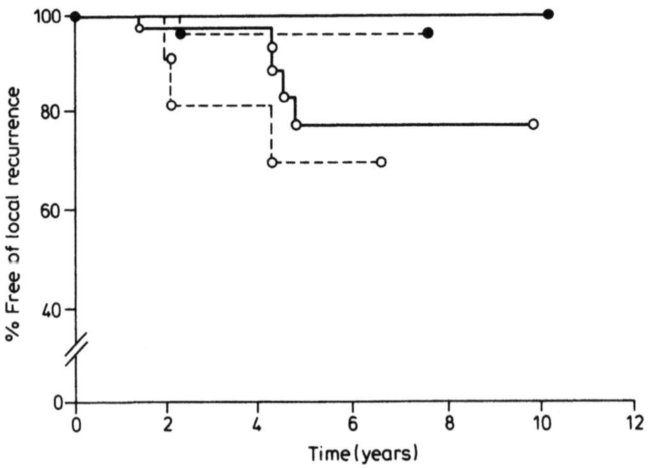

Fig. 1. The effect of a delay in the initiation of primary radiotherapy on the local recurrence rate. The patients with limited and extensive intraductal carcinoma on histologic evaluation were evaluated separately. Limited intraductal cancer: ●——●, < 4 weeks to initiation of radiotherapy ($n = 65$); ●----●, ⩾ 5 weeks to the initiation of radiotherapy ($n = 34$; $p = 0.17$). Extensive intraductal cancer: ○——○, < 4 weeks to initiation of radiotherapy ($n = 42$); ○----○, ⩾ 5 weeks to initiation of radiotherapy ($n = 11$; $p = 0.26$). (Joint Center for Radiation Therapy)

relapse rate of 9% among the patients randomized to radiotherapy after chemotherapy in years 2–8 is not significantly different from the 4% local recurrence rate among the patients who elected to receive mastectomy and radiotherapy prior to chemotherapy in the first year of the study.

One hundred twenty-three patients were randomized following the completion of adjuvant chemotherapy (Table 1). One of the patients randomized to have no radiotherapy subsequently elected to have radiotherapy in spite of the randomization. Twenty of the patients randomized to receive radiotherapy subsequently declined to receive the therapy. The study has been analyzed as patients were randomized and as they were treated. The results are the same. The local recurrence rate among patients randomized to receive radiotherapy was one-third of that observed in the patients not randomized to radiotherapy ($p = 0.03$). However, there was no statistically significant difference in the frequency of local recurrence among patients who had their adjuvant radiotherapy delayed for 15 weeks compared to those who had a delay of 30 weeks. In fact, in the analysis based on the actual treatment received there was a trend toward better local control among the patients with a delay of 30 weeks. The data from this trial utilizing adjuvant radiotherapy after mastectomy suggests that it may be inappropriate to assume that delays of up to 30 weeks in the initiation of radiotherapy while adjuvant therapy is being given will compromise local control.

Table 1. The effect of a delay in adjuvant radiotherapy on the local recurrence rate

	Local recurrence rate		*p*
Randomization			
No radiotherapy	12/60	20%	0.03
Radiotherapy after chemotherapy	4/63	6%	
Radiotherapy delayed			
15 weeks	2/36	6%	1.00
30 weeks	2/27	7%	
Treatment			
No radiotherapy	12/59	20%	0.007
Radiotherapy after chemotherapy	1/43	2%	
Radiotherapy delayed			
15 weeks	0/27	0%	0.37
30 weeks	1/16	6%	

The Effect of Adjuvant Chemotherapy on Cosmesis

Synergistic interactions between chemotherapy and radiotherapy have been frequently reported, especially toxic synergy in normal tissues. Methotrexate and doxorubicin are among the drugs known to augment the response to radiation therapy [16,36]. Both of these drugs are very effective in the treatment of breast cancer and have been used successfully in a number of adjuvant chemotherapy programs. Local skin reactions are observed more frequently and with greater intensity when adjuvant radiotherapy and adjuvant chemotherapy are administered concurrently. A statistically significant increase in erythema and skin edema was observed among the 26 patients given both adjuvant radiotherapy and CMF compared to the 43 patients treated with adjuvant radiation therapy and no adjuvant chemotherapy [20]. Skin reaction subsided 4–6 weeks after the completion of the radiation therapy. No long-term sequelae were observed.

At the JCRT 49 patients received both adjuvant chemotherapy and primary radiotherapy between 1976 and 1980. During the same period, 206 patients were treated with primary radiotherapy and no adjuvant chemotherapy. Adjuvant chemotherapy was administered concurrently or after radiotherapy and consisted of one of the following: either the original CMF regimen or some minor modification of it in 37 patients, MF without cyclophosphamide in seven patients, and CA in five patients. Cosmesis of the radiated breast was evaluated at regular intervals, and the degree of breast edema, breast retraction, and telangiectasia was systematically evaluated. Patients were also examined for evidence of arm edema, and an overall cosmetic score was assigned using a scoring system previously developed for evaluating cosmesis in patients who had received no adjuvant chemotherapy [23]. Patients were considered to have an excellent cosmetic result if the treated breast appeared nearly identical to the untreated breast. Patients with a good cosmetic result had slight differences between the treated and untreated breast, and patients were scored as having a fair result if the two breasts were clearly different but the treated breast was not seriously distorted. If there was serious distortion of the breast contour the patient was considered to have had a poor result.

At 6 months of follow-up there was little difference in the cosmetic results achieved in patients treated with adjuvant chemotherapy compared to those given primary radiotherapy and no adjuvant chemotherapy [3]. With longer follow-up there was more rapid deterioration of the cosmetic results among women given adjuvant chemotherapy than among those given radiotherapy alone (Fig. 2). Most of the shift in score was from an excellent to a good cosmetic result in the patients given adjuvant chemotherapy. For example, at 2 years of follow-up 24% of the patients given adjuvant chemotherapy had an excellent cosmetic result compared to 64% of those given primary radiotherapy without adjuvant chemotherapy. However, the percentage of patients with *either* a good or an excellent result at 2 years and 4 years of follow-up was almost the same. By 4 years there was a nonsignificant trend toward an increased incidence of fair or poor cosmetic results among those given adjuvant chemotherapy. Forty percent of the patients given adjuvant chemotherapy but only 22% of those given primary radiotherapy and no adjuvant chemotherapy had a fair or poor cosmetic result ($p = 0.47$). The major reason for an increased incidence of a fair or poor result among patients given adjuvant chemotherapy was increased breast retraction.

Other investigators have found similar results. The National Cancer Institute (NCI) studied 28 patients, 10 given adjuvant chemotherapy and 18 treated with primary radiation therapy and no adjuvant chemotherapy [32]. These patients were enrolled in a randomized trial comparing mastectomy with primary radiotherapy. Only patients with histologically involved nodes received adjuvant chemotherapy.

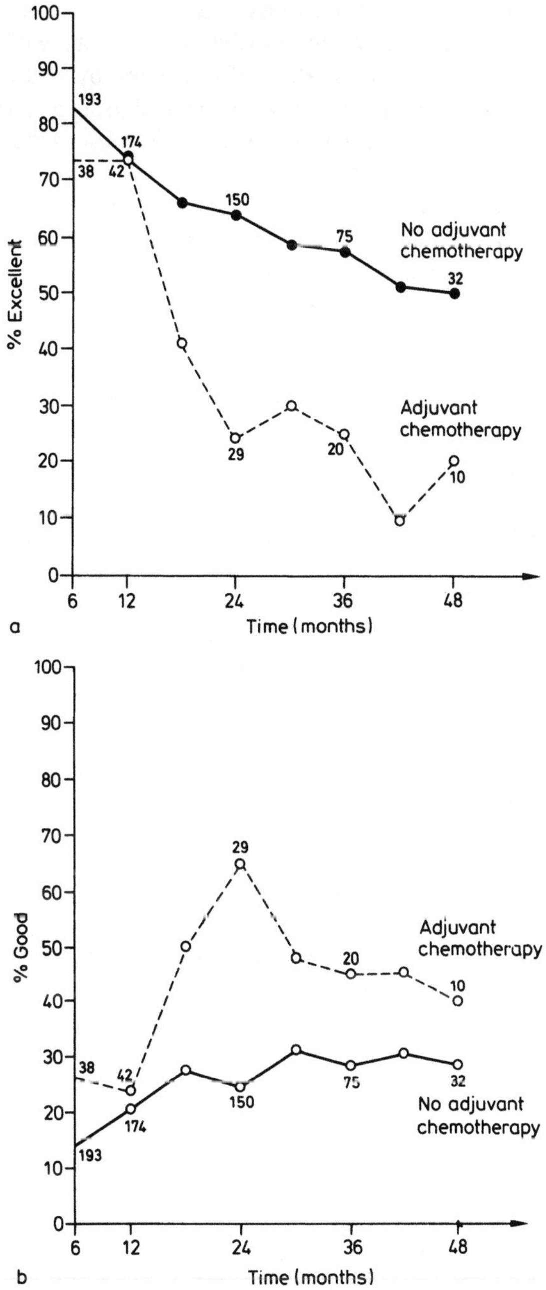

Fig. 2a,b. The effect of adjuvant chemotherapy on the cosmetic results after primary radiotherapy. **a** Percentage of patients receiving radiotherapy without adjuvant chemotherapy (——) or both primary radiotherapy and adjuvant chemotherapy (----) scored as having an excellent cosmetic result (see text for definitions). **b** Percentage of patients with a good cosmetic result. (Joint Center for Radiation Therapy 1976–1980)

Thus, this is a comparison of the cosmetic results obtained in node-positive patients with those in node-negative patients as well as a comparison of cosmesis following a combination of radiotherapy and chemotherapy with radiotherapy alone. Cosmetic scores were assigned using a system very similar to that employed at the JCRT. At the time of analysis, most of these patients had been observed for only 1-2 years. As in the JCRT study, there was primarily a shift in results from excellent to good. Seventy percent of the patients treated with both chemotherapy and radiotherapy had either a good or an excellent result; 78% of the patients who received radiotherapy alone had a good or excellent result. However, only 10% of the chemotherapy-treated patients, in contrast to 39% of the patients treated without chemotherapy, had an excellent result.

At the University of Pennsylvania, 27 patients treated with chemotherapy [18 treated concomitantly with CF followed by CMF + prednisone (CMFP) after completion of radiotherapy and nine treated with CMF only after completion of radiotherapy] were compared to 19 patients with similar clinical characteristics who were treated with primary radiation therapy and no chemotherapy during the same period of time [19]. In this series the early cosmetic results (median follow-up of 24-26 months) appeared to be almost identical. Excellent cosmesis was observed in 58% of the patients treated with radiotherapy alone and 63% of those treated with both radiotherapy and adjuvant chemotherapy. Eighty-nine percent of the patients treated with radiotherapy alone had either good or excellent results, compared to 81% of those treated with both modalities.

Sequential Versus Concomitant Chemotherapy and Radiotherapy

The cosmetic results from primary radiotherapy may be worse when adjuvant chemotherapy is given concomitantly rather than sequentially. This trend was seen in the University of Pennsylvania series [12]. Although the number of patients treated concomitantly with chemotherapy and radiotherapy was small, of nine, four of them (44%) had an excellent result and six (67%) had either an excellent or a good result. In contrast, 13 of the 18 patients (72%) treated with sequential chemotherapy after completion of all radiation therapy had an excellent result; 16 (89%) had either a good or an excellent result.

Ninety patients have been treated at the JCRT with adjuvant chemotherapy and primary radiotherapy: 47 were given concomitant chemotherapy and 43 patients were given sequential chemotherapy. The longest follow-up is in excess of 3 years. At 6 months there appeared to be a marked difference in the cosmetic results achieved in these two groups of patients (Fig. 3). More than 70% of the patients treated with sequential chemotherapy had an excellent result, compared to only 30% of the patients treated with concomitant chemotherapy and radiotherapy. Most of the shift in score was from an excellent to a good result. However, among the patients given concomitant chemotherapy and radiotherapy, there were seven fair or poor results among 40 breasts which could be evaluated at 6 months. None of the 32 breasts treated with sequential radiation and chemotherapy had a fair or poor result. Five of the seven fair or poor results at 6 months were due to moderate

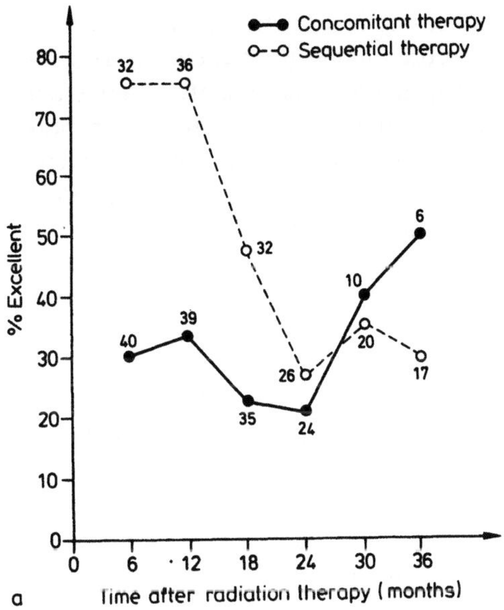

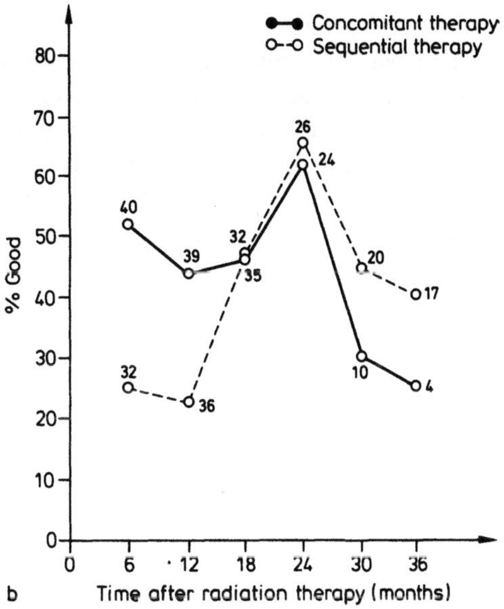

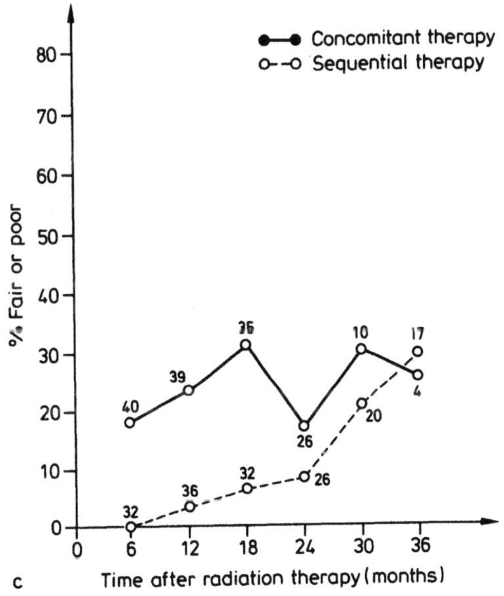

Fig. 3a-c. Effect of adjuvant chemotherapy timing on cosmetic result. **a** Percentage of patients achieving an excellent cosmetic score during 30 months of follow-up. All patients had primary radiotherapy and adjuvant chemotherapy: ——, both modalities given concomitantly, -----, the two modalities given sequentially, usually radiotherapy first. **b** Percentage of patients achieving a good cosmetic result. **c** Percentage of patients with a fair or poor result. Joint Center for Radiation Therapy 1978–1982

or severe skin hyperpigmentation. Three of the patients had breast retraction, one with skin hyperpigmentation as well. One patient had moderate or severe skin hyperpigmentation and breast edema. The overall difference in the cosmetic scores of patients in these two groups was less evident by the 2nd year of follow-up. At the 30th month there were 10 breasts evaluable for a cosmetic score among those treated with concomitant therapy and 20 among those who were treated with sequential therapy. The number with a fair or poor result was three of the 10 (33%) given concomitant therapy and four of the 20 (20%) given sequential therapy. In both cases the major reason for a fair or poor cosmetic result was breast retraction. This was the only cause for a fair or poor score among the patients given concomitant therapy. Among those given sequential therapy, one had breast retraction alone, one had breast retraction plus edema, one had breast retraction plus telangectasia, and one had only telangectasia as the cause for a fair or poor cosmetic result. Further follow-up of these patients will be required to assess more accurately the relative effects of sequential and concomitant chemotherapy on the cosmetic outcome.

We feel that these data provide convincing evidence that the use of adjuvant chemotherapy in patients treated with primary radiotherapy is likely to result in a small but measurable compromise of breast cosmesis. In the JCRT series this has been characterized primarily by a shift in cosmetic score from excellent to good but has not resulted in a marked distortion of the breast. This cosmetic compromise may be acceptable if it is accompanied by prolongation of survival as a result of adjuvant chemotherapy. However, it remains to be seen whether careful coordination of the timing of radiotherapy and chemotherapy will result in better cosmesis. Our own data suggest that the sequential use of these two modalities may be preferable to concomitant administration.

Delaying Chemotherapy: Effect on Survival

Adjuvant chemotherapy trials initiated in the 1950s anticipated that chemotherapy would be effective in destroying those cancer cells released at or just before the time of mastectomy. For this reason the perioperative chemotherapy courses were of very short duration. In one of these studies six daily doses of intravenous cyclophosphamide improved the survival of all treated patients: premenopausal and postmenopausal women, node-positive and node-negative patients [37]. These studies have been reported with more than 15 years of follow-up and continue to show a statistically significant benefit from this short course of chemotherapy. The second generation of adjuvant chemotherapy studies utilized intermittent courses of chemotherapy for periods of 1–2 years. This change in experimental design resulted from the recognition that patients die of well-established micrometastases which are implanted months to years prior to diagnosis and initiation of therapy.

In these later studies it was assumed that micrometastases should be treated with the same chemotherapy regimens used for clinically apparent metastases. However, the effectiveness of the perioperative cyclophosphamide regimen suggests that some cells are freshly implanted in distant sites immediately following mastectomy and that these cells may be very sensitive to the effects of chemotherapy. NISSEN-MEYER, the principle investigator of this study, has hypothesized that a delay of even 2 weeks might be critical [38,39]. Eleven separate hospitals were involved in Nissen-Meyer's study, and a treatment benefit was observed in most of these. While in several centers the number of accrued patients was too small to produce meaningful results, no improvement in disease-free survival and no statistically significant improvement in overall survival was observed in one of the hospitals with a large number of patients. This hospital contributed 110 of the 1136 patients entered into the study. A careful analysis of patient characteristics failed to reveal any particular reason why this one hospital should have had less significant results than the others. The one identifiable difference in the pattern of care in this hospital compared to all others was the fact that most of the patients were referred to this center, a radiotherapy clinic, 2–4 weeks after initial surgical therapy had been completed in other hospitals. Both chemotherapy and radiotherapy were initiated an average of 21 days postoperatively. NISSEN-MEYER speculated that this 2–3 week delay may have accounted for the different results between the hospitals. This analysis has been accepted by many oncologists as evidence that the time when chemotherapy is initiated is important.

NISSEN-MEYER et al.'s [38] hypothesis has not been confirmed or refuted since its first publication in 1978. Five groups of investigators have performed retrospective analyses of their data to determine whether a relationship between disease-free survival and the timing of adjuvant chemotherapy is evident. However, the "short" interval in these studies varies from 2 to 10 weeks, whereas in NISSEN-MEYER's study the "short" interval was the day of surgery. These other investigators have evaluated delays of 3 to 18 weeks [7,8,11,18,45], but NISSEN-MEYER's longest delay was 4 weeks. Other studies have used disease-free survival as an endpoint of analysis; NISSEN-MEYER, however, used both disease-free survival and survival as an endpoint. Three of the studies have failed to find any evidence of a relationship between disease-free survival and the time at which adjuvant chemotherapy is initiated [8,18,45].

Two studies have been interpreted by their authors as providing support for the NISSEN-MEYER hypothesis. In one of these studies, 158 patients were randomized to one of four treatment groups following mastectomy: L-PAM alone, L-PAM plus adjuvant radiotherapy, CMF alone, or CMF plus radiotherapy [11]. Adjuvant chemotherapy was delayed until the completion of adjuvant radiotherapy among the patients randomized to receive both adjuvant radiotherapy and chemotherapy. The relapse rate was 14% among the patients treated with CMF alone and 31% among the patients treated with both CMF and radiotherapy ($p=0.04$). The authors speculated that this difference between CMF alone and CMF plus radiotherapy might be due to the delay in the initiation of CMF. However, in the same study a similar pattern of recurrence was not seen in the comparison of patients randomized to either L-PAM alone or L-PAM plus radiotherapy. The recurrence rate was 33% among the patients treated with L-PAM alone and 24% among those treated with both modalities ($p=0.85$). The only other study that suggests there is a relationship between the timing of the initiation of adjuvant chemotherapy and disease-free survival is a retrospective analysis of 169 patients, 75 of whom had a 4-week delay in the initiation of chemotherapy [7]. There was no evidence of a relationship between this delay and disease-free survival among all treated patients. However, for the subset of patients with one to three positive nodes (85 patients), the 4-year disease-free survival was 85% among those treated within the first 4 weeks post mastectomy compared to 59% in the patients treated more than 4 weeks after mastectomy ($p=0.02$). Neither of these studies was specifically designed to investigate the NISSEN-MEYER hypothesis, and the conclusions of the authors must be considered tenuous.

Although the timing of adjuvant chemotherapy is widely accepted as important in the use of adjuvant chemotherapy, there are few data to justify this notion. No randomized control trials testing this concept have yet been published, but the Ludwig Breast Cancer Study Group has recently completed accrual to a study in which two-thirds of the patients were randomized on the day of mastectomy to receive immediate CMF; the remaining one-third began CMF treatment after a 1-month delay. This study includes premenopausal and postmenopausal, node-negative and node-positive women. When published, this study should provide the strongest available evidence to either confirm or refute the NISSEN-MEYER hypothesis.

Effect of Radiotherapy on Chemotherapy Dose

It is possible that the use of radiotherapy prior to or concomitant with adjuvant chemotherapy might compromise the dose of chemotherapy which may be given. Many studies have shown that medical oncologists frequently reduce adjuvant chemotherapy doses when prior adjuvant radiotherapy or primary radiotherapy has been given (Table 2). In an NCI study comparing primary radiotherapy with mastectomy, the average dose of cyclophosphamide or doxorubicin given to patients after mastectomy was only slightly higher than that given to patients who had excision and radiotherapy [33]. This difference was not statistically significant. However, only 13 of the 27 patients (48%) treated with primary radiotherapy and adjuvant chemotherapy received more than 95% of the scheduled doxorubicin (i.e., the dose recommended in the protocol). This was in contrast to 22 of 29 patients (76%) treated with mastectomy. In a study from Stanford, 42 patients who were

Table 2. Adjuvant chemotherapy dose reduction in patients treated with either primary or adjuvant radiotherapy

			Patients (%) above scheduled dose level		
Study	*n*	Dose level	Chemotherapy only	Chemotherapy + radiotherapy	*p*
National Cancer Institute* [33]	56	>95%	76	48	
Stanford+ [31]	84	>85%	19	2	< 0.02
Marshfield, Wisconsin+ [2]	45	>70%	84	50	0.029
Joint Center for Radiation Therapy [10]	50	>85%	–	88	
University of Pennsylvania	101	>85%	88	87,73	0.16
Georgetown [19]	64	>85%	29	53	>0.1

*Randomized trial
+All or some patients had postmastectomy radiotherapy

treated with either postoperative radiotherapy (29 patients) or primary radiotherapy (13 patients) were compared restrospectively to a group of 42 patients treated with mastectomy and no radiation therapy during the same time period [31]. CMF adjuvant chemotherapy was given to both groups. Patients treated with adjuvant CMF and radiotherapy received an average of 60% of the maximally prescribed dose of drug compared to 74% for patients given only adjuvant CMF ($p < 0.001$). In this study only 2% of the patients treated with both chemotherapy and radiotherapy received more than 85% of the prescribed doses compared to 19% of the patients treated with adjuvant CMF alone.

Other investigators have not observed such a significant reduction in chemotherapy dose when radiotherapy is given. In an analysis from the Beth Israel Hospital and the JCRT, it was observed that 88% of the patients given adjuvant CMF and concomitant radiotherapy tolerated more than 85% of the prescribed dose [10]. At the University of Pennsylvania, patients were initially treated with CF (i.e., without methotrexate) while primary radiotherapy was given and with CMFP when radiotherapy was completed [17]. Of the 61 patients who completed the first two cycles of CF, 87% tolerated more than 85% of the recommended dose. Of 41 patients given primary radiotherapy who later completed six cycles of CMFP, 73% tolerated more than 85% of the recommended dose. These dose reductions were not significantly greater than those in 40 matched patients treated with mastectomy only during the same time period. Eighty-eight percent of the mastectomy patients tolerated more than 85% of the prescribed CMF dose. In another study, patients given a combination of chemotherapy and radiotherapy actually tolerated chemotherapy better than those patients given chemotherapy following mastectomy [19].

Reductions in chemotherapy dose are not based on uniform criteria, and it is possible that many patients in these studies would have tolerated higher doses than those given. Investigators from Stanford calculated a "prescribable" CMF dose for each patient included in their study [31]. In their retrospective analysis the investigators felt the drug dose should have been based on the following dose reduction schema: total leukocyte count $\geq$ 3500, 100% of protocol doses; leukocyte count of 3000–3500, 50% reduction in the dose of methotrexate and 5-fluorouracil but not cyclophosphamide; leukocyte count of 2000–2900, 50% reduction of all drugs; leukocyte count of < 2000, no drug. Based on these criteria, patients receiving both chemotherapy and radiotherapy would still have received a significantly lower dose of chemotherapy. The mean "prescribable" dose of CMF was 83% for those given CMF plus radiotherapy and 91% for those given CMF alone ($p < 0.001$).

In practice, medical oncologists utilize the total leukocyte count to determine drug dosage. Generally this is not a problem, because the fall in leukocyte count associated with chemotherapy administration usually results primarily from a fall in the granulocyte count. However, for reasons that are not entirely known, radiotherapy has a differential lymphocytic effect. For example, in one study the granulocyte count, the lymphocyte count, and the band count were determined serially in 10 patients [9]. The first leukocyte count was obtained before mastectomy, the second immediately after mastectomy, the third before radiotherapy, the fourth following the completion of radiotherapy, the fifth at 6 months of follow-up, and the final count at 1 year of follow-up. Over this period of time there was remarkably little fall in the total granulocyte count; the lowest nadir occurred immediately following the completion of adjuvant radiotherapy. In contrast, the lymphocyte count fell steadily from its preoperative level, and when adjuvant radiotherapy was completed the total lymphocyte count was less than 50% of the preoperative value. At 1 year of follow-up, the lymphocyte count was still depressed even though it had begun to return to normal. Thus, chemotherapy dose reductions based on total leukocyte count may be inappropriate in patients who have received prior radiotherapy.

Because of this selective effect of radiation on lymphocytes, the Stanford group performed a third calculation on their data and determined the prescribable dose utilizing the granulocyte count, rather than total leukocyte count, to determine the maximal dose of adjuvant chemotherapy which might have been given [31]. It was assumed in these calculations that patients with a granulocyte count between 1000 and 1900 should have had a 50% reduction in drug dose and that those patients with a granulocyte count below 1000 should have received no adjuvant therapy. Using the granulocyte count as a basis for determining the mean prescribable chemotherapy dose, the mean dose which might have been administered to the patients treated with both radiotherapy and chemotherapy was 91.8% compared to 91.7% for the patients treated with chemotherapy only.

In the NCI randomized trial comparing mastectomy and primary radiotherapy, serial total white blood counts, granulocyte counts, and lymphocyte counts were recorded throughout the time adjuvant chemotherapy was given. There was a slight tendency for the nadir granulocyte counts to be lower in the patients receiving radiotherapy, but there was a marked reduction in lymphocyte count among the patients receiving radiotherapy compared to those given only mastectomy [33].

A potential confounding variable which has not been analyzed in chemotherapy dose reduction studies is radiotherapy technique. The amount of sternal and thoracic bone marrow treated with radiotherapy may be much greater in centers where radiotherapy is used to treat the internal mammary nodes than in those units that use only tangential fields to treat the breast.

Is the Dose of Chemotherapy Important in Determining Patient Survival?

It is a fundamental principle of medical oncology that the chemotherapy used in any treatment program should be at the maximum tolerated dose. It has been shown in other tumor types and in experimental animal models that dose may be a critical factor in determining both response to therapy and survival [15]. In 1981, BONADONNA and VALAGUSSA [4] published a retrospective analysis of the relationship between dose and survival among patients randomized in the original Milan trial to receive adjuvant CMF. Patients were divided into three groups: those who had received 85% or more of the optimal calculated doses, those who had received 65% to 84%, and those who had been given less than 65% of the CMF doses required by the protocol. Only 22% of the premenopausal women and 11% of the postmenopausal women actually received an average of more than 85% of optimal calculated doses. However, for these patients there was significantly better disease-free survival and overall survival advantage than for the control population. At 5 years disease-free survival was 79% among the premenopausal women given the highest doses, 56% for those receiving the middle doses, and 46% for those with the lowest doses. The disease-free survival difference between those patients who received the highest CMF doses and patients in the control population was highly significant ($p < 0.0001$). The disease-free survival for postmenopausal women in the three dosage groups was 75%, 56%, and 49% respectively. The difference in the disease-free survival of the postmenopausal women given the highest dose and the mastectomy-only control patients was also statistically significant ($p = 0.03$). After 10 years of follow-up, for those patients given the highest dose of CMF there is still a disease-free survival advantage (56% vs 39%, $p = 0.006$) and an overall survival advantage. While 66% of the patients given the highest dose were still alive at 10 years, 47% of those given less than 65% of optimal doses survived ($p = 0.04$).

Similar retrospective analyses have been performed by other investigators, but an improvement in overall survival among the patients receiving the highest dose was seen in only one of the studies. In the Swiss OSAKO trial, there was a marginally significant advantage for patients who received more than 90% of optimal LMF (chlorambucil, methotrexate, and 5-fluorouracil) ($p = 0.08$) [44]. There was a trend toward improved disease-free survival for patients receiving the highest dose of drug in three studies [27,46,48], but no relationship at all was found between disease-free survival and dose in three other studies [6,18,34]. Two trial groups observed a negative relationship between dose and disease-free survival [1,41], but this trend was statistically significant in only one of these two studies [41] ($p = 0.005$).

There are several methodological problems in retrospective studies of this type. The initial division of patients into three groups given $\geq$ 85%, 65%–84% and $\leq$ 65% of optimal dose is data-derived, i.e., these are the dose groupings which resulted in the greatest survival differences in the Milan trial. Although most investigators have used the same groupings, several have not. The OSAKO group divided their patients into two dose levels: $\geq$ 90% and $<$ 90% of optimal calculated dose [44]. The Southeastern Cancer Study Group compared patients who had received $>$85% and those who had received $\leq$ 85% of the optimal calculated dose [46], and the Danish Group compared patients given $\geq$ 75% of optimal dose and those given $<$ 75% [6]. The Southwest Oncology Group (SWOG) compared the mean drug dose administered to patients who were disease-free and to those who had relapsed [18]. Since no statistically significant differences in the mean drug dose were found, these investigators concluded there was no dose effect.

It is likely that patients able to tolerate higher doses of chemotherapy are also more likely to survive longer regardless of their response to chemotherapy, and this is an important bias in all retrospective analyses of this question. However, the Ludwig Breast Cancer Study Group has unintentionally performed a prospective, randomized trial with a significant difference in dose between the two treatment arms [34]. Premenopausal women with one to three histologically involved axillary nodes were randomized to receive either CMF or CMFP. In an unanticipated development, the patients given prednisone were able to tolerate more CMF. An average of 83% of full CMF doses were given to the CMFP patients compared to an average of 72% of full CMF doses in the patients randomized to CMF without prednisone ($p = 0.001$). No significant differences in disease-free survival or overall survival have been observed thus far among the patients given the higher doses of CMF as part of the CMFP regimen. This study avoids some of the bias of the retrospective analyses.

The methodologic problems associated with retrospective analyses of dose have been reviewed, and a number of different methodologies have been proposed for evaluating this problem [41]. However, these authors conclude that none of these methods represents an optimal approach. Some methodologies are even consistent with a possible placebo dose response. This is not inconsistent with other randomized trials, such as those evaluating tolbutamide for diabetes and clofibrate for coronary heart disease. In both of these studies "compliant" patients who regularly took their placebo in the control population (i.e., those treated with placebo) were observed to do better than control patients who were "non-compliant" [41].

The importance of chemotherapy dose is currently being evaluated in a prospective randomized trial by the Cancer and Leukemia Group B (CALGB). Patients are treated after mastectomy or excisional biopsy with four courses of CAF (cyclophosphamide, doxorubicin, 5-fluorouracil). Patients randomized to receive high-dose or intensive CAF are given cyclophosphamide 600 mg/m^2 on day 1, doxorubicin 60 mg/m^2 on day 1, and 5-fluorouracil 600 mg/m^2 on days 1 and 8. Patients randomized to low-dose CAF are treated with exactly 50% of these doses on the same treatment schedule. Patients treated with primary radiotherapy are given radiation after the completion of either the high or low dose of adjuvant chemotherapy. No results from this trial are available yet.

The importance of radiotherapy in determining chemotherapy dose and the importance of dose in determining patient survival are both reasonable subjects for further study. Preliminary data suggest the possibility that full doses of adjuvant chemotherapy may be given with or after primary radiotherapy, particularly when the granulocyte count is used to make close adjustment, but is it not established that dose is a critical factor in determining the effectiveness of adjuvant chemotherapy.

Other Side Effects from Concomitant Chemotherapy and Radiotherapy

Side effects which occur infrequently with either radiotherapy or chemotherapy may occur with increased frequency or with greater intensity when both modalities are used. It has been reported in one study that the incidence of arm edema may be increased when both modalities are administered. In this study, six of 27 patients (22%) given both adjuvant CMFP and radiotherapy developed mild to moderate edema (two mild and four moderate). In contrast, none of the patients treated with only radiotherapy in the same time period developed arm edema [12]. Others have not always observed a similar increase in arm edema. In the NCI study, one of 10 patients (10%) receiving adjuvant chemotherapy and radiotherapy developed arm edema compared to four of 18 patients (22%) given radiotherapy alone [32]. At the

JCRT, the actuarial risk of arm edema at 6 years was found to be principally related to the extent of axillary dissection. The risk of arm edema was 31% among patients treated by full dissection and chemotherapy compared to 32% for patients treated by full dissection without chemotherapy, and 8% for patients treated by limited dissection and chemotherapy compared to 6% for patients treated by limited dissection without chemotherapy [29].

Radiotherapy to the left hemithorax has been shown in one series to be associated with an increased incidence of cardiotoxicity in those patients receiving doxorubicin chemotherapy [28]. For this reason, it might be anticipated that patients treated with adjuvant chemotherapy regimens which include doxorubicin and who have left-sided lesions treated with radiotherapy will have an increased incidence of doxorubicin-induced cardiotoxicity. In the DFCI/JCRT adjuvant study described above, the overall incidence of cardiotoxicity among 280 patients given adjuvant doxorubicin was 4%. In the subset of 44 patients receiving both adjuvant radiotherapy and adjuvant doxorubicin there were two (5%) cases of cardiotoxicity, 0/20 among those with right-sided lesions and 2/24 (8%) among those with left-sided lesions ($p = 0.49$). Although the subgroups are small and the difference non-significant, these data suggest there might be an increased incidence of cardiotoxicity as a result of using both modalities together for a left-sided breast cancer. However, as in the study of myelosuppression, the radiotherapy techniques used and the fields included may have an important role in determining the frequency with which cardiotoxicity is seen.

Brachial plexopathy was observed in eight of 565 (1.4%) patients treated at the JCRT with primary radiotherapy [42]. Although this syndrome is usually characterized by hand and forearm paresthesias, mild to moderate axillary pain, and mild finger weakness, two of these eight patients developed nearly complete paralysis and atrophy of the involved arm. However, all patients eventually had full return of normal function. The etiology of this brachial plexopathy is not entirely clear. A plausible hypothesis is that it is related to the use of axillary dissection, but only four of the eight patients underwent such dissection. There was a much better correlation with the administration of adjuvant chemotherapy. Seven of the eight patients with brachial plexopathy had adjuvant chemotherapy, and in six of these seven the appearance of the syndrome followed the initiation of adjuvant chemotherapy.

With time and the accruing of larger numbers of patients treated with both of these modalities, other unusual toxicities may be observed or there may be a slight increase in uncommon toxicities. It is possible that some patients may undergo profound or prolonged myelosuppression, a rare event when chemotherapy is used alone. It is also possible that the incidence of pneumonitis, rib fractures, or secondary leukemia may increase with combined therapy. However, the reported results of combined radiation and chemotherapy trials have not yet shown an associated increase in the frequency of such complications [30].

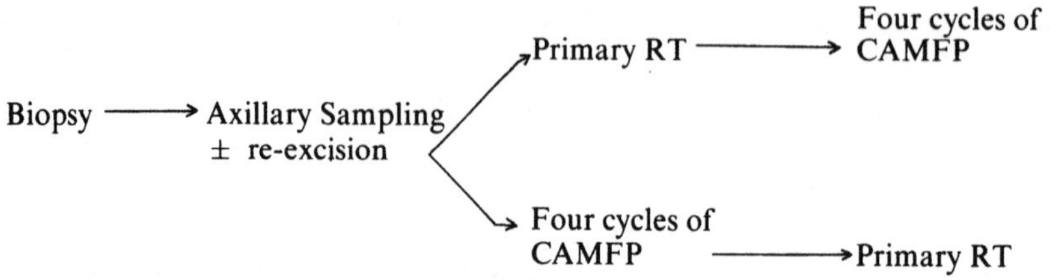

Fig. 4. Schema of ongoing adjuvant chemotherapy/primary radiotherapy protocol at the Joint Center for Radiation Therapy/Beth Israel Hospital/Dana-Farber Cancer Institute. Patients are randomized to receive chemotherapy either before or after primary radiotherapy. (See text for details of the chemotherapy regimen)

Conclusions

The proper integration of radiotherapy and chemotherapy to achieve optimal local control of breast cancer, excellent cosmesis, and prolonged survival for the patients is still unknown. In our opinion, this is an appropriate subject for prospective, randomized controlled trials. To evaluate systematically the impact of radiotherapy on the maximum tolerated dose of chemotherapy and to determine whether a delay in the initiation of radiotherapy will compromise local control, we have initiated a trial in which patients with histologically involved nodes are randomized to receive chemotherapy before or after primary radiotherapy (Fig. 4). Patients entered onto this study may have clinical T_{1-3}, N_{0-1} disease as long as the lesion fulfills the usual criteria of operability. All patients must have a node dissection with demonstration of histologically involved nodes. Treatment is initiated within 4 weeks of the node sampling. Because of the demonstration that short courses of chemotherapy are as effective as a more prolonged course of therapy [26], all patients receive four cycles of chemotherapy. Each cycle consists of an intensive program of cyclophosphamide 500 mg/m^2 on day 1, doxorubicin 45 mg/m^2 on day 3, methotrexate with leukovorin rescue 200 mg/m^2 on days 1 and 15, 5-fluorouracil 500 mg/m^2 on day 1, and prednisone 40 mg/m^2 orally on days 1–5.

Prospective controlled trials of this type are the only alternatives to the continued use of the unfounded assumptions outlined near the end of the Introduction above. Primary radiotherapy and adjuvant chemotherapy each offer the patient important benefits. It is now time to determine the best means of integrating these two treatment modalities.

References

1. Ahmann D, O'Fallon J, Scanlon P, Payne WS, Bisel H, Edmonson J, Frytak S, et al. (1982) A preliminary assessment of factors associated with recurrent disease in a surgical adjuvant clinical trial for patients with breast cancer with special emphasis on the aggressiveness of therapy. Am J Clin Oncol 5:371–381

2. Banerjee TK, Hoehn JL, Greenlaw RH, Jacoby C (1984) Chemotherapy drug dose alteration due to radiation therapy in an adjuvant situation in breast cancer. Am J Clin Oncol 7:437–442
3. Beadle GF, Harris JR, Come S, Henderson IC, Silver B, Hellman S (1984) Effect of adjuvant chemotherapy on the cosmetic results after primary radiation treatment for early stage breast cancer. Int J Radiat Oncol 10:2131–2137
4. Bonadonna G, Valagussa P (1981) Dose-response effect of adjuvant chemotherapy in breast cancer. N Engl J Med 304:10–15
5. Bonadonna G, Valagussa P, Rossi A, Tancini G, Brambilla C, Zambetti M, Veronesi U (1985) Ten-year experience with CMF-based adjuvant chemotherapy in resectable breast cancer. Breast Cancer Res Treat 5:95–115
6. Brincker H, Mouridsen HT, Rank F, Rose C, Andersen KW (1985) Evidence of a castration-mediated effect of adjuvant chemotherapy (CT) in a randomized trial of cyclophosphamide monotherapy versus CMF in premenopausal stage II breast cancer. Proc Am Soc Clin Oncol 4:56
7. Brooks RJ, Jones SE, Salmon SE, Chase EM, Davis SL, Moon TE, Giordano GF, et al. (1983) Improved outcome with early treatment in an adjuvant breast cancer program. Proc Am Soc Clin Oncol 2:110
8. Buzdar AU, Smith TL, Powell KD, Blumenschein GR, Gehan EA (1982) Effect of timing of initiation of adjuvant chemotherapy on disease-free survival in breast cancer. Breast Cancer Res Treat 2:163–169
9. Byfield JE (1984) Hemotologic parameters in the adjustment of chemotherapy doses in combined modality treatments involving radiation. Am J Clin Oncol 7:371–374
10. Come S, Botnick L, Lange R, Goldstein M, Tishler S, Schnipper L (1983) Concurrent radiation therapy (RT) and chemotherapy (CT) in the primary management of pathologic stage II breast cancer. Proc Am Soc Clin Oncol 2:99
11. Cooper R, Rhyne AL, Muss HB, Ferree C, Richards FI, White DR, Stuart JJ, et al. (1981) A randomized comparative trial of chemotherapy and irradiation therapy for stage II breast cancer. Cancer 47:2833–2839
12. Danoff BF, Goodman RL, Glick JH, Haller DG, Pajak TF (1983) The effect of adjuvant chemotherapy on cosmetics and complications in patients with breast cancer treated by definitive irradiation. Int J Radiat Oncol Biol Phys 9:1625–1630
13. Fisher B, Fisher ER, Redmond C (1986) Ten year results from the NSABP clinical trial evaluating the use of L-phenylalanine mustard (L-PAM) in the management of primary breast cancer. J Clin Oncol 4:929–941
14. Fisher B, Bauer M, Margolese R, Poisson R, Pilch Y, et al. (1985) Five-year results of a randomized clinical trial comparing total mastectomy and segmental mastectomy with or without radiation in the treatment of breast cancer. N Engl J Med 312:666–673
15. Frei E III, Canellos GP (1980) Dose: A critical factor in cancer chemotherapy. Am J Med 69:585–594
16. Fu KK (1985) Biological basis for the interaction of chemotherapeutic agents and radiation therapy. Cancer 55:2123–2130
17. Glick JH, Danoff B, Haller D, Weiler C, Hurwitz S, Richter M, Goodman R (1984) Integration of adjuvant chemotherapy with definitive radiotherapy for primary breast cancer. In: Jones SE, Salmon SE (eds) Adjuvant therapy of cancer IV. Grune and Stratton, Orlando
18. Glucksberg H, Rivkin SE, Rasmussen S, Tranum B, Gad-el-Mawla N, Costanzi J, Hoogstraten B, et al. (1982) Combination chemotherapy (CMFVP) versus L-phenylalanine mustard (L-PAM) for operable breast cancer with positive axillary nodes: A Southwest Oncology Group Study. Cancer 50:423–434
19. Goldberg R, Byrne P, Feller W, Harter K, Ueno W, Dritschilo A (1984) A comparison of adjuvant chemotherapy in lumpectomy-primary breast radiation and mastectomy patients. Proc Am Soc Clin Oncol 3:126
20. Hahn P, Hallberg O, Vikterlof KJ (1978) Acute skin reactions in postoperative breast cancer patients receiving radiotherapy plus adjuvant chemotherapy. AJR 130:137–139
21. Harris JR, Abram R, Schnitt S, Connolly J, Silver B, Come S, Henderson IC (1985) Current status of conservative surgery and radiotherapy as primary local treatment for early carcinoma of the breast. Breast Cancer Res Treat 5:245–255

22. Harris JR, Connolly JL, Schnitt SJ, Cady B, Love S, Osteen RT, Patterson WB, et al. (1985) The use of pathologic features in selecting the extent of surgical resection necessary for breast cancer patients treated by primary radiation therapy. Ann Surg 201:164–169
23. Harris JR, Levene MB, Svensson G, Hellman S (1979) Analysis of cosmetic results following primary radiation therapy for stages I and II carcinoma of the breast. J Radiat Oncol Biol Phys 5:257–261
24. Harter K, Goldberg R, Bryne P, Lee T, Smith F, Dritschilo A (1984) Local recurrence of breast cancer following therapy in patients receiving adjuvant chemotherapy prior to definitive breast irradiation. Proc Am Soc Clin Oncol 3:125
25. Henderson IC (1987) Adjuvant systemic therapy for early breast cancer. Curr Probl Cancer, (in press)
26. Henderson IC, Gelman RS, Harris JR, Canellos GP (1986) Duration of therapy in adjuvant chemotherapy trials. NCI Monogr 1:95–98
27. Howell A, Bush H, George WD, Howat JMT, Crowther D, Sellwood RA, Rubens RD, et al. (1984) A controlled trial of adjuvant chemotherapy with cyclophosphamide, methotrexate and fluorouracil for breast cancer. Lancet 2:307–311
28. Kinsella TJ, Ahmann DL, Giuliani ER, Lie JT (1979) Adriamycin cardiotoxicity in stage IV breast cancer: possible enhancement with prior left chest radiation therapy. Int J Radiat Oncol Biol Phys 5:1997–2002
29. Larson D, Weinstein M, Goldberg I, Silver B, Recht A, Cady B, Silen W, Harris JR (1986) Edema of the arm as a function of the extent of axillary surgery in patients with stage I-II carcinoma of the breast treated with primary radiotherapy. Int J Radiat Oncol Biol Phys 12:1575–1582
30. Levitt SH (1985) Primary treatment of early breast cancer with conservation surgery and radiation therapy: the effect of adjuvant chemotherapy. Cancer 55:2140–2148
31. Levine JF, Coleman CN, Cox RS, Ray GR, Rogoway WM, Martinez A, Stockdale FE (1984) The effect of postoperative and primary radiation therapy on delivered dose of adjuvant cyclophosphamide, methotrexate, and 5-fluorouracil (CMF) chemotherapy in breast cancer. Cancer 53:237–241
32. Lichter AS, Lippman ME, Gorrell CR, d'Angelo TM, Edwards BK, deMoss EV (1983) Adjuvant chemotherapy in patients treated primarily with irradiation for localized breast cancer. In: Harris JR, Hellman S, Silen WJB (eds) Conservative management of breast cancer. Lippincott, Philadelphia
33. Lippman ME, Lichter AS, Danforth D, Ellenberg S, D'Angelo T, Gorrell C (1984) The influence of primary breast cancer treatment – mastectomy or excisional biopsy plus radiation – on the ability to deliver adjuvant chemotherapy. In: Jones SE, Salmon SE (eds) Adjuvant therapy of cancer IV. Grune and Stratton, Orlando
34. Ludwig Breast Cancer Study Group (1985) A randomized trial of adjuvant combination chemotherapy with or without prednisone in premenopausal breast cancer patients with metastases in one to three axillary lymph nodes. Cancer Res 45:4454–4459
35. Meeting Report London (1984) Review of mortality results in randomised trials in early breast cancer. Lancet 2:1205
36. Muggia FM, Cortes-Funes H, Wasserman TH (1978) Radiotherapy and chemotherapy in combined clinical trials: Problems and promise. Int J Radiat Oncol Biol Phys 4:161–171
37. Nissen-Meyer R, Host H, Kjellgren K, Mansson B, Norin T (1984) Scandinavian trials with one single postoperative course vs 12 courses. Recent Results Cancer Res 96:48–54
38. Nissen-Meyer R, Kjellgren K, Malmio K, Mansson B, Norin T (1978) Surgical adjuvant chemotherapy. Cancer 41:2088–2098
39. Nissen-Meyer R, Kjellgren K, Mansson B (1982) Adjuvant chemotherapy in breast cancer. Recent Results Cancer Res 80:142–148
40. Peters MV (1977) Wedge resection with or without radiation in early breast cancer. J Radiat Oncol Biol Phys 2:1151–1156
41. Redmond C, Fisher B, Wieand HS (1983) The methodologic dilemma in retrospectively correlating the amount of chemotherapy received in adjuvant therapy protocols with disease-free survival. Cancer Treat Rep 67:519–526

42. Salner AL, Botnick LE, Herzog AG, Goldstein MA, Harris JR, Levene MB, Hellman S (1981) Reversible brachial plexopathy following primary radiation therapy for breast cancer. Cancer Treat Rep 65:797–802
43. Sarrazin D, Le M, Rouesse J, Contesso G, Petit JY, Lacour J, Viguier J, Hill C (1984) Conservative treatment versus mastectomy in breast cancer tumors with macroscopic diameter of 20 millimeters or less. Cancer 53:1209–1213
44. Senn HJ, Jungi WF, Amgwerd R, Hochuli E, Ammann J, Engelhart G, Heinz C, et al. (1984) Adjuvant chemoimmunotherapy with LMF+BCG in node-negative and node-positive breast cancer: 8 year results. Recent Results Cancer Res 96:90–101
45. Taylor SG, Kalish LA, Olson JE, Cummings F, Bennett JM, Falkson G, Tormey DC, Carbone PP (1985) Adjuvant CMFP versus CMFP plus tamoxifen versus observation alone in postmenopausal, node-positive breast cancer patients: Three-year results of an Eastern Cooperative Oncology Group Study. J Clin Oncol 3:144–154
46. Velez-Garcia E, Moore M, Vogel CL, Marcial V, Ketcham A, Raney M, Smalley R (1984) Post surgical adjuvant chemotherapy in women with breast cancer and positive axillary nodes: The Southeastern Cancer Study Group (SECSG) experience. In: Jones SE, Salmon SE (eds) Adjuvant therapy of cancer IV. Grune and Stratton, New York
47. Veronesi U, del Vecchio M, Greco M, Luini A, Muscolino G, Rasponi A, Saccozzi R, Zucali R (1983) Results of quadrantectomy, axillary dissection, and radiotherapy (QUART) in T1N0 patients. In: Harris JR, Hellman S, Silen WJB (eds) Conservative management of breast cancer. New surgical and radiotherapeutic techniques. Lippincott, Philadelphia
48. Wallgren A, Baral E, Beling U, Carstensen J, Friberg S, Glas U, Kaigas M, Skoog L (1984) Tamoxifen and combination chemotherapy as adjuvant treatment in postmenopausal women with breast cancer. Recent Results Cancer Res 96:

Adjuvant Endocrine Treatment With and Without Simultaneous Adjuvant Chemotherapy

H. MAASS

Endocrine treatment procedures are effective particularly in metastatic breast cancer. In patients with hormone-sensitive tumors long-term remissions and a definitive gain in survival are observed. Based on the pioneer work of JENSEN [6] we are able to select patients for endocrine therapy versus chemotherapy.

The challenging problem is the treatment of primary breast cancer. On one hand we perform conservative surgery in the early stage of the disease and on the other we try to increase the survival rate by means of systemic measures. The effectiveness of systemic therapy in the metastatic state of breast cancer is one of the presuppositions for the application in the adjuvant situation. Endocrine measures as well as chemotherapy are effective in the metastatic state. Regarding remission rates, endocrine treatment procedures are comparable to chemotherapy in selected patients. The best situation is the combination of a steroid receptor-rich status and favorable clinical criteria, such as slow tumor growth or osseous or locoregional metastases (low-risk situation). The overall remission rate achieved by endocrine therapy in patients with known receptor status, summarized from many publications, is shown in Table 1. Receptor-positive patients not only show higher remission rates but have definitively longer survival. Our experience is shown in Fig. 1 [19]. Four years after the first diagnosis of metastasis, the proportion of patients surviving is double that of patients with receptor-negative tumors.

In the following we will present: (a) a discussion of new methods for selecting hormone-sensitive breast cancer patients; (b) a brief overview of major publications concerning the clinical value of adjuvant endocrine therapy and combined chemohormone therapy; (c) the data from the Gynecological Adjuvant Breast Group (GABG) trial.

Table 1. Metastasized breast cancer: endocrine therapy remission rates (%)

Without selection	20–35
ER+	50–60
ER+ LOW RISK	-80
ER+ PR+	65–70
ER+ PR−	30–40
ER− PR+	~50
ER− PR−	<10

ER, estrogen receptor; PR, progesterone receptor

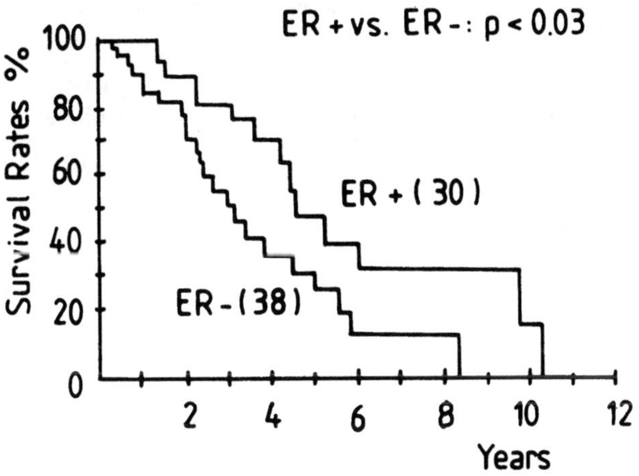

Fig. 1. Metastasized breast cancer: results of endocrine and cytostatic therapy. ER, estrogen receptor (From STOLZENBACH et al. 1982)

New Methods for Selection

The availability of monoclonal antibodies against receptor proteins makes it possible to estimate the receptor status of tumors by immunohistochemical methods. The advantage is that we need less tumor tissue and gain an impression of the distribution of receptor-positive tumor cells in the specimen. The disadvantage is the subjectivity of the method.

The experience so far shows quite good correlation between the biochemical and the histochemical determination of estrogen receptor. Clinical data for the progesterone receptor are not yet available. It is now under investigation whether histochemical estimation of the receptor status is suitable as a prediction test compared with biochemical measurement of receptor content.

The data gathered so far are shown in Table 2 [3, 5, 6, 8, 12, 15]. Patients with receptor-poor tumors as measured with the estrogen receptor immunocytochemical assay (ERICA) method responded in only 8% of cases to endocrine therapy compared with 70% of those patients with receptor-rich tumors. Compared with the data measured biochemically the histochemical assay seems to be superior. Besides the improvement of methods for receptor determination, in future we expect more possibilities for selecting patients with the aid of proliferation markers, growth factors and other autocrine factors.

Present Knowledge of Adjuvant Endocrine and Combined Chemohormone Therapy

Besides better selection parameters, new therapy concepts are under study. Regarding the adjuvant situation, experience with so-called prophylactic castration and, recently, with tamoxifen has been reported. In the case of antiestrogen

Table 2. Response to endocrine therapy in advanced breast cancer; predictive value of ERICA

Author	*n*	ERICA positive	ERICA negative
Pertschuk (1985)	43	9/16	2/27
Coombs (1985)	56	21/29	1/27
McCarty (1985)	23	13/14	1/9
Jonat (1985)	20	6/11	1/9
(1986)	10	5/7	1/3
TOTAL	152	54/77 70%	6/75 8%
Conventional assays (Bethesda 1979)	1336	480/852 56%	27/484 6%

substances, investigations have been performed to synthesize substances with lower estrogen activity. This is important especially for premenopausal patients. So far knowledge is scanty on the suitable dose of tamoxifen in premenopausal patients. The collected data on metastatic breast cancer patients show that tamoxifen, mostly in doses of 30–40 mg/day, gives remission rates similar to those yielded by ovariectomy. This is confirmed by one randomized study [2]. On the other hand the data are not sufficient to recommend generally the application of tamoxifen in the premenopause.

At present tamoxifen is the most important drug in adjuvant endocrine studies. Prospective studies on the efficacy of surgical or radiological castration have shown different results. With the sole exception of the LUDWIG study [11], the receptor status was not available. At present ovariectomy is no alternative to the application of tamoxifen in the adjuvant situation.

In all seven adjuvant trials comparing tamoxifen-treated patients with untreated controls in node-positive postmenopausal patients [13], the recurrence-free survival rate could be elevated by the application of tamoxifen, generally at a dose of 20 or 30 mg/day, for 1 or 2 years after randomization. Only the Nolvadex Adjuvant Trial Organisation (NATO) trial could demonstrate an effect of the tamoxifen treatment on the overall survival [1].

Unfortunately, in all studies the receptor status was known only in subsets of patients. In patients with known estrogen receptor status, there was a correlation in six of seven trials. In two trials – albeit only with a higher receptor content – more than 100 fmol/mg protein could be measured [17,18]. The NATO study shows absolutely no correlation to the receptor status, which was measured in about half of the patients. That means that receptor-negative patients also benefited from tamoxifen treatment. The NATO investigators offer some explanations [1]; however, others point out that there may be methodological problems in the NATO study. Thus, the rate of patients with receptor-negative findings below 5 fmol/mg is relatively high. That means that there may be some false-negative determinations. On the other hand there are some uncertainties regarding the correlation of estrogen receptor status to the outcome of patients in adjuvant trials. The Danish group [17] reported that a positive correlation was found only if the tumor contains more than 100 fmol/mg; in the group of 10–99 fmol/mg there is a negative correlation. This is due especially to a relatively high disease-free survival rate in the control group. A similar observation was made by the investigators of the Scottish trial [18].

To draw definitive conclusions we have to wait for long-term results. We know that receptor-positive patients without any adjuvant treatment have a better prognosis within 5 years after primary treatment. Longer observation times reveal equal prognosis for receptor-positive and -negative patients. Thus the difference between the controls and the tamoxifen-treated group could be reduced after a longer observation time in the receptor-positive control group.

In five of the seven trials the data were analyzed regarding the site of metastases. These data are summarized in Table 3. It is obvious that in the tamoxifen-treated group of patients local as well as distant metastases could be reduced. This was not observed in the LUDWIG trial [11]. Possibly this is one of the reasons for the smaller difference between the control and tamoxifen groups concerning distant and local metastasis.

Table 3. Adjuvant tamoxifen therapy: site of metastases (five trials)

Local		Distant	
Control	Tamoxifen	Control	Tamoxifen
227	124	493	397

In contrast to the results of the LUDWIG trial the Christie Hospital tamoxifen trial [16] shows a considerable effect in reducing the number of distant metastasis in postmenopausal women.

So most of the trials show an effect of endocrine treatment procedures in the adjuvant situation on reducing the rate of distant metastases. To answer the question of whether an adjuvant chemotherapy can be replaced by endocrine measures, we have to analyze the extent of the effects of different procedures regarding recurrence-free and overall survival. We have learned that up to now only one prospective trial shows a significant reduction of the overall survival. Thus it is questionable whether we can yet give a definitive answer to this essential question. Nevertheless, by collecting all data PETO calculated the gain of survival on the basis of all published results of the ongoing prospective trials. The results of this calculation are well known [10]. Concerning the results of adjuvant tamoxifen trials, we can conclude that patients below 50 years of age currently show no benefit, while older patients have a significant improvement of overall survival.

It is remarkable that the chemotherapy trials show the same low benefit in postmenopausal women. Compared with the efficacy of an adjuvant chemotherapy observed in premenopausal patients the effect of tamoxifen is relatively small.

Combination of Adjuvant Chemotherapy and Tamoxifen

Besides trials which compare tamoxifen with an untreated control, there are studies with longer observation times in which the effect of tamoxifen in addition to chemotherapy was investigated. The results are summarized in Table 4. The longest observation time is reported by the Case Western study [14] comparing cyclophosphamide + methotrexate + 5-fluorouracil (CMF) chemotherapy with CMF + tamoxifen. Regarding the recurrence-free survival an improvement is effected by tamoxifen in receptor-positive postmenopausal patients. This effect of adding tamoxifen to standard chemotherapy was especially observed in high-risk patients with a poor prognosis due to the nodal status. Similar but less impressive results were observed in the ECOG study [21]. It should be mentioned that in this latter study there is no effect of tamoxifen at all compared to the two chemotherapy arms, and also no effect of chemotherapy compared with the observation group. The only group of patients who benefited from the adjuvant treatment were patients with receptor-negative tumors. But in this case the recurrence rate in the control group is very high, so that we are faced with the same problems that we discussed before.

The most impressive correlation to estrogen and progesterone receptor contents is shown by the NSABP-09 trial comparing chemotherapy with phenylalanine mustard + 5-fluorouracil with and without tamoxifen. At 4 years this is true only for recurrence-free survival, not for overall survival. It is important to consider that in this trial the addition of tamoxifen to the chemotherapy reduces the recurrence-free survival in premenopausal patients with receptor-negative tumors.

Table 4. Adjuvant therapy: chemotherapy vs chemotherapy plus Tamoxifen

Case-Western	CMF vs CMF+TAM	Recurrence-free survival IER$^+$ post menopausal N $\geqslant$ 4
ECOG post menopausal	Control vs CMFP vs CMFP+TAM	TAM no effect
NSABP–09	PF vs PF+TAM	↑ER$^+$↑ ↑PgR$^+$ post menopausal ↓ pre menopausal ER$^+$
GABG high risk	AC vs AC+TAM	↑post menopausal ER$^+$

CMF, cyclophosphamide + methotrexate + 5-fluorouracil; TAM, tamoxifen; CMFP, CMF + prednisone; PF, phenylalanine mustard + 5-fluorouracil; AC, adriamycin + cytoxan; ER, estrogen receptor; PR, progesterone receptor; N, nodes

Results from the Gynecological Adjuvant Breast Group I Trial

The discussion of adjuvant treatment in breast cancer is focussed on the question of whether, for selected subgroups, aggressive chemotherapy can be replaced by endocrine treatment procedures with low short-term and long-term side effects. This question is currently under investigation in a multicenter prospective trial in Western Germany. The design is shown in Fig. 2. We compared a low-risk and a high-risk group of patients. All patients were treated by radical mastectomy and axillary node dissection without radiotherapy. Low risk was defined as one to three positive nodes and a positive estrogen and/or progesterone receptor status. High-risk subjects are node-positive patients with receptor-negative tumors and patients with more than four involved nodes regardless of receptor status.

The data after a follow-up of 54 months are shown in Table 5. The most interesting group is the so-called low-risk group, for which there are no differences between standard chemotherapy with CMF and therapy with tamoxifen alone. It is remarkable that at present there is no difference between pre- and postmenopausal patients. As in other trials with tamoxifen, it is possible that tamoxifen has a delaying effect on the manifestation of metastases, so a deviation of the two curves after longer follow-up is possible.

The high-risk group was treated with a very aggressive chemotherapy: eight cycles of adriamycin + cytoxan with and without tamoxifen. The results are

Fig. 2. Design of GABG study. *receptor positive (≥ 20 fmol/mg cytosol protein by dextran-coated charcoal method); AC, doxorubicin and cyclophosphamide; CMF, cyclophosphamide, methotrexate, 5-fluorouracil; ER, estrogen receptor; PR, progesterone receptor

Table 5. GABG I results after 54 months: metastases

	Low risk, % Tamoxifen	CMF	High risk, % AC	AC+Tamoxifen
Locoregional	4.0%	7.3%	12.9%	7.2%
Distant [+/–loc. reg.]	5.1%	5.9%	17.0%	15.4%
Total	9.1%	12.8%	30.0%	22.7%

AC, adriamycin-cytoxan

comparable with the Case-Western and the ECOG study. We found a significant reduction of recurrences due to the addition of tamoxifen. There is a correlation to the receptor status but this effect is not very impressive. One possible explanation could be that the adriamycin-containing chemotherapy eliminates especially receptor-negative clones of the tumor, so that in a heterogeneous tumor population receptor-positive cells survive and can be attacked by tamoxifen. This hypothesis is supported by the fact that we found a change of receptor status from negative to positive in patients who had been treated by adjuvant chemotherapy.

Comparable to the results of the Case-Western trial, we observed in our trial a remarkable effect of the additional application of tamoxifen to the chemotherapy in patients with very poor prognosis, having more than 10 involved nodes.

Summary

From the literature data and our own results of the GABG I trial, we can summarize our present state of knowledge regarding adjuvant endocrine therapy with or without chemotherapy as follows:

1. Adjuvant endocrine therapy is effective regarding the increase of recurrence-free survival and possibly overall survival.
2. A receptor-positive primary tumor is a precondition.
3. We do not yet know the extent of the efficacy. Based on the present data the effect of endocrine methods is smaller regarding the overall survival, especially for some subgroups.
4. Probably only postmenopausal patients have a benefit. Therefore endocrine procedures are justified and have to be recommended, with the precondition of a positive receptor status.
5. The effect of adjuvant endocrine measures is probably independent of the nodal status.
6. Combination of adjuvant chemotherapy and tamoxifen seems to be effective in high-risk patients, but generally is not to be recommended.
7. The optimal duration of adjuvant endocrine therapy with tamoxifen is not known. It should last at least 2 years, probably longer.
8. Patients with receptor-negative primary tumors, and especially premenopausal patients independent of receptor status, should have adjuvant chemotherapy.

References

1. Baum M, Brinkley DM, Dossett A, McPherson K, Patterson JS, Rubens RD, Smiddy FG, et al. (1985) Controlled trial of tamoxifen as single adjuvant agent in management of early breast cancer. Analysis at six years by Nolvadex Adjuvant Trial Organisation. Lancet 1:836–840
2. Buchanan RB, Williams CJ, Hall V, Blamey RW, Webster DJ (1985) Tamoxifen versus surgical oophorectomy in premenopausal women with advanced breast cancer. Proc Am Soc Clin Oncol 4:59

3. Coombs RC, McClelland RA, Berger U, Müller L, Jensen E, Neville AM (1984) Use of an enzyme linked immunocytochemical assay (ERICA) utilizing a monoclonal antibody to estrogen receptor (ER) in predicting response to endocrine therapy in advanced breast cancer patients. Symposium on Estrogen Receptor Determination with Monoclonal Antibodies, Monte Carlo
4. Fisher B, Wolmark N (1985) Adjuvant tamoxifen and chemotherapy in stage II breast cancer: interim findings from NSABP Protocol B-09. In: Stoll BA (ed) Endocrine-related cancer. [Suppl] 17, p 51 ICI Pharmacent Div, Cheshire England
5. Greene GL, Nolan C, Engler JP, Jensen EV (1980) Monoclonal antibodies to human estrogen receptor. Proc Natl Acad Sci USA 77:5115–5119
6. Jensen EV (1970) The pattern of hormone receptor interaction. In: Some aspects of aetiology and biochemistry of prostatic cancer. Griffiths K, Pierrepoint CG (eds). 151–169, Alpha Omega Alpha, Cardiff, 1970
7. Jensen EV (1985) Immunochemical detection and measurement of estrogen receptors. In: Jonat W, Kaufmann M, Kubli F, Maass H (eds) Prätherapeutische Tumortestung. Zukschwerdt, Mūnich
8. Jonat W, Stegner HE, Maass H (1985) Immunhistochemische Bestimmung von Östrogenrezeptoren in Mammakarzinomgeweben mittels monoclonaler Antikörper. Erste Ergebnisse. Geburtshilfe Frauenheilkd. 45:473–476
9. Jonat W, Stegner HE, Maass H (1986) Immunohistochemical measurement of estrogen receptor in breast cancer tissue samples. Cancer Res 46:4296–4298
10. Kaufmann M, Kubli F, Caffier H, Jonat W, Maass H (1985) Adjuvante Chemo-Hormontherapie des Mammakarzinoms. Neue Ergebnisse zur Mortalität. Dtsch Med Wochenschr 110:1009–1010
11. Ludwig Breast Cancer Study Group (1984) Randomised trial of chemo-endocrine therapy, endocrine therapy, and mastectomy alone in postmenopausal patients with operable breast cancer and axillary node metastasis. Lancet 1:1256–1260
12. McCarty KS Jr., Miller L, Cox EB, Flowers JC, Budwit DA, Szabo E, Snowhite JC, et al. (1984) Clinical and histological correlation of estrogen receptor distribution as determined by immunohistochemistry using monoclonal antibody. Symposium: on Estrogen Receptor Determination with Monoclonal Antibodies, Monte Carlo
13. Mouridsen HT (1985) Review lecture: anti-hormones in primary breast cancer. Rev Endocrine Related Cancer [Suppl] 17:81 p 4
14. Pearson OH, Hubay CA, Gordon NH, Marshall JS, McGuire WL, et al. (1985) Eight-year follow up of adjuvant therapy for Stage II breast cancer. Rev Endocrine Related Cancer [Suppl 17] p 71
15. Pertschuk LP, Eisenberg KB, Carter AC, Feldmann JG (1985) Immunohistologic localization of estrogen receptors in breast cancer with monoclonal antibodies. Cancer 55:1513
16. Ribeiro G, Swindell R (1985) The Christie Hospital tamoxifen (Nolvadex) adjuvant trial for operable breast carcinoma – 7-yr results. Eur J Cancer Clin Oncol 21 (8):897–900
17. Rose C, Andersenn KW, Mouridsen HT, Thorpe SM, Pedersen BoV, Blichert-Toft M, Rasmussen B (1985) Beneficial effect of adjuvant tamoxifen therapy in primary breast cancer patients with high oestrogen receptor values. Lancet 1 pp 16–19
18. Stewart HJ, Prescott R (1985) Adjuvant tamoxifen therapy and receptor levels. Lancet 1:573
19. Stolzenbach G, Jonat W, Maass H, Strohmeier E, Trams G (1982) Relationship between estrogen receptor values and survival in patients with advanced breast cancer. In: Georgii (ed) Solide Tumoren und Metastasierung. Fischer, Stuttgart, p 214 (Verhandlungen der deutschen Krebs gesellschaft, vol 3)
20. Taylor SG, Olsen JE, Cummings FJ, Knuiman M (1985) Observation compared to adjuvant chemo-hormonotherapy in postmenopausal breast cancer: the ECOG trial. Proc Am Soc Clin Oncol 4:61
21. Tormey DC, Holland JF, Weinberg V, Weiss R, Falkson G, Glidewell O, Leone L, Perloff M (1983) 5 drugs vs 3 drug post operative chemotherapy for mammary carcinoma. In: Salmon SE, Jones SE (eds) Adjuvant therapy of cancer II. Grune and Stratton, New York, pp 377–384

Additional GABG Participants

M. Kaufmann, K.D. Buse, F. Kubli	Heidelberg
W. Jonat, H. Maass	Bremen/Hamburg
H. Caffier, K.H. Wulf	Würzburg
F. Melchert, R. Kreienberg, V. Friedberg	Mainz
J. Hilfrich	Hannover
M. Mahlke, P. Knapstein	Krefeld
U. Stosiek, K. Gumbrecht	Karlsruhe
K. Brunnert, P. Dördelmann	Karlsruhe
W. Kleine, A. Pfleiderer	Freiburg
H. Schorscher, D. Langnickel	Bremen
P. Hohlweg-Majert, P. Stoll	Mannheim
R. Stiglmayer, O. Fettig	Karlsruhe
H.F. Wander, G. Nagel	Göttingen

Complication Rates of Radiotherapy with Adjuvant Chemotherapy for Conservative Treatment

M. BAUER, D. VON FOURNIER, F. KUBLI, H. SCHMID, and R. SCHULZ-WENDTLAND

Introduction

Over the last 30 years, it has not been possible to bring about any decisive improvements in the prognosis of carcinoma of the breast with radical treatment methods, since by the time most women with breast cancer undergo primary treatment they are already suffering from systemic tumor disease that can no longer be controlled by locoregional therapy. FISHER et al. [12] and VERONESI et al. [35] have shown that the results of less radical, breast-conserving treatments are no worse than those of the conventional radical treatment as far as DFS and OAS are concerned; FISHER bases this conclusion on a follow-up period of 5 years, while VERONESI had followed his patients for 10 years. In both cases, this proved true even for patients in whom histological examination had revealed positive lymph nodes. Nonetheless, we feel that adjuvant chemotherapy is essential when positive lymph nodes are present, at least for premenopausal women [27]. This raises the question of the tolerance of a combination of radiotherapy and adjuvant chemotherapy, especially as experimental studies conducted by PHILLIPS et al. [28], REDPATH [31], and COLLINS and STEEL [10] have indicated that when radiotherapy is combined with chemotherapeutic regimens including cyclophosphamide and adriamycin the toxicity is synergistic.

In this paper, we compare the tolerance of the combined-modality therapy and of postoperative radiotherapy alone and the effectiveness of the combined-modality therapy and radical surgery with reference to patients treated at the University Hospital for Women in Heidelberg.

Patients, Treatment Regimens, Methods

Patients

From January 1975 to June 1986 a total of 426 women with carcinoma of the breast received primary organ-conserving treatment. Up to December 1985, 275 case histories were available for evaluation. A follow-up period of at least 12 months was

Abbreviations: AC, adriamycin + cyclophosphamide; AV, adriamycin + vincristine; CMF, cyclophosphamide + methotrexate + 5-fluorouracil; CMFP, cyclophosphamide + methotrexate + 5-fluorouracil + prednisolone; LF, leukeran + 5-fluorouracil; NSABP, National Surgical and Adjuvant Breast Project; DFS, disease-free survival; OAS, overall survival

Table 1. Features defining a "typical" conservative treatment of breast carcinoma

1.	Size of tumor up to 3 cm
2.	Segmental resection/quadrantal resection and axillary lymphadenectomy
3.	Dissection of eight or more axillary lymph nodes
4.	Radiotherapy of the residual breast + boost with 45-65 Gy
5.	Definitive operation and irradiation

set as the criterion for evaluability. There were 212 women who fulfilled the criteria of a "typical" treatment (Table 1). Their average age was 48 years, the average observation period, 38 months; 57 women (25%) had histologically confirmed positive lymph nodes, and 41 received adjuvant chemotherapy.

Treatment Regimens

The surgical intervention took the form of quadrantal or segmental resection of the primary tumor with relatively radical lymphadenectomy (an average of 17 lymph nodes being removed).

Percutaneous radiotherapy of opposing tangential fields was started 3 weeks after surgery. Cobalt-60 gamma-irradiation was used. A computer-assisted method based on three horizontal CT sections was used to plan radiotherapy (Fig. 1). Up to 1981 a dose of 60-65 Gy was administered, while since 1981 a dose of 50-55 Gy has been given, referred to the midplane of the residual breast. (The target mass comprises the whole of the breast, including the underlying chest wall and extending 1 cm into the lung; the reference point for determination of the dose is in

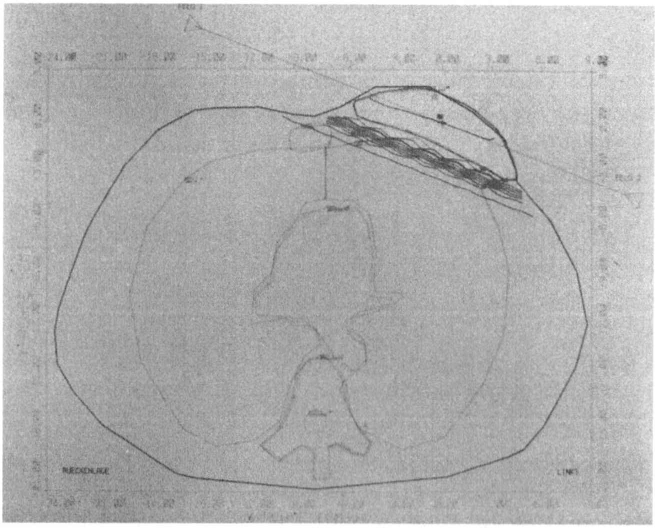

Fig. 1. Dose distribution over opposing tangential fields (relative isodoses as percentages) following conservative treatment of breast carcinoma

the middle of the breast about 2 cm below the skin.) In case of unfavorable histology (lymphangitis carcinomatosa, histologic grade III, surgical tumor margins not definitely known to be free or tumor invading the ducts with noninvasive ductal tumor parts) a boost dose of 5–10 Gy was given to the tumor bed. The total dose, including that to the tumor bed, now no longer exceeds 60 Gy. A weekly dose of 10 Gy is given in fractions of 2 Gy.

Adjuvant chemotherapy was administered to 28 premenopausal and 13 postmenopausal women shown by histologic examination to have positive lymph nodes. The chemotherapy was started as soon as possible after surgery, and in any case before the 12th postoperative day. After two or three treatment cycles followed by a treatment-free interval of 14 days the residual breast was irradiated; after a further 14-day treatment-free interval the chemotherapy was then completed. The chemotherapy regimens shown in Table 2 were used. In the event of poor local tolerance of the radiotherapy, poor general tolerance or bone marrow depression, the dose was reduced in the early years; since 1984 we have preferred to interpolate a longer chemotherapy interval.

Table 2. Adjuvant chemotherapy in conservative treatment of carcinoma of the breast

Drug	Dosage
LF regimen (Kaufmann et al. 1978)	
Leukeran	0.07 mg/kg b.w. p.o., days 1–14
5-Fluorouracil	10 mg/kg b.w. p.o., days 1, 8 and 15
	Repeated every 42 days
Modified CMF regimen (Bonadonna et al. 1977)	
Cyclophosphamide	500 mg/m² i.v., days 1 and 8
Methotrexate	40 mg/m² i.v., days 1 and 8
5-Fluorouracil	600 mg/m² i.v., days 1 and 8
	Repeated every 28 days
Modified AC regimen (Salmon and Jones 1975)	
Adriamycin	30 mg/m² i.v., day 1
Cyclophosphamide	300 mg/m² i.v., days 1 and 8
	Repeated every 21 days

Methods

To test the combined-modality treatment (surgery, irradiation of the residual breast, and adjuvant chemotherapy), women with positive nodes who underwent breast-conserving treatment were compared with patients who had undergone modified radical mastectomy. The extent of axillary lymphadenectomy performed was identical in the two groups. The groups being compared were matched for tumor stage, lymph node status (N_{1-3} $N \geqq 4$), age (± 3 years), date of operation (± 2 years) and estrogen receptor status (ER+, ER−). The mean age was 48 years

Table 3. Matched groups of node-positive patients treated with conservative and with radical therapies

Therapy	Matched pairs	
	Conservative therapy	Radical therapy
Patient group (*n*)	57	57
Mean age (years)	48	49
Mean observation period (months)	40	42
Adjuvant chemotherapy	41 (72%)	40 (70%)
CMF	26	18
AC	9	18
LF	6	4

in the conservative treatment group and 49 years in the radical treatment group, and the mean observation periods were 40 and 42 months respectively. Adjuvant chemotherapy had been administered in 72% of women in the conservative treatment group and in 70% of the women who had undergone modified radical mastectomy (Table 3).

The results were evaluated with reference to local recurrences, DFS and OAS. The rates take account of the KAPLAN and MEIER [21] estimation of error. The life-table analyses obtained were compared with the log-rank method of PETO et al. [26].

To test the local and general tolerance of the combination of radiotherapy and chemotherapy, women who had undergone conservative therapy with and without chemotherapy were separated into matched groups for comparison (Table 4). The criteria on which the patients were matched were tumor size (± 0.5 cm, max. 3 cm),

Table 4. Matched groups of women receiving conservative treatment with and without chemotherapy

	NO+R	NO+R+CH
Patients (*n*)	41	41
Mean age of patients at time of surgency (years)	45	46
Mean follow-up (months)	40	39
Radiation = 45 Gy	41	41
Radiation = 60 Gy	20	20

NO, nonradical operations; R, radiotherapy to the residual breast; CH, adjuvant chemotherapy age (± 3 years), date of surgery (± 3 years) and reference dose of irradiation (± 5 Gy). Local and general tolerance was tested with reference to the following points: (1) redness of the skin/telangiectasia; (2) hyperpigmentation; (3) palpably increased density of the breast tissue on clinical examination; (4) signs of fibrosis visualized by mammography; (5) pulmonary reaction to irradiation visualized by X-ray examination; (6) general subjective tolerance.

The basic examinations for purposes of comparison were conducted not less than 12–18 months after completion of the radiotherapy. The patients were examined and assessed separately by two experienced specialists. For assessment of the pulmonary reaction to radiotherapy a chest X-ray taken 6–12 months after the radiotherapy was compared with the X-ray findings before therapy by two radiologists with experience in roentgenological diagnostic procedures. The frequency of local and general subjective side effects of the combined-modality therapy and of the treatment with no adjuvant chemotherapy was compared with the aid of the χ^2 test [32]. A p value of less than 0.05 was considered to be significant.

Results

Comparison of the Effectiveness of Breast-Conserving Combination Treatment and Radical Therapy

Table 5 shows both the absolute and the relative frequencies of local recurrences, axillary recurrences, distant metastases, contralateral breast carcinomas and deaths in the matched groups compared. In addition, the patients who had died with local recurrences are listed. Figures 2, 3, and 4 allow a comparison of local recurrences, DFS and OAS in the matched groups of patients. The differences between the groups are not significant for local recurrences, DFS or OAS.

Table 5. Effectiveness of conservative and radical treatment of breast carcinoma in node-positive patients

	Matched pairs	
	Conservative treatment	Radical treatment
Patients (n)	57	57
Local recurrence	4 (7%)	4 (7%)
Axillary recurrence	2 (3.5%)	1 (1.8%)
Carcinoma of contralateral breast	3 (5.3%)	2 (3.5%)
Distant metastasis	8 (14%)	7 (12.3%)
Death	4 (7%)	5 (8.8%)
With local recurrence	1	2

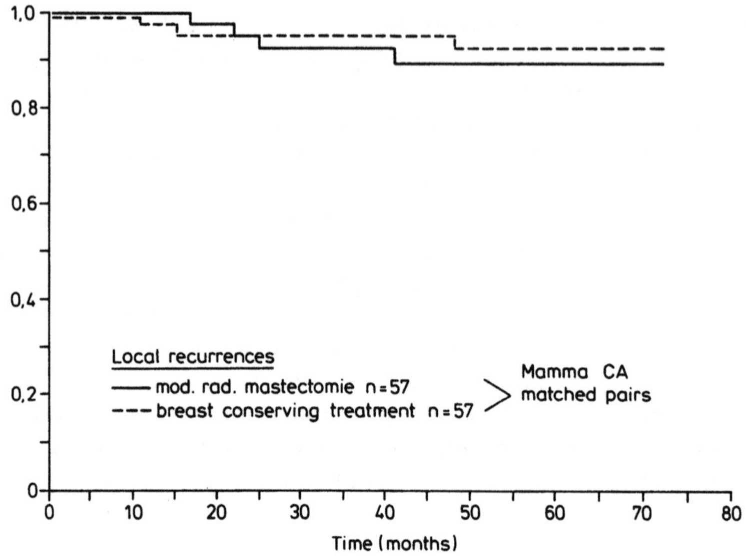

Fig. 2. Comparative incidence of local recurrences in the matched patient groups. The curves correspond to the error estimations of Kaplan and Meier; the life-table analyses obtained were compared by means of the log-rank method. No significant difference

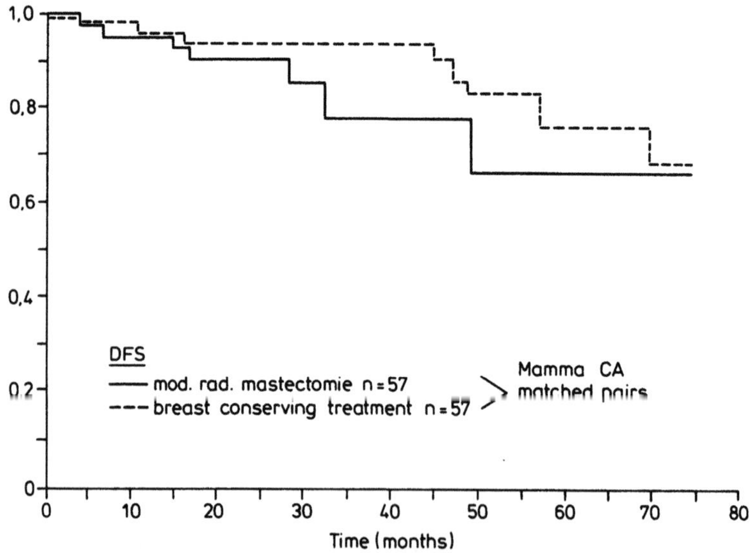

Fig. 3. Comparative DFS in the matched patient groups. The curves correspond to the error estimations of Kaplan and Meier; the life-table analyses obtained were compared by means of the log-rank method. No significant difference

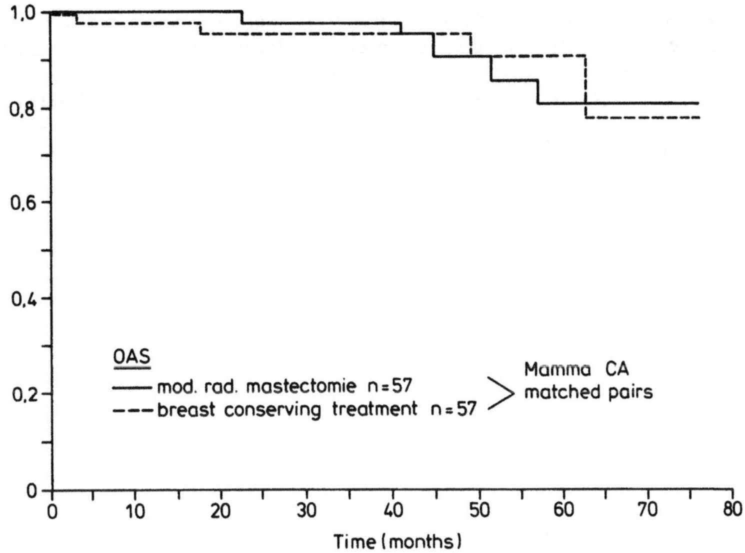

Fig. 4. Comparative OAS in the matched patient groups. The curves correspond to the error estimations of Kaplan and Meier; the life-table analyses were compared by means of the log-rank method. No significant difference

Local and General Tolerance of the Combined-Modality Treatment

Redness and telangiectasia of the skin (Table 6) were observed in 10 of the 41 patients (24%) who received no adjuvant chemotherapy. The frequency of cutaneous reactions was higher, with 30%, following a dose of over 60 Gy. Following combined-modality treatment the cutaneous changes were 5% or 10% more frequent overall. In view of the small numbers of patients this result is not significant, but there is a clearly recognizable tendency to more pronounced cutaneous reactions after combination treatment. An example of marked telangiectasia 4 years after the primary treatment is shown in Fig. 5.

Table 7 compares the occurrence of local cutaneous reactivity, taking the form of hyperpigmentation (Fig. 6), in the two groups. Hyperpigmentation was observed in 34% of cases without chemotherapy and in 41% with chemotherapy. These cutaneous changes increase clearly in frequency with increasing radiation dose (from 34% to 45% without chemotherapy and from 41% to 55% with chemotherapy). Here, too, is a tendency for the cutaneous changes to be more marked following the combination treatment (34% as against 41% and 45% as against 55% following a dose of over 60 Gy), but the difference is not statistically significant.

A clinically palpable increase in the density of the breast tissue (Table 8) was observed in 41% of patients who received no adjuvant chemotherapy and rather less frequently, in 36% of the patients, in the chemotherapy group. Following a dose of over 60 Gy this change was found in half the women in each group. Pronounced

Table 6. Redness of the skin/telangiectasia following combination treatment or postoperative radiotherapy alone after conservative treatment of breast carcinoma

	Doses (Gy)	*n*	Total	Discrete	Moderate	Marked
NO+R	≧45	41	24.4% (10)	14.6% (6)	7.3% (3)	2.4% (1)
	≧60	20	30.0% (6)	15.0% (3)	10.0% (2)	5.0% (1)
NO+R+CH	≧45	41	29.3% (12)	12.2% (5)	12.2% (5)	4.9% (2)
	≧60	20	40.0% (8)	20.0% (4)	15.0% (3)	5.0% (1)

Abbreviations: see Table 4

Table 7. Hyperpigmentation following combination treatment or postoperative radiotherapy alone after conservative treatment of breast carcinoma

	Dose (Gy)	*n*	Total	Discrete	Moderate	Marked
NO+R	≧45	41	34.1% (14)	14.6% (6)	14.6% (6)	4.9% (2)
	≧60	20	45.0% (9)	20.0% (4)	15.0% (3)	10.0% (2)
NO+R+CH	≧45	41	41.5% (17)	14.6% (6)	17.1% (7)	9.8% (4)
	≧60	20	55.0% (11)	25.0% (5)	20.0% (4)	10.0% (2)

Abbreviations: see Table 4

Table 8. Incidence of clinically palpable increase in density of breast tissue following combined radio- and chemotherapy after conservative treatment of breast carcinoma

	Dose (Gy)	*n*	Total	Discrete	Clear	Massive
NO+R	≧45	41	41.5% (17)	22.0% (9)	14.6% (6)	4.9% (2)
	≧60	20	50.0% (10)	25.0% (5)	20.0% (4)	5.0% (1)
NO+R+CH	≧45	41	36.6% (15)	12.2% (5)	17.1% (7)	7.3% (3)
	≧60	20	50.0% (10)	20.0% (4)	20.0% (4)	10.0% (2)

Abbreviations: see Table 4

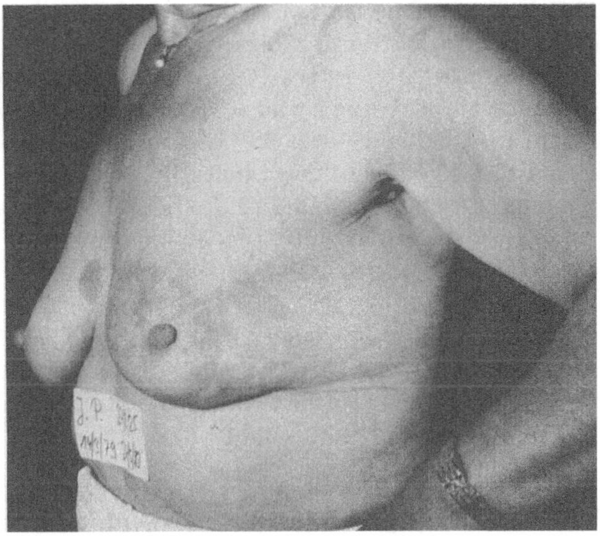

Fig. 5. Carcinoma of left breast: $T_1N_0M_0$. Quadrantal resection upper left, percutaneous radiotherapy to residual breast with 65 Gy + 5 Gy boost dose to tumor bed. Pronounced telangiectasia 4 years after primary treatment

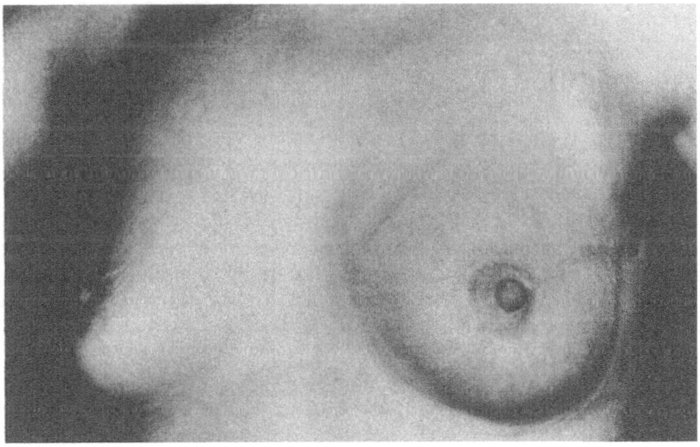

Fig. 6. Carcinoma of left breast: $T_1N_+M_0$. Segmental resection upper left, percutaneous radiotherapy to residual breast with 60 Gy + 10 Gy boost dose to tumor bed. Hyperpigmentation 5 years after primary treatment

fibrotic changes detectable on clinical examination were observed in less than 10%. Fibrocystic disease recognizable by mammography (Table 9) is more common than a clinically palpable increase in density, being found in 51% of cases with chemotherapy and in 54% with adjuvant chemotherapy, and 55% of cases in both groups with a dose of over 60 Gy. Pronounced fibrotic changes visualized by mammography are also rare (under 1%). There was no difference between the combined treatment group and the radiation only group. Figure 7 shows the pronounced fibrosis visualized by mammography of the left breast after organ conservation in comparison with the nontreated breast 1 year after primary treatment.

Table 10 displays the changes in the lung (Fig. 8) on X-ray examination (reaction to radiation), without chemotherapy. Fibrosis of the ipsilateral lung segments peripherally irradiated in the ventral and ventrolateral parts was observed in barely

Table 9. Incidence of fibrosis of the breast visualized by mammography following combined radio- and chemotherapy after conservative treatment of breast carcinoma

	Dose (Gy)	*n*	Total	Discrete	Clear	Massive
NO+R	≧45	41	51.2% (21)	24.4% (10)	22.0% (9)	4.9% (2)
	≧60	20	55.0% (11)	25.0% (5)	20.0% (4)	10.0% (2)
NO+R+CH	≧45	41	53.7% (22)	26.8% (11)	17.1% (7)	9.8% (4)
	≧60	20	55.0% (11)	20.0% (4)	25.0% (5)	10.0% (2)

Abbreviations: see Table 4

Table 10. Incidence of pulmonary changes observed on X-ray examination following combined radio- and chemotherapy after conservative treatment of breast carcinoma

	Dose (Gy)	*n*	Total	Fibrosis Discrete	Marked
NO+R	≧45	41	9.8% (4)	9.8% (4)	–
	≧60	20	10.0% (2)	10.0% (2)	–
NO+R+CH	≧45	41	22.0% (9)	17.1% (7)	4.9% (2)
	≧60	20	30.0% (6)	20.0% (4)	10.0% (2)

Abbreviations: see Table 4

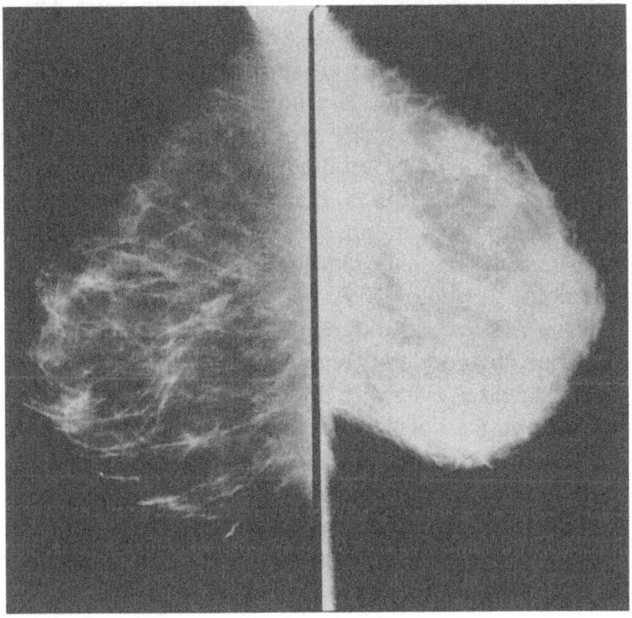

Fig. 7. Mammography of both breasts at follow-up examination 1 year after conservative treatment of carcinoma of left breast: $T_1N_0M_0$. Percutaneous radiotherapy to residual breast with 55 Gy. Clearly visible fibrotic changes in left breast

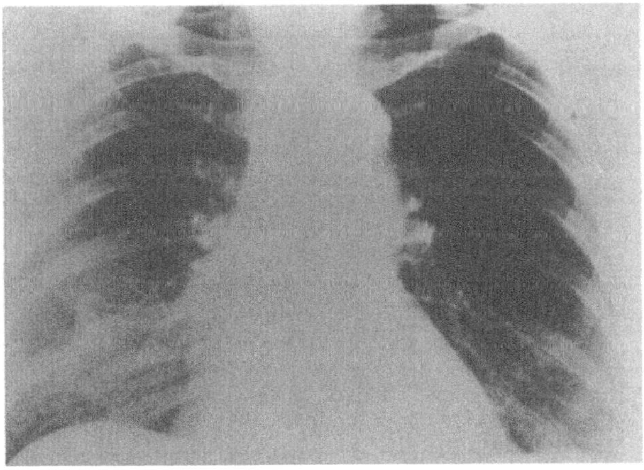

Fig. 8. Carcinoma of right breast: $T_1N_+M_0$. Adjuvant chemotherapy (2×CMF), percutaneous radiotherapy to residual breast with 55 Gy, chemotherapy (4×CMF). Chest X-ray on follow-up after 12 months: pronounced fibrotic changes in right breast

10%; in all cases this was clinically asymptomatic. The relative proportion was no higher following a dose of over 60 Gy. In the case of the combined-modality treatment, however, we were surprised to find that the X-ray examination revealed an irradiation reaction in nine of the 41 patients, or 22%. In this group, too, the reactions were clinically asymptomatic, but in contrast to the postoperative radiotherapy only group, there were two women in whom the fibrosis was very pronounced. In addition, the incidence of roentgenological pulmonary changes was higher in the combined treatment group with 30%, following a dose of over 60 Gy. Both the patients who had pronounced reactions to radiation had received chemotherapy with CMF.

There were clear differences in subjective general tolerance between the two adjuvant chemotherapy regimens (Table 11). The radiotherapy was well tolerated in 90% of cases, even with doses of over 60 Gy. Tolerance of the radiotherapy was never poor (Karnofsky index below 70%) in any case. Only six of 41 patients showed good tolerance of the adjuvant chemotherapy (Karnofsky index 90%–100%). This treatment was poorly tolerated in 51%, tolerance of both chemotherapy regimens, CMF and AC, being approximately equally poor (61.5% and 55.5% respectively). Chlorambucil and 5-fluorouracil were clearly better tolerated; none of the six patients had a Karnofsky index lower than 80%.

Table 11. Subjective general tolerance of adjuvant chemotherapy regimens following conservative treatment of breast carcinoma

Tolerance	Good	Moderate	Poor
Karnofsky index	90%–100%	80%	≦ 70%
Radiotherapy ($n=41$)	90.3% (37)	9.7% (4)	–
Chemotherapy ($n=41$)	17.1% (6)	31.7% (14)	51.2% (21)
LF ($n=6$)	50.0% (3)	50.0% (3)	–
CMF ($n=26$)	7.7% (2)	30.8% (8)	61.5% (16)
AC ($n=9$)	11.1% (1)	33.3% (3)	55.5% (5)

Discussion

Following a mean observation period of 40 months, there was no significant difference between the matched groups (organ conservation vs radical treatment, N+) in our own patient sample in frequency of locoregional recurrences, axillary recurrences or contralateral breast carcinoma, DFS or OAS.

HAYWARD [17] and ATKINS et al. [3] report a significantly higher rate of locoregional recurrences in clinically node-positive breast cancer patients treated by conservative methods (wide excision and radiation of the residual breast with lymph drainage regions) than in node-positive women who have undergone radical treatment (radical mastectomy with radiotherapy excluding the lymph drainage regions). The follow-up period for these patients was between 11 and 21 years. It should be remarked at this point that the conservative treatment did not include axillary lymphadenectomy, so that no information on histologic lymph node status was available. In addition, the radiotherapy to the residual breast, with 38 Gy, and to the untreated axilla, with 30 Gy, was underdosed and the radiation technique was also not comparable to the more modern methods in use today. This explains the high incidence of axillary recurrences observed (21%). The difference in distant metastasization was not significant, and the OAS was better in patients who had undergone radical treatment ($p \leqq 0.05$).

FISHER et al. [12] observed 1843 patients with breast cancer in the NSABP study who were randomized to organ conservation (segmental resection and axillary dissection) with and without radiotherapy to the residual breast (groups SM and SM + RTX) or total mastectomy with axillary dissection (group TM). These women had tumors up to 4 cm in size, and the histologic lymph node status was disregarded. The average observation period was 39 months. Women known to have positive lymph nodes received adjuvant chemotherapy (melphalan and 5-fluorouracil). The 5-year life-table analyses yielded no differences between groups TM and SM in DFS and OAS. The DFS obtained in group SM + RTX was significantly better than that achieved in group TM ($p=0.04$) or group SM ($p=0.02$). This trend can still be recognized when the patients are broken down into node-positive and node-negative groups. FISHER et al. [12] observed recurrences in the residual breast following conservative treatments with radiotherapy of the residual breast in 27.9% of cases, as against 7.7% following conservative treatment with radiotherapy. This highly significantly ($p< 0.001$) better result in the patients who received adjuvant radiotherapy is even more pronounced in node-positive women.

VERONESI et al. [35] report on a randomized study including 701 patients with tumors up to 2 cm in size. In this study organ conservation (quadrantal resection plus axillary dissection and radiotherapy of the residual breast) was compared with radical treatment in the form of HALSTED's operation. Women with positive nodes also received adjuvant chemotherapy (CMF) as a matter of policy. The observation period was between 3 and 10 years. Life-table analyses revealed that OAS was the same in both groups, DFS was slightly better in the conservative treatment group and the local recurrence rate was the same in both groups. The differences are still not significant if they are divided for node-negative and node-positive women.

Comparison of VERONESI's and FISHER's studies with our own results allows us to say, at least, that DFS and OAS are no worse in any of these studies after conservative treatment with radiotherapy to the residual breast than after radical treatment. According to FISHER's study, only more local recurrences must be expected if the recurrences in the residual breast are also taken into account. FISHER suggests that a recurrence in the residual breast which can be operated upon cannot necessarily be compared with a recurrence in the chest wall after radical treatment, since in this case a radical secondary ablation still leads to good long-term results [16]. HAYWARD's study does not seem so important, because the operative technique used (without axillary dissection) and the irradiation technique are inadequate by modern standards.

In our own patients we observed more local cutaneous reactions following the combination of radiotherapy and adjuvant chemotherapy (redness and telangiectasia in 29.3% as against 24.4%, hyperpigmentation in 41.5% as against 34.1%). These observations are confirmed by the studies of BOTNICK et al. [8] and DANOFF et al. [11]. BOTNICK et al. [8] began radiotherapy and adjuvant chemotherapy (CMF) simultaneously about 2 weeks after surgery and avoided dose reductions whenever possible. The volume of tissue irradiated was greater than in our hospital in Heidelberg, since in addition to irradiation of the residual breast, the supra-infraclavicular, axillary and parasternal lymph drainage regions were irradiated with doses of 45–50 Gy. BOTNICK observed increased cutaneous toxicity in 80.6% of the patients, in some cases taking the form of weeping epitheliolysis. DANOFF et al. [11] report increased cutaneous toxicity with deterioration of the cosmetic result, but without the fatal combination effects observed by BOTNICK. This study also involved additional irradiation of the lymph drainage regions, but the chemotherapy with CMFP initiated in parallel to the radiotherapy was reduced to CF for the duration of the irradiation. In addition, the doses of chemotherapeutic preparations were reduced to 50% as soon as incipient leukopenia was observed. RAY et al. [30] and BEADLE et al. [4] also report increased cutaneous reactions and cosmetic detriment with additional adjuvant chemotherapy. The changes described in the last studies cited are not serious, and they weigh about as heavily in the overall quality of the result as the cutaneous reactions observed in our own patients. Other authors [1,5,12,25] report no increased local cutaneous reactions.

The frequency of a clinically palpable increase in the density of the breast tissue was no greater after combination treatment in our own patients (clinical fibrosis in 36.6%, as against 41.5% without chemotherapy). This is true for radiation doses both over and under 60 Gy. The increased density seems to depend exclusively on an increased irradiation dose. This is in agreement with the data of PIERQUIN [29] and KURTZ et al. [24]. Roentgenologically apparent fibrotic change or increased density of the breast tissue was more common and more pronounced in our own patients than was clinically palpable fibrosis, but X-ray examination also revealed no significant difference or any tendency for fibrosis to be more frequent following combination treatment (54% after combination treatment as against 51% without chemotherapy). Thus, our results do not confirm the data of RAY et al. [30], who reported clinical fibrotic changes of the breast in 8% of cases after postoperative radiotherapy alone, as against 22% following irradiation and chemotherapy. This low percentage could result from different, subjectively selected grading criteria.

Following surgery and irradiation by means of the technique described, two opposing tangential fields being irradiated with cobalt-60 gamma rays, clinically asymptomatic, discrete irradiation fibrosis of the lung was observed on X-ray examination in a bare 10% of cases. With adjuvant chemotherapy in addition, the frequency was 22%, and the fibrosis was clearly pronounced in 5%, though all cases were clinically asymptomatic. BOTNICK et al. [8] also reported increased pulmonary toxicity, which was even clinically symptomatic (cough and fever) in 9% of cases. ALLEN et al. [1] found a raised incidence of roentgenologically confirmed asymptomatic pulmonary fibrosis after combination treatment. The adjuvant chemotherapy comprised adriamycin + endoxan.

With reference to the pathogenesis the reader is referred to the experimental studies of PHILLIPS et al. [28], REDPATH [31], and COLLINS and STEEL [10]; we must assume that chemotherapy regimens including cyclophosphamide and adriamycin potentiate the pulmonary toxicity of radiation when a combined-modality treatment with radiotherapy is used. One factor that should not be underestimated in this is the treatment regimen: with sequential treatment, as in our patients, the trauma resulting from the combination could be relatively slight, while more intense reactions must be expected with simultaneous administration of both treatment modalities [2,8]. The interval after chemotherapy and before the start of radiotherapy should be 14 days when adriamycin is given, in any case at least 1 week, since the long biological half-life [22] means that radiosensitizing doses must still be expected to be present in the tissues after up to 14 days [14]. In 91% of the patients who underwent conservative treatment, the radiotherapy was tolerated well or very well (Karnofsky index 90%–100%). In contrast to this, tolerance of the adjuvant chemotherapy was poor (Karnofsky index less than 70%) in 55%–62% of cases when CMF or AC was used.

There is still no uniform opinion about the best relative timing of radiotherapy and adjuvant chemotherapy for combined-modality treatment of carcinoma of the breast. The data relating to the possible necessity for reducing the doses of chemotherapeutic agents, which can put the effectiveness of treatment in question [6,18,34], vary considerably. ALLEN et al. [1] reported that in the case of a sequential combination treatment with AC and radiotherapy it was necessary to reduce the doses in over 29% of cases, mainly because of leukopenia and occasionally because of hyperemesis. LICHTER et al. [25] indicated increased local reactions necessitating dose reduction with sequential combination treatment including AV chemotherapy (in 27% of cases, as against 12% without radiotherapy). LICHTER draws attention to a practically equivalent neutrophil titer in both groups, while the lymphocyte counts were clearly lowered in the group of patients who received radiotherapy. This has also been confirmed by our own investigations [19]. LICHTER suggests that the neutrophil count should be used for clinical application, since then dose reduction would not so often be necessary. In the NSABP study [12] the combination treatment was carried out in a sequential manner. Increased toxicity was not observed with the combination treatment. BONADONNA et al. [5] report on the simultaneous use of both adjuvant treatment modalities; in the radiotherapy group thrombopenia was observed more frequently, but seldom necessitated dose reduction. GLICK et al. [13] reported slight bone marrow toxicity following CMF chemotherapy with or without radiotherapy. In this study methotrexate was omitted from the CMF regimen in the first two chemotherapy cycles at the time of radiation. BOTNICK et al. [8], who, as already mentioned, preferred simultaneous administration of both modalities, reported increased cutaneous and increased pulmonary toxicity, though with extensive irradiation volumes. In clinical practice, this has meant that BOTNICK now administers only two cycles of chemotherapy during the radiotherapy, as opposed to four.

Concerning the treatment regimen in node-positive women, with reference to adjuvant chemotherapy, we prefer to give preference to systemic adjuvant chemotherapy, since the patient's fate is decided by whether or not distant metastases are present. With this in mind, chemotherapy should be started before the 12th postoperative day at the full doses [5]. This is also in keeping with the model of GOLDIE and COLDMAN [15], according to whose hypothesis an increased number of primarily chemotherapy-resistant cells must also be expected as the number of tumor cells increases. This is similar to the mutation theory for bacteria. Once three cycles of adjuvant chemotherapy have been administered the radiotherapy should be given–especially as it has still not been shown scientifically whether three cycles of adjuvant chemotherapy really are effective as part of an adjuvant treatment [7,9,20]. Delaying percutaneous irradiation while giving adjuvant chemotherapy can be justified by saying that a local treatment effect is also expected of the adjuvant chemotherapy.

The present study has led us to adopt the following attitude to combination treatment with radiotherapy and chemotherapy for conservative treatment of carcinoma of the breast: There are no apparent differences in the effectiveness between the combination treatment and radical therapy; it must be borne in mind that the observation period is still short, with an average of 41 months, and the number of patients is small ($n=57$). The local tolerance of the combination treatment tends to be worse (redness of the skin, telangiectasia, hyperpigmentation), but there is no difference in clinically palpable increased density of the breast tissue or fibrosis visualized by mammography. The pulmonary irradiation reactions seen on X-ray pictures are not significant, but the absolute figures for incidence show clear differences to the detriment of the combination treatment.

Despite local side effects of the breast-conserving combination therapy, just over 90% of these women are satisfied with the cosmetic result of the treatment (Fig. 9).

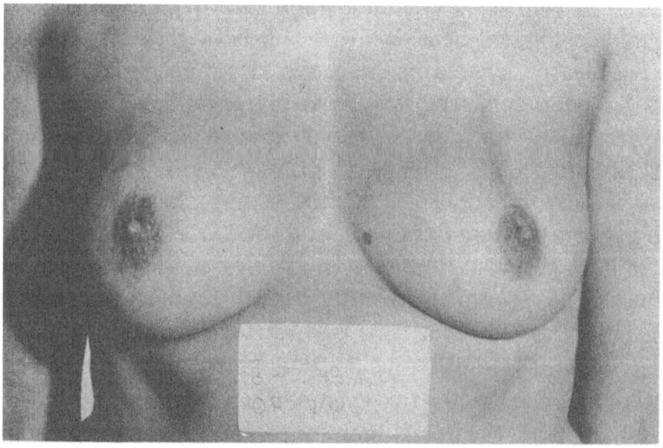

Fig. 9. Carcinoma of left breast: $T_2N_0M_0$. Upper inner quadrantal resection and axillary dissection, percutaneous radiotherapy to residual breast with 55 Gy. Good cosmetic result despite unfortunate tumor site

References

1. Allen H, et al. (1981) Adjuvant treatment for stage II (node positive) breast cancer with adriamycin-cyclophosphamide (AC) + radiotherapy (XRT). In: Salmon SE, Jones SE (eds) Adjuvant therapy of cancer III. Grune and Stratton, New York, pp 453–462
2. Aristizabal SA, et al. (1979) Combined radiation-adriamycin effects on human skin. Front Radiat Ther Oncol 13:103–112
3. Atkins H, Hayward JL, Klugman BL, Wayte AB (1972) Treatment of early breast cancer: a report after ten years of a clinical trial. Br Med J 2:423–429
4. Beadle GF, et al. (1984) The effect of adjuvant chemotherapy on the cosmetic results after primary radiation treatment of early stage breast cancer. Int J Radiat Oncol Biol Phys 10:2131–2137
5. Bonadonna G, Valagussa P (1983) Chemotherapy of breast cancer: Current views and results. Int J Radiat Oncol Biol Phys 9:279–297
6. Bonadonna G, et al. (1977) The CMF program for operable breast cancer with positive axillary nodes. Updated analysis on the disease-free interval, site of relapse and drug tolerance. Cancer 39:2904–2915
7. Bonadonna G, et al. (1983) Feasibility of adjuvant chemotherapy plus radiotherapy in operable breast cancer. In: Harris RJ, Hellman S, Silen W (eds) Conservative management of breast cancer. Lippincott, Philadelphia, pp 329–336
8. Botnick LE, et al. (1983) Primary breast irradiation and concomitant adjuvant chemotherapy. In: Harris RJ, Hellman S, Silen W (eds) Conservative management of breast cancer. Lippincott, Philadelphia, pp 321–328
9. Cavalli F (1983) Die adjuvante Chemotherapie beim Mamma-Karzinom: Ist eine Schlußbeurteilung schon möglich? In: Kubli F, Nagel GA, Kadach U, Kaufmann M (eds) Neue Wege in der Brustkrebsbehandlung. Zuckschwerdt, München, pp 168–178
10. Collins CH, Steel GG (1983) Lung damage in mice from cyclophosphamide and thoracic irradiation: the effect of timing. Int J Radiat Oncol Biol Phys 9:685–689
11. Danoff BF, et al. (1983) The effect of adjuvant chemotherapy on cosmetic and complications in patients with breast cancer treated by definitive irradiation. Int J Radiat Oncol Biol Phys 9:1625–1630
12. Fisher B, et al. (1985) Five-year results of a randomized clinical trial comparing total mastectomy and segmental mastectomy with or without radiation in the treatment of breast cancer. N Engl J Med 312:665–673
13. Glick JH, et al. (1983) Adjuvant chemotherapy in patients undergoing definitive irradiation for primary breast cancer. The University of Pennsylvania experience In: Harris RJ, Hellman S, Silen W (eds) Conservative management of breast cancer. Lippincott, Philadelphia, pp 311–320
14. Göhde W, et al. (1975) Synchronisation von Tumorzellen durch Adriamycin – Möglichkeiten der Kombinationstherapie. In: Ghione M, Fetzer G, Maier H (eds) Ergebnisse der Adriamycin-Therapie. Adriamycin Symposium Frankfurt/Main 1974. Springer, Berlin Heidelberg New York, pp 14–23
15. Goldie JH, Coldman AJ (1979) A mathematical model for relating the drug sensitivity of tumor to their spontaneous mutation rate. Cancer Treat Rep 63:1727–1733
16. Harris JR, Hellman S (1983) The results of primary radiation therapy for early breast cancer at the Joint Center for Radiation Therapy. In: Harris JR, Hellman S, Silen W (eds) Conservative management of breast cancer. Lippincott, Philadelphia, pp 47–52
17. Hayward JL (1983) The Guy's Hospital trial on breast conservation. In: Harris JR, Hellman S, Silen W (eds) Conservative management of breast cancer. New surgical and radiotherapeutic techniques. Lippincott, Philadelphia, pp 77–90
18. Holland JF, et al. (1980) Adverse effect of radiotherapy on adjuvant chemotherapy for carcinoma of the breast. Surg Gynecol Obstet 150: 817–821
19. Job G, et al. (1984) The influence of radiation therapy on T-Lymphocyte subpopulations defined by monoclonal antibodies. Int J Radiat Biol Phys 10:1–5
20. Jungi WF, et al. (1981) Short- or long-term adjuvant chemotherapy for breast cancer. In: Salmon SE, Jones SE (eds) Adjuvant therapy of cancer III. Grune and Stratton, New York, pp 395–402

21. Kaplan EL, Meier P (1958) Non-parametric estimation from incomplete observation. J Am Stat Assoc 53:457–482
22. Kaufman SD, Weitzman S (1980) The clinical pharmacology of anticancer drugs. In: Sokol GH, Maickel RP (eds) Radiation-drug interactions in the treatment of cancer. Wiley, New York, pp 63–77
23. Kaufmann M, et al. (1978) Zur adjuvanten (prophylaktischen) postoperativen Chemotherapie beim Mammakarzinom. Dtsch Med Wochenschr 103:1881–1887
24. Kurtz JM, et al. (1984) Radiation therapy after breast-conserving surgery for stage I and II mammary carcinoma. Results of the Marseille experience 1961–1976. Strahlentherapie 160:239–243
25. Lichter AS, et al. (1983) Adjuvant chemotherapy in patients treated primarily with irradiation for localized breast cancer. In: Harris RJ, Hellman S, Silen W (eds) Conservative management of breast cancer. Lippincott, Philadelphia, pp 299–310
26. Peto R, et al. (1977) Design and analysis of randomized clinical trials requiring prolonged observation of each patient. II. Analysis and examples. Br J Cancer 35:1–39
27. Peto R, et al. (1985) Adjuvante Hormon- und Chemotherapie beim Mammakarzinom. Bericht über das 4. Consensus-Treffen zum Thema "Mammakarzinom" am National Institute of Health, Washington D.C. Dtsch Arztebl 83:32–34
28. Phillips TL, et al. (1975) Modification of radiation injury to normal tissues by chemotherapeutic agents. Cancer 35:1678–1684
29. Pierquin B (1985) Conservative treatment of breast cancer: experience at the Mondor Hospital, Créteil. In: Zander J, Baltzer J (eds) Early breast cancer: histopathology, diagnosis and treatment. Springer, Berlin Heidelberg New York, pp 276–284.
30. Ray GR, et al. (1984) Impact of adjuvant chemotherapy on cosmetic and complications in stages I and II. Carcinoma of the breast treated by biopsy and radiation therapy. Int J Radiat Oncol Biol Phys 10:837–841
31. Redpath JL (1978) The effect of adriamycin on radiation damage to mouse lung and skin. Int J Radiat Oncol Biol Phys 4:229–232
32. Sachs L (1974) Angewandte Statistik. Planung und Auswertung, Methode und Modelle. Springer, Berlin Heidelberg New York, pp 357–366
33. Salmon SE, Jones SE (1975) Studies of the combination of adriamycin and cyclophosphamide (alone or with other agents) for the treatment of breast cancer. Oncology 36:40–47
34. Stjernswärd J (1977) Can survival be decreased by postoperative irradiation? Int Radiat Oncol Biol Phys 2:1171–1175
35. Veronesi U, et al. (1983) Results of quadrantectomy, axillary dissection and radiotherapy (QUART) in T_1N_0 patients. In: Harris RJ, Hellman S, Silen W (eds) Conservative management of breast cancer. Lippincott, Philadelphia pp 91–99

VIII. Strategies for the Prevention of Invasive Breast Cancer: Treatment of Mastopathic, Precancerous and Non-Invasive Lesions

Diagnosis and Classification of Benign Breast Diseases (Mastopathy)

H. JUNKERMANN, D. VON FOURNIER, E. WEBER, and B. ARABIN

Benign breast diseases originating from proliferation of epithelial and connective tissue (mastopathy) will be discussed in this chapter. Inflammatory lesions will not be included.

Clinical Classification

From a clinical point of view a classification of mastopathic benign breast disorders according to the following symptoms and their severity seems advisable:

- Cyclical pronounced mastodynia
- Diffuse or localized nodules
- Pathological secretion

Often these symptoms are combined. Their intensity is usually dependent on the phase of the menstrual cycle, with the peak shortly before menstrual flow begins.

Mastodynia

The hormone-dependent cyclical pronounced mastodynia is by far the most frequent form. It is important to discriminate this condition from other forms of mastodynia (Table 1). Non-cyclical mastodynia may result from inflammatory disorders or localized thrombophlebitis (MONDOR's syndrome), may follow surgery or other trauma or may be the first sign of a mammary carcinoma [18]. Patients may refer to pain originating from the chest or the chest wall as breast pain. Often the cause of non-cyclical mastodynia cannot be found. The reason why it is important to discriminate cyclical mastodynia from non-cyclical mastodynia and pain not originating from the breast itself is that only cyclical mastodynia is amenable to hormonal measures.

Nodules

The painful nodular breast is the typical clinical picture of mastopathy. As well as cases of mastodynia of the cyclical variety without significant nodularity, there are also nodular breasts without mastodynia. Nodules may pose great problems to both

Table 1. Mastodynia and non-breast pain

Syndrome	Origin
Cyclical or cyclically pronounced mastodynia	In the scar after surgery
Hormonal	Traumatic (hematoma, fat necrosis)
Non-cyclical mastodynia	Chronic inflammation (periductal mastitis)
	Mammary carcinoma
	Mondor's disease
	Idiopathic
Pain originating from chest or chest wall	Tietze syndrome
	Cardiac pain
	Pleural pain
	Intercostal neuralgia

Modified from [16]

physician and patient. While after the appropriate clinical evaluation patients with breast pain can in most cases be assured of the benign nature of the condition, uncertainty may remain when the patient presents with increased nodularity. Though clinical investigation can give important hints as to the benign or malignant nature of the nodules, paraclinical methods should be employed to make the diagnosis as sure as possible. While it is good policy to excise every isolated nodule except a cyst, which can be aspirated, this procedure is not possible in cases of severe nodularity with multiple nodules. In certain very severe cases even prophylactic subcutaneous mastectomy may be a reasonable procedure for diagnosis and treatment.

Pathological Secretion

In cases of pathological secretion a thorough clinical evaluation is necessary in order to decide the diagnostic steps to be taken. Bilateral, milky secretion from several ducts may be a symptom of a generalized hormonal disorder and the blood prolactin level should be determined. In cases involving one duct system only, often with serous or bloody secretion, a morphological lesion in this duct system must be suspected and radiological localization and histopathological diagnosis must be pursued.

The main concern of most patients with benign breast disease is whether they have cancer or whether they are cancer prone. Patients with benign breast disease and pronounced objective breast alterations, especially in conjunction with a family history, seem to have an elevated risk for the development of invasive cancer. We therefore find useful a classification of mastopathy (Table 2) which is based on the results of clinical evaluation as well as paraclinical methods [10].

It is useful to discriminate between those cases where subjective complaints, like pain and tenderness, are conspicuous with little or no objective change, and those case where objective changes like nodularity and pathological secretion are the

Table 2. Clinical and paraclinical classification of mastopathy

Mild mastopathy	Severe mastopathy
– Slight radiological dysplasia (Fig. 1) – Slight induration or nodularity with no evidence of proliferative changes, premenstrual engorgement – Premenstrually abnormal thermography – Premenstrual mastodynia	– Pronounced radiological dysplasia, often with diffuse microcalcifications (Fig. 2) – Pronounced induration or nodularity which impairs clinical assessment – Abnormal thermography throughout the cycle – Mastodynia throughout the cycle, usually more pronounced before menstruation

Fig. 1. Slight radiological dysplasia

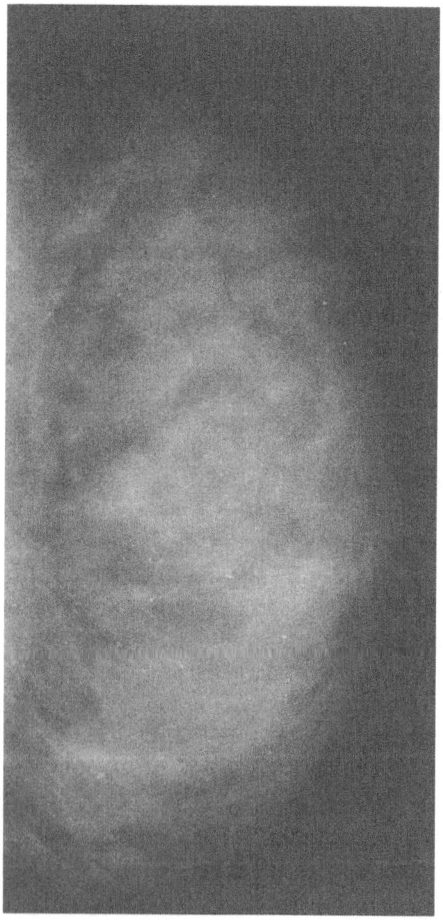

Fig. 2. Severe radiological dysplasia with diffuse microcalcifications

main manifestation. While in the first case adequate information of the patient about the benign nature of the complaint is often sufficient, the second group may be problematic from the diagnostic as well as from the therapeutic point of view.

Mastodynia shows only a very loose correlation with objective changes [7]. Patients with severe objective changes may not complain at all about mastodynia. Those patients,however, who have severe pain for a substantial part of the cycle usually also show objective changes.

Classification According to Morphological Criteria

The pathomorphological basis of benign breast diseases comprises progressive and regressive changes of the different tissues constituting the breast. The development of a uniformly accepted classification has been hampered by the fact that several pathomorphological entities may coexist in the same breast specimen. Most authors today find useful a classification which is based on the presence and degree of intraductal proliferations. BÄSSLER [2], referring to PRECHTEL [17], described three groups of *mastopathy* based on the degree of intraductal proliferation which correlate with the risk for developing subsequent invasive carcinoma (Table 3).

Table 3. Histopathological classification of mastopathy according to cancer risk

Grade	Histology	Risk Factor
I	Without intraductal proliferations	0.86
II	Intraductal proliferations without atypia	2.43
III	Intraductal proliferations with cellular atypia	5–11

Data from [2,4,17]

According to [BÄSSLER] cases of painful breasts without the full picture of mastopathy are classified as *mastodynia*. These are cases where only an exaggeration of the normal hormone-dependent cyclical response of the breast is found. In *mazoplasia* a localized induration of breast tissue with abnormal differentiation of the glandular tissue is found. Rarer forms of benign breast disease are *fibrosis*, a sequel of abnormal proliferation of the collagenous tissue of the breast, and *sclerosing adenosis*, which is produced by proliferation of the myoepithelial cells. Sclerosing adenosis may form a tumor or, more often, it can be found in a multilocular diffuse form as an element of mastopathy. Some cases of sclerosing adenosis are difficult to differentiate from carcinoma, especially in frozen sections. MEYER (1957) reported from Basel about 61 women between 25 and 35 years of age who had been treated for mammary carcinoma. In 12 of these cases the diagnosis had to be revised retrospectively as these women actually had sclerosing adenosis only.

Papillary tumors, if centrally located, are usually detected after the finding of bloody or serous secretion from the mammary duct system. It is controversial whether or not intraductal papilloma predisposes to subsequent invasive carcinoma [2,8]. Papillary cyst adenomas or multiple papillomas are found in mastopathy.

Fibroadenoma is a separate entity of usually solitary tumors which consist of abnormally proliferated mesenchymal and epithelial elements of the breast. Multiple fibroadenoma may be present, however, in certain cases of mastopathy. Fibroadenoma usually does not predispose to the development of carcinoma. Fibroadenoma in older women, however, may show increased proliferation of the epithelial component and in such cases may represent the origin of an invasive carcinoma.

Classification on the Basis of Paraclinical Methods: Sonography, Thermography, Mammography

Sonography

Paraclinical methods allow us a further discrimination of benign breast diseases. Sonography, in recent years, has become a valuable adjunctive method in the diagnosis of benign breast diseases for its power to differentiate gross cystic disease from microcystic or non-cystic forms of mastopathy (Fig. 3). It is possible to visualize macrocysts bigger than 3-5 mm in diameter [22]. Isolated palpable tumors and mammographically discernible lesions can be aspirated after sonographic verification of their cystic nature – if necessary under direct sonographic guidance. Thus the tumor is removed and its cystic nature is ascertained. According to HAAGENSEN et al. [9] clinically symptomatic gross cystic disease carries an approximately threefold cancer risk. It is not known whether this is also true for sonographically detected asymptomatic gross cystic disease. Others question the relation between cyst size and cancer risk [2]. Until now there have been no attempts to define sonographic risk categories. At present it is not possible to detect minimal cancers routinely in the screening situation using ultrasound.

Thermography

Thermography has been not proven useful for the detection of minimal cancers in screening programs. Claims of the prospective value of thermography for the detection of risk groups [6] were not substantiated by other studies [14,23]. The value of thermography for the detection of cancer risk in unselected patient groups cannot be determined definitely on the basis of published data [19].

Mammography

Mammography is the most important method for differentiation between benign and malignant breast lesions. Using modern equipment the sensitivity of this method in symptomatic women is about 90% [5]. In severe cases of mastopathy, however, mammography is of less value. Though it is possible to discriminate

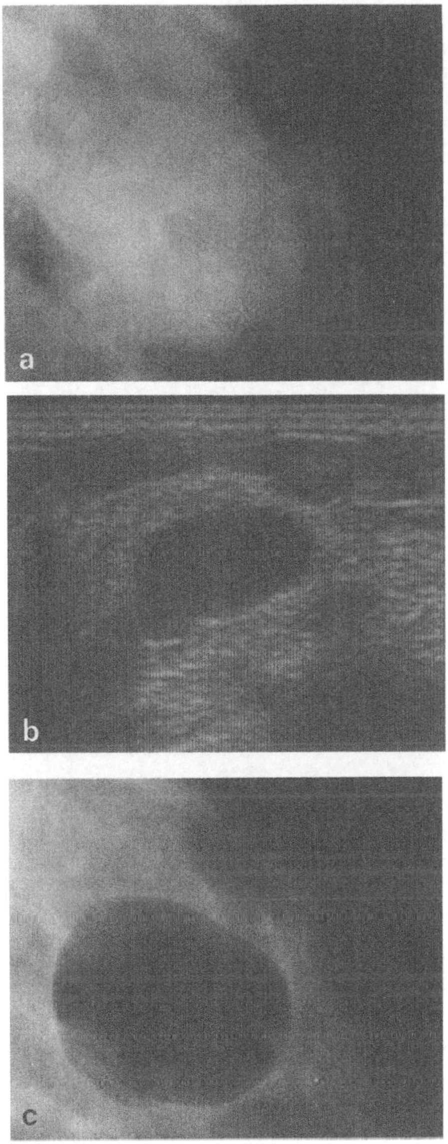

Fig. 3. a Round, smoothly rimmed opacification. **b** Sonographical diagnosis of its cystic nature. **c** Radiological confirmation after aspiration and injection of air

between benign and malignant lesions with a high degree of certainty, it is not possible to set out a radiological classification that reflects histological classification, as differentiation between different pathomorphologically defined benign diseases is only seldom possible. By mammographic means it is not possible, for instance, to discriminate between solid and cystic lesions.

Certain types of calcifications, however, are pathognomonic for distinct types of benign disease. Fibroadenomas show typical coarse calcifications (Fig. 4). Milk of calcium-containing cysts can be identified by the teacup phenomenon (Fig. 5). Plasma cell mastitis has a distinctive linear calcification pattern (Fig. 6). In most

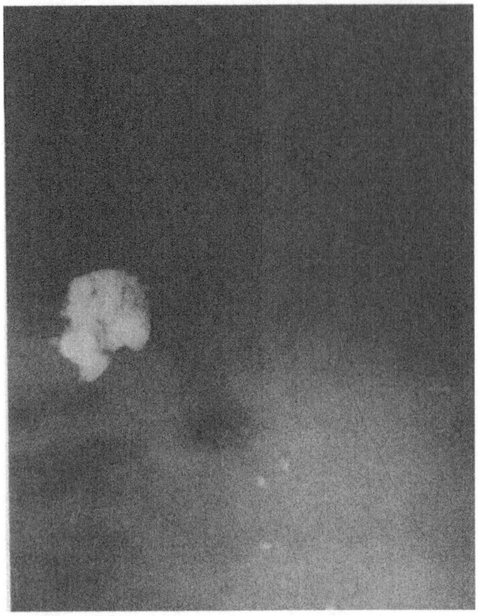

Fig. 4. Typical coarse calcification in a fibroadenoma

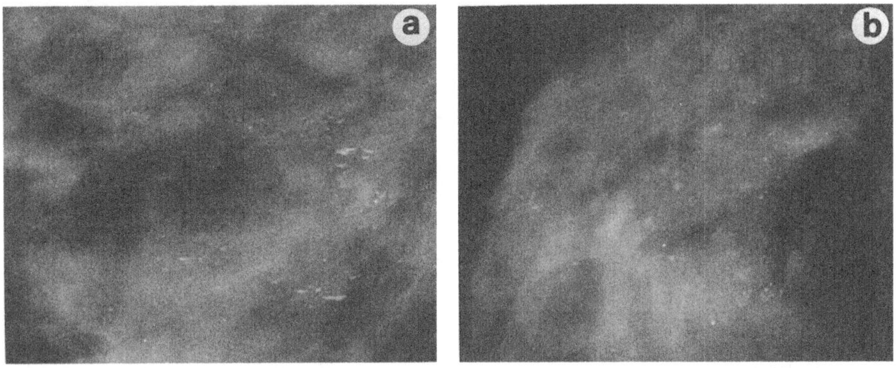

Fig. 5a,b. Milk of calcium-containing cysts exhibiting the teacup phenomenon. **a** Horizontal view showing calcium-containing fluid at the bottom of small cysts. **b** Craniocaudal view with typical soft round opacities

cases microcalcifications can be classified as either intraductal or lobular [12,21]. While lobular calcifications are of a benign nature, intraductal calcifications (Fig. 7) accompany both benign and malignant lesions and histological diagnosis is usually necessary.

Concerning the determination of risk factors it is an advantage of mammography that the whole breast can be evaluated, while histological diagnosis usually concentrates on a small piece of tissue.

On the basis of mammography it is possible to define risk factors for the development of invasive carcinoma of the breast (Table 4). Up to 37-fold risk was

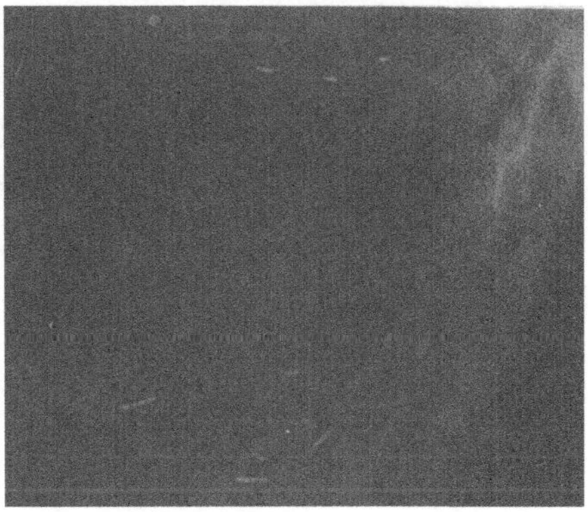

Fig. 6. Typical linear calcifications in plasma cell mastitis

Fig. 7. Intraductal calcifications in an intraductal cancer in situ

Table 4. Cancer risk according to mammographic findings

Author(s)	Classification	Risk factor
Wolfe (1976)	Parenchymal patterns	Up to 37
Tabár and Dean (1982)	Wolfe's criteria	5.9
Boyd et al. (1982)	Extent of dysplasia	5.7
Arabin et al. (1985)	Degree of dysplasia	Significant correlation

estimated by WOLFE [24] using criteria of extensive prominent duct pattern and dysplasia. The severity of radiological dysplasia [1] and its extent [3] have also been shown to correlate with breast cancer risk. Prospective studies have confirmed that WOLFE's classification is able to select risk groups [20]. The practical value for screening strategies has been doubted, however, as most cancers develop in patients who do not belong to mammographic risk groups. In individual cases, however, mammographic risk factors in combination with clinical risk factors and positive family history may have considerable impact on the treatment of these patients. In such patients we found a more than 30% incidence of preinvasive or early invasive lesions after prophylactic subcutaneous mastectomy [15].

References

1. Arabin B, von Fournier D, Kubli F, Müller A, Weber E (1985) Probleme und Grenzen der mammographischen Karzinomdiagnostik: Vergleich der präoperativen radiologischen Diagnose mit dem histologischen Befund bei 335 Patientinnen mit subkutaner Mastektomie. Geburtshilfe Frauenheilkd 45:595–603
2. Bässler R (1978) Pathologie der Brustdrüse. In: Doerr W, Seifert G, Mehlinger E (eds) Spezielle pathologische Anatomie, vol 11. Springer, Berlin Heidelberg New York
3. Boyd NF, O'Sullivan B, Campbell JE, Fishell E, Simor I, Cooke G, Germanson T (1982) Mammographic signs as risk factors for breast cancer. Br J Cancer 45:185
4. Dupont WD, Page DL (1985) Risk factors for breast cancer in women with proliferative breast disease. N Engl J Med 312:146–151
5. Frischbier HJ, Lohbeck HU (1977) Frühdiagnostik des Mammakarzinomes. Thieme, Stuttgart, p 105
6. Gautherie M, Gros CM (1980) Breast thermography and cancer risk prediction. Cancer 45:51–56
7. Goodson WH, Mailman R, Jacobson M, Hunt TK (1985) What do breast symptoms mean? Am J Surg 150:271–274
8. Haagensen CD (1971) Diseases of the breast, 2nd edn. Saunders, Philadelphia
9. Haagensen CD, Bodian C, Haagensen DE Jr (1981) Breast carcinoma: risk and detection. Saunders, Philadelphia
10. Junkermann H, Eggert-Kruse W, Teubner J, Kubli F, von Fournier D (1985) A useful clinical classification of benign breast disease. In: Baum M, George WD, Hughes LE (eds) Benign breast disease. The Royal Society of Medicine, London (Royal Society of Medicine International Congress and Symposia series no 76)
11. Kubli F, Lorenz U, Müller A, Weiger H (1984) Die subkutane Mastektomie; Komplikationen und Indikatonen. In: Kubli F, von Fournier D (eds) Neue Konzepte der Diagnostik und Therapie des Mammakarzinoms. Springer, Berlin Heidelberg New York, p 69
12. Lanyi M (1985) Morphologic analysis of microcalcifications. A valuable differential diagnostic system for early detection of breast carcinomas and reduction of superfluous exploratory excisions. In: Zander J, Baltzer J (eds) Early breast cancer. Springer, Berlin Heidelberg New York, pp 113–135
13. Meyer P (1957) Über das Vorkommen von myoepithelialen Tumoren bzw. von Fibrosing adenosis der Brustdrüse bei Frauen von 20–35 Jahren. Beobachtungen der Jahre 1938–1954 des Pathologischen Instituts Basel. Oncologia 10:254–271
14. Moskowitz M, Fox SH, Brun del Re R, Milbrath JR, Bassett LW, Gold RH, Shaffer KA (1981) The potential value of liquid-crystal thermography in detecting significant mastopathy. Radiology 140:659–662
15. Müller A, Tschahargane C, Bothmann GA, Kubli F (1980) Morphologische Befunde bei subkutanen Mastektomien. Untersuchungen an 200 Patienten. 1. Internationaler Kongreß für Senologie, Hamburg
16. Peters F (1986) Prolaktin und Erkrankungen der Brust. Urban and Schwarzenberg, Munich
17. Prechtel K (1972) Beziehungen der Mastopathie zum Mammakarzinom. Fortschr Med 90:43–45
18. Preece PE, Braun M, Mansel RE, Webster DJT, Fortt RW, Gravelle IH, Hughes LE (1982) Importance of mastalgia in operable breast cancer. Br Med J 284:1299–1300
19. Sickels EA (1985) Breast imaging: a view from the present to the future. Diagn Imag Clin Med 54:118–125
20. Tabár L, Dean PB (1982) Mammographic parenchymal patterns: risk indicator for breast cancer? JAMA 247:185–189
21. Tabár L, Dean PB (1985) Lehratlas der Mammographie. Thieme, Stuttgart
22. Teubner J, van Kaick G, Junkermann H, Pickenhan L, Wesch H, Eggert-Kruse W, Müller A, Tschahargane C, von Fournier D, Kubli F (1985) 5MHz Realtime-Sonographie der Brustdrüse. Teil 2. Untersuchungstechnik und diagnostische Wertigkeit. Radiologe 25:457–467

23. Threatt B, Norbeck JM, Ullmann NS, Kummer R, Roselle PF (1980) Thermography and breast cancer: an analysis of a blind reading. Ann NY Acad Sci 335:501–509
24. Wolfe JN (1976) Breast patterns as an index of risk for developing breast cancer. AJR 126:1130–1139

Fibrocystic Disease, Precancerous Lesions, and Carcinoma In Situ: Characteristic Morphology and Risk of Malignant Degeneration

K. Prechtel

Introduction

Carcinoma of the breast is the most common malignant growth in women, and the breast is an increasing source of risk with advancing age.

A breakdown of the diagnoses possible on the basis of pathologic anatomy shows three main conditions, with a clear development in their predominance in the course of life: fibroadenoma, fibrocystic disease, and carcinoma. The shift in predominance over time must not, however, be prematurely interpreted as an indication that fibrocystic disease is a precursor of carcinoma (Fig. 1).

As mammogenesis is hormonally controlled, and the hormonal balance, especially of the ovarian steroids, is by no means constant, phases of disturbance reflected in the morphology are only to be expected. A complex microscopic picture is known to reflect hormonal imbalance, although we do not yet have any detailed knowledge of whether the causation lies in an imbalance in the hormones supplied or in impaired responsiveness of the receptors in the target organ.

Fibrocystic Disease

The term "fibrocystic disease" is applied to any condition that on microscopic examination gives the impression of abnormal, but not malignant restructuring and alterations in the layering of the actual parenchyma. It is a familiar fact that this term is used somewhat loosely when the results of examination are recorded – rather too loosely in view of the serious nature of the condition. There are various reasons for this, not the least of which are the wish to oblige and consideration for the colleague who is actually treating the patient and who has requested the histological examination.

What does this mean? The person conducting the examination – in many cases the patient herself performs the initial examination – notices a circumscribed alteration, which gives rise to feelings of uncertainty and insecurity. The process of diagnosis is set in motion and grinds on to culminate in the operation room with the surgeon's knife. The biopsy specimen taken is analyzed by pathologists, who may find, for example, atrophic epithelial segments with fibrous replacement. They breathe a sigh of relief and record a diagnosis of fibrous or fibrocystic breast disease: there is a name for what they have observed, a diagnosis. We are aware from postmortem examinations, however, that it is practically unknown for any breast to

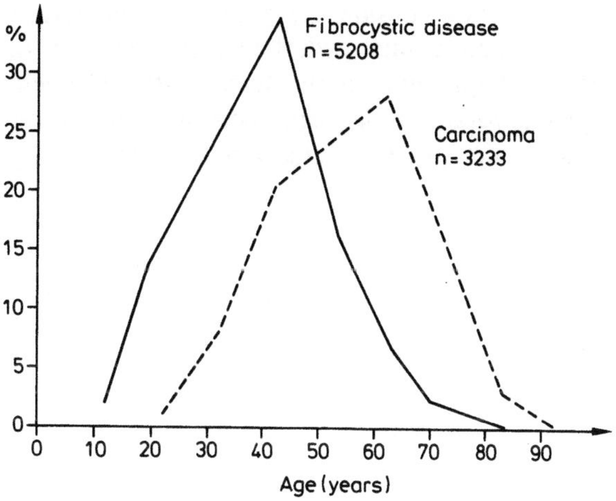

Fig. 1. Nonstandardized distribution of fibrocystic disease and breast carcinoma by age in patients whose condition was diagnosed by biopsy (1965–1975)

be consistently perfect in its histology and that some area justifying a diagnosis of fibrocystic disease can be found in almost any breast without illness necessarily being present. Every woman has latent or occult fibrocystic disease. It depends on the manner in which the examination is conducted whether a diagnosis of fibrocystic disease is recorded, and this will continue to be so as long as pathologists cannot bring themselves to refer to nonpathologic findings, i.e., findings that fall within the bounds of the normal when considered in light of the patient's age.

Up to this point, Hutter's valediction, "Goodbye to fibrocystic disease" can be tolerated.

However, fibrocystic disease means more than fibrosis or ectasia or a cyst in the ductal system of the gland. We subsume under fibrocystic disease those alterations that are not neoplastic in nature, which is why "dysplasia" was the preferred term for some time. This includes such detailed observations as blunt or sclerosing adenosis, radial scar, or intracanalicular epithelioses. There are many individual conditions that can be reflected simultaneously or in succession in the body of the breast and are offered as specific diagnoses. The terms used for them are specialty-oriented and give rise to difficulties in communication with the people who, while not immediately concerned with morphology, nonetheless have to introduce the name of the condition diagnosed into the treatment setting.

Pathologists should summarize their observations in a few words and make sure they sum them up in a key word or phrase that will be immediately comprehensible to their listeners without the necessity for questions about what is really meant.

Risk Inherent in Fibrocystic Disease

The term "fibrocystic disease" is familiar in interdisciplinary communication. It should be retained and merely qualified by adjectives to differentiate the various forms. In addition, however, an observation that it does not rank as an illness should be recorded in the report if appropriate.

Let us now consider the question of the nature or degree of fibrocystic disease. For anyone familiar with the histomorphology of the breast, an unusual proliferation of epithelium in the ductal system is much more a reason for disquiet than is a disproportion between ductal and lobular development, which was seen in a study which I carried out as a reason for dividing cases of fibrocystic disease into three subgroups:

Grade I (simple): abnormal alterations in the body of the breast with no concomitant increase in intracanalicular cell proliferation

Grade II (proliferating, without atypia): obvious epitheliosis within the ducts and/or ductules in addition, but with no characteristic signs of atypia in the syplasm

Grade III (proliferating, with atypia): atypia of the proliferating epithelium in addition, but with preservation of the dual cell pattern (atypical epitheliosis of the borderline type)

In a retrospective/prospective study, 1300 women were followed up for several years after diagnosis, in biopsy specimens, of fibrocystic disease classified according to the above schedule referred to the cell status. The purpose of the study was to find how often there were recurrences and how often carcinomas would be discovered. It turned out that the incidence really did vary in the different groups (Fig. 2). It

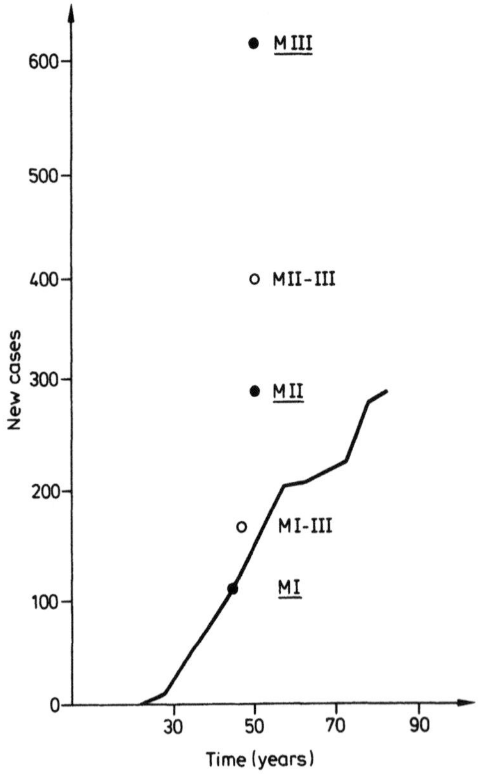

Fig. 2. Incidence of first appearance of breast carcinoma (per 100 000 per year) compared with probable risk after fibrocystic disease grades I–III confirmed by biopsy

Table 1. Risk of invasive breast carcinoma in women around 50 years of age after operation of fibrocystic disease or carcinoma in situ

Disease	Risk Factor[a]
Fibrocystic disease I	1
Fibrocystic disease II	2
Fibrocystic disease III	4
Carcinoma lobulare in situ	10 (?)
Carcinoma ductale in situ	30 (?)

[a]Risk Factor 1 = approximately 150 per 100 000 per year (normal incidence)

seems that women with grade I fibrocystic disease remain in the normal range so far as the risk of developing carcinoma is concerned, while in women with grade II the risk is twice as high (following conversion to correspond to a 1-year observation period) and in women with grade III (atypical) fibrocystic disease the risk of developing carcinoma is 4 times the normal risk.

This relatively low risk of malignant degeneration (Table 1) does not justify the conclusion that proliferating fibrocystic disease should be categorized as a precancerous lesion, especially as the simultaneous occurrence of atypical epitheliosis and carcinoma can be observed only in a minority of cases. In view of the slightly elevated risk, however, we are justified in placing women for whom a diagnosis of fibrocystic disease grade III is recorded, in the sense of a condition predisposing to carcinoma, in a risk group to be particularly carefully monitored, in the hope that if carcinoma does subsequently develop it will be discovered earlier, with correspondingly hopeful implications for prognosis and therapy.

In a small percentage of cases (fibrocystic disease grade III, representing about 5% of cases diagnosed by biopsy), fibrocystic disease is an indirect trace leading to carcinoma. It is possible that it merely progresses in parallel with a carcinoma, rather than being an immediate precursor. We cannot, however, exclude the possibility that atypical epitheliosis is a borderline type with facultative potential malignity.

Noninvasive Carcinoma of the Breast (Carcinoma In Situ)

According to the latest WHO classification, noninvasive carcinoma, which really means nothing more nor less than not yet invasive carcinoma, falls into two subtypes (Fig. 3): carcinoma ductale in situ (CDIS) and carcinoma lobulare in situ (CLIS). There have recently been problems with determination of the significance of CLIS with its risk factor of about 10, which is not very high (Table 1). Discussion is beginning over whether CLIS, which was initially made a great deal of, has adequate malignant potential to be transformed often enough into a fully developed invasive carcinoma or whether it just has to be considered as a high-risk indicator of carcinoma and in this sense perhaps as a precancerous lesion. On

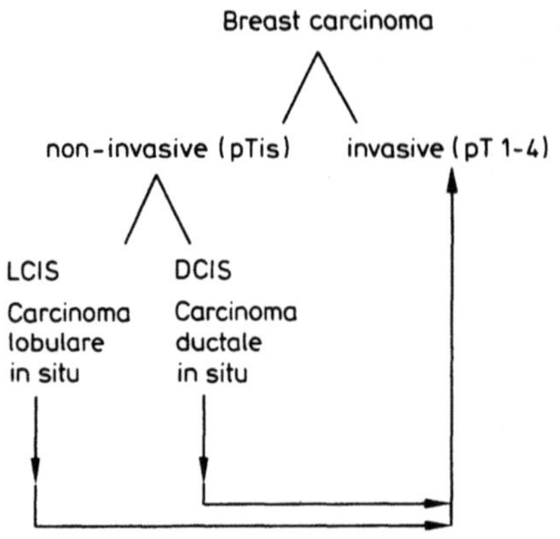

Fig. 3. Histologic classification of carcinoma according to WHO

contemplation of the risk factor given (Fig. 3) there is no need for any discussion in the case of CDIS: a malignant cell alone is present, with initially unresisted extension within the ductal system and invasion of the stroma after an unknown latent period and with no apparent reason. Two subgroups can be distinguished, a monomorphous and a polymorphous form (Table 2), the latter being more frequently discovered because of its particular predilection for calcification. The monomorphous type can be difficult to distinguish from atypical epitheliosis (fibrocystic disease grade III).

Table 2. Characteristics of carcinoma ductale in situ of the breast

Histological characteristics	cell type	
	Monomorphous	Polymorphous
Localization relative to mamillary region	Usually more distant	Usually closer
Structure	Tubular Cribriform Pseudopapillary	clinging Solid
Cell size	Medium	Large
Calcification	Fairly infrequent	Common

Multicentricity of Ductal Carcinoma in Situ

M. Reitzenstein, A. H. Tulusan, N. Bauer, and G. Ronay

The increasing treatment of breast cancer with breast-conserving surgery has reopened the discussion of multicentricity in breast cancer. To help answer this question we made a careful histological examination of 192 breasts with either invasive cancer or ductular carcinoma in situ (CDIS) using the radial technique of whole-organ sectioning [4]. The frequency of multicentricity was estimated in 104 invasive breast cancers, 20 microinvasive cancers and 68 cases of CDIS.

Multicentricity was diagnosed when – excluding the primary tumor – more than one quadrant was affected by invasive cancer or CDIS. In contrast, we defined multifocal involvement as several lesions (invasive or in situ) lying closely together but separate within one quadrant only.

The figures on multicentricity in the literature vary [1–3]. Multicentricity is quoted in these papers as having an incidence as low as 13.4% and as high as 74%. This is probably accounted for by differences in histological preparation and examination technique of the breast tissue. The latest figures from our study [4] support the results obtained by Lagios et al. [3] using similar histological techniques. Our results show multicentricity in 33% of 210 patients with breast cancer, Lagios et al. demonstrated it in 28% of 246 patients. In 79 cases of breast cancer we were able to exactly measure the extent of spread of the tumor in all directions. No direct relationship between tumor size and multicentricity could be found for tumors smaller than 3 cm.

Forty-one percent of 68 cases treated by modified radical mastectomy showed multicentricity. A closer analysis of these cases shows several factors which have an obvious influence on the probability of multicentricity. One very important parameter indeed is the extension of the CDIS. For this reason we differentiated between those specimens with occasional CDIS lesions (+) and those where up to half of the biopsy tissue was affected with CDIS lesions (+ +). Both of these groups were compared with biopsies where more than half of the biopsy tissue was affected by CDIS (+ + +). Twenty-nine percent of the cases with limited extension (+) showed multicentricity. Those with moderate extension (+ +) showed multicentricity in 34% of cases. However, in contrast to these first two groups we found multicentricity in 59% (10/17) of cases displaying wide extension of CDIS (+ + +). These results are similar to those obtained by Lagios et al. [3]. He showed that CDIS extensions of more than 25 mm are associated with a frequency of multicentricity significantly greater than CDIS lesions of smaller size.

However, other factors unrelated to extension also affect multicentricity. For instance, the histological type appears to be important. Cribriform and cribriform-papillary types of CDIS, with 60% show a markedly high frequency of multicentric lesions. Furthermore, the family history is important. Women without breast cancer in the family have, with 39% (24/62), considerably fewer multicentric lesions than women with breast cancer in the family (67%; 4/6 cases). Also, premenopausal women up to the age of 49 years were affected more often by multicentric lesions than women older than 50 years. Multicentricity of CDIS in the upper-outer quadrant is less frequent (27%) than in other quadrants. Presumably this depends on the glandular distribution in the four quadrants.

In order to prove whether the invasion affects multicentricity we compared 20 microinvasive cancers (invasive cancer smaller than 5 mm) with 33 cases of CDIS with comparable histological classification and extension. The incidence of multicentricity was similar, at 50% (10/20) and 48% (16/33) respectively. Thus invasion does not appear to influence the frequency of multicentric lesions.

As a result of these investigations we can state that patients with CDIS can be treated with breast-conserving surgery according to the same indications as patients with invasive cancer. In order to make an exact judgement of the remaining risk to the affected breast, careful histological examination and evaluation of the resected quadrant is necessary.

References

1. Fisher ER, Gregorio RM, Fisher B (1975) The pathology of invasive breast cancer. A syllabus derived from findings of the National Surgical Adjuvant Breast Project (protocol no 4). Cancer 36:1
2. Gallager HS, Martin JE (1969) Early phases in the development of breast cancer. Cancer 24:1170
3. Lagios JD, Westdahl PR, Margolin FR, Rose MR (1982) Duct carcinoma in situ: relationship of extent of non-invasive disease to the frequency of occult invasion, multicentricity, lymph node metastases, and short-term treatment failures. Cancer 50:1309
4. Tulusan AH, Egger H, Schneider ML, Willgeroth F (1982) A contribution to the natural history of breast cancer. IV. Lobular carcinoma in situ and its relation to breast cancer Arch Gynecol 231:219

Precancerous Lesions and Carcinoma In Situ: Problems of Treatment from the Morphological Viewpoint

H.-E. STEGNER

In theory there seem to be three ways in which carcinoma of the breast could develop:

1. De novo development with an intermediate noninvasive stage, i.e., a ductal or lobular carcinoma in situ
2. Development from primarily benign hyperplasia of the ducts and lobules of the mammary gland
3. Development from primarily atypical epithelial hyperplasia

One of the most important advances in the histopathologic examination of breast tumors is the more precise definition of noninvasive carcinoma. The confusion of noninvasive carcinomas with various forms of atypical epithelial hyperplasia of the mammary gland has led to mistaken assessments of the risk of malignant degeneration of hyperplastic processes in older statistics relating to the course of disease, not uncommonly followed by the initiation of overtreatment.

According to the WHO classification of 1981, in situ carcinomas can be divided into two types: noninfiltrating ductal carcinomas and noninfiltrating lobular carcinomas (carcinoma lobulare in situ). This division into two classes gives the impression that we are dealing here with two sorts of lesion that are comparable in their potential for malignant degeneration and differ only in the topography of the development. In fact, however, noninfiltrating carcinomas of the breast vary over a spectrum of manifestations with involvement of both the ductal and lobular compartments, and there are differences in the potential for malignant degeneration depending on type. A precise distinction of the different types of noninvasive carcinomas from the various forms of epithelial hyperplasia considered to be high-risk changes is extremely important from the clinical aspect, because of the implications for selection of the most suitable therapy. Overestimation of the risk involves the danger of unnecessarily radical treatment, while underestimation involves the risk of throwing away the advantage won by early diagnosis.

Noninfiltrating Intraductal Carcinoma

Intraductal carcinomas (IDC) are cancers that have developed within the glandular ducts and are growing in situ with solid, comedo-type, cribriform, or papillary differentiation. Another variant is the clinging type defined by AZZOPARDI [2].

Secretory or mucinous reactions can cause further changes in the presentation. The comedo type with typical central formation of detritus and calcification is the most common of the various forms of IDC. The sites of predilection for development are the extra- and intralobular sections of the terminal ducts [28]. The lobules of the gland can be involved by the neoplasia as a result of segmental spread (so-called lobular cancerization). Extension toward the nipple and infiltration of the mamillary epidermis lead to the clinical picture of Paget's disease. All types of IDC are characterized by the absence of destructive stromal infiltration. In the case of "pure" IDC the myothelial compartment is conserved according to immuno-histochemical and electron-microscopic investigations, and the basal laminae appear to be intact on electron-microscopic examination, as does the basement membrane on light-microscopic examination. Transformation to destructive stromal infiltration is a multifocal process. Early stromal invasion is difficult to interpret morphologically. Infiltration is preceded by loss of myothelial cells and breaks in the basal laminae and in discontinuities of the histochemically demonstrable membrane proteins [27]. The question of whether tumor cells are able to cross an intact basement membrane is speculative. The demonstration of gaps in the basal laminae on electron microscopic investigation and cytoplasmic protrusions of tumor cells in these regions have been interpreted by some authors as a sign that tumor cells similar to lymphocytes and leucocytes are able to pass the "open barrier" between epithelium and stroma in certain conditions [11,17,18].

In about 25% of cases, IDC develops in multiple sites in the same breast. The larger the primary focus of disease, the higher the probability of a multifocal development and also of unrecognized invasion (occult invasion). The histological diagnosis of IDC can therefore be made only with reservations, even after the most careful preparation of excised tissue, as clinical experience has clearly shown. Regional lymph node metastases are found in 4%–6% of cases of IDC diagnosed by histologic means and distant metastases with about the same frequency [3,5,10,24]. A palpable tumor can be the first indication of IDC. This is caused by expansion of the ducts, proliferation of connective tissue around the ducts (desmoplastic reaction) and lymphoid cell infiltration. The most important sign for clinical diagnosis, however, is the presence of microcalcification seen on mammography. It must be added that this sign restricts the mammographic diagnosis only for the types of IDC associated with calcium precipitation, especially the comedo type, more rarely the cribriform or the clinging type. In our own material approximately 85% of cases of IDC have been discovered by mammography. When the typical segmental arrangements of the calcifications is seen, the total extention of the process can be estimated by mammography. With increasing use of mammographic techniques, the chances of discovering ductal carcinomas while they are still in a noninvasive stage have risen.

There is still a great deal of lively controversy about the most suitable therapy. What are the implications of a histologically confirmed diagnosis of IDC? Intraductal carcinomas do not merely entail the risk of malignancy; rather they *are* cancers, growing in situ, usually with aneuploid DNA distribution and all the characteristics of cancerized cells. When IDC has been confirmed by excision biopsy and no further treatment has been given, in 75%–85% of cases an ipsilateral carcinoma of the same type develops, usually after a latency period of 6–10 years and usually in the same quadrant [4,8,19]. Complete local clearance is therefore just as important in the case of IDC as in the case of a frankly obviously invasive tumor. There is no doubt but that mastectomy continues to offer the best chance of a cure. Owing to the possibility of occult invasion, this should always be associated with dissection of proximal axillary lymph nodes to improve prognosis.

This recommendation of complete mastectomy for IDC may seem contradictory and out of proportion in view of the increasingly more generous indications adopted for breast-conserving treatment of invasive carcinoma. This apparent incongruity can be understood, however, if we bear in mind the way the methods of differential diagnosis have developed. Pathologists long regarded comedocarcinoma as a separate entity, without dividing it into noninfiltrating and infiltrating types. Only since the introduction of mammography has it been possible to recognize purely intraductal early lesions more frequently. Radiologists, balancing the benefits and risks, were very hesitant for a long time about delivering curative doses of irradiation to noninvasive stages of carcinoma. In isolated cases attempts led to negative results and reinforced the opinion that IDC was less sensitive to irradiation than invasive forms of the same type. MONTAGUE, in 1984, reported the results of conservative treatment of 34 noninvasive IDC. Her results do not allow any adequate conclusions about the effectiveness of radiotherapy of IDC. FISHER et al. report in protocol 6 of the National Surgical and Adjuvant Breast Project Study on 51 patients in this randomized study who underwent lumpectomy with or without radiotherapy. Within an average follow-up period of 53 months, 7% of patients in the radiotherapy group developed local recurrences as opposed to 23% in the group without radiotherapy. The authors see these results as an indication that IDC do not basically respond differently to radiotherapy than invasive carcinomas. It must be pointed out that their follow-up period is still not so long as the average latency periods known from earlier studies for the appearance of recurrences after excision biopsy.

Even if the sensitivity of IDC to radiotherapy should be confirmed in later studies, the same difficulties will persist in placing IDC anywhere in the current concept of conservative treatment. Conservative surgery is only possible when complete lumpectomy is performed. The more sharply circumscribed a tumor is, the easier it is to perform complete lumpectomy. But IDC has a segmental pattern of extension, following the course of the duct system. This means that it is impossible for the pathologist to decide whether the tumor has been completely resected, that is with a safe margin of healthy tissue, even on examination of subgross sections prepared from the whole of the excised tissue. The probability of persistent residual structures in the breast is therefore almost certainly higher than in the case of circumscribed and nodular tumors. The risk of persistent residual structures in the parenchyma falls with increasingly generous execution of the primary excision [15]. Wide excision, quadrantectomy, and subcutaneous mastectomy, in that order, offer increasing safety margins as primary surgical methods of treatment. The more extensive the primary tumor resection has to be, however, the more the actual point of conservative treatment, that is conservation of the organ to the greatest possible degree, is missed.

According to the principle accepted in our hospital, noninfiltrating IDCs with an extension of more than 20 mm are not suitable for conservative procedures. In the case of IDCs with an extension of up to 20 mm, wide excision with axillary lymphadenectomy is performed with no subsequent radiotherapy. Mammography is performed to allow preoperative planning and determination of tumor size. We do not yet have adequate data from this controlled clinical study.

Noninfiltrating Lobular Carcinoma (Carcinoma Lobulare In Situ)

The second main type of noninvasive breast carcinoma is the so-called carcinoma lobulare in situ (CLIS). It does not occur in so many forms as IDC. A monomorphic type A is differentiated from a more polymorphic (incohesive) type B. It is not uncommon for the two types to appear together. Clear differentiation is not always possible. Ultramicroscopic examinations show a relatively wide variation in form [25,26]. In the differential diagnosis it is important to distinguish CLIS from the lobular cancerization that occurs in IDC. The latter is characterized by its pleomorphic character with large cells and by combination with other forms of IDC. In addition, CLIS can proceed along a segmental course into the adjacent extralobular duct segments in forms of so-called intramural spread, as a small-cell variant of an IDC or as so-called pagetoid spreading. The sequence of progression of CLIS up to infiltrating carcinoma is less clear than that of IDC. The cumulative risk of malignant degeneration is beyond all doubt, and transformation of the in situ lesion to infiltrating lobular carcinoma in the form of microglandular or mono-cellular buddings is occasionally observed. The latency period before occurrence of subsequent carcinomas, at 15–24 years, is clearly longer for CLIS, however, than for IDC (6–10 years). Subsequent carcinomas occur in the ipsilateral and the contralateral breast with approximately the same frequency. They are not consistently cancers of the infiltrating lobular carcinoma type, but can be any of a wide variety of types of malignant breast tumors [1,6,12,13,22,23,29].

In our own sample of 94 cases recurrences were recorded in 16, e.g. 17%, of cases in an observation period of 12 years at most. The new cancer was CLIS in six cases, a variant of IDC in five, and invasive carcinoma in five further cases, the lobular type being found in only three of these. If the basic and concomitant structures are examined in CLIS, atypical ductal and also lobular forms of epithelial hyperplasia are found in almost 50%. Thus, CLIS is seen to be an indicator of an elevated risk of malignant degeneration rather than a true in situ carcinoma. The persistent hesitation in acceptance of the concept of carcinoma in situ and the preference for less prejudicial designations, such as lobular neoplasia, are therefore justified. A prospective wait-and-see attitude is becoming more and more widely adopted in the treatment strategy. This seems justified if the patient is cooperative, if the anatomy of the mammary glands makes them suitable for mammographic monitoring, and if there are no other cumulative e.g., epidemiological, risk factors. If surgical prophylaxis is decided upon, the frequent multifocal and bilateral development means that the appropriate alternatives are bilateral mastectomy with reconstruction and, as a means of reducing the risk of malignancy, bilateral subcutaneous mastectomy.

Atypical Epithelial Hyperplasia

Compared with the clear definition of ductal and lobular carcinoma in situ, the so-called atypical forms of epithelial hyperplasia of the mammary gland are still very much open to subjective interpretation. "Atypical hyperplasia" is the term used when, as a working hypothesis, we class together all pathologic proliferations of ductal epithelia that differ in cellular atypia from the forms of benign hyperplasia (epithelioses) regularly seen in the context of fibrocystic disease (cystic mastopathy) but in which the degree of atypia is not so extreme as in IDC or CLIS. In the presence of atypical ductal hyperplasia the epithelial is made up of several layers, and can form pseudopapillary buds, and epithelium bridges, which do not, however, have the rigid character of IDC. As in benign forms of hyperplasia, ultramicroscopy and immunohistochemistry allow a distinction between two cell types characterized by secretory and myothelial differentiation. The dual cell character, with involvement of cells with myoepithelial differentiation in the proliferation, should be regarded as a sign of benignity. The atypical forms of epithelial hyperplasia are obviously the decisive tissue component in grade III fibrocystic disease of the mammary gland according to PRECHTEL. Their role as an intermediate stage in the formal histogenesis of breast carcinoma is so far unconfirmed, but their significance as a risk indicator has been confirmed many time [7,20]. Grade III fibrocystic disease accounts for approximately 5%–10% of the entire group of cystic mastopathy if the cytomorphologic criteria are strictly observed. The risk of malignant degeneration to carcinoma, according to the results of numerous retrospective and prospective studies, is 2.5–4.5 times as high as the incidence of carcinoma that has to be expected otherwise in women aged 45–50 years [20,21]. The extrapolated risk of carcinoma in women with so-called grade III fibrocystic disease, is high enough to warn the patients of the advisability of regular monitoring with the diagnostic methods now available. It does not, however, give any statistical justification for general application of prophylactic surgery. Surgical treatment does not seem justified unless there is a cumulation of risk factors. The decision for ablation should be made only with caution, with full knowledge of all the facts, and jointly by of pathologist and clinicians after consideration of individual factors. Standardized treatment is simple and convenient, but it does not do justice to the complex clinical picture of atypical hyperplastic lesions. KONJETZNY, in his book on pathology, clinical features and treatment of fibrocystic disease, which appeared in 1942, wrote: "In view of the many forms the clinical picture of fibrocystic disease can take, the indications for surgical intervention cannot be fitted into any one system. It is only possible to give more or less general pointers, and it is only possible to follow these, when proceeding in full awareness of the histology and the clinical features of the particular case of fibrocystic disease concerned."

This statement is still true today. Those specialized in morphology have learned in past years, however, to consider the broad spectrum of manifestations in a more critical manner and to differentiate early stages of carcinoma and risk indicators more precisely. This learning process is still in progress. It will help us to decide on the correct prophylactic or therapeutic action for the individual case.

References

1. Andersen JA (1977) Lobular carcinoma in situ of the breast. An approach to rational treatment. Cancer 39:2597–2602
2. Azzopardi JG (1979) Problems in breast pathology. Saunders, London
3. Bahnsen J, Warneke B, Frischbier H-J, Stegner H-E (1985) Das intraduktale Mammakarzinom. Klinische röntgenologische und histologische Befunde und ihre therapeutischen Konsequenzen. Geburtshilfe Frauenheilk 45:488–493
4. Betsill WL, Rosen PP, Liebermann PH, Robbins GF (1978) Intraductal carcinoma. Long-term follow-up after treatment by biopsy alone. JAMA 239:1863–1867
5. Carter D, Smith RR (1977) Carcinoma in situ of the breast. Cancer 40:1189–1193
6. Curletti E, Giordano J (1981) In situ carcinoma of the breast. Arch Surg 116:309–310
7. Dupont WD, Page DL (1985) Risk factors for breast cancer in women with proliferative breast disease. N Engl J Med 312:136
8. Farrow JH (1970) Current concepts in the detection and treatment of the earliest of the early breast cancers. Cancer 25:468–477
9. Fisher ER, Sass R, Fisher B, Wickerham L, Pai SM, et al. (1986) NSABP Investigators: Pathologic findings from the National Surgical Adjuvant Breast Project (Protocol 6) I. Intraductal carcinoma (DCIS). Cancer 57:197–208
10. Gallager HS (1980) The developmental pathology of breast cancer. Cancer 46:905–907
11. Gould VW, Snyder RW (1974) Ultrastructural features of papillomatosis and carcinoma of the nipple ducts. The significance of myoepithelial cells and basal lamina in benign, "questionable" and malignant lesions. Pathol Annu 9:441
12. Haagensen CD, Lane N, Lattes R, Bodian C (1978) Lobular neoplasia (so-called lobular carcinoma in situ) of the breast. Cancer 42:737–769
13. Hutter RVP, Foote F (1969) Lobular carcinoma in situ. Cancer 24:1081–1085
14. Konjetzny GE (1942) Pathologie, Klinik und Behandlung der Mastopathie. Enke, Stuttgart
15. Lagios MD, Westdahl PR, Margolin FR, Rose MR (1982) Duct carcinoma in situ: relationship of extend of noninvasive disease to the frequency of occult invasion, multicentricity, lymph node metastases and short-term treatment failures. Cancer 50:1309–1314
16. Montague ED (1984) Conservation surgery and radiation therapy in the treatment of operable breast cancer. Cancer 53:700–704
17. Ozzello L (1971) Ultrastructure of intraepithelial carcinomas of the breast. Cancer 28:1508–1515
18. Ozzello L, Sanpitak P (1970) Epithelial-stromal junction of intraductal carcinoma of the breast. Cancer 26:1186–1198
19. Page DL, Dupont WD, Rogers LW, Landenberger M (1982) Intraductal carcinoma of the breast: follow-up after biopsy only. Cancer 49:751–758
20. Page DL, Dupont WD, Rogers LW, Rados MS (1985) Atypical hyperplastic lesions of the female breast. A long-term follow-up study. Cancer 55:2698–2708
21. Prechtel K, Geiger G (1985) Langzeitbeobachtung von Frauen mit bioptisch gesicherter Mastopathie. Dtsch Med Wochenschr 110:1883–1888
22. Rosen PP, Liebermann PH, Braun DW Jr, Kosloff C, Adair F (1978) Lobular carcinoma in situ of the breast: detailed analysis of 99 patients with average follow-up of 24 years. Am J Surg Pathol 2:225–251
23. Rosen PP, Senie R, Schottenfeld D, Ashikari R (1979) Non-invasive breast carcinoma: frequency of unsuspected invasion and implications for treatment. Ann Surg 189:377–382
24. Rosen PP, Braun DW, Kinne DE (1980) The clinical significance of pre-invasive breast carcinoma. Cancer 46:919–925
25. Stegner H-E (1985) Ultrastruktur und elektronenmikroskopische Klassifikation nicht-invasiver und invasiver Mammakarzinome. Verh Dtsch Ges Pathol 69:74–87
26. Stegner H-E (1986) Histopathologie der Mammatumoren. Licht- und elecktronenmikroskopischer Atlas. Enke, Stuttgart

27. Tulusan AH, Grünsteidel W, Ramming I, Egger H (1982) A contribution to natural history of breast cancer. III. Changes in the basement membrane in breast cancer with stroma microinvasion. Arch Gynecol 231:209–218
28. Wellings SR, Jensen HM, Marcum RG (1975) An atlas of subgross pathology of the human breast with special reference to possible precancerous lesions. JNCI 55:231–273
29. Wheeler JE, Enterline HT, Roseman JM, Tomasulo JP, Macilvaine GH, Fitts WT, Kirshenbaum J (1974) Lobular carcinoma of the breast. Cancer 34:554–563
30. WHO (1981) International classification of tumours, no 2. WHO, Geneva

Endocrinological Profiles in Benign Breast Disease

R. E. MANSEL

The structural and pathological changes that occur in the human female breast are often labelled as benign breast disease (BBD), although it is evident that many of the changes are in fact aberrations of normal development and involution. Since these developmental and involutional changes are under direct hormonal control, it would be expected a priori that BBD would be related to hormonal changes. There are certainly epidemiological correlations between BBD and oral contraceptive use and obesity, both being protective [3]. Also a previous history of both benign and malignant breast disease and small breast size increase the risk of subsequent benign breast biopsy [15]. Further circumstantial evidence of a hormonal aetiology is suggested by the fact that conditions such as fibroadenoma and cystic disease occur in age ranges that correspond with particular phases of ovarian function. Despite these epidemiological associations and the development of accurate estimations of hormones by radioimmunoassay, a clear abnormality of any single hormone has not been found in patients with BBD. One of the major difficulties in all the studies published is the definition of the term "BBD". The condition is very heterogeneous and different terms are used to describe the same patient group in different countries. The endocrine defect, if it exists, is likely to be subtle and may only be present in certain subgroups of BBD. Many of the published studies do not describe their BBD patients accurately and so it is not possible to know whether the patients have been diagnosed by clinical examination alone or by pathology after a biopsy. Further methodological problems have been caused by assay differences and sampling differences between studies. It is therefore not surprising that no definite reproducible defect has been demonstrated in most cases of BBD.

Ovarian Hormones

Ovarian hormones have been known to be important in the growth of hormone-dependent breast cancer ever since the classic work of BEATSON demonstrating regression of these tumours after oophorectomy, and early workers investigating BBD suggested ovarian hypersecretion as an aetiological factor. Both ATKINS [1] and GESCHICKTER [12] suggested this mechanism but were unable to directly measure the hormones involved. When direct assay of serum oestradiol became possible in the early 1970s, several reports describing these measurements in patients with BBD were published but gave conflicting results. ENGLAND et al. [7] reported that daily blood sampling in patients with painful lumpy breasts and patients with cystic disease showed normal levels of oestradiol in the former group but elevated luteal levels in patients with macroscopic cysts. However, another study using random sampling showed no difference between normal controls and a group of biopsied BBD [38]. In general this situation of some studies showing increased oestrogen levels, but most showing normal oestrogen levels has continued and no clear abnormality has emerged. A recent study [32] has shown normal plasma levels of oestradiol and oestrone in the plasma but an increase in the unbound or free oestradiol in patients with BBD. This finding may be of importance as the unbound fraction represents the biologically active steroid.

An alternative explanation for the normal oestradiol levels found in most studies could be a deficiency of progesterone leading to a relative hyperoestrogenism as proposed by SHERMAN and KORENMAN [35]. Support for this hypothesis came from a study by SITRUK-WARE et al. [36] in which they demonstrated gross luteal deficiency in women with mastodynia, cysts, fibrocystic disease, fibroadenomas and nodularity when random sampling of basal progesterone was undertaken. In this study the plasma oestradiol was found to be normal or elevated in two of the subgroups but the ratio of luteal oestradiol to progesterone (PEL) was < 1 in the patient groups. Several further studies have lent support to the French group [5,23,25,34] in variously defined patients with BBD, although two of these studies came from the same group in Paris.

However, the case for luteal deficiency has not been proven as there are large numbers of studies showing no defect in progesterone levels in the luteal phase of the cycle. SWAIN et al. [38], ENGLAND et al. [8], GELLER et al. [11] and WALSH et al. [39] all showed normal progesterone levels in carefully sampled, well-defined patients. These studies included similar subgroups of BBD as in the MAUVAIS-JARVIS study and the complete lack of correlation is surprising, but again some of the differences could be explained by the heterogeneity of the clinical presentation of BBD. Recent studies of salivary progesterone levels performed by two groups in Britain have also shown normal levels of the steroid in the saliva of patients with BBD [20,31]. Both of these studies collected daily salivary samples and thus gave an estimate of the biological or free fraction of progesterone in the saliva. The Glasgow study [31] compared biopsied BBD showing epithelial hyperplasia with normal controls, while the Cardiff study [20] investigated patients with cyclical mastalgia, and both of these subgroups of BBD showed normal levels of salivary progesterone. It thus appears clear that luteal deficiency is not a universal phenomenon and does not appear to be a major aetiological factor in BBD. It is possible that luteal deficiency may be important in a minority of patients and the epidemiological evidence suggesting a relative hyperoestrogenism is fairly strong. These inconsistencies may be resolved by estimations of free oestradiol in the serum of carefully defined BBD subgroups.

Pituitary Hormones

The principal hormones controlling ovarian function are luteinizing hormone (LH) and follicle-stimulating hormone (FSH) and many studies have been undertaken to investigate a possible role of these hormones in the aetiology of BBD. Again there are sampling problems, as the levels of these hormones vary widely at different times in the menstrual cycle. As with oestradiol and progesterone, no clear abnormality has been identified, with some studies showing elevated levels of LH [13,37] while other show a normal level [16,24]. Studies of FSH levels have shown normal levels of this hormone in most BBD cases.

Most attention has been focused on the primary lactogenic hormone prolactin, secreted by the anterior pituitary. As lactation depends on the presence of prolactin, it was naturally assumed that this hormone would be important in the aetiopathology of BBD. Once a reliable radioimmunoassay had been established some 10 years ago, many investigators set out to measure this hormone in normal and diseased states. The sampling problem in prolactin estimations is formidable, as the hormone has a marked circadian secretion with a peak of secretion in the early hours of the morning [26]. In addition, the hormone is released under stressful conditions and this gives rise to transient fluctuations in the level throughout the day. In view of this problem it is not surprising that a large number of studies where random single samples were taken showed no differences from normal controls [40]. This lack of difference persisted even when 24-h blood sampling was used [24]. Thus the basal levels of prolactin did not appear to be different in BBD.

However, studies of stimulated levels of prolactin conducted by several different investigators have shown definite differences in patients with BBD. Due to the sampling problems inherent in a hormone with rapidly fluctuating levels, some investigators have examined the control mechanisms of prolactin secretion. Prolactin secretion is normally under tonic inhibition from the pituitary via dopaminergic mechanisms, but several substances are known to release the hormone from the pituitary. Most work has been done with thyrotropin-releasing hormone (TRH) [21], but other agents such as sulpiride [22], domperidone and metaclopramide [4], also produce a large rise in serum prolactin which occurs within 90 min of injection with a peak secretion at around 45–60 min post injection. These effects are probably due to dopaminergic blockade. PETERS et al. [27], using TRH as the stimulating agent, and BOHNET et al. [2], using metaclopramide, demonstrated an increased release of prolactin in cases of mastodynia, breast hypertrophy and fibroadenomata. Two further studies in carefully defined women with cyclical mastalgia have shown a significantly enhanced response to TRH stimulation [18,28] in the luteal phase of the menstrual cycle. DÖGLIOTTI et al. showed that a similar enhanced response to TRH was also seen in the follicular phase of cycle in women with gross cystic disease, as defined by sonography [6]. WATT-BOOLSEN et al. [41] examined the response to both TRH and metaclopramide in women with cyclical mastalgia and showed an enchanced response to TRH, in agreement with the previous studies, but a normal response to metaclopramide, thus suggesting that the enhanced TRH response is not due to a primary decreased dopaminergic tone. Recent evidence of the value of these pituitary stimulation tests and their clinical relevance comes from a report by PETERS et al. [29] demonstrating correlation of therapeutic response with normalization of the exaggerated TRH peak and a report by KUMAR et al. [19] correlating peak prolactin response to TRH/domperidone with therapeutic response to endocrine agents.

These studies show a considerable degree of consistency and suggest that there may be an increased release of prolactin in patients with cyclical mastalgia and nodular breasts. No studies of these dynamic tests have been carried out in other subgroups of BBD.

Other Hormones

Several studies have examined the role of androgens in BBD, but despite claims of increased androgen levels [9,13,14,17], the consensus view is that serum androgens are normal in BBD, but RANNEVIK et al. [30] have reported abnormally high levels of sex hormone-binding globulin in "fibrocystic disease" and suggest that this abnormality may reflect abnormalities in the androgen/oestrogen balance. ROLLAND et al. [33] have suggested that prostaglandins may play a role in BBD and have found elevated plasma levels of prostaglandin E2 in patients with BBD during both phases of the menstrual cycle, but no other reports of prostaglandins in BBD have emerged.

Thyroid hormones have also been suggested to be abnormal in BBD, but most reports have examined the epidemiological relationship, and detailed studies of thyroid function in BBD have shown no real differences from controls. The thyroid-stimulating hormone response to the TRH test gives a sensitive indicator of thyroid function and was found to be normal in the studies of KUMAR et al. [18], DOGLIOTTI et al. [6] and WATT-BOOLSEN et al. [41]. However, ESTES [10] has claimed that administration of thyroid hormone does improve the symptoms of BBD, and PETERS et al. [29] have shown that administration of thyroid hormone does normalise the exaggerated prolactin response to TRH seen in patients with cyclical mastalgia, perhaps suggesting the mechanism of action of thyroid hormone in the relief of mastalgia.

Conclusions

The overall conclusion must be that no specific abnormality of hormone levels has been found in BBD in general, and it is clear that no gross defect of any single hormone is present. However, there are interesting abnormalities such as the enhanced prolactin response to TRH, which suggests that subtle changes may be present in the relationships between the principal ovarian and pituitary hormones. These changes appear to be reproducible between well-defined subgroups of BBD, and correlation of these changes with subsequent therapeutic responses supports their validity. Careful study of these small abnormalities and measurement of the biologically active fractions of the relevant hormones in well-documented cases of BBD should define the hormonal basis of BBD in the future.

References

1. Atkins HJB (1940) Treatment of chronic mastitis. Lancet 2:411
2. Bohnet HG, Gabel AK, Kreutzer P (1980) Prog Reprod Biol 6:172
3. Brinton LA, Vessey MP, Flavel R, et al. (1981) Risk factors for benign breast disease. Am J Epidemiol 113:203
4. Brouwers JRBJ, Assies J, Wiersinga WM, Huizing G, Tytgat GN (1980) Plasma prolactin levels after acute and subchronic oral administration of domperidonone and of metodopramide: A cross-over study in wealthy volunteers. Clin Endocrinol 12:435
5. De Boever J, Vanderkerckhove D (1982) J Steroid Biochem 113
6. Dogliotti L, Fagginulo, Ferruso A, et al. (1985) Prolactin and Thyrotropin response to Thyrotropin-releasing hormone in premenopausal women with fibrocystic disease. Horm Res 21:137
7. England PC, Skinner LG, Cottrell KM, Sellwood RA (1974) Sex hormones in breast disease. Br J Cancer 30:571
8. England PC, Skinner LG, Cottrell KM, Sellwood RA (1975) Sex hormones in breast disease. Br J Surg 62:806
9. England PC, Sellwood RA, Khyba RE, Irvine JDB (1981) Serum androgen levels and the menstrual cycle in women with benign or malignant breast disease. Clin Oncol 7:213
10. Estes NC (1981) Mastodynia due to fibrocystic disease of the breast controlled with thyroid hormone. Am J Surg 142:746
11. Geller S, Grenier J, Nahoul K, Scholler R (1979) Ann Endocrinol (Paris) 40:45
12. Geschickter CF (1945) Diseases of the breast 2nd edn. Lippincott, Philadelphia
13. Golinger RC, Krebs J, Fisher ER, Danowski TS (1978) Hormones and the pathophysiology of fibrocystic mastopathy: Elevated luteinizing hormone levels. Surgery 84:212
14. Grattarola R (1978) Anovulation and increased androgenic activity as breast cancer risk in women with fibrocystic disease of the breast. Cancer Res 38:3051
15. Hislop TG, Elwood JM (1981) Risk factors for benign breast disease: a 30-year cohort study. Can Med Assoc J 124:283
16. Jones MK, Ramsay ID, Collins WP (1979) Clin Oncol 5:305
17. Jones MK, Dyer GI, Ramsay ID, Collins WP (1981) Studies on apparent free cortisol and testosterone in plasma from patients with breast tumors. Postgrad Med J 57:89
18. Kumar S, Mansel RE, Hughes LE, et al. (1984) Prolactin response to Thyrotropin-releasing hormone stimulation and dopaminergic inhibition in benign breast disease. Cancer 53:1311
19. Kumar S, Mansel RE, Hughes LE, Edwards CA, Scanlon MF (1985) Prediction of response to endocrine therapy in pronounced cyclical mastalgia using dynamic tests of prolactin release. Clin Endocrinol 23:699
20. Kumar S, Mansel RE, Wilson DW, Read GF, Truran PL, Hughes LE, Griffiths K (1986) Daily salivary progesterone levels in cyclical mastalgia patients and their controls. Br J Surg 73:260
21. L'Hermite M, Vanhaelst L, Copinschi G, et al. (1972) Prolactin release after injection of thyrotrophin releasing hormone in man. Lancet 1:763
22. L'Hermite M, Danayer P, Golstein J, et al. (1978) Acute endocrine profile of sulpiride in the human. Clin Endocrinol 9:195
23. London RS, Sundaram GS, Schultz M, Nair PP, Goldstein PJ (1981) Endocrine parameters and a Tocopherol therapy of patients with mammary dysplasia. Cancer Res 41:3811
24. Malarkey WB, Schroeder LL, Stevens VC, James AG, Lanese RR (1977) Twenty-four hour preoperative profiles in women with benign and malignant breast disease. Cancer Res 37:4650
25. Martin PM, Kuttenn F, Serment H, Mauvais-Jarvis P (1978) J Steroid Biochem 9:1251
26. Nokin J, Vekemans M, L'Hermite M, Robyn C (1972) Circadian periodicity of serum prolactin concentration in man. Br Med J 3:561
27. Peters F, Pickardt CR, Zimmerman G, Breckwoldt M (1981) PRL, TSH, and thyroid hormones in benign breast diseases. Klin Wochenschr 59:403

28. Peters F, Schuth W, Scheurich B, Breckwoldt M (1984) Serum prolactin levels in patients with fibrocystic breast disease. Obstet Gynaecol 64:383
29. Peters F, Pickardt CR, Breckwoldt M (1985) Normalization of exaggerated prolactin responsiveness to thyrotropin-releasing hormone. Cancer 56:1082
30. Rannevik G, Doberl A, Gershagen S, et al. (1983) Elevated serum concentrations of sex hormone binding globulin in fibrocystic breast disease. In: Angeli A, et al. (eds) Endocrinology of cystic breast disease. Raven, New York, pp 127–133
31. Read GF, Bradley JA, Wilson DW, George WD, Griffiths K (1985) Evaluation of luteal-phase salivary progesterone levels in women with benign breast disease or primary breast cancer. Eur J Cancer Clin Oncol 21:9
32. Reed MJ, Cheng RW, Noel CT, Dudley HAF, James VHT (1983) Plasma levels of estrone sulfate and estradiol and the percentage of unbound estradiol in postmenopausal women with and without breast disease. Cancer Res 43:3940
33. Rolland PH, Martin PM, Rolland AM, Bourry M, Serment H (1979) Benign breast disease: Studies of prostaglandin E2, steroids, and thermographic effects of inhibition of prostaglandin biosynthesis. Obstet Gynaecol 54:715
34. Rolland PH, Martin PM, Bourry M, Rolland AM, Serment H (1980) Adv Prostaglandin Thromboxane Res 6:581
35. Sherman BM, Korenman SG (1974) Inadequate corpus luteum function: A pathophysiological interpretation of human breast cancer epidemiology. Cancer 33:1306
36. Sitruk-Ware R, Sterkers N, Mauvais-Jarvis P (1979) Inadequate corpus luteal function in women with benign breast diseases. Obstet Gynaecol 53:457
37. Sundaram GS, London R, Margolis S, Wenk R, et al. (1981) Serum hormones and lipoproteins in benign breast disease. Cancer Res 41:3814
38. Swain MC, Hayward JL, Bulbrook RD (1973) Plasma oestradiol and progesterone in benign breast disease (1973) Eur J Cancer 9:553
39. Walsh PV, Wang DY, McDicken I, Stell PM, Bulbrook RD, George D (1984) Serum progesterone concentration during the luteal phase in women with benign breast disease. Eur J Cancer Clin Oncol 20:1339
40. Wang DY, Fentiman IS (1985) Epidemiology and Endocrinology of benign breast disease. Breast Cancer Res Treat 6:5
41. Watt-Boolsen S, Eskildsen PL, Blaehr H (1985) Release of prolactin, thyrotropin and growth hormone in women with cyclical mastalgia and fibrocystic disease of the breast. Cancer 56:500

Endocrinology of Benign Breast Disease in Relation to the Severity of Radiological Dysplasia

H. JUNKERMANN, K. KLINGA, E. WEBER, and D. VON FOURNIER

Attempts to relate benign breast disease with a hormonal disbalance have had inconsistent results (MANSEL, this volume). One reason for this may be the lack of a generally accepted classification. Some authors have even denied the existence of such a disease entity [3].

The main concern of most women who seek advice because of benign breast disease is the risk of development of mammary carcinoma. Apart from histological parameters and family history [2], mammographic parenchymal pattern is the most accepted risk indicator [1,5,6].

We studied endocrinological parameters in 148 women with different degrees of radiological dysplasia who attended our breast clinic either for noncancerous symptoms or for screening purposes. Blood was taken in the early follicular phase (days 4–7 of the cycle) as well as three times during the luteal phase (days 5, 7 and 9 after ovulation as determined from the basal body temperature record).

In each case a standardized history was taken. Each mammogram was graded according to the severity and extent of radiological dysplasia (Tables 1, 2).

Table 1. Grading according to severity of radiological dysplasia

Grade	Radiological Findings
0	No radiological dysplasia
1	Nodular or trabecular densities of low degree, or homogenous shadowing. No microcalcifications
2	Nodular or trabecular densities of medium degree often with benign scattered microcalcifications
3	Irregular nodular or trabecular densities usually combined with diffuse scattered microcalcifications whose nature is difficult to evaluate

Table 2. Grading according to extent of radiological dysplasia

Grade	Radiological Findings
0	No dysplasia present
A	Dysplasia covering less than 25% of the mammogram
B	Dysplasia covering 25%–50% of the mammogram
C	Dysplasia covering 50%–75% of the mammogram
C	Dysplasia covering over 75% of the mammogram

Four groups have been formed on the basis of these gradings of radiological dysplasia:

1. No dysplasia, or low-grade dysplasia covering less than 50% of the mammogram (severity grade 0–1, extent grade A or B; $n=46$)
2. Low-grade dysplasia covering more than 50% of the mammogram (1, C or D; $n=12$)
3. Moderate to high-grade dysplasia covering less than 50% of the mammogram (2–3, A or B; $n=27$)
4. Moderate to high-grade dysplasia covering more than 50% of the mammogram (2–3, C or D; $n=63$)

The evaluation of some epidemiological factors revealed the following:

- Patients in group 4 were significantly older (mean 40.0 years) than patients in group 1 (mean 36.6 years), thus proving that degree of dysplasia can be differentiated from the juvenile density of the breast.
- The length of the follicular as well as the luteal phase as judged from basal body temperature curve was not different between the groups. However, women in group 3 (21%) and group 4 (18%) reported more irregularities of their menstrual cycle than women in group 1 (7.3%) and group 2 (10%). These differences were not significant.
- There were no differences in the frequency of nulliparity among the four groups. However, women in dysplasia group 4 were significantly older at their first pregnancy (mean 24 years) and especially at the birth of the first living child (mean 25 years) than women in dysplasia group 1 (means 22 and 22 years).

The evaluation of estradiol and progesterone during the luteal phase revealed no differences between dysplasia groups (Figs. 1, 2). Sex hormone-binding globulin (SHBG)-binding capacity in the luteal phase was significantly elevated above the values of the follicular phase. The SHBG-binding capacity was slightly higher in dysplasia group 4 than group 1 ($p<0.05$) (Fig. 3).

On the basis of the pain charts a mastodynia score was computed by adding the degree of mastodynia recorded for each day of the luteal phase. No correlation of mastodynia with progesterone, estradiol, or SHBG-binding capacity (Fig. 4) could be detected.

Clinical observation indicates that benign breast disease is hormone-dependent. Despite extensive research the exact nature of the endocrinological disturbance has not been conclusively elucidated. RANNEVIK et al. [4] were the first to describe elevated SHBG values in patients with symptomatic benign breast disease. These results were interpreted as an indication of enhanced biological estrogen activity in these women. Our results show that elevated SHBG-binding capacity is correlated with the severity of radiological dysplasia irrespective of subjective symptoms. It remains to be elucidated whether physicochemically increased bioavailability of estradiol or some other mechanism is the basis of this increased estrogen effect.

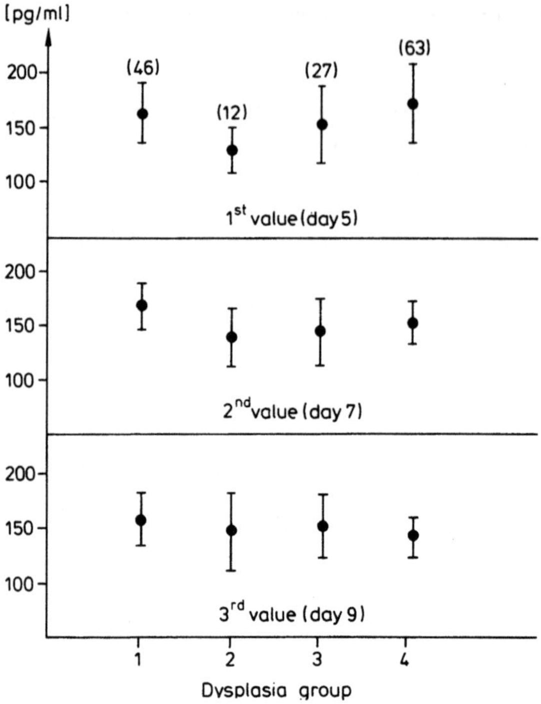

Fig. 1. Estradiol blood levels on three days of the luteal phase in 148 women with different degrees and extension of radiological dysplasia. Shown are the mean and 95% confidence interval

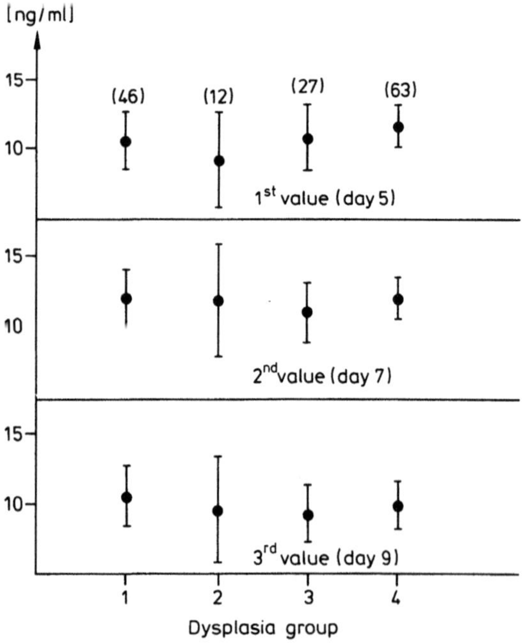

Fig. 2. Progesterone blood levels on three days of the luteal phase in 148 women with different degrees and extension of radiological dysplasia. Shown are the mean and the 95% confidence interval

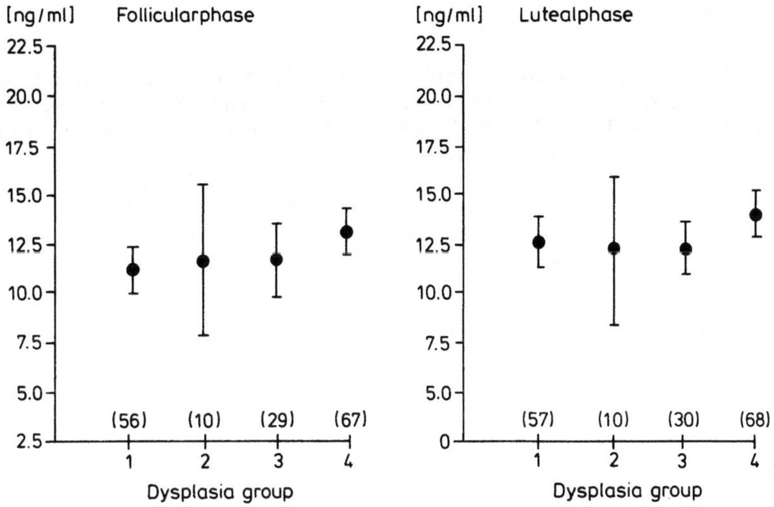

Fig. 3 SHBG-binding capacity in the follicular phase ($n = 162$) and the luteal phase ($n = 165$) in women with different degrees of radiological dysplasia. The luteal phase value was determined at the day of the highest progesterone value. Mean and 95% confidence interval are shown. The values during the luteal phase are significantly higher than those in the follicular phase ($p < 0.05$). SHBG-binding capacity is higher in patients with extensive radiological dysplasia (group 4) than in patients with no or little dysplasia (group 1) ($p < 0.05$)

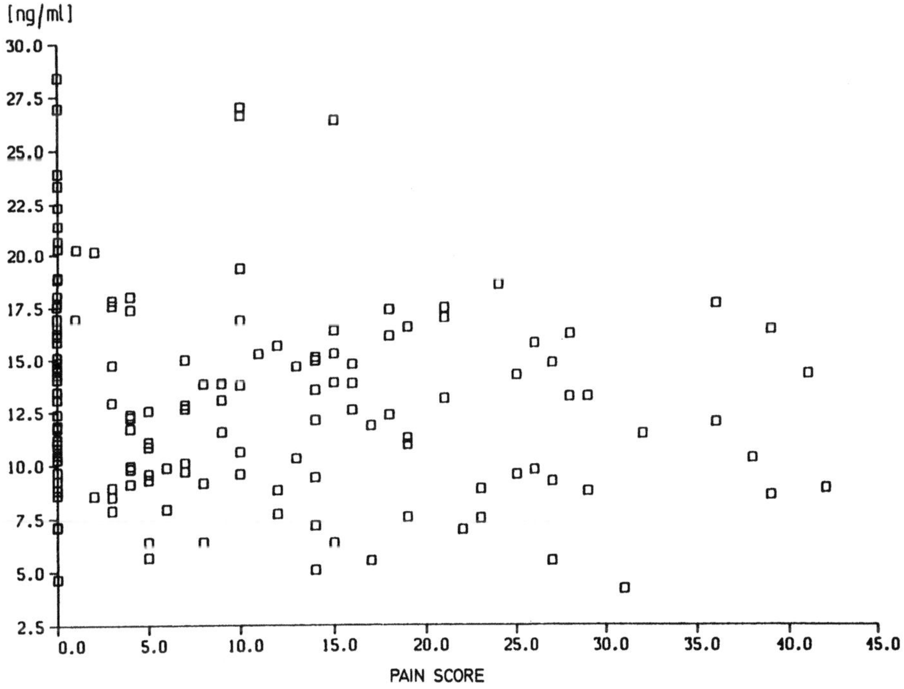

Fig. 4. Relation between SHBG-binding capacity in the luteal phase and the mastodynia pain score. No significant correlation can be found

References

1. Boyd NF, O'Sullivan B, Campbell JE, Fishell E, Simor I, Cooke G, Germanson T (1982) Mammographic signs as risk factors for breast cancer. Br J Cancer 45:185
2. Dupont WD, Page DL (1985) Risk factors for breast cancer in women with proliferative breast disease. N Engl J Med 312:146–151
3. Hutter RVP (1985) Goodbye to "fibrocystic disease". N Engl J Med 312:179
4. Rannevik G, Döberl A, Gershagen S, Rasmussen TH, Tobiassen T (1983) Elevated serum concentrations of the sex hormone binding globulin in fibrocystic breast disease. In: Angeli A, Bradlow HL, Dogliotti L (eds) Endocrinology of cystic breast disease. Raven, New York, pp 127–134
5. Tabár L, Dean PB (1982) Mammographic parenchymal patterns. Risk indicator for breast cancer. JAMA 247:185–189
6. Wolfe JN (1976) Breast patterns as an index of risk for developing breast cancer. AJR 126:1130–1139

Hormonal and Non-Hormonal Medical Therapy of Benign Breast Disease

D. VON FOURNIER, H. JUNKERMANN, U. WARENDORF, E. WEBER, E. KRAPFL, and U. ABEL

For the treatment of the nodular painful breast (mastopathy), a variety of non-hormonal and hormonal measures have been proposed.

Non-Hormonal Therapy

Non-hormonal measures for the treatment of mastopathy include the following: cooling ointments/local alcohol; plant extracts; diuretics; acupuncture; methylxanthine withdrawal (coffee, tea, chocolate); vitamins (B1, E). Few data exist to prove the effectiveness of these measures, though they are widely used. In the evaluation of therapeutic effectiveness of measures for the treatment of the subjective complaints of mastopathy, a large unspecific (placebo) effect has to be taken into account. Because of their relatively low cost and lack of undesirable side effects, however, such treatments can be used as the first step in cases where the subjective complaint prevails.

Alcoholic ointments improve subjective symptoms in about 50% of cases (Table 1) irrespective of the severity of objective changes.

Plant extracts are widely used in Germany. KUBISTA et al. (1984) have found them effective in a double-blind placebo-controlled study. PREECE (this volume) found a plant extract (oil of evening primrose) effective in a placebo-controlled double-blind study. The exact mechanisms by which these preparations are effective remain to be elucidated. *Diuretics* have been proposed on the assumption that a general hormone-induced retention of water is the cause of cyclical mastodynia. PREECE et al. [20], however, demonstrated that this is not the case. Because of general effects on electrolyte composition and rebound effects after withdrawal, we do not recommend the application of diuretics for mastodynia. BAUER et al.

Table 1. Results of non-hormonal treatment of symptomatic mastopathy

Therapy	Degree of mastopathy	n	Subjective improvement (%) Complete	Partial	None
Alcoholic ointment	Mild	250	14.4	39.2	46.4
	Severe	100	18.0	34.0	48.0
Acupuncture	Mild	40	49.8	35.2	15.0
	Severe	90	48.1	37.2	14.7

(1981) from our group found very good results with *acupuncture*. Verification with a placebo-controlled group is lacking, and would be difficult with this treatment. MINTON et al. (1982) proposed that withdrawal of *methylxanthines* is helpful. The proposed mechanism is that methylxanthines enhance cyclic AMP in breast cells and thus promote proliferation. In a placebo-controlled study, however, only a minimal effect of this treatment could be found [9]. *Vitamin B1* was said to promote detoxification of estrogens in the liver [14]. Recently SUNDARAM et al. [22] proposed *vitamin E*; however, they were not able to demonstrate any effect in a placebo-controlled study.

Hormonal Therapy

The following agents have been proposed for hormonal treatment of mastopathy: androgens; thyroid hormones; local progesterone; systemic progestogens; estrogen-progestogen combinations; prolactin inhibitors; antiestrogens; danazol (impeded androgen, antigonadotropin).

In the early days of hormone therapy *androgens* or androgen-progestogen combinations were proposed and were found effective in the treatment of mastopathy [4]. Unwanted side effects – sometimes persisting androgenization – have, however, made this treatment obsolete.

Thyroid hormones were proposed by PETERS et al. [19], based on the finding that subclinical thyroid disfunction is often detectable in patients with benign breast diseases. In a small group of our patients with exaggerated TSH stimulation the effect of thyroid hormone substitution was disappointing (Table 2).

The application of *progesterone* in an alcoholic gel preparation has been proposed by MAUVAIS-JARVIS et al. [17]. Penetration of progesterone in small

Table 2. Results of hormonal treatment of symptomatic mastopathy

Therapy	Severity of Mastopathy	N	Subjective improvement (%) Complete	partial	none
Tamoxifen	Mainly severe	49	51% (23)	37% (20)	12% (9)
Danazol	Mainly severe	50	59% (27)	32% (17)	9% (5)
Local progesterone		42	41%(17)	21%(9)	38%(16)
Carrier gel only		52	34%(18)	29%(15)	37%(19)
Progestogens	Mild	140	49%	30%	21%
	Severe	130	42%	33%	25%
Thyroxine		10	10% (1)	30% (3)	60% (6)

amounts through the skin has been demonstrated. Progesterone in breast tissue and fat is elevated after local application [6]. After unilateral application, however, the concentration is elevated in both breasts (unpublished results). It seems that progesterone accumulates via the blood stream. In a placebo-controlled double-blind study we could not find any effect of the progesterone-containing preparation greater than that of the alcoholic carrier gel.

Progestogens have been widely propagated on the basis of the luteal insufficiency hypothesis of GESCHICKTER [11]. We used 5 mg medroxyprogesterone or medrogestone from the 15th to the 25th day of the cycle and had subjective improvement in about 70% of the patients. Only one placebo-controlled study has been published, by COLIN et al. [7], who showed an effect of cyclical lynestrenol. They could demonstrate a difference only after correcting the responders on the basis of thermography: on the basis of subjective responses alone no significant differences could be demonstrated. *Estrogen-progestogen* combinations using high-dose hormonal contraceptives were proposed by ARIEL [2] on the basis of an uncontrolled study.

The effectiveness of *bromocriptine* has been shown in several double-blind placebo-controlled studies [see PREECE, this volume].

Danazol must be regarded as the most effective agent for the treatment of benign breast diseases. Its effect has been documented in numerous uncontrolled and several placebo-controlled double-blind studies [1,3,8,12,15,16]. We have compared danazol in an open randomized study with tamoxifen. In the meantime a double-blind placebo-controlled study has also proved the effectiveness of tamoxifen [10].

In our study we used 200 mg danazol/day continuously or 10 mg tamoxifen from the 5th to the 25th day of the cycle [21]. Subjective complaints were improved under both treatments in 80%–90% of patients. After 3 months of therapy danazol seems to be slightly more effective than tamoxifen (Table 2). In those patients where treatment was continued for 6 months treatment results improved further (Table 3).

In about two thirds of patients a softening of the breast tissue was noted by the physician (Table 4). Progressive improvement of the induration after 6 months of therapy was also seen under tamoxifen and danazol (Table 5).

Table 3. Subjective improvement after 3 and 6 months of tamoxifen or danazol

Drug	Improvement		
	Complete	Partial	None
Tamoxifen ($n=40$)			
3 months	45%(18)	38%(15)	17%(7)
6 months	58%(23)	40%(16)	2%(1)
Danazol ($n=37$)			
3 months	59%(22)	33%(12)	8%(3)
6 months	65%(24)	32%(12)	3%(1)

Table 4. Clinical improvement after treatment with tamoxifen or danazol

Therapy	Improvement	No change
Tamoxifen ($n=49$)	67% (33)	33% (16)
Danazol ($n=48$)	64% (31)	36% (17)

Table 5. Clinical improvement after 3 and 6 months of tamoxifen and danazol

Drug	Improvement		
	Complete	Partial	None
Tamoxifen ($n=39$)			
3 months	–	64%(25)	36%(14)
6 months	–	77%(30)	23%(9)
Danazol ($n=37$)			
3 months	3%(1)	59%(22)	38%(14)
6 months	5%(2)	73%(27)	22%(8)

Objective regression of mastopathic densities in the mammogram could be documented in 40%–50% of the cases by blind reading of mammograms before and after a 6-month course of treatment with tamoxifen or danazol (Fig. 1,2). Patients who were treated with an alcoholic gel preparation in a parallel study did not improve (Table 6).

Both tamoxifen and danazol were associated with a significant number of side effects. In general the side effects were slight to moderate and were well tolerated by the patients if they had been informed about their harmlessness. Only a very small number of patients had to discontinue the medication because of the severity of side effects (Table 7).

After stopping the treatment the pain did not resume immediately but with a latency period of about 1 year. One year after both treatments one-third of the patients remained symptom-free (Fig. 3).

According to our experience danazol and tamoxifen are two very effective treatments for benign breast diseases. Unfortunately these agents both carry a substantial risk of subjectively unpleasant, although not dangerous, side effects. This limits their widespread use. After withdrawal the complaints will recur in the majority of the patients after several months, although at a more tolerable intensity.

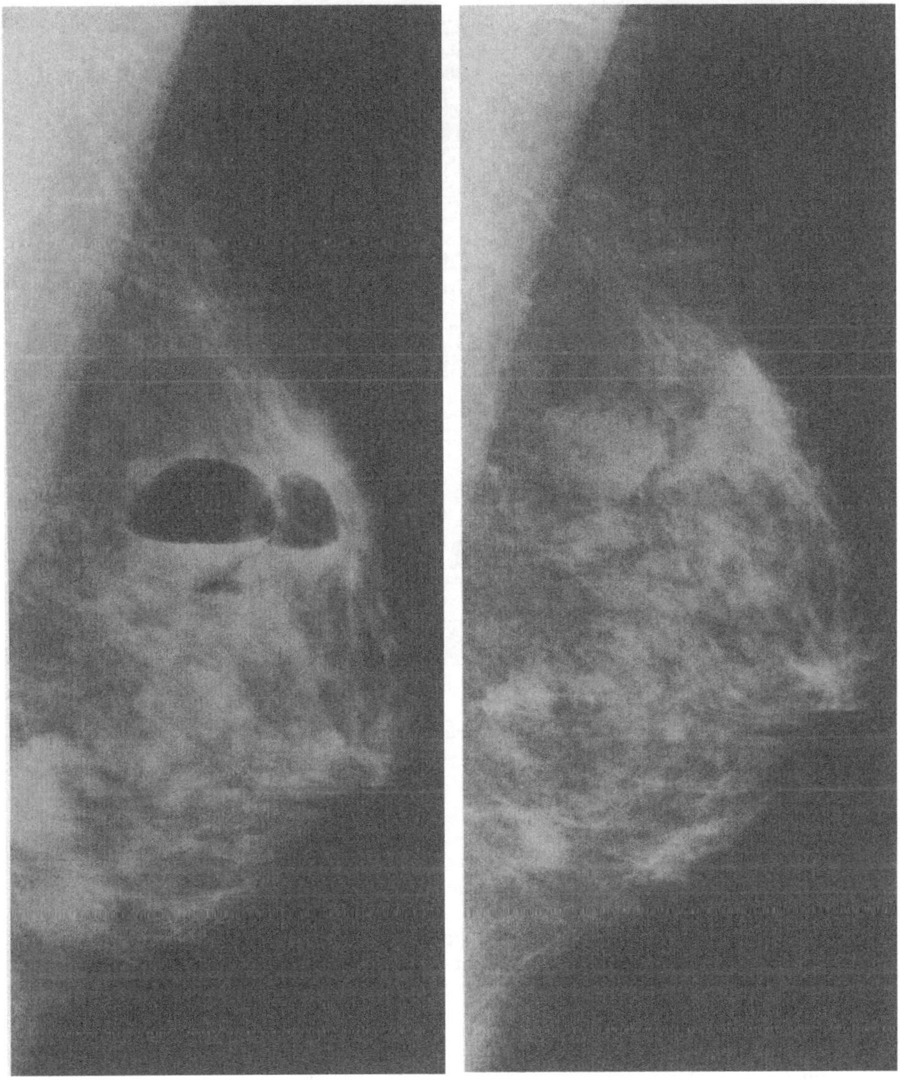

Fig. 1. Marked improvement of mammographic densities after 6 months of 10 mg tamoxifen/day (right side)

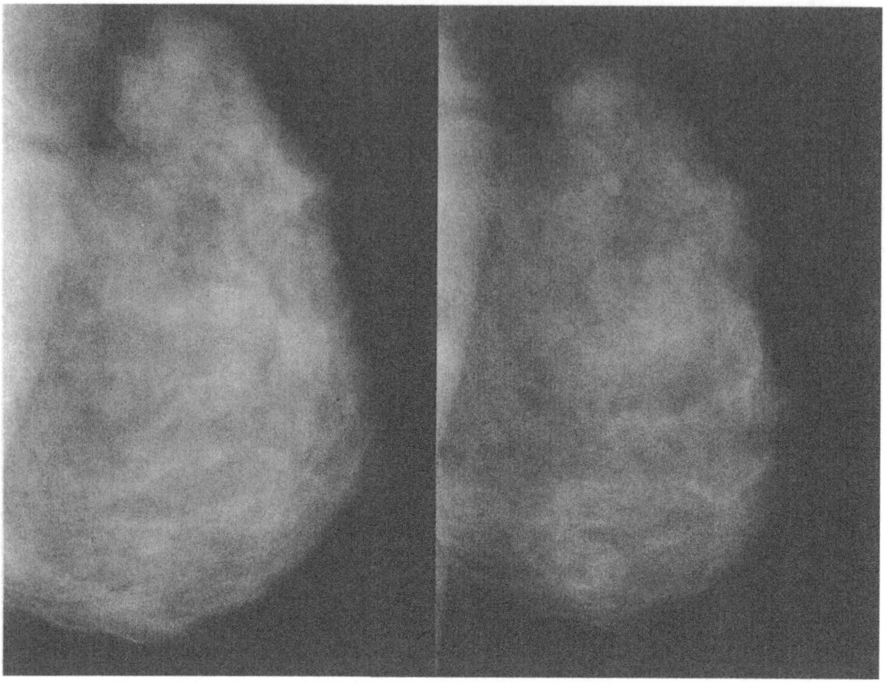

Fig. 2. Marked improvement of mammographic densities after 6 months of 200 mg danazol/day (right side)

Table 6. Regression of mastopathic densities as detected by mammography

Therapy	Improvement Marked	 Slight	None	Deterioration
Tamoxifen (*n* = 17)	41% (7)	18% (3)	35% (6)	6% 1
Danazol (*n* = 16)	31% (5)	31% (5)	38% (6)	
Alcoholic gel (*n* = 28)	–	18% (5)	75% (21)	7% (2)

Table 7. Side effects of tamoxifen and danazol

Side effects		Tamoxifen 10 mg/day ($n=53$)		Danazol 200 mg/day ($n=55$)
None		23		27
Mild				
	Hot flushes	9	Acne	6
	Nausea	5	Irregular menses	4
	Acne	3	Nausea	1
	Spotting	1	Varicosis	1
Marked				
	Fatigue	4	Weight gain >4 kg	9
	Amenorrhea	4	Amenorrhea	3
	Weight gain>4 kg	3	Hoarseness	4
	Hot flushes	2	Muscle cramps	2
	Loss of hair	1	Loss of hair	3
	Pruritus vulvae	3	Acne	1
	Ovarian cysts	1	Fatigue	1
	Decreased libido	1	Varicosis	1
	Vertigo	1	Vertigo	1
Severe (therapy discontinued)				
	Nausea/gastric pain	2	Nausea and depression	2
	Headache	1	Gastric pain	1
	Intestinal cramps	1	Muscle cramps	1
			Exanthema	1

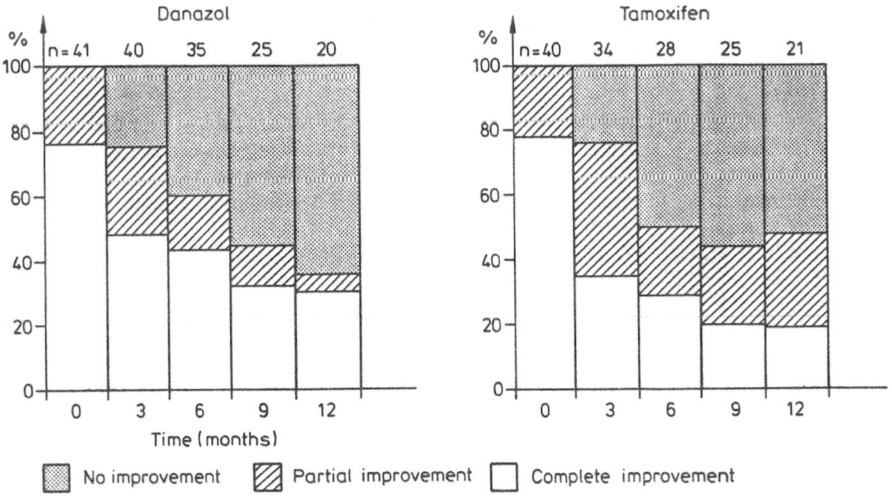

Fig. 3. Delayed recurrence of mastodynia after a course of 3–6 months tamoxifen or danazol

References

1. Aksu MF, Tzingounis VA, Greenblatt RB (1978) Treatment of benign breast disease with danazol: a follow-up report. J Reprod Med 21:181–184
2. Ariel IM (1973) Enovid therapy (norethynodrel with mestranol) for fibrocystic disease. Am J Obstet Gynecol 117:453–459
3. Asch RH (1977) The use of an impeded androgen-danazol – in the management of benign breast disorders. Am J Obstet Gynecol 127:130–134
4. Atkins HJB (1949) The effect of endocrines on fibro-adenosis. Br Med J:750–752
5. Bauer M, von Fournier D, Späh U, Kubli F, Jansa J (1982) Behandlungsergebnisse bei der Mastopathie. In: Frischbier HJ (ed) Die Erkrankungen der weiblichen Brustdrüse. Thieme, Stuttgart
6. De Boever J, Verheugen C, van Maele G, Vandekerckhove D (1983) Steroid concentrations in serum glandular breast tissue, and breast cyst fluid of control and progesterone-treated patients. In: Angeli A, Bradlow HL, Dogliotti L (eds) Endocrinology of cystic breast disease. Raven, New York, pp 93–99
7. Colin C, Graspard U, Lambotte R (1978) Relationship of mastodynia with its endocrine environment and treatment in a double blind trial with lynestrenol. Arch Gynakol 225:7–13
8. Dhont M, Delbeke L, VanEyck J, Voorhoof L (1979) Danazol treatment of chronic cystic mastopathy; a clinical and hormonal evaluation. Postgrad Med J 55:66–70
9. Ernster VA, Mason L, Goodson WH, Sickles EA, Sacks ST, Seloin S, Dupny ME, Hawkinson J and Hunt TK (1982) Effects of caffeine-free diet on benign breast disease. A randomized trial. Surgery 91:263–267
10. Fentiman IS, Caleffi M, Brame K, Chaudary MA, Hayward JL (1986) Double-blind controlled trial of tamoxifen therapy for mastalgia. Lancet I:287–288
11. Geschickter CF (1948) Diseases of the breast: diagnosis, pathology, treatment, 2nd edn. Lippincott, Philadelphia
12. Greenblatt B, Ben-Nun I (1980) Danazol in the treatment of mammary dysplasia. Drugs 19:349–355
13. Kubista E, Müller G, Spona J (1986) Behandlung der Mastopathie mit zyklischer Mastodynie: Klinische Ergebnisse und Hormonprofile. Gynäk Rundsch 26:65–79
14. Lang WR, Renwick S, Johnson L, Wyse E (1972) Benign mammary dysplasia. Med J Aust 2:147–149
15. Lauersen NH, Wilson KH (1976) The effect of danazol in the treatment of chronic cystic mastitis. Obstet Gynecol 48:93–98
16. Mansel RE, Wisbey JR, Hughes LE (1982) Controlled trial of the antigonadotropin danazol in painful nodular benign breast disease. Lancet 1:928–930
17. Mauvais-Jarvis P, Kuttenn F, Ohlgiesser C (1974) Résultats du traitement des mastodynies et des mastopathies par la progestérone percutanée. Nouv Presse Med 16:1027–1028
18. Minton JP, Abou-Issa H, Reiches N, Roseman JM (1981) Clinical and biochemical studies on methylxanthine-related fibrocystic breast disease. Surgery 90:299–304
19. Peters F, Pickardt CR, Breckwoldt M (1983) Hormonal status of women with benign cystic breast disease: clinical implications. In: Angeli A, Bradlow HL, Dogliotti L (eds) Endocrinology of cystic breast disease. Raven, New York, pp 113–122
20. Preece PE, Richards AR, Owen GM, Hughes LE (1975) Mastalgia and total body water. Br Med J 4:498–500
21. Ricciardi I, Ianniruberto A (1979) Tamoxifen-induced regression of benign breast lesions. Obstet Gynecol 54:80–84
22. Sundaram GS, London R, Margolis S, Wenk R, Lustgarten J, Nair PP, Goldstein P (1981) Serum hormones and lipoproteins in benign breast disease. Cancer Res 41:3814–3816

Medical Treatment of Benign Breast Disease

P.E. PREECE

Since there is no internationally accepted terminology for benign diseases of the breast, it is essential to describe the conditions to which this chapter refers. Recently there has been debate as to whether some of these conditions are "diseases" at all. For practical purposes, benign breast diseases can be defined as "those conditions of the breast which cause patients to experience symptoms which are not malignant in their behaviour or natural history".

There are only five symptoms relating to the breast. These are:

- Lump
- Nipple discharge
- Nipple retraction
- Pain
- Skin changes

A classification of benign breast disease can be constructed using these symptoms as its basis (Table 1).

For clinicians who regard the treatment of the symptoms of our patients as the most important objective, this classification has the virtue that it guides us to think

Table 1. Classification of benign breast disease

Type	Symptoms				
	Lump	Discharge	Retraction	Pain	Skin
Congenital			√		
Cyst	√				
Eczema					√
Fibroadenoma	√				
Galactocoele	√				
Galactorrhoea		√*			
Mastopathy	√*			√*	
Mondor's disease	√			√	
Papilloma		√			
Periductal mastitis	√	√	√	√*	√
Scar/trauma	√		√	√*	√
Sclerosing adenosis	√			√	
Tietze syndrome	√			√*	

*Amenable to medical (rather than surgical) treatment

about the aetiology, i.e. the pathological precursor of each particular symptom in each individual patient.

For the purpose of this chapter, of the conditions generally accepted as being medically treatable, hormonal mastopathy causes both lumpiness and pain: periductal mastitis can cause any one of the five symptoms (although not all of these can be remedied by medical means). Of the three remaining, galactorrhoea, scar pain and Tietze syndrome, each is a single clinically distinguishable entity for which particular management is appropriate.

Hormonal Mastopathy

Hormonal mastopathy, which causes lumpiness and pain, often does so in a cyclical pattern, the signs and symptoms being at their peak in the luteal, especially late luteal phase of each menstrual cycle. Although the symptom of pain is poorly localised, the lumpiness detected on palpation is frequently maximal in the upper outer quadrant of the breast, where the tenderness to touch is also most pronounced. The pain may radiate to the ipsilateral arm and even on occasion to the neck (Fig. 1).

Periductal Mastitis

Pain caused by or in association with this disorder does not have a regular time pattern, i.e. it is spasmodic. It is most commonly located in inner quadrants or deep to the areola, and it is frequently described as "burning". The distinctive features of this pain are illustrated in Fig. 2.

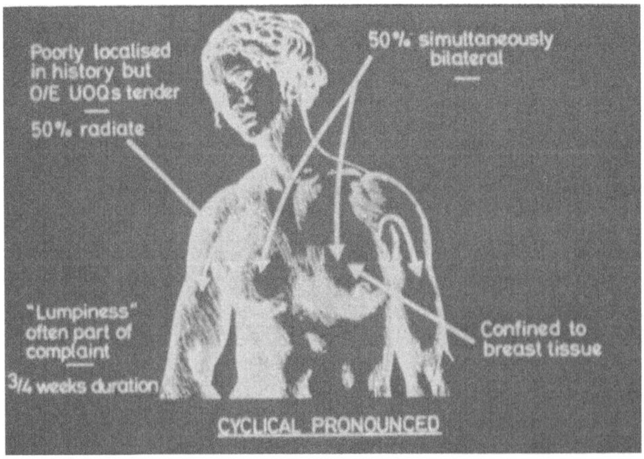

Fig. 1. Features of cyclical pronounced mastalgia

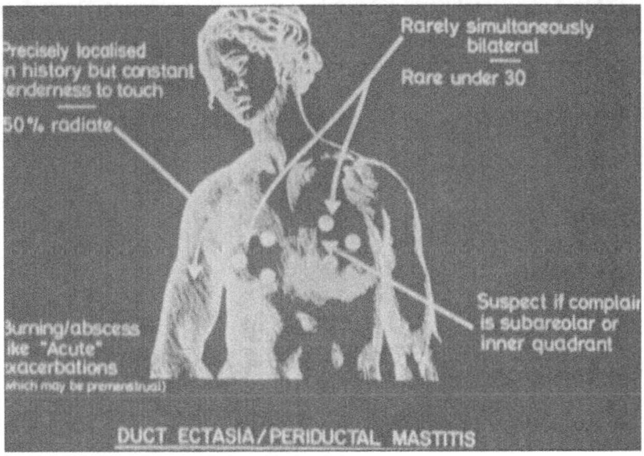

Fig. 2. Distinctive features of breast pain associated with periductal mastitis

Medical Treatment of Cyclical Breast Pain and Lumpiness

The medicaments available for these symptoms of which I have personal experience are bromocriptine (Parlodel), danazol (Danol) and oil of evening primrose (Efamol-G). Placebo-controlled trials have been conducted of all three, and the results of one such trial with bromocriptine in the non-cyclical group are shown in Table 2. Although clinicians' assessment of tenderness and nodularity showed a trend towards reduction being reduced, this was not statistically significant.

Using the patients' own assessment of their symptoms, measured by visual linear analogues, it was evident that those with cyclical symptoms were those who were being relieved to a significant extent on bromocriptine (Table 3). For this reason, the trial of danazol was limited to women whose symptoms were cyclical. This was checked in the pre-trial period by asking them to fill in a breast pain chart, as illustrated in Fig. 3.

Placebo produced a reduction in symptoms, but danazol, a significant improvement (Fig. 4).

A fascinating hypothesis about the possible role of dietary essential fatty acids in the aetiology of these symptoms led to a placebo-controlled trial of oil of evening primrose. The cumulative visual linear analogue results are summarised in Fig. 5,

Table 2. Tenderness and nodularity scores and prolactin levels in the non-cyclical group in late cycle: bromocriptine vs placebo

	Tenderness Mean ± SE	Nodularity Mean ± SE	Plasma prolactin Mean ± SE (mU/100 ml)
Pre-trial ($n=8$)	2.01 ± 0.09	1.63 ± 0.21	20.7 ± 2.9
Placebo ($n=10$)	1.95 ± 0.12	1.58 ± 0.13	17.5 ± 2.3
Bromocriptine ($n=13$)	1.76 ± 0.13	1.24 ± 0.19	19.6 ± 5.9
Bromocriptine vs placebo	n.s.*	n.s.*	n.s.**

*Wilcoxon's signed rank test
**Student's t test

Table 3. Cyclical pain group: linear analogue results. Numbers of patients favouring either treatment

Breast symptoms	Better on bromocriptine	Better on placebo	No change
Pain	14*	2	5
Heaviness	16*	4	1
Tenderness	18*	1	2
Soreness	14*	5	2
Interference with sex life	12*	0	1 (8 not sexually active)

*Wilcoxon's signed rank test

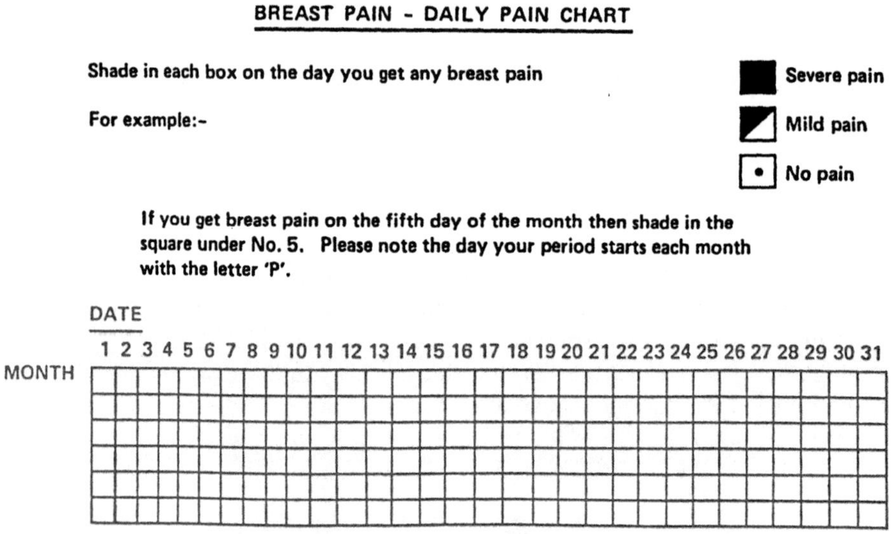
BREAST PAIN - DAILY PAIN CHART

Shade in each box on the day you get any breast pain

For example:-

Severe pain

Mild pain

No pain

If you get breast pain on the fifth day of the month then shade in the square under No. 5. Please note the day your period starts each month with the letter 'P'.

DATE

1 2 3 4 5 6 7 8 9 10 11 12 13 14 15 16 17 18 19 20 21 22 23 24 25 26 27 28 29 30 31

MONTH

Fig. 3. Chart for determining pattern of mastalgia before medical treatment

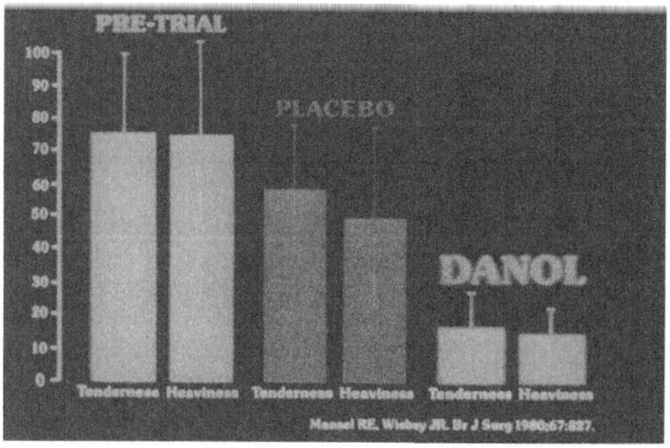

Fig. 4. Responses in danazol trial for tenderness and heaviness

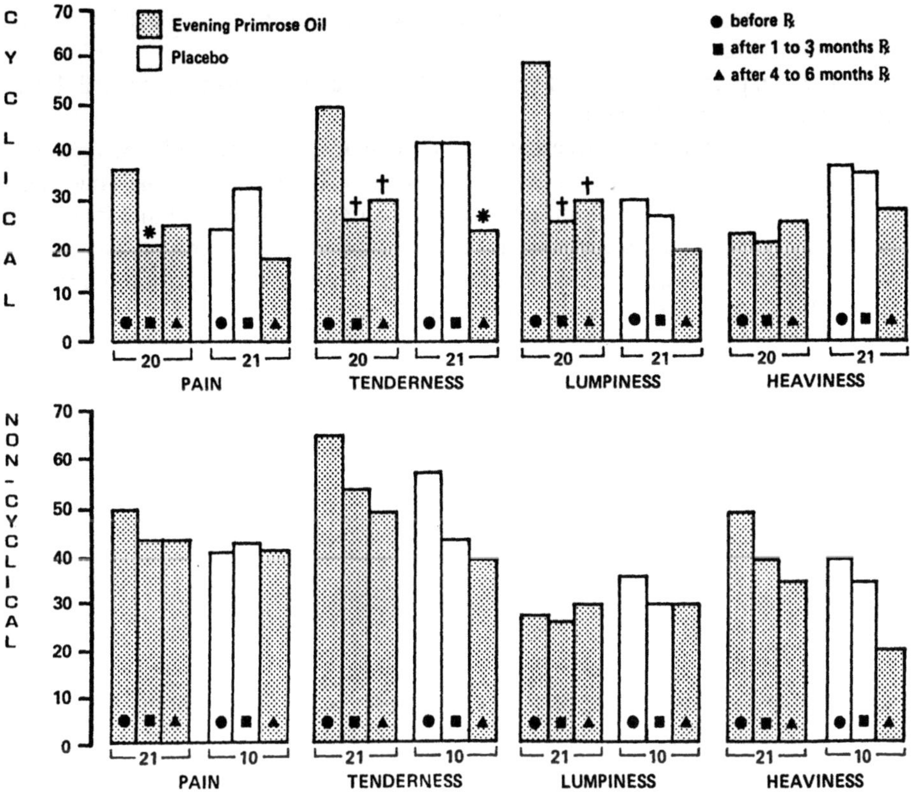

Fig. 5. Evening primrose oil: visual linear analogue results for 72 patients with mastalgia

Table 4a. Trial of evening primrose oil (Efamol) for painful lumpy breasts: Palpable nodularity in patients with cyclical symptoms after 3 months treatment

Score	I	II	III		Score	I	II	III	
Pretreatment	4	10	6	20	Pretreatment	8	10	3	21
After 3/12 Efamol	9	10	1	20	After 3/12 placebo	11	7	3	21
	13	20	7			19	17	6	
	$p < 0.025$					n.s.			

Table 4b. Trial of evening primrose oil for painful lumpy breasts: Palpable tenderness in patients with non-cyclical symptoms after 3 months treatment

Score	I	II	III		Score	I	II	III	
Pretreatment	1	12	8	21	Pretreatment	3	6	1	10
After 3/12 Efamol	7	10	4	21	After 3/12 placebo	4	2	4	10
	8	22	12			7	8	5	
	$p < 0.025$					n.s.			

I, none; II, some; III, marked
Analysed by X^2 for trend

which shows that again significant benefit occurred for those with cyclical symptoms, but not for the others.

Table 4 expresses the same results for the clinicians assessment of nodularity and tenderness on palpation.

Finally, since two of the three agents which can be regarded as influencing breast symptoms by hormonal means have no effect on non-cyclical symptoms, how might such symptoms be treated? Although no trial has been completed of this, it appears that anti-inflammatory drugs, such as non-steroidal anti-inflammatory agents, are helpful in relieving pain from periductal mastitis, although for the other symptoms caused by this condition, the only treatment is surgery.

In Situ Carcinoma of the Female Breast: Frequency, Growth Pattern and Biologic Significance

J.A. ANDERSEN, J.M. NIELSEN, G.L. OTTESEN, and J.L. THOMSEN

Carcinoma in situ is an essential stage in the natural history of breast cancer. Knowledge of its incidence and growth pattern contributes considerably to better explanation of findings in the individual patient and also improves the teamwork between surgeons, radiologists, and pathologists. Furthermore, the almost disregarded growth patterns of carcinoma in situ are probably related to differences in tumor biology.

Present knowledge of the biologic significance of lobular carcinoma in situ (LCIS) and ductal carcinoma in situ (DCIS) has been derived only from retrospective studies and is insufficient, especially with regard to the ductal type. Consequently, prospective trials are extremely difficult to plan. Progress in breast-preserving treatment will therefore be slow – progressing step by step for a long time to come. It is our intention to review current knowledge of the incidence, growth pattern, and biologic significance of carcinoma in situ, on the basis of literature and our own ongoing studies.

Frequency

In old surgical materials representing women who were more or less self-selected, the reported frequency of carcinoma in situ was about 4% that of invasive carcinoma (IC) [6,33]. LCIS predominated, and the ratio between LCIS and DCIS was 3:1, the reverse of the ratio between the IC types. The high reported frequency of LCIS has been explained as being due to its minor biologic significance, and to the very short in situ stage that the ductal type was presumed to have [33]. These explanations completely lack supportive evidence.

The frequency of carcinoma in situ reported in old surgical materials is primarily dependent on the degree of scrutiny applied in histopathologic investigation [22], especially with respect to the microfocal type. Palpable tumor-forming carcinomas in situ generally selected themselves for discovery. Furthermore, after the beautiful presentation of FOOTE and STEWART in 1947 [15], very small LCIS lesions were accepted as real carcinomas in situ, whereas minimal mastopathic lesions of the ductal type were not. They were probably mostly overlooked or misinterpreted as benign or atypical lesions because of their small size and innocent nuclear appearance, which were very different characteristics from those of the well known carcinomas. These factors most likely explain the ratio between LCIS and DCIS found in old surgical materials.

In the 1960s and 1970s, the introduction of mammography changed the situation completely, especially in connection with screening for IC. The reported incidence of carcinoma in situ increased by a factor of 3–4 or even 6, this being related to the number of screenings. Mammography also changed the recognized ratio between LCIS and DCIS to 1:3, due to the fact that microcalcification and abnormal density, which mammography demonstrates, characterizes DCIS rather than LCIS [7,24].

It is generally accepted that IC passes through either a short, or more often a long, in situ stage. The frequency of carcinoma in situ (4%–25% of ICs, which would correspond to only 0.3%–2% in all women) is certainly not in agreement with the fact that about 8% of all women develop IC [11]. From this it may be deduced that surgeons and radiologists only discover a very small and selected proportion of carcinomas in situ, and that most in situ lesions are not palpable and also lack significant microcalcification. They are simply occult lesions which presently can be discovered only by very careful histopathologic investigation. When we started our autopsy studies, we assumed that most carcinomas in situ were very small, probably 5 mm or less. The frequency of carcinoma in situ would have to be higher than the frequency of IC (8%), most likely being about 25% in all women. This very high incidence was assumed on the basis of current knowledge of the biologic significance of carcinoma in situ, which indicated that less than one-third of women with biopsy-treated carcinoma in situ later develop IC. Consequently, the frequency of carcinoma in situ would be approximately the frequency of IC at all ages (i.e., about 8%) multiplied by a factor of 3.

We have performed three autopsy studies. Two were intended to represent the general female population [26,27], and one represented women with clinical carcinoma [25].

The two groups representing the general female population were 83 elderly women who had died in a general hospital and 110 unselected forensic autopsy cases. The third group consisted of 84 unselected women who had been treated for clinical IC. At autopsy, total mastectomy was performed in all groups, bilaterally in the first two groups, and unilaterally (on the contralateral side) in the women treated for IC. All breast tissue was sliced, embedded in paraffin, and stained for histologic examination. More than 100 000 tissue blocks were prepared.

In the groups representing the general female population, we found that among the elderly women (Table 1) exactly 25% had or had had carcinoma in situ, and most cases were first discovered by the extensive autopsy investigation [26]. Among the

Table 1. Lifelong cumulative occurrence of breast carcinoma in 83 women

IC	7[a]
DCIS	8
LCIS	3
DCIS, LCIS	3
Total	21 (25%)

IC, invasive carcinoma; DCIS, duntal carcinoma in situ; LCIS, lobular carcinoma in situ
[a]Of these, six were diagnosed prior to death

younger women, the frequency of carcinoma in situ was 20%, but this was age-dependent. Among women less than 40 years of age, the frequency was only 5%, whereas it was 37% for women 40–55 years of age [27]. In all, the frequency of carcinoma in situ in the general female population was very high, and most appeared after the age of 40 years, i.e., 15–20 years before the mean age at which IC appeared clinically. The ratio between LCIS and DCIS was 1:4, in agreement with both mammography findings and the known ratio between lobular and ductal IC. Among the 84 women with clinical cancer, 33% had a new IC in the contralateral breast. A further 34% had only carcinoma in situ, predominantly DCIS [25].

Growth Pattern

A few years ago we presented our initial investigations of the growth pattern of carcinoma in situ [1,2]. We distinguished between three patterns of growth: microfocal, tumor-forming, and diffuse. The microfocal type is a very small lesion less than 5 mm in largest diameter, and usually less than 1 mm (Fig. 1). Microfocal lesions occupy one or a few lobules, and therefore are first discovered by careful histologic investigation. Few cases have altered density and/or sufficient micro-calcification for mammographic demonstration. In the clinical situation, the microfocal type is predominantly discovered in biopsy material removed from benign lesions, such as fibroadenoma, papilloma, and fibrocystic disease.

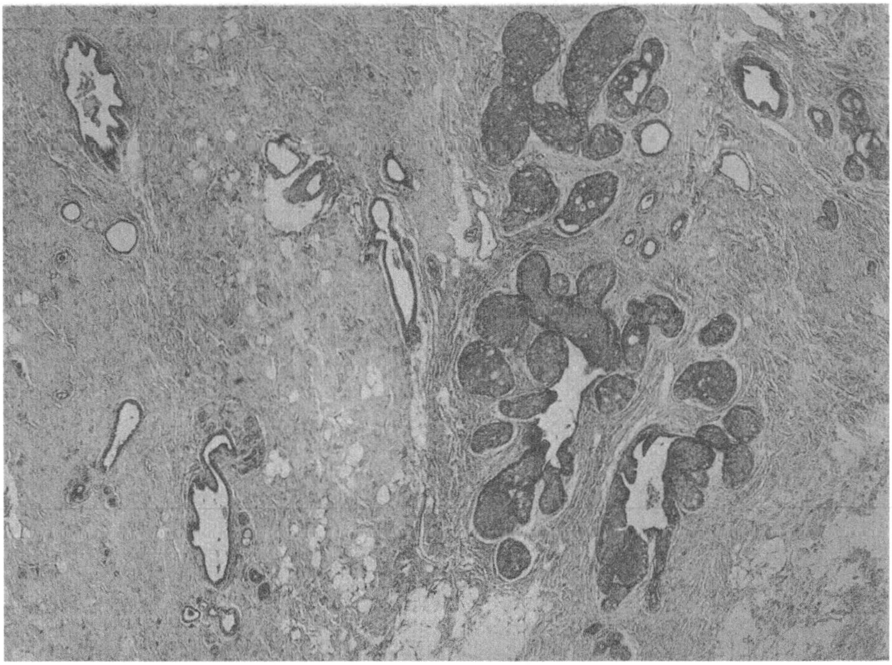

Fig. 1. Typical microfocal ductal carcinoma in situ found only in two lobules. The largest diameter was 2 mm. Haematoxylin-eosin (H-E) × 46

The tumor-forming type is a more or less circumscribed tumor which is usually diagnosed on clinical examination and/or mammography.

The diffuse growth pattern, in contrast, consists of dispersed in situ lesions within a small or often a large, segmental, part of the breast. It has no abnormalities of density, but very often shows typical casts and branching calcification, which are recognized easily on mammography. A few cases are discovered because of bleeding from the nipple. Combinations of the growth patterns are very common: the tumor-forming types, particularly, may be surrounded by diffuse carcinoma in situ (Fig. 2). Figure 3 summarizes these growth-pattern types. We have found the establishment of growth-pattern types essential for collaboration between the surgeon, the radiologist, and the pathologist, because they explain why some lesions go unrecognized despite clinical examination or mammography. They are also valuable in planning treatment [1] and probably also reflect differences in tumor biology.

All our autopsy cases of in situ carcinoma in the two groups representing the general female population were of the microfocal type [26,27]. A few cases of clinical IC had in situ lesions of the diffuse type [25]. In contrast, among mammography-selected clinical cases (Table 2), nearly one-third had tumor-forming and/or diffuse in situ lesions, but in the microfocal type still predominated [1]. This classification of growth patterns is most useful for DCIS lesions, simply because most LCIS lesions are microfocal [1].

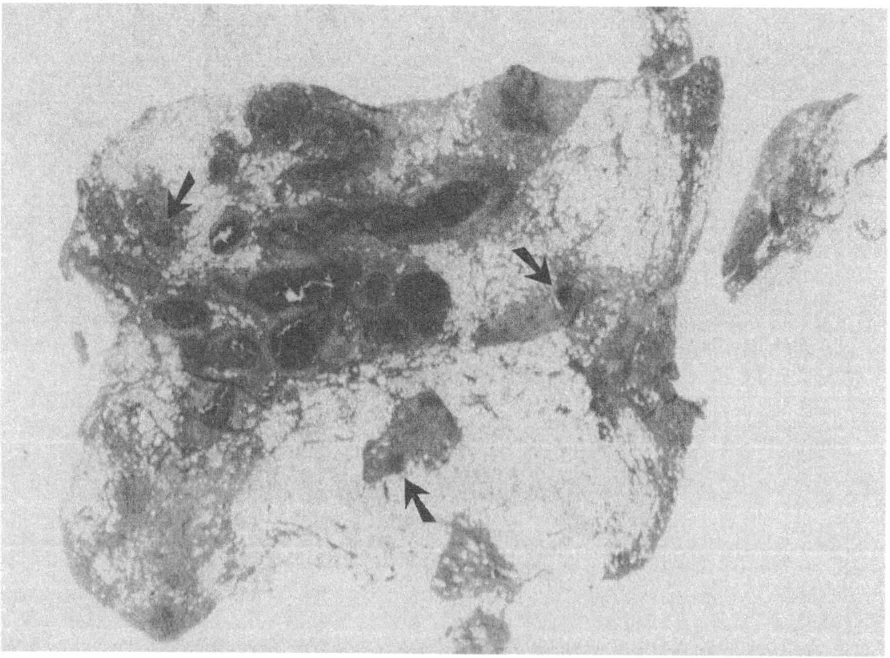

Fig. 2. Combined tumor-forming and diffuse growth pattern. On the *left* is a tumor with a diameter of about 10 mm. Some of the diffuse lesions are marked by *arrows*. H-E × 7

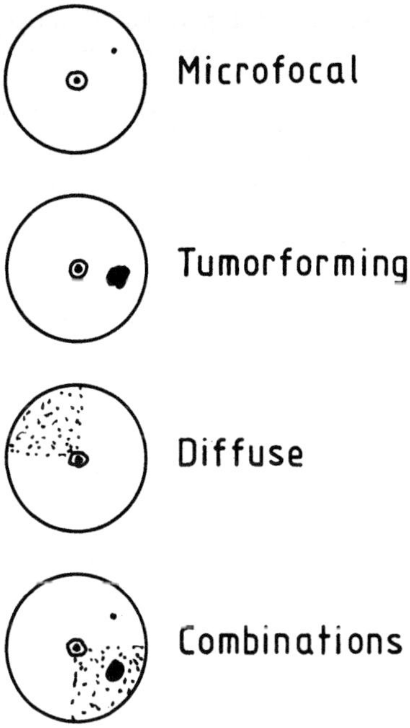

Fig. 3. Growth-pattern types of carcinoma in situ; at the *top*, the microfocal type appears as a *dot* representing lesions of often 1 mm or less. Below this can be seen the tumor-forming and the diffuse, mostly segmental, types. *At the bottom*, the frequent combinations of the growth-pattern types are shown

Table 2. Type and growth pattern of 40 mammography-selected carcinomas in situ

Growth pattern	Type LCIS	DCIS
Microfocal	13	11
Tumor-forming	–	6
Diffuse	–	3
Tumor-forming and diffuse	–	7

Biologic Significance

A vital aspect of carcinoma in situ, its biologic significance, has been evaluated in retrospective studies only, but a few prospective trials are in progress. We will have to wait more than 10 or even 20 years for results. Meanwhile, we are dependent on retrospective studies for planning of prospective trials and therefore certainly need new investigations.

Knowledge of the biologic significance of LCIS is summarized in Tables 3 and 4. These three histologically comparable sets of data [5,18,32] indicate that about 25% of LCIS cases treated only by biopsy develop into IC, with approximately equal frequency in both breasts. In 1980, death from metastatic disease was proven in only 7% of all the cases studied during a very long follow-up period.

Table 3. Development of IC among biopsy-treated cases of LCIS (1980)

	No. of patients	Invasive carcinoma	Average follow up (years)
Rosen et al. [32]	99	32	24
Haagensen et al. [18]	211	36	13
Andersen [5]	52	17	25[a]
Total	362	85(23%)	

[a] Average follow-up for women alive without IC

Table 4. Development of invasive carcinoma among 362 cases of LCIS treated only by biopsy, related to side of appearance

Ipsilateral	Contralateral	Bilateral
37	27	12

Previous Danish surgical records [4] were even reevaluated by (for practical purposes) lifelong follow-up. More than half of the women had died, and the mean age of the women still alive was more than 76 years. This study showed that the risk of both later development of IC and death from metastatic disease is increased by a factor of 4 compared with the general female population. With lifelong follow-up, IC was shown to develop significantly more frequently in the ipsilateral than in the contralateral breast.

Knowledge of the biologic significance of LCIS is therefore sufficient for the planning of prospective trials. We recommend careful continuous follow-up only. However, if for some reason a woman prefers surgery to lifelong follow-up, we advocate the treatment recommended by the Memorial Sloan-Kettering Cancer Institute, New York, USA, [31] which is ipsilateral mastectomy with simultaneous biopsy from the upper-outer quadrant of the contralateral breast.

Knowledge about the biologic significance of DCIS is insufficient, and the literature, furthermore, extremely difficult to evaluate. Most DCIS cases are still treated by mastectomy. Many follow-up studies of mastectomy-treated cases have been published (Table 5) [8,9,13,16,23,34]. They indicate that very few recurrences develop. Furthermore, less than 1% develop IC in the contralateral breast within a follow-up period of 1–10 years or even longer. Consequently, the biologic significance of DCIS must be elucidated from cases treated only by biopsy where the ipsilateral breast is preserved for follow-up.

Table 6 shows 31 cases of selected, probably large, DCIS lesions [12,17,19,20]. They indicate that most cases develop IC in the ipsilateral breast. Studies of mastectomy specimens after biopsy-confirmed DCIS [10,21] show that about 20% have invasive foci left in the breast. Unfortunately, it is impossible from the published results to evaluate the localization of these invasive foci in relation to the

Table 5. History of breast carcinoma in 426 women treated by mastectomy for DCIS, all of whom were selected for previous or simultaneous IC

	n	Follow-up (years)	Local recurrence	Node metast.	Distant metast.	Contralateral DCIS	Breast IC
Gillis et al. [16]	36	5–15	0	1	0	NM	NM
Farrow [13]	180	5–20	2	0	4	4	6
Ashikari et al. [8]	82	1–10	0	1	1	1	3
Millis and Thynne [23]	28	2–10	2	0	1	2	—
Westbrook and Gallager [34]	64	5–25	1	1	1	5	3
Brown et al. [9]	36	1–15	0	1	0	NM	1
Total	426		5	4	7	12	13

n, no. of patients; metast., metastasis; NM, not mentioned
IC: invasive breast cancer
DCIS: ductal carcinoma in situ

Table 6. Published reports of DCIS treated only by biopsy

	n	Type	IC (%)
Dean and Geschickter [12]	8	Comedo carcinoma	75
Kiaer [19]	8	Unspecified	75
Kraus and Neubecker [20]	4	Papillary	50
Haagensen [17]	11	Papillary	73
Total	31		67

primary biopsy. Some of these cases with invasive foci could therefore be incisional biopsies of carcinomas, with predominance of carcinoma in situ. Furthermore, some of the invasive carcinomas are certainly cases with microinvasion, which may be extremely difficult to evaluate. In our experience, the figure of 20% with invasive foci is remarkably high, and new studies are needed before the result can find general acceptance.

Only three, rather large follow-up studies of DCIS cases treated only by biopsy are available (Table 7) [21,28,30]. They include smaller in situ lesions, many of which were originally unrecognized or misinterpreted. The study of ROSEN et al. is of little value, as 15 of the 30 cases were lost to follow-up. The study of LAGIOS et al. has a very short follow-up period, making conclusions impossible at present. We must wait for further follow-up results of this unique study, which includes mammography-selected cases.

We have recently collected new data [3] from 30 DCIS cases that were discovered retrospectively from 3299 consecutive biopsies from 1942 to 1961 – all were originally interpreted as benign. After approximately lifelong follow-up, the Danish Cancer Registry discovered that only eight cases (26%) later developed nine IC's, a figure in agreement with a study by PAGE et al. [28]. A few investigations are available in which women with DCIS have been treated by tumorectomy and irradiation [14,29]. The very short follow-up periods make conclusions impossible. The study of FISHER et al. [14], furthermore, is invalidated by the retrospective selection of cases from among patients with IC. Their 51 cases of tumor-forming DCIS were classified as IC on original histologic examination, but the diagnosis was reviewed to DCIS only.

Our total knowledge of the biologic significance of DCIS is inconclusive. The study of PAGE et al. [28] and our most recent study [3] may show that later

Table 7. Development of IC following DCIS treated only by biopsy

	n	IC	Average follow up (years)
Rosen et al. [30]	30	8	24
Page et al. [28]	28	7	16
Lagios et al. [21]	20	1	5

development of IC after excisional biopsy of DCIS is rather rare. These two studies speak in favor of breast-preserving treatment for DCIS, providing the patients are included in careful follow-up programs.

Conclusion

Our autopsy studies, which cannot be compared with other studies, and the follow-up studies available, seem clearly to indicate that carcinoma in situ very frequently occurs in women after the age of 40 years without causing any symptoms of cancer or breast disease at all. Most cases run a silent course, but some patients develop IC. Soundly based follow-up studies of LCIS indicate that the risks of both later development of IC and death from metastatic disease are increased by a factor of 4 compared with the risks for the general female population. The biologic significance of DCIS is still inadequately understood. Follow-up studies of mastectomy-treated patients clearly show that women with DCIS almost never develop IC in the contralateral breast. A few, rather limited, follow-up studies of patients treated with excisional biopsy show that only 25% later develop IC. Together, these studies provide a foundation for planning of trials to evaluate breast-preserving treatment, but new retrospective follow-up studies, especially of the ductal type, are still required.

References

1. Andersen JA, Blichert-Toft M, Dyreborg U (1987) In situ carcinomas of the breast: Types, growth pattern, diagnosis and treatment. Eur J Cancer Clin, 13:105–111
2. Andersen JA, Nielsen M, Christensen L (1985) New aspects of the natural history of in situ and invasive carcinoma in the female breast: Results from autopsy investigations. Verh Dtsch Ges Pathol 69:88–95
3. Andersen JA, Ottesen GL (1987) Ductal carcinoma in situ: A lifelong follow-up of 30 biopsy treated cases, (in preparation)
4. Andersen JA, Ottesen GL (1987) Lobular carcinoma in situ: Results of lifelong follow-up of 46 cases. (submitted)
5. Andersen JA (1982) Pathologie und Prognose des Carcinoma lobular in situ. In: Frischbier H-J (ed) Die Erkrankungen der weiblichen Brustdrüse. Thieme, Stuttgart, pp 54–58
6. Andersen JA, Schiødt T (1980) On the concept of carcinoma in situ of the breast. Pathol Res Pract 166:407–414
7. Andersson I (1981) Radiographic screening for breast carcinoma. II. Prognostic considerations on the basis of a short-term follow-up. Acta Radiol [Diagn] 22:227–233
8. Ashikari R, Hajdu SI, Robbins GF (1971) Intraductal carcinoma of the breast. Cancer 28:1182–1187
9. Brown PW, Silverman J, Owens E, Tabor DC, Lawrence W (1976) Intraductal "noninfiltrating" carcinoma of the breast. Arch Surg 111:1063–1067
10. Carter D, Smith AL (1977) Carcinoma in situ of the breast. Cancer 40:1189–1193
11. Danish Cancer Registry (1980) Cancer incidence in Denmark 1978, 1979 and 1980. Danish Cancer Society, Copenhagen
12. Dean L, Geschickter CF (1938) Comedo carcinoma of the breast. Arch Surg 36:225–234

13. Farrow JH (1970) Current concepts in the detection and treatment of the earliest of the early breast cancers. Cancer 25:468–477
14. Fisher ER, Sass R, Fisher B, Wickerham L, Paik SM, et al. (1986) Pathologic findings from the National Surgical Adjuvant Breast Project (protokol no 6). I. Intraductal carcinoma (DCIS). Cancer 57:197–208
15. Foote FW, Stewart FW (1941) Lobular carcinoma in situ: A rare form of mammary cancer. Am J Pathol 17:491–495
16. Gillis DA, Dockerty MB, Glagget OT (1960) Preinvasive intraductal cancer. Surg Gynecol Obstet 110:555–562
17. Haagensen CD (1971) Diseases of the breast, 2nd edn. Saunders, New York, pp 528–544, 586–590
18. Haagensen CD, Lane N, Lattes R, et al. (1978) Lobular neoplasia (so-called lobular carcinoma in situ) of the breast. Cancer 42:737–769
19. Kiaer W (1954) Relation of fibroadenomatosis ("chronic mastitis") to cancer of the breast. Munksgaard, Copenhagen
20. Kraus FT, Neubecker RD (1962) The differential diagnosis of papillary tumours of the breast. Cancer 15:444–455
21. Lagios MD, Westdahl PR, Margolin FR, Rose MR (1982) Duct carcinoma in situ: Relationship of extent of noninvasive disease to the frequency of occult invasion, multicentricity, lymph node metastases and short-term treatment failures. Cancer 50:1309–1314
22. Lambird PA, Shelley WM (1969) The spatial distribution of lobular in situ mammary carcinoma. JAMA 210:689–693
23. Millis RR, Thynne GS (1975) In situ intraduct carcinoma of the breast: A long term follow-up study. Br J Surg 62:957
24. Moskowitz M (1981) Mammographic screening: Significance of minimal breast cancers. AJR 136:735–738
25. Nielsen M, Christensen L, Andersen JA (1986) Contralateral cancerous breast lesions in women with clinical invasive breast carcinoma. Cancer 57:897–903
26. Nielsen M, Jensen J, Andersen JA (1984) Precancerous and cancerous breast lesions during lifetime and at autopsy: A study of 83 women. Cancer 54:612–615
27. Nielsen M, Thomsen JL, Primdahl S, Dyreborg U, Andersen JA (1987) Breast cancer and atypia among young and middle-aged women: A study of 110 medicolegal autopsies, (in preparation)
28. Page DL, Dupont WD, Rogers LW, Landenberger M (1982) Intraductal carcinoma of the breast: Follow-up after biopsy only. Cancer 49:751–758
29. Recht A, Danoff BS, Solin LJ, Schnitt S, Connolly J, Botnick L, Goldberg I, Goodman RL, Harris JR (1985) Intraductal carcinoma of the breast: Results of treatment with excisional biopsy and irradiation. J Clin Oncol 3:1339–1343
30. Rosen PP, Braun DW, Kinne DE (1980) The clinical significance of pre-invasive breast carcinoma. Cancer 46:919–925
31. Rosen PP, Braun DW, Lyngholm B, Urban JA, Kinne DW (1981) Lobular carcinoma in situ of the breast: Preliminary results of treatment by ipsilateral mastectomy and contralateral breast biopsy. Cancer 47:813–819
32. Rosen PP, Lieberman PH, Braun DW, Kosloff FA (1978) Lobular carcinoma in situ of the breast: Detailed analysis of 99 patients with average follow-up of 24 years. Am J Surg Pathol 2:225–251
33. Rosner D, Bedwani RN, Vana J, Baker HW, Murphy GP (1980) Noninvasive breast carcinoma: Results of a national survey by the American College of Surgeons. Ann Surg 192:139–147
34. Westbrook KO, Gallager HS (1975) Intraductal carcinoma of the breast: A comparative study. Am J Surg 130:667–670

DNA Synthesis Rate and Ploidy in Precancerous and Non-Invasive Lesions of the Breast

G. E. FEICHTER and I. A. BORN

Prognostic evaluations and classifications of mastopathic breast disease based on morphologic criteria are not completely satisfactory. Measurement of the proliferative activity of the tumor cells by means of autoradiography or by DNA flow cytometry (FCM) has proved to be of major prognostic value in human tumors and especially in breast cancer [6,8,9]. DNA aneuploidy is also of prognostic relevance [1,3] and furthermore a precious help in detection of malignancy [2].

A comparison of the advantages and shortcomings of autoradiography, DNA FCM and single-cell photometry is given in Table 1. The main advantage of FCM consists in the ability to carry out, fairly easily and at the same time, cell cycle analysis and measurement of DNA ploidy of a tumor sample.

As far as fibrocystic disease is concerned, few autoradiographic [7] or DNA FCM studies [10] are available in the literature. The present study was carried out in order to find correlations between histopathologic classes of mastopathy and the percentage of cells in the S phase and DNA ploidy. With a similar intention, 10 cases of ductal carcinoma in situ were examined by means of DNA FCM.

Table 1. Comparison of different methods for the determination of DNA content, ploidy and S phase fractions

Method	Advantages	Shortcomings
Autoradiography	Accuracy	Time-consuming examinations No information on DNA ploidy
Chromosome counting	Accuracy	Time-consuming examination No information on S phase fractions or other kinetic parameters
Flow cytometry	Rapid examination High numbers of cells Sufficient accuracy Measurement of both ploidy and S phase fractions	Measurement without visual control of the cells Admixture of non-neoplastic cells to the sample
Single-cell cytophotometry	Measurement of exactly identified cells Accuracy of the ploidy measurements, especially of small hypertetraploid subpopulations	Low numbers of cells Inaccurate quantitation of S phase fractions

Altogether, 99 tissue samples were classified into the following histopathologic groups: fibroadenoma (18), fibrocystic mastopathy without signs of proliferation (49), mastopathy with proliferation but without cellular atypia (16), proliferative mastopathy with atypia (6) and ductal carcinoma in situ (10). The results were compared with those of DNA FCM measurements of invasive breast cancer which is a part of a prospective study running since 1980 [5]. More details to this point are given in the chapters 4, 8 and 9 and KAUFMANN in this volume. The method of DNA FCM as carried out in our laboratory has been described in detail elsewhere [4]. It is based on mechanical disaggregation and digestion by pepsin, staining with diamidophenylindole (DAPI), measurement of pulses with an ICP 22 cytometric device and computer-assisted evaluation of the DNA histograms using the rectangular model and a background correction for unspecific background pulses. The final evaluation of the DNA histogram gives two independent figures which are the percentage of S phase fractions and DNA ploidy.

The results are summarized in Table 2. The percentage of S phase fractions was generally low. It increased continuously from fibroadenoma and fibrocystic mastopathy towards proliferative mastopathy with atypia ($p < 0.05$). All cases of fibroadenoma and mastopathy without proliferation had a diploid DNA distribution of the cells in the $G_{0/1}$ phase. In contrast to this, a small aneuploid peak ("irregular S phase") was found in one case of proliferative mastopathy without atypia and in four of six cases of proliferative mastopathy with atypia (Fig. 1).

Table 2. DNA ploidy and mean percentages of S phase fractions in fibroadenoma, mastopathy, ductal carcinoma in situ and invasive carcinoma of the breast

Histologic Classification	Number of cases	DNA*Ploidy Diploid		Aneuploid		S phase fractions (%; mean, SD)	
		n	(%)	*n*	(%)	1.74	(1.09)
Fibroadenoma	18	18	100	0	0	1.74	(1.09)
Fibrocystic mastopathy without proliferation	49	49	100	0	0	1.49	(0.97)
Proliferative mastopathy	16	15	93.7	1*	6.3	2.01	(0.91)
Proliferative mastopathy with atypia	6	2	33.3	4*	66.6	2.46	(0.85)
Ductal carcinoma in situ	10	4	40	6	60	5.35	(3.75)
Invasive carcinoma	300	113	37.6	187	62.4	4.83	(3.65)

*, small aneuploid peaks, e.g., subpopulations in addition to a diploid DNA stemline

The results in ductal carcinoma in situ were similar to those of invasive carcinoma. The percentages of S phase fractions were significantly higher than in mastopathy ($p < 0.01$), and in six of 10 cases a clear-cut aneuploid stemline could be identified in the histogram (Fig. 2).

In conclusion, it is probable that DNA FCM may be of value in the attempts to classify mastopathy into proliferative and non-proliferative types. Furthermore, DNA FCM may identify aneuploid cellular subpopulations, which otherwise cannot be detected by light microscopy. As known from the literature [2], aneuploidy is a strong indicator of malignancy. The identification of aneuploid sub-

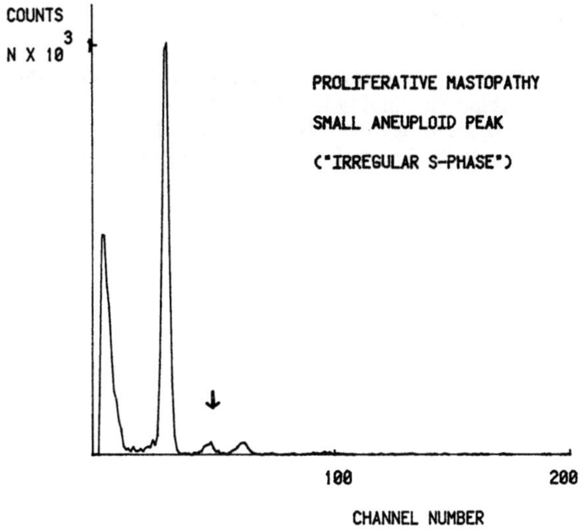

Fig. 1. DNA histogram obtained from proliferative mastopathy; diploid main peak and additionally a small aneuploid peak indicating the existence of a small aneuploid subpopulation (coefficient of variation 3.75%)

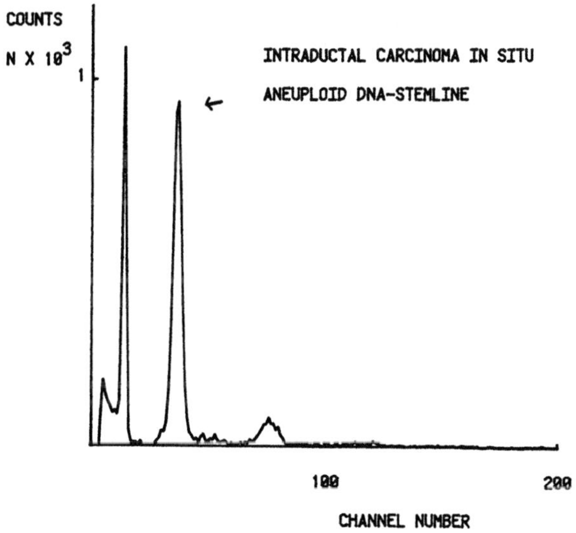

Fig. 2. DNA histogram obtained from intraductal carcinoma in situ: clear-cut aneuploidDNA stemline with a DNA index of 2.6, and 6.4% S phase fractions (coefficient of variation 4.04%)

populations could lead to classification of these lesions as precancerous states. Similar observations have been published by UCCELLI et al. [10]. Further DNA FCM studies on larger groups of proliferative mastopathy with and without atypia, including follow-up data, should be carried out.

References

1. Auer GU, Caspersson TO, Wallgren AS (1980) DNA content and survival in mammary carcinoma. Anal Quant Cytol 2:161–165
2. Barlogie B, Raber MN, Schumann J, Johnson TS, Drewinko B, Swartzendruber DE, Göhde W, Andreeff M, Freireich EJ (1983) Flow cytometry in clinical cancer research. Cancer Res 43:3982–3997
3. Coulson PB, Thorntwaite JT, Woolley TW, Sugarbaker EV, Seckinger D (1984) Prognostic indicators including DNA histogram type, receptor content, and staging related to human breast cancer patient survival. Cancer Res 44:4187–4196
4. Feichter GE, Kühn W, Czernobilsky B, Müller A, Heep J, Abel U, Haag D, et al. (1985) DNA flow cytometry of ovarian tumors with correlation to histopathology. Int J Gynecol Pathol 4:336–345
5. Feichter GE, Müller A, Kaufmann, M, Haag D, Born I, Kubli F, Goerttler K (1985) DNA-Ploidy, DNA synthesis, histological grading, stage and steroid receptor content of breast cancer. Verh Dtsch Ges Pathol 69:143–144
6. McDivitt RW, Stone KR, Craig B, Palmer JO, Meyer JS, Bauer WC (1986) A proposed classification of breast cancer based on kinetic information derived from a comparison of risk factors in 168 primary operable breast cancers. Cancer 57:269–276
7. Meyer JS, Connor RE (1982) Cell proliferation in fibrocystic disease and postmenopausal breast ducts measured by thymidine labeling. Cancer 50:746–751
8. Meyer JS, Lee Y (1980) Relationships of S-phase fraction of breast carcinoma in relapse to duration of remission, estrogen receptor content, therapeutic responsiveness, and duration of survival. Cancer Res 40:1890–1896
9. Tubiana M, Pejovic MH, Chavaudra N, Contesso G, Malaise EP (1984) The long term prognostic significance of the thymidine labeling index in breast cancer. Int J Cancer 33:441–445
10. Uccelli R, Calugi A, Forte D, Mauro F, Polonio-Balbi P, Vecchione A, Vizzone A, de Vita R (1986) Flow cytometrically determined DNA content of breast carcinoma and benign lesions: correlations with histopathological parameters. Tumori 72:171–177

Pathoanatomical Findings in Subcutaneous Mastectomy Specimens Referred to the Indications for Surgery

A. Müller

Subcutaneous mastectomy (SCM) is the subject of some controversy in the literature. While some authors deny that this operation is ever indicated [12, 14] others maintain that it is worthwhile from the aspects of prophylaxis [16] and diagnosis [11]. Owing to the relatively short follow-up periods so far, it is not yet possible to make any precise statement on the prophylactic value, i.e., the level of certainty that the operation can prevent the development of invasive carcinomas. The diagnostic value of the operation, in contrast, can be assessed from the frequency with which examination of SCM specimens reveals carcinomas that were not detectable by clinical and radiological examination. The pathoanatomical findings depend on the reason for the operation, the surgical technique and the intensity of the histological examination [10]. With the intention of making it possible to assess the influence of the indications adopted for the operation, we examined SCM specimens taken from the 250 patients who underwent comparably radical surgery at the University Hospital for Women in Heidelberg between 1978 and 1987. During this period the surgical specimens were uniformly prepared by the same histopathological technique, which was more elaborate and thorough than those normally used.

Patients and Methods

The study concerns SCM specimens from 250 patients who underwent surgery at the University Hospital for Women in Heidelberg from 1978 to 1987. The age range was 24–65 years (mean 46 years). We divided the patients into three groups, depending on the reasons for operation.

Group I. This group consisted of 111 patients who had undergone SCM because of problems with diagnosis by means of clinical or radiological examination. Problems with clinical diagnosis were the main source of difficulty in 33 patients, problems with radiological diagnosis, in 13 patients (Table 1). There were seven patients who already had had four or more biopsy specimens taken, all of which had been found to indicate benign conditions. In the remaining 58 patients in this group there were problems with both clinical and radiological diagnosis. Among these 58 women, 21 (36%) were known to have a genetic predisposition to carcinoma of the breast.

Table 1. Indications for subcutaneous mastectomy ($n=250$)

Group	Indication		No. of patients
Group I ($n=111$)	Diagnostic problems	Clinical only	33
		Radiological only	13
		Clinical and radiological	58
	More than four biopsies		7
Group II ($n=41$)	Invasive carcinoma of contralateral breast		41
Group III ($n=98$)	Proliferating fibrocystic disease with epithelial atypia		30
	Carcinoma lobulare in situ		28
	Carcinoma ductale in situ		40

Group II. All 41 patients in this group had already undergone ablation of the contralateral breast for invasive carcinoma. If there were problems with clinical or radiological diagnosis in the remaining breast in addition, SCM was carried out during the same operative session as the reconstruction on the contralateral side. In this group there were 10 women who had a genetic predisposition to carcinoma of the breast.

Group III. All 98 patients in this group underwent SCM because of pathoanatomical findings documented by biopsy. In 30 patients (11 with a genetic predisposition to carcinoma of the breast) proliferative fibrocystic disease with epithelial atypia was present. In a total of 28 cases (including four patients with a genetic predisposition) carcinoma lobulare in situ (CLIS) had been diagnosed before the performance of SCM. The SCM was carried out because of histologically documented carcinoma ductale in situ (CDIS) in 40 patients (nine with genetic predisposition).

Techniques Applied in Histopathological Examination

The surgical specimens were fixed in 4% formalin and then cut and laminated into 2.5-mm-thick slices. These lamellae were X-rayed. The tissue slices were subjected to full histological examination, except for a few tissue regions that obviously contained fat. Documentation of the tissue block removed on the X-ray pictures of the specimens made retrospective topographic allocation of the pathoanatomical findings possible. We have described the preparation technique in detail elsewhere [10].

Results

Group I

Among the total of 46 patients in whom there were problems exclusively with the clinical or exclusively with the radiological diagnosis, on examination of the SCM specimens only one was found to have non-invasive lobular carcinoma and one, proliferative fibrocystic disease with epithelial atypia. Among the cases in which both clinical and radiological diagnosis was problematic (58 patients), in contrast, we found occult invasive carcinoma in 4 (6.9%) and occult non-invasive carcinoma in eight (14%). In a further 15% of the patients in this subgroup we found fibrocystic disease with atypical epithelial proliferation (Table 2).

Among the 21 patients in whom clinical and radiological diagnosis was problematic and a genetic predisposition to carcinoma was present, when all the pathoanatomical findings were taken into account we diagnosed non-invasive carcinoma in five cases and proliferative fibrocystic disease with epithelial atypia in six cases. The four instances of invasive carcinoma were also all discovered in patients with a genetic predisposition (Table 7).

Table 2. Histological findings in subcutaneous mastectomy specimens from patients selected on basis of clinical *and* radiological diagnostic problems

Histological findings[a]	Patients *n*	Patients %	
Proliferating fibrocystic disease with epithelial atypia	9	15.5	36.2%
Carcinoma lobulare in situ	5	8.6	
Carcinoma ductale in situ	3	5.2	
Invasive carcinoma	4	6.9	
Proliferating fibrocystic disease without epithelial atypia, fibrosis, fibroadenoma, adenosclerosis	37	63.8%	
Total	58	100%	

[a]The case of any patient in whom more than one kind of pathologic change was observed is classed under the more/most serious diagnosis; for example, a patient with invasive carcinoma and concomitant CLIS is entered only under invasive carcinoma

Group II

Among the 41 patients known to have had invasive carcinoma of the contralateral breast we found occult invasive carcinoma in four patients' SCM specimens, CLIS in three and CDIS in one. Proliferative fibrocystic disease with epithelial atypia (Table 3) was found in two cases. Among the 10 women in this group who had a genetic predisposition to carcinoma of the breast, three were found to have invasive carcinoma and three each to have non-invasive carcinoma and proliferative fibrocystic disease with epithelial atypia. Among the remaining 31 patients we found only one case of invasive and three of non-invasive carcinoma (Table 7).

Table 3. Histological findings in subcutaneous mastectomy specimens from patients in whom SCM was performed together with reconstruction following ablation of the other breast

Histological findings[a]	Patients *n*	Patients %	
Proliferating fibrocystic disease with epithelial atypia	2	4.9	24,4%
Carcinoma lobulare in situ	3	7.3	
Carcinoma ductale in situ	1	2.4	
Invasive carcinoma	4	9.8	
Fibrocystic disease without epithelial atypia, fibrosis, fibroadenoma, adenosclerosis	31	75.6%	
Total 41		100%	

[a]See footnote to Table 2

Group III

Among the 30 patients in whom fibrocystic disease with epithelial atypia had already been histologically confirmed in one breast, four were found to have invasive and a further four, non-invasive, carcinoma in the same breast. In a further nine patients there were additional focuses of disease with atypical proliferative fibrocystic disease. Examination of the contralateral breast revealed fibrocystic disease with epithelial atypia in eight women and non-invasive carcinoma in two. In all, then, carcinoma or premalignant lesions were found in the contralateral breast in 33% of these patients and in the same breast in 57% (Table 4). Among the 11 patients in this subgroup who had a genetic predisposition to carcinoma of the

Table 4. Histological findings in ipsilateral and contralateral mastectomy specimens from patients operated on because of proliferating fibrocystic disease with epithelial atypia confirmed by biopsy

Histological findings[a]	Ipsilateral *n*	Ipsilateral %		Contralateral *n*	Contralateral %	
Proliferating fibrocystic disease with epithelial atypia	9	30	57%	8	27	33%
Carcinoma lobulare in situ	2	7		1	3	
Carcinoma ductale in situ	2	7		1	3	
Invasive carcinoma	4	13		–	–	
Fibrocystic disease without epithelial atypia, fibrosis, fibroadenoma, adenosclerosis	13	43%		20	67%	
Total	30	100%		30	100%	

[a]See footnote to Table 2

breast, when all the pathoanatomical findings were taken into account we diagnosed invasive carcinoma in two and non-invasive carcinoma in five. The SCM specimens from six of the 11 genetically predisposed patients were found to contain areas of fibrocystic disease with epithelial atypia (Table 7). Among the 28 patients with histologically confirmed CLIS in one breast the same breast was found to be affected by non-invasive carcinoma in seven patients and by invasive carcinoma in one patient. A further three patients had fibrocystic disease with epithelial atypia. Non-invasive carcinoma of the contralateral breast was found in seven of these patients and fibrocystic disease of the contralateral breast with epithelial atypia in three. In all, then, 39% of the patients were found to have carcinoma or premalignant lesions in the same breast and 36%, in the contralateral breast (Table 5).

We found evidence of fibrocystic disease with epithelial atypia in the SCM specimens from all four patients with previously confirmed CLIS and a genetic predisposition to carcinoma of the breast. In two of these women non-invasive carcinoma was discovered in addition. Among the remaining 24 patients we found invasive carcinoma in only one and non-invasive carcinoma in six (Table 7).

Table 5. Histological findings in ipsilateral and contralateral mastectomy specimens from patients operated on because of previously confirmed non-invasive lobular carcinoma

Histological findings[a]	Ipsilateral *n*	Ipsilateral %		Contralateral *n*	Contralateral %	
Proliferating fibrocystic disease with epithelial atypia	3	11	39%	3	11	36%
Carcinoma lobulare in situ	3	11		1	3	
Carcinoma ductale in situ	4	14		6	22	
Invasive carcinoma	1	3		–	–	
Fibrocystic disease without epithelial atypia, fibrosis, fibroadenoma, adenosclerosis	17	61%		18	64%	
Total	28	100%		28	100%	

[a]See footnote to Table 2

In 40 cases, SCM was performed because non-invasive intraductal carcinoma was confirmed by biopsy. We found invasive carcinoma in the ipsilateral SCM specimens from six of these patients and non-invasive carcinoma in those from 17. Ipsilateral fibrocystic disease with epithelial atypia was present in four patients. Examination of SCM specimens from these patients' contralateral breasts revealed invasive carcinoma in two, non-invasive carcinoma in 10, and fibrocystic disease with epithelial atypia in seven patients. Overall, then, carcinoma or premalignant disease was present in the SCM specimen in the same breast in 67.5% of cases and in the contralateral breast in 47.5% of cases following biopsy confirming CDIS (Table 6).

Table 6. Histological findings in ipsilateral and contralateral subcutaneous mastectomy specimens from patients operated on because of noninvasive ductal carcinoma previously confirmed by biopsy

Histological findings[a]	Ipsilateral *n*	Ipsilateral %		Contralateral *n*	Contralateral %	
Proliferating fibrocystic disease with epithelial atypia	4	10	67.5%	7	17.5	77.5%
Carcinoma lobulare in situ	2	5		1	2.5	
Carcinoma ductale in situ	15	37.5		9	22.5	
Invasive carcinoma	6	15		2	5.0	
Fibrocystic disease without epithelial atypia, fibrosis, fibroadenoma, adenosclerosis	13	32.5%		21	52.5%	
Total	40	100%		40	100%	

[a]See footnote to Table 2

Among the nine patients in this subgroup who had a genetic predisposition to carcinoma of the breast, when all the pathoanatomical findings were taken into account we diagnosed invasive carcinoma in two and non-invasive carcinoma in seven. Among the patients who did not have any genetic predisposition, invasive carcinoma was found in six cases and non-invasive carcinoma in 13 (Table 7).

Discussion

After SCM, cosmetically satisfactory results are obtained in only about two-thirds of cases [8,9]. In addition, there is very often a loss of sensitivity in the area of the nipple and the skin of the breast. Critics of SCM also point out that even with the best surgical techniques, only about 90%–95% of the mammary gland tissue can be removed [3] – a fact that increases in significance especially when premalignant or preinvasive changes are being treated.

We would certainly not do justice to patients' individual situations if SCM were completely rejected because of these problems. On the other hand, however, it is necessary to apply strict standards in checking whether SCM is indicated, in order to keep the number of operations subsequently recognized as unnecessary as low as possible. At present, the number of cases of clinically and radiologically undetected premalignant disease and non-invasive/invasive carcinoma revealed by SCM is the only measure of whether this intervention should be performed as a matter of urgency. Among the 111 patients in our study group who underwent SCM because there were problems with the diagnosis, the number in whom this applied was only 23 (20%). This result underscores the fact that SCM should be used as a method of diagnosis only with serious reservations. When there are problems with both

Table 7. Histological findings[a] in subcutaneous mastectomy specimens, referred to the indications for SCM and the genetic predisposition to carcinoma of the breast in each case ($n = 197$)[b]

Indications	Genetic predisposition	Occult invasive carcinoma		Noninvasive carcinoma		Proliferating fibrocystic disease with epithelial atypia		Other, benign, findings	
Problems with clinical and radiological diagnosis $n=58$	Yes ($n=21$)	4	19%	5	24%	6	28%	11	52%
	No ($n=37$)	0	0	5	14%	6	16%	27	73%
Carcinoma of contralateral breast $n=41$	Yes ($n=10$)	3	30%	3	30%	3	30%	5	50%
	No ($n=31$)	1	3%	3	10%	2	6%	26	84%
Proliferating fibrocystic disease with epithelial atypia $n=30$	Yes ($n=11$)	2	20%	5	40%	6	50%	2	18%
	No ($n=19$)	2	10%	1	5%	8	42%	10	53%
Carcinoma lobulare in situ $n=28$	Yes ($n=4$)	–	(0%)	2	(50%)	4	(100%)	0	(0%)
	No ($n=24$)	1	4%	6	25%	2	8%	16	67%
Carcinoma ductale in situ $n=40$	Yes ($n=9$)	2	(22%)	7	(77%)	6	(66%)	2	(22%)
	No ($n=31$)	6	19%	13	42%	6	19%	9	29%
Totals		21	11%	50	25%	49	25%	108	55%

[a]In contrast to the classification method used in the previous tables, in this one, if several pathoanatomical findings were observed in any one SCM specimen they have all been entered, except for the nonmalignant findings e.g., fibrocystic disease without epithelial atypia, fibrosis, fibroadenoma, sclerotic adenosis

clinical and radiological diagnosis and there is also a familial predisposition to carcinoma of the breast, in our opinion SCM should be performed. We found premalignant disease or invasive or preinvasive carcinoma in 48% of the patients in whom this combination prevailed. According to the studies published by ARABIN et al. [2] there is also a correlation between the number of cases in which occult carcinoma is found and the degree of dysplasia diagnosed from the preoperative X-ray. Thus, the degree of dysplasia can be used as an additional aid in deciding whether or not SCM is indicated. Among those of our patients who had contralateral invasive carcinoma and a genetic predisposition to carcinoma we found premalignant, preinvasive and invasive alterations in 50% of cases. In 70% of these patients there were radiological signs of increased risk, such as grade II or III dysplasia and correspondingly poor assessability.

DUPONT and PAGE [5] state unequivocally that the risk of invasive carcinoma after histological confirmation of proliferating fibrocystic disease with epithelial atypia is a function of genetic predisposition to carcinoma. With a corresponding risk situation, even at the point when fibrocystic disease was diagnosed we found invasive carcinoma in 20% of cases and non-invasive carcinoma in 40%. In these circumstances we feel SCM is even more urgently indicated if a fairly high-grade dysplasia is recognized on X-ray at this time, as such dysplasia could prevent the early diagnosis so essential for successful treatment of these cases of carcinoma.

The forms of therapy recommended in the literature after histological confirmation of CLIS range from closely coordinated clinical monitoring [1,7] to simple mastectomy with selective lymphadenectomy [15].

We have discovered non-invasive or invasive carcinoma after biopsy removal of CLIS in 28% of cases in the same breast and in 25% in the contralateral breast. It was not possible to check the influence of genetic predisposition in this subgroup, because of the small number of patients concerned. In view of the risk of malignant degeneration (approximately 30% within about 20 years) after histological confirmation of CLIS [15], the decision to perform SCM should be made dependent on the patient's age, the clinical and radiological assessability of the gland, and the patient's readiness to accept the risk. Following the confirmation of non-invasive ductal carcinoma by biopsy, further surgery should certainly be performed, because the risk of malignant degeneration is estimated to be higher [4]. In view of the number of cases in which we discovered invasive or non-invasive carcinoma (ipsilateral 57%, contralateral 30%), it is more appropriate to ask whether SCM constitutes an adequate therapy or whether it would not be preferable to perform a full mastectomy. The results achieved so far with segmental resection and subsequent irradiation to the residual breast [6,13] certainly need to evaluate with caution at present, bearing in mind the short follow-up periods and the long latency periods of non-invasive carcinoma. We believe that it is permissible to carry out SCM following confirmation of CDIS if the primary tumor is not too large and there is a sufficiently large distance between it and the nipple, the subcutis and the pectoral fascia. The surgical technique must allow complete removal of the glandular body as far as possible. The pathologist concerned should apply an exceptionally thorough preparation technique when processing the primary tumor and the SCM specimen, so that it will be possible not only to detect any occult carcinoma but also to construct a topographic picture of any carcinoma present.

Conclusions

There is no condition that constitutes an absolute indication for SCM. The decision as to whether or not this operation should be performed must always depend on the patient's individual situation. We are of the opinion that SCM is contraindicated when invasive carcinoma has already been confirmed and in situations where both clinical and radiological examination indicate that this should be suspected. In such cases a biopsy should first be taken and examined. Our results can only suggest situations in which the operation should be carried out as a matter of urgency. These indications include:

1. The body of the gland is difficult to monitor by clinical and radiological examination, severe dysplasia is seen on radiological examination and the patient has a genetic predisposition to carcinoma of the breast.
2. The body of the gland is difficult to monitor by clinical and radiological examination; in addition, the patient has a genetic predisposition and is also known to have carcinoma of the contralateral breast.
3. Non-invasive lobular carcinoma is present and the body of the gland is difficult to monitor; perhaps also when non-invasive lobular carcinoma is present and there is a genetic predisposition.
4. Non-invasive ductal carcinoma has been histologically confirmed and the size and site of the primary tumor are appropriate; particular care must taken in removal of the body of the gland and in the histopathological preparation of the resected tissue.

References

1. Andersen JA (1977) Lobular carcinoma in situ of the breast. Cancer 39:2597
2. Arabin B, Fournier DV, Kubli F, Müller A, Weber E (1985) Probleme und Grenzen der mammographischen Karzinomdiagnostik: Vergleich der präoperativen radiologischen Diagnosen mit dem histologischen Befund bei 335 Patientinnen mit subkutaner Mastektomie. Geburtsh. u. Frauenheilk. 45:595
3. Bohmert H (1984) Präinvasive Tumoren und Präkanzerosen der Mamma: subkutane Mastektomie und Wiederaufbauplastik. Chirurg 55:152
4. Büchels H, Thaler C, Bohmert H, (1982) Ein Beitrag zum Problem des Entartungsrisikos der Präkanzerosen, In: Brustkrebs und Brustrekonstruktion, Hrsg. von Bohmert, H., Thieme, Stuttgart
5. Dupont WD, Page DL (1985) Riskfactors for breast cancer in women with proliferative breast disease. N Engl J Med 312:146
6. Fisher ER, Sass R, Fisher B, Wickenham W, Puick SM (1986) Pathologic findings from the national surgical adjuvant breast project (protocol 6). I. Intraductal carcinoma (DCIS). Cancer 57:197–208
7. Haagensen CD, Lane M, Lathes R, Bodian C (1978) Lobular neoplasia (so-called lobular carcinoma in situ) of the breast. Cancer 42:737
8. Hirsch HA (1977) Die operative Behandlung des invasiven Mammakarzinoms. Gynäkologe 10:160
9. Kubli F, Lorenz U, Müller A (1981) Die subkutane Mastektomie. Gynäkologe 14:30
10. Müller A, Tschahargane C, Kubli F (1984) Zum Problem der subkutanen Mastektomie. Die Bedeutung der histopathologischen Aufarbeitung des Mastektomiepräparates. Dtsch Med Wochenschr 109:50

11. Ober KG (1979) Operative Behandlung der frühen Neoplasie und der frühen Karzinome der weiblichen Brust. In: Frühe Tumoren in Diagnostik und Therapie. Edited by A. Georgii, Fischer, Stuttgart
12. Olbrich RR (1981) Gibt es noch Indikationen zur subkutanen Mastektomie? Chirurg 52:467
13. Recht A, Danoff BS, Solin LJ, Schnitt S, Conolly J, Botnick L, Goldberg J, Goodman RL, Harris JR (1985) Intraductal carcinoma of the breast: Results of treatment with excisional biopsy and irradiation. J Clin Oncol 3:1339
14. Redfern AB, Hoopes JE (1978) Subcutaneous mastectomy: A Plea for conservatism Pl Reconstr Surg 62:706
15. Rosen PP, Lieberman PH, Braun DW, Kosloff C, Adair F (1978) Lobular carcinoma in situ of the breast. Am J Surg Path 2:225
16. Stegner HE (1977) Indikationen zur subkutanen Mastektomie. Arch Gynäk 224:302

Subject Index

A

Academic cancer 88, 166
Accelerator 248
Activity, mitotic 29
-, proliferative 29
Acute effects, late changes 361
Adaptation of gland 231
Adequate radiation therapy 225
Adjuvant chemotherapy 71–74, 160, 161, 163–169, 181–182, 185, 416, 419, 422, 463, 440, 442, 447–448, 456, 458, 459
--, disease free survival 290
Adjuvant endocrine therapy 182–183
Adjuvant hormone therapy 245
Adjuvant radiotherapy after mastectomy 241
Adjuvant systemic therapy 181–183
Advanced carcinomas 184 ff
Advanced stages 158–169
Afterloading 263
-, remote-controlled 267
Aggressiveness, of cancer 174
Air Kerma rate 269
Amplification, oncogene 75
Amputation 209, 210
-, with reconstruction 211
Analysis, cell cycle 43
Anaplastic tumor 24
Anatomical extension 170
A. Anderson Hospital 263
Anesthesia 197
Aneuploidy 71,171
Antibody, cytokeratin 38
-, monoclonal 31, 32, 34
Antiestrogens 19,167, 181, 245
Antiestrogen therapy 182, 183
Anxieties, patient 214
Armfunction, impaired 392
Aspiration drain 199
Asymmetry 235
Atypical epithelial hyperplasia 485
---, surgical treatment 485
Auchincloss-Madden 200
Autopsies 167
Autoradiography 43
Axilla, access to 227
-, apex 204
-, involvement 244
-, irradiation of 179, 243, 245
-, radiological clearance 179
-, surgical clearance 179
Axillary dissection 264
Axillary fatty tissue 244
Axillary lymphadenectomy 185, 198, 243
Axillary Lymph Nodes 179–180
---, groups I, II, II 179
Axillary node dissection 203–204, 207
Axillary recurrence 241, 243, 262
-, seroma 228
-, vein 202, 204, 227

B

Bardenheuer incision 195
Basel protocol new guidelines 340
Benign breast disease
---, acupuncture 500
---, alcoholic ointments 499
---, androgens 491
---, androgen treatment 500
---, bromocriptin 501
---, classification 507
---, danazol 501
---, diagnosis and classification 464–473
---, diuretics 499
---, estrogen-progestogen treatment 501
---, follicle stimulating hormone 489
---, hormonal mastopathy 508
---, hormonal treatment 500
---, luteal deficiency 489
---, luteinizing hormone 489
---, medical therapy 493
---, medical treatment 507
---, methylxanthines 500
---, non-cyclical symptoms 511
---, oestradiol 488
---, ovarian hormones 488–489
---, periductal mastitis 508
---, pituitary hormones 489
---, plant extracts 499
---, progesterone levels 489
---, progesterone treatment 500
---, progestogen treatment 501
---, prolactin 490
---, sex hormone – binding globulin 491
---, stimulated levels of prolactin 490
---, tamoxifen 501
---, tamoxifen, side effects 502
---, thyroid hormones 491
---, thyroid hormones treatment 500
---, treatment mammogram 502
---, vitamin B_1 500
---, vitamin E 500
Bilateral breast cancer 56, 59
Biological expression 170

Biologic treatment planning 271
Biologic predeterminism 163, 169
Biology of the breast 308
Biology of breast cancer 24
Biology, cell 62
Biopsy 57
-, aspiration 37
-, drill 190–191
-, fine needle 119
-, punch 190–191
Bolus material 249, 264
Boost of electrons
---, fibrosis 361
---, indurations 361
---, teleangiectasia 361
Boost radiation therapy 225, 226, 250–251
Brachial plexus damage 391
---, adjuvant chemotherapy
Breast conserving therapy 48, 50, 157, 185, 205–208, 209–217
---, advantages 283, 318
---, Basel Lumpectomy protocol 329–342
---, Berlin study 324
---, criteria 253, 278, 330
---, contraindications 282
---, comparison of results 276–283
---, extramammary complications 327
---, German breast cancer study 343–357
---, history of 1–5
---, local recurrence 278, 292–300
---, long term survival 276–283
---, maximal tumor diameter 330
---, opponents 283
---, radiotherapy in 246–261
---, retrospective studies 246, 276
---, secondary mastectomy 324
---, stages III and IV 279
---, survival 324
Breast Cancer Detection and Demonstration Project (BCDDP) 102
Breast conserving surgery 178–179, 416
Breast conserving treatment
---, long-term complications 328–342
Breast edema 306
---, extent of lymphadenectomy 326
Breast irradiation alone 246–247
Breast-preserving surgery 24
Breast-preserving therapy
---, prospective studies 247
Breast reconstruction 216, 319
Breast size 216, 231

C

Cancer risk, of mastopathy 467
Cancer of the uterine corpus, estrogen treatment for breast cancer and ovarian radiotherapy 364
Capsular contraction 183
Carcinogens 94
Carcinoma ductale in situ 477–478
Carcinoma in situ 481–488, 513–523
---, biologic significance 513, 517
---, frequency 513
---, frequency, age-dependence 515
---, growth pattern 515
---, WHO-classification 481
Carcinoma lobulare in situ 477–478, 484
Carcinoma in situ, risk of malignant degeneration 477–478
Castration 160, 161, 181, 182, 183
Cell death 97
--, dormancy 97
--, loss 101
--, replication 97
Cellular effects 271
Central location 205
Charcoal method 34
Chemotherapy 165–169
-, adjuvant endocrine and combined 437
-, with breast preservation 265
-, for patients over 50 years 289
Chemotherapy, randomized adjuvant trials 74
Chest wall, radiotherapy 185
Choice of treatment 174–187
Classification of primary tumors 310
Clavicular lymph nodes 244
Clinical examination 189
Clinical stages I 277 ff, 299
--, II 278–279
Clip 204, 227
-, at apex 265
CMF 160, 303, 225
Cobalt 248, 264
Columbia clinical classification 156
Combination radiotherapy with chemotherapy 245
Combined chemohormonal therapy 289
Complete cure 160, 165
Complications
-, duration 328
-, of breast cancer 389
Complications of breast-conserving therapy 389

Complications
-, of Surgery and irradiation 324–328
Complications, radiological 391
Cyclical breast pain 509
Computed dosimetry 267, 269
Concept of conservative treatment 226
Concomitant chemotherapy 422, 423, 430
Concomitant invasive breast cancer 56
Conservative therapy, results 282
--, local recurrences 301–307
Contact therapy, advantages 267
Contraindications 219
Contralateral adjustment 210
Contralateral breast cancer 296
Controlled studies 178, 179
Control window (ccw) 99
Cosmetic aspects of breast conserving therapy 402, 479, 420
Cosmetic complications 236, 237
Cosmetic results 178, 183, 195, 197, 199, 205, 208, 210, 211, 216, 225, 230, 340
--, adjuvant chemotherapy 410
--, booster techniques 352
--, conserving treatment 339, 319–320
--, cesium irradiation 352
--, cutaneous changes 405
--, close 350
--, external tumor boost 409
--, incision 407, 408
--, interstitial irradiation boost 409
--, irradiation 407, 409
--, one-stage or two-stage surgery 406
--, quality of radiation beam 351
--, scar formation 405, 408
--, shape of the breast 403
--, site of the tumor 406, 408
--, size of the breast 406, 407
--, time factor 411, 412
Curative therapy 171
Curie Institute 263
Curvilinear incision 231, 232, 234
Cyclophosphamide 160
Cyst 189
Cytodifferentiation 100
Cytokeratin 25
Cytokinetics 97
Cytological examination 189, 190
Cytology 163
-, of breast cancer 147
-, of fine-needle aspirate 145, 230
-, ex-foliative 146–151
-, puncture 143
Cytostatics 31

D

Dana Farber Institute 246
Décollettage 233
Defect 231, 234
Deformity 234
Delaying Chemotherapy 424
Diagnosis, cytologic 143
-, early 93
Demineralization of bone 391
Diploid 170
Disease-free survival 181, 223, 289, 316
Disease, multicentric 48, 49
Dissection
-, level I 219
-, levels I and II 219
Dissemination 174
Distant metastases 165–169, 262
DNA-index 171
DNA synthesis rate, precancerous and non-invasive lesions 523–526
Dose of chemotherapy 426, 428
Dose of Ir-implant 270
Dose rate 269
Dose-volume curve of irradiation 249
----, large breasts 250
Doubling times 108, 168–169
Drainage 202, 204, 228
-, suction 227, 228
Ductal invasive carcinoma 148
Dysplasia, radiological 466

E

Early breast cancer 158
Early detection 159, 168
Early dissemination 161
Early stromal invasion 482
Edema, of arm 327
-, in the breast 390
Effect of radiotherapy on thoracic wall 243
Efficacy of breast conserving therapy 313–322
Efficacy of irradiation 240
Electron field 264
Electrons 225, 251
Employment disability 318
Endocrinological profiles in benign breast disease 488–493
Endocrinology of benign breast disease 494
EORTC trial 225, 314, 318
--, 10801, phase III 315

Epidemiology, of breast cancer 13
Epidermal growth factor 31, 33
Epidermal growth factor receptor (EGFR) 76
Estrogens 19
-, endogenous substitution 19
-, exogenous substitution 19
Examination of tumor 207
Excision
-, adequate 219
-, under local anesthesia 300
Excisional biopsy 197, 218, 292
--, probability of local recurrence 293
Excision line 206
Exponential growth 168–169

F

Fast-growing tumors 43, 92, 163, 169
Fat-dermis flap 236, 237
Fibrocystic disease, atypia 476
--, risk of malignant degeneration 474–478
Fibrosis 318
Fibrosis of breast
---, smoking 339
Fibrosis, radiogenic 390
Fibrotic nodules 306
Fibrotic tissue formation in the breast 390
Flow cytometry 523
"Foreign body" response 216
Frozen section 200, 230
--, of dissected axilla 358

G

Galactography 194, 117
German Breast Cancer Study 342
----, cosmetic results 349
----, irradiation technique 344
----, late sequelae 349
----, patient recruitment 347
----, quality of radiation therapy 347–348
----, randomization 343
----, study design 343
Grade
-, histological 68
-, nuclear 75
Granulomas 306
Growth of breast cancer 100
Growth behavior 12, 78–79, 163–173
--, implications for staging 156–173
--, implications for treatment 156–173
Growth fraction 30, 169
Growth, Gompertzian 101
Growth of multicentric tumor 50
Growth, neoplastic 43
Growth rate 81, 86, 100–101
Growth rate of cell colony 101
Growth, very slow 170
-, very fast 171
Guide needles 267
Guy's Hospital study 178, 222–226, 262, 276, 282

H

Halsted mastectomy 2, 158, 204, 301
Halsted-Meier 313
Halsted-Rotter operation 156–176
Harvard Joint Center for Radiation Therapy 292
Hayward, thesis 259, 308
Heidelberg University Hospital 308
Hematoma 227, 228
Hematoxylin-eosin 254
--, staining 254
Hemostasis 197, 199, 227
Heterogeneity 100, 168
High dose rate 251
Histogram 43
-, DNA 44–45
Histological investigation 253–255
Homogenous irradiation of breast 248
Hormonal stimulus 167
Hormonal therapy 31, 160–161, 167, 438, 450
Hormones 19
Hostfactor 170
Host-tumor relationship 158
Humerus, fracture of 391
Hybridization 65–66
Hyperchromatism 27
Hyperpigmentation 237

I

Immune status 174
Immunological defense 174
Impairment by therapy 212
Implanted needles 271
Implants 269
-, iridium 225, 264
-, of 192-Ir wires 267, 269
-, silastic 183
Improvement in survival 160–169, 240
Inactive guide 269
Inadequate control of tumor 308

Inadequate treatment 174
Incidence 167–168
Incision, circular or radial 359
-, choice of 196
-, insufficient 250
-, of skin 201, 202
Index
-, labelling 71
-, mitotic 75
Indigo blue 193, 195
Inflammatory carcinoma 163, 171
Informed consent 316
Inoperable carcinoma 171
Intercostobrachial nerve 221
Interpectoral lymph nodes 203
Internal mammary field 264
Internal mammary nodes 264
---, irradiation of 264
---, metastases to 284, 305
Interstitial afterloading for breast-conserving therapy 267–274
Interstitial brachy-therapy 361
Interstitial iridium boosting 250, 353
Interstitial implantation 207
Interstitial irradiation 247
Interval surfacing breast cancer 103–104
Intracutaneous alignment 199
Intracystic carcinoma 151
Intraductal carcinoma 297–298, 311
--, conservative treatment 483
--, excision biopsie 482
--, latency period 483
--, local recurrence 483
--, regional lymph node metastases 482
--, therapy 482
Intraoperative processing 199
Invasion, stromal 27
Invasive carcinoma 53, 252
Invasive ductal carcinoma 32, 38
Ionization chamber 269, 272
Ionizing radiation 20
Ipsilateral carcinomas
--, new primary 301–307
--, second 304
Iridium-192 247
Irradiation
-, all fields daily 351, 361
-, dose to lymph node regions 245
-, dose to thoracic wall 245
-, techniques 248–251
Irradiation of clavicular lymph nodes 244
Irradiation of ovaries 245
Irradiation of remaining breast tissue 248
Irradiation of sternal lymph vessels 244
Isocentric stereoradiograph 267
Israelitisches Krankenheim 1

J

Joint Center for Radiation Therapy 263

K

Keloid 233
King's Cambridge trial 175

L

Labelling index 163–169, 170–171
Laminin 29
-, receptors 29
Langer's lines 195, 196, 231
Large breast 205, 226, 249
Large tumors, risk of local failure 306
Late changes, percutaneous radiation 361
Laterally placed tumors 285
Latissimus dorsi muscle 183, 202, 204, 227
Lead-time bias 163–164
Length-time bias 159, 163–164
LHRH analogs 181–182
Life expectancy 165–169
Lifting 216
Limited resection 218
Linear accelerator 264
Lobular breast cancer 27, 32
Lobular cancerization 482
Lobular invasive carcinoma 148
Local failure 252, 259
--, by type of biopsy 294–295
Local control 174, 223–224, 262
--, inadequate 209
Local excision 218
Localization 192
Local treatment failure, pathoanatomical characteristics 308–312
Loco-regional clearance 308
Loco-regional eradication 245
Loco-regional irradiation 245
Loco-regional recurrence 23, 158, 179, 282, 287, 292, 301–307, 310–312, 358, 418
--, chemotherapy 245–246

--, chemotherapy and radiotherapy 289
--, influence on survival 301, 304-305
--, risk of 304
Local recurrence rate in breast conserving treatment 336
Loco-regional recurrence free survival
---, Basel protocol 336
Loco-regional spread 158
Loco-regional treatment 158, 166, 174, 176-180
--, variations 285
Location, unfavorable 219
Long-term survival 162-169, 158-159, 282
Long thoracic nerve 202, 221, 227
Low axilla 204
Leukemia following chemotherapy and radiotherapy 364
Lumpectomy 205
Lung fibrosis 339
Lymphangiosis carcinomatosa 250, 309, 310
--, peritumoral 311
Lymphangiosarcoma 363
Lymphedema 243
-, of arm 277, 230, 393
-, axillary lymph node dissection 395-398
-, definition 393
-, number of lymphnodes 340
-, risk of 398
-, score 393
Lymph node involvement 158
--, number 179
--, status 76
--, irradiation 241
Lymphadenectomy, subradical 179
Lymphocytes 44, 65-66
Lymphoma, malignant 27

M

Macrometastases 69, 70
Macrophage 65-66
Magnification technique 133-134
Malignant potential 163
Malignant tumor 43
Malignant degeneration 311
Mammoplasty reduction 57
Mammary gland 202
Mammography 112, 122, 127, 152, 192
-, baseline 116
-, calcifications 469, 470
-, cancer risk 471
-, film 131
Manchester study 174, 241, 242
Margins, involved 219
Margin of resection 248, 250
Marital relationship 318
Marking of occult lesions 192
Marseille Cancer Institute 276, 278
Mastodynia 464
Mastopathy, diagnosis and classification 464-473
Medially located tumors 244
Medroxyprogesterone 245
Medullary carcinoma 68, 148
Megavoltage radiotherapy 276
Metastasis, spread of 94
Metastatic potential 163-169
Microcalcifications 205, 219
Micrometastases 62, 69, 70, 289
Microscopic investigation 254
Microselectron 271
Milan Cancer Institute 301
Milan study 178, 181, 224, 245, 247, 276, 302
Milk ducts 193-194
"Minimal" breast cancer 79
Minimal local surgery 225-226
Mitosis 102
-, rate 163-169
Mitotic index 250
Mitoxantrone 74
"Mix-and-match techniquc" 264
Mobilization of breast tissue 234, 235
Modified radical mastectomy 1, 57, 176-177, 185, 201-204, 202
Morphological examination 309
--, characteristics of primary tumor 310
Mortality 174, 224
Multicenter studies 315
Multicentric carcinomas 250, 48, 53, 57, 59, 61, 252-261
Multicentricity of ductal carcinoma in sity 479-480
------, family history 480
------, histological type 479
------, invasion 480
------, premenopausal women 480
------, extension 479
Multicentric subclinical lesions 248
Multicentric tumor 257-259
--, definition 256
--, development 50
--, volume after segment resection 257
Multifocal cancer 205, 311, 479
Multiple primary cancers, etiologic factors 363
Mutants 65

N

Natural folds of skin 227
Necrosis 236, 237
Nipple location 318
New primary carcinomas 305
Node-negative breast cancer 71–74
Node-positive breast cancer 71–74
Nodules, benign 464
Nolvadex 182
Noncontrolled studies 313–314
Non-infiltrating intra-ductal carcinoma, clinging type 481
---, comedo-type 481
Non-infiltrating lobular carcinoma 484
---, latency 484
---, recurrence 484
NSABP (National Surgical Adjuvant Breast Project) study 174, 181, 182, 241, 247, 251, 252, 262, 276, 278, 282, 285–291

O

Occult cancer 166–167
Oncogene 163–169
Oophorectomy 160, 182
Opponent fields 248
Orthovoltage techniques 263
Ovariectomy 181, 245
Overall survival 158–161
--, corrected 279
--, stage I-III 280–281
Overlapping fields 264
Overtreatment 186

P

Paget's disease 205, 482
Pain 318
Parasternal lymph nodes 175, 180, 185
Paris system 267
Partial mastectomy 209, 218
Partnership 213
Patey 201
Pathological secretion 465
Pathologic review 220
Patient's complaints 216
Pectoral fold 227
Pectoral muscles 179
Pectoral fascia 202
Pectoralis major muscle 183, 185, 203, 216, 227
Pectoralis minor muscle 179, 203, 227
Pendulous breasts 234, 236
Periareoar incision 195
Perimamillary incision 194
Perioperative clarification 189–199
Peritumoral intraductal tumor extensions 308
Physical appearance, acceptance of 213
Plastinated breast slice 253
Plastination 51–53, 253
Ploidy 43, 163–169
-, DNA 43
-, status 72
-, poly 89
Ploidy in precancerous and non-invasive lesions of the breast 523–526
Pneumocystography 189
Pneumonitis, radiation induced 392
Polymorphism 27
Polyploidy 250
Positioning of patient 201
Postmenopausal patients 167, 181, 182
Precancerous lesions 481–488
--, risk of malignant degeneration 474–478
Premenopausal patients 161, 167, 181, 182
Preoperative examinations 191 ff
-, irradiation 241, 244
Primary tumor 67, 78–79
--, size 306
Professional situation 214
Progesterone 19
Prolactin 19
Prognostic factors 163, 170–171, 174, 176
Progression of breast cancer 99
Proliferation rate 163–169
Prophylactic locoregional irradiation 241
Prosthesis acceptance 216
-, dislocation 216
Protein, antigenic nuclear 29
Psychological care of cancer patients 383
Psychological problems 376
--, aftercase strategy 380
--, theories of illness 382
Psychological status 318
Psychological impairment 212
Psychosocial problems 209, 210, 212–217
Pulmonary fibrosis 327
--, radiation induced 392
Puncture 189

Q

Quadrantectomy 57, 205, 218, 224, 263
Quadrant resection 252, 259
Quality of life 282, 318
QUART 301

R

Radial incision 194, 196, 197, 231, 232, 233
Radical mastectomy 204
Radiation 20
Radiation exposure 131
Radiation-induced breast cancer 371, 336
--, side effects 329
Radiation pneumonitis 339
Radiation reaction 225
Radiation of regional lymph nodes 264
Radiation techniques and cosmetic results 350–354
Radiation therapy 354
-, field junction 354
--, quality 347
Radical surgery 175
--, failure 283
Radical therapy 449, 262
Radicality 174
-, of treatment 175
-, locoregional 175
-, declining 175
Radio-insensitive tumor 226
Radiological dysplasia,
--, estradiol 494
--, progesterone 495
--, sex hormone-binding globulin 495
Radiotherapy 240–274, 416, 417, 419, 426, 430, 445
-, adjuvant 457
-, with adjuvant chemotherapy 246
-, arrangement of fields 248
-, bilateral breast cancer 364
-, insufficient 278
-, initiation of 208
-, percutaneous 446
-, concept, modified, Basel protocol 341
-, primary 418, 432
Radiotherapy in breast conserving therapy 330
---, axillary and supraclavicular lymphnodes 332
---, internal mammary lymphnodes 332
---, regional lymphnodes 331
Radiotherapy and survival 285
Radium dose 3
-, implant 240, 263
Readaptation of breast tissue 232
Receptor
-, analysis 37
-, epidermal growth factor (EGF) 31, 75
-, estrogen (ER) 31, 46, 69, 89, 289
-, estrogen status 31
-, estrogen-negative cases 34
-, immunohistochemical analysis 34
-, progesterone (PR) 69, 89, 289
-, status 24, 37
-, steroid 46
-, steroid hormone 69
Receptor content 163–169, 170–171, 182
Reconstruction 183–184, 185, 202, 209, 210, 211, 216, 235
-, of gland body 36, 360
-, gel prosthesis 210
Rectus abdominal muscle 183
Recurrence 50, 53, 174
-, axillary 305
-, circumscribed 50
-, diagnosis 311
-, distant 3
-, fear of 214
-, local 3, 50, 308, 451
-, probability of 245
-, rate 348
-, retrosternal 244
-, spatially limited 50
Recurrence after mastectomy, distant failure 298–299
Reduction mammaplasty 206, 249
Reexcision 199, 206, 219, 304
Reference dose rate 269, 271
Relapse, contralateral breast 336
-, local 75
-, pattern of first 336
-, pathologic tumour stage 336
-, postmastectomy 426
Reoccurrence 316–317
Resection line 177
Resection margins 197, 201, 263, 292, 310
Residual breast 208
Residual tumor 206, 252–261
--, after segmental resection 256, 257
--, cell 241
--, definition 256
--, primary 256–259
--, radioresistant 311
Resistance to chemotherapy 161
Response to radiotherapy 240–241

Resting cells 169
Results, short-term 184
Retraction 234, 235
Rib fractures 391
--, adjuvant chemotherapy 391
Risk
-, factors 10, 14, 67
-, group 10, 174, 182
-, of local recurrence 250, 293
-, psychological 17
-, of radiation 124
Rotter 204
Rotter's lymph nodes 203

S

Salvage mastectomy 287
Sample sizes, insufficient 315
Scandinavian trial 181
Scar 231
-, appearance 318
Scirrhous carcinoma 148
Screening 112, 159, 166, 169
-, mammography 113, 114, 115, 122
Second cancer, risk of 364
Second posttreatment decade 282
Second primaries 166
Second primary cancers associated with irradiation 363
Secondary carcinomas 181
Secondary resection 259, 312
Second decade 281
--, mortality 281
Secretions breast 146
Segmental mastectomy 218, 197
Segmental resection, simulated 254–255
Segmental tissue margins 309–319
Segmentectomy 197, 218
Sequelae, irradiation 326
-, postoperative 325
-, secondary mastectomy 326
Sequential chemotherapy 422–423
Serial mammographies 165, 170
Seroma 227
Sexual problems 318
Shieldhing of organs 248
Shoulder mobility, restricted 392
Side effects, breast-conserving therapy 389
--, radiological 391
Simultaneous radiotherapy-hormone therapy 245
Skin creases 227
-, color 318
-, dose 264
-, mobilisation 231
-, recurrences 297
Skip metastases 204
Slowly growing tumors 43, 92, 163–169
Small-to-medium breasts 226
Socioeconomic factors 17
Solid nodes 190
Sonography 117, 119
-, for benign breast diseases 468
Speed of growth 163–169
S-phase fractions 163–169, 171, 524
Spread, metastatic 78
Stage distribution
-, Basel protocol 335
Staging 170–171
--, preoperative 170
-, postoperative 170
Status, menopausal 73
Steinthal clinical classification 156, 157, 168
Sternal field 248
Stockholm study 180, 241
Subclavius muscle 204
Subclinical metastases 241
Subcutaneous alignment 199
Subcutaneous fat 197
Subcutaneous mastectomy 57, 237
--, cosmetic results 532
--, pathoanatomical findings 525
Submammary fold 210, 227
Submamillary tumor localisation 360
Superradical mastectomy 285
Supraclavicular lymph node metastases 240, 244, 305
---, irradiation of 264
Supra and infraclavicular field 248
Surgical complications 222–238
Surgical techniques 220–221
--, of breast preservation 218–221
--, definition of terms 218–219
--, less radical 259
Surgical treatment 201–207
Survival rates 158–159
--, according to first unfavorable event 305
--, according to tumour location 287
--, 20-year 279, 280
Survival, disease-free 70, 73, 75
-, long-term 1
-, recurrence free 2, 182
-, relapse-free 181, 182
Systemic disease 158–161
Systemic therapy 160

T

Tamoxifen 183
-, treatment 73, 74, 245, 289
Tangential fields 264
Target volume 248
Teleangiectasia 318
Templates 267
Therapeutic consequences 170–171
Therapeutic guidelines 184–188
Thermography 119, 188
-, cancer risk 468
Thio-TEPA 160
Thoracic wall, irradiation of 241
Thoracic wall recurrence 241, 243
Thoracodorsal nerve 202, 221
Three dimensional treatment 248
Thromboembolism 228
Time-effect correction factor 271
Tissue expander 216
-, wasting 318
Thymidine labelling 169–170
TNM Staging 157, 158, 170
Tolerance dose 271
Toxicity, short-term 181
-, long-term 181
Transposition of nipple-areola complex 236, 237
Treatment
-, adjuvant 67
-, adjuvant endocrine 436
-, combination 449
-, combined-modality 447, 451
-, palliative 67
-, regimens 446
-, time 269, 271
-, satisfaction 318
Treatment failure, local 177
Treatment side effects
-, Basel protocol 336
Trials
-, randomized clinical 314–316
-, multicenter 314, 315
-, unicenter 315
-, phase III 316
Tumor bed 227, 250
-, burden 161
-, control 263
-, diameter 82
-, diversification 64
Tumorectomy 198, 205, 218
-, bilateral 234, 235
-, and radiotherapy 246
Tumor grading 27, 89
--, II 171
--, III 171
--, Steinthal 2
Tumor growth 70, 83, 84
Tumor, histological types 226
Tumor-host relationship 174
Tumor metastasis formation 62
Tumor progression 64, 65
Tumor proliferation 70
Tumor remnants 248, 250
Tumor response 163
Tumor size 68, 113, 226, 231
Tumor-sterilizing dose 250
Tumor variants 65, 66
Tumor volume 105
Two-step procedure 200, 207

U

Underdosing 264
Undertreatment 186
Unicenter trials, disadvantage 315
Untreated patients 158–159

V

Value of irradiation in breast cancer 247
Variations in trial procedures 315
Volume of breast cancer 98, 254
Volume defect 197
Volume of residual 252

W

Wedges 249
Wide excision 197, 198, 205, 206–207, 218, 225, 252, 278
World Health Organization Trial 276
Wound closure 199, 202, 207
Wound infection 227, 229
Wrinkles 197

X

Xeromammography 131

Z

Zoladex 182, 245

GPSR Compliance

The European Union's (EU) General Product Safety Regulation (GPSR) is a set of rules that requires consumer products to be safe and our obligations to ensure this.

If you have any concerns about our products, you can contact us on ProductSafety@springernature.com

In case Publisher is established outside the EU, the EU authorized representative is:

Springer Nature Customer Service Center GmbH
Europaplatz 3
69115 Heidelberg, Germany

Batch number: 10838062

Printed by Printforce, the Netherlands